Sports Medicine

Sports Medicine
Study Guide and Review for Boards

Mark A. Harrast, MD
Director, Sports Medicine Fellowship
Clinical Associate Professor of Rehabilitation Medicine
Orthopaedics and Sports Medicine
University of Washington
Seattle, Washington

Jonathan T. Finnoff, DO
Associate Professor
Assistant Fellowship Director, Sports Medicine Fellowship
Department of Physical Medicine and Rehabilitation
Mayo Clinic Sports Medicine Center
Rochester, Minnesota

Editors

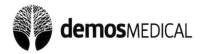

Visit our website at www.demosmedpub.com

ISBN: 978-1-9362-8723-9
E-book ISBN: 978-1-6170-5053-4

Acquisitions Editor: Beth Barry
Compositor: Techset

Medicine is an ever-changing science. Research and clinical experience are continually expanding our knowledge, in particular our understanding of proper treatment and drug therapy. The authors, editors, and publisher have made every effort to ensure that all information in this book is in accordance with the state of knowledge at the time of production of the book. Nevertheless, the authors, editors, and publisher are not responsible for errors or omissions or for any consequences from application of the information in this book and make no warranty, express or implied, with respect to the contents of the publication. Every reader should examine carefully the package inserts accompanying each drug and should carefully check whether the dosage schedules mentioned therein or the contraindications stated by the manufacturer differ from the statements made in this book. Such examination is particularly important with drugs that are either rarely used or have been newly released on the market.

Library of Congress Cataloging-in-Publication Data

CIP data is available from the Library of Congress

Special discounts on bulk quantities of Demos Medical Publishing books are available to corporations, professional associations, pharmaceutical companies, healthcare organizations, and other qualifying groups. For details, please contact:

Special Sales Department
Demos Medical Publishing
11 West 42nd Street, 15th Floor
New York, NY 10036
Phone: 800-532-8663 or 212-683-0072
Fax: 212-941-7842
E-mail: rsantana@demosmedpub.com

Printed in the United States of America by Bang Printing.

11 12 13 14 / 5 4 3 2 1

Contents

Contributors

Venu Akuthota, MD Department of Physical Medicine and Rehabilitation, University of Colorado Medical School, University of Colorado Denver, Department of Physical Medicine and Rehabilitation, Aurora, Colorado

Irfan M. Asif, MD Department of Family Medicine, University of Washington, Seattle, Washington

Darryl E. Barnes, MD Medical Director of Sports Medicine and Physical Therapy, Department of Orthopedics and Sports Medicine, Austin Medical Center, Mayo Clinic Health System, Austin, Minnesota

Holly J. Benjamin, MD Associate Professor of Pediatrics and Surgery, Section of Academic Pediatrics and Section of Orthopedic Surgery and Rehabilitation Medicine, Director of Primary Care Sports Medicine, University of Chicago, Chicago, Illinois

Larry Leone Benson, MD, CAQ Primary Care Sports Medicine, CJW Sports Medicine, LLC, CJW Medical Center HCA Healthcare, Team Physician, Longwood University, Chester, Virginia

Omar Bhatti, MD Resident Physician, Department of Physical Medicine & Rehabilitation, Milwaukee, Wisconsin

Joanne Borg-Stein Medical Director, Spaulding Wellesley, Chief, Physical Medicine & Rehabilitation Newton-Wellesley Hospital, Medical Director, Newton-Wellesley Hospital Spine Center, Assistant Professor, Department of Physical Medicine and Rehabilitation, Harvard Medical School, Wellesley, Massachusetts

Gary P. Chimes, MD, PhD Fellowship Director, Musculoskeletal Sports and Spine Fellowship, Assistant Professor, Department of PM&R, University of Pittsburgh Medical Center, Pittsburgh, Pennsylvania

John C. Cianca, MD Medical Director, Chevron Houston Marathon, Adjunct Associate Professor of Physical Medicine & Rehabilitation, Baylor College of Medicine, Human Performance Center, Houston, Texas

Daniel V. Colonno, MD Sports Medicine Fellow, University of Washington Physical Medicine and Rehabilitation, Department of Rehabilitation Medicine, University of Washington, Seattle, Washington

Leah G. Concannon, MD Department of Rehabilitation Medicine, University of Washington, Seattle, Washington

Katherine Louise Dec, MD, CAQ Medical Director, Women's Sports Medicine, CJW Sports Medicine, LLC, CJW Medical Center HCA Healthcare, Team Physician, Longwood University, Midlothian, Virginia

Robert J. Dimeff, MD Professor of Orthopaedic Surgery, Pediatrics, and Family Medicine, Director of Primary Care Sports Medicine, University of Texas Southwestern Medical Center, Dallas, Texas

Jonathon A. Drezner, MD Department of Family Medicine, University of Washington, Seattle, Washington

Michael Esrick, MD Resident Physician Combined Internal Medicine and Pediatrics, UMDNJ-NJMS Newark, Newark, New Jersey

Jonathan T. Finnoff, DO Associate Professor, Assistant Fellowship Director, Sports Medicine Fellowship Department of Physical Medicine and Rehabilitation, Mayo Clinic Sports Medicine Center, Rochester, Minnesota

Ryan Foreman, MD Memorial Sports Medicine Institute, South Bend, Indiana

Cassandra Forsythe-Pribanic, PhD, RD, CSCS, CISSN Cassandra Forsythe, LLC, Broad Brook, Connecticut

Jason Friedrich, MD Department of Physical Medicine and Rehabilitation, University of Colorado Medical School, University of Colorado Denver, Department of Physical Medicine and Rehabilitation, Aurora, Colorado

Christopher A. Gee, MD, FACEP Assistant Professor, Division of Emergency Medicine, University of Utah, Salt Lake City, Utah

Paul Gerrard, MD Resident Physician, Spaulding Rehabilitation Hospital/Department of Physical Medicine and Rehabilitation, Harvard Medical School, Boston, Massachusetts

Andrew John Maxwell Gregory, MD, FAAP, FACSM Assistant Professor of Orthopaedics and Paediatrics, Vanderbilt University School of Medicine, Medical Center East, South Tower, Nashville, Tennessee

Mederic M. Hall, MD Clinical Assistant Professor, University of Iowa Institute for Orthopaedics, Sports Medicine and Rehabilitation Iowa City, IA

Kimberly G. Harmon, MD Clinical Professor, University of Washington, Seattle, Washington

Mark A. Harrast, MD Director, Sports Medicine Fellowship, Clinical Associate Professor of Rehabilitation Medicine, Orthopaedics and Sports Medicine, University of Washington, Seattle, Washington

Michael Henrie, DO Clinical Instructor, University of Utah Orthopaedic Center, Division of Sports Medicine, Salt Lake City, Utah

Marni G. Hillinger, MD Resident, Physical Medicine and Rehabilitation, New York Presbyterian Hospital-Columbia and Cornell, New York, New York

Anne Z. Hoch, DO Director, Women's Sports Medicine Fellowship, Professor, Sports Medicine Department of Orthopaedic Surgery, Milwaukee, Wisconsin

Kerry L. Hulsing, MD Assistant Professor, Department of Neurology, University of Michigan, Michigan

Devyani Hunt, MD Washington University School of Medicine, Section, Physical Medicine and Rehabilitation, Department of Orthopaedic Surgery, One Barnes Jewish Hospital Plaza, St. Louis, Missouri

Joseph Michael Ihm, MD Attending Physician, Rehabilitation Institute of Chicago, Assistant Professor, Department of Physical Medicine and Rehabilitation, Northwestern University Medical School and Rehabilitation Institute of Chicago, Chicago, Ilinois

David Jewison, MD Sports Medicine Fellow, MacNeal Medical Center, Department of Family Medicine, Chicago, Illinois

Marla S. Kaufman, MD Clinical Assistant Professor, Department of Rehabilitation Medicine, Department of Orthopaedics & Sports Medicine, UW Medicine Sports & Spine Physicians, University of Washington Medical Center, Seattle, Washington

Susan M. Kleiner, PhD, RD, FACN, CNS, FISSN High Performance Nutrition, LLC, Mercer Island, Washington

Jeffrey S. Kutcher, MD Director, Michigan NeuroSport, Clinical Assistant Professor, Department of Neurology, University of Michigan, Ann Arbor, Michigan

Kelli M. Kyle, ATC, ATR Mayo Clinic Sports Medicine Center, Rochester, Minnesota

Scott R. Laker, MD Department of Rehabilitation Medicine, Department of Orthopedics and Sports Medicine, University of Washington, Seattle, Washington, scott.r.laker@gmail.com

Mark E. Lavallee, MD, CSCS, FACSM Memorial Sports Medicine Institute, South Bend, Indiana

Constance Marie Lebrun, MDCM, MPE, CCFP, Dip Sport Med, FACSM Associate Professor, Faculty of Medicine and Dentistry, Glen Sather Sports Medicine Clinic, E-05 Van Vliet Centre, University of Alberta, Edmonton, Alberta, Canada

Gerard Malanga, MD New Jersey Sports Medicine, Summit, New Jersey

Bryan Mason, MD Memorial Sports Medicine Institute, South Bend, Indiana

Kenneth R. Mautner, MD Director, PM&R Sports Medicine Fellowship, Assistant Professor of Rehabilitation Medicine, Orthopaedics and Sports Medicine, Emory University, Emory Sports Medicine Center, Atlanta, Georgia

Matthew D. Maxwell, MD Resident Physician, Department of PM&R, University of Pittsburgh Medical Center, Pittsburgh, Pennsylvania

Joanna L. McKey MD Pediatric Department, University of Texas Southwestern Medical Center, Childrens Medical Center, Dallas, Texas

John P. Metzler, MD Assistant Professor, Washington University School of Medicine, Department of Orthopaedic Surgery, Physiatry Section, St. Louis, Missouri

Nicole Detling, Miller, PhD, CC-AASP Assistant Professor (Lecturer), Department of Exercise and Sport Science, University of Utah, Salt Lake City, Utah

Lucinda T. Myers, MD PGY-3 Resident, Department of Physical Medicine and Rehabilitation, University of Utah, Salt Lake City, Utah

Darlene R. Nelson, MD Pulmonary/Critical Care Fellow, Division of Pulmonary and Critical Care Medicine, Mayo Clinic, Rochester, Minnesota

Jerome T. Nichols, MD Physical Medicine and Rehabilitation Resident, Emory University, Atlanta, Georgia

Megan L. Noon, MD Associate Director, Women's Sports Medicine Fellowship, Assistant Professor, Sports Medicine, Department of Orthopaedic Surgery, Milwaukee, Wisconsin

John W. O'Kane Jr, MD Associate Professor Orthopaedics and Sports Medicine, Adjunct Associate Professor Family Medicine, Head Team Physician, University of Washington, Seattle, Washington

Somnang Pang, DO Resident, Department of Physical Medicine & Rehabilitation, University of Pennsylvania, Philadelphia, Pennsylvania

Christopher T. Plastaras, MD Director, Penn Spine Center, Director, Spine, Sports & Musculoskeletal Medicine Fellowship, Assistant Professor of PM&R, University of Pennsylvania, Philadelphia, Pennsylvania

Heidi Prather, DO Washington University School of Medicine, Section, Physical Medicine and Rehabilitation, Department of Orthopaedic Surgery, St. Louis, Missouri

Cara C. Prideaux, MD Fellow, Sports Medicine, Department of Physical Medicine and Rehabilitation, University of Utah Orthopaedic Center, 590 Wakara Way, Salt Lake City, UT 84108, 801-587-5458, cara.prideaux@hsc.utah.edu; cara.prideaux@gmail.com

Ashwin Rao, MD Clinical Assistant Professor, Department of Family Medicine, Hall Health Sports Medicine, University of Washington, Seattle, Washington

Tracy R. Ray, MD Director, Primary Care Sports Medicine Fellowship, American Sports Medicine Institute, Birmingham, Alabama

Paul D. Scanlon, MD Professor of Medicine, Division of Pulmonary and Critical Care Medicine, Mayo Clinic, Rochester, Minnesota

Michael P. Schaefer, MD Assistant Professor of Physical Medicine and Rehabilitation, Case Western Reserve University, Director of Musculoskeletal PM&R, Cleveland Clinic Foundation, Cleveland, Ohio

Jacob L. Sellon, MD Chief Resident, Department of Physical Medicine and Rehabilitation, Mayo Clinic, Rochester, Minnesota

Abbie E. Smith, PhD, CSCS, CISSN Applied Physiology Laboratory, Department of Exercise and Sport Science, University of North Carolina Chapel Hill, Chapel Hill, North Carolina

Jay Smith, MD Professor of Physical Medicine and Rehabilitation, Mayo Clinic Sports Medicine Center, Rochester, Minnesota

William J. Sullivan, MD Associate Professor, Site Fellowship Director, Pain Medicine Fellowship, Director of Medical Student Education, Clinical Block Director, Musculoskeletal Block, Department of Physical Medicine and Rehabilitation, University of Colorado School of Medicine, Aurora, Colorado

Cameron L. Trubey, MD Memorial Sports Medicine Institute, South Bend, Indiana

Ricardo Vasquez-Duarte, MD New Jersey Sports Medicine Fellow, Summit, New Jersey

Christopher J. Visco, MD Assistant Professor of Clinical Rehabilitation, Assistant Residency Program Director, Department of Rehabilitation and Regenerative Medicine, Columbia University College of Physicians and Surgeons, New York Presbyterian Hospital, New York, New York

Brandee Waite, MD Co-Director, PM&R Sports Medicine Fellowship, Assistant Professor Dept. of Physical Medicine and Rehabilitation, University of California Davis Health System, Sacramento, California

Brian P. Williams, MD Pulmonary/Critical Care Fellow, Division of Pulmonary and Critical Care Medicine, Mayo Clinic, Rochester, Minnesota

Stuart Willick, MD Associate Professor, Sports Medicine Fellowship Director, University of Utah Orthopaedic Center, Division of Sports Medicine, Salt Lake City, Utah

Steve J. Wisniewski, MD Assistant Professor, Department of Physical Medicine and Rehabilitation, Mayo Clinic, Rochester, Minnesota

D. Harrison Youmans, MD Primary Care Sports Medicine Fellow, American Sports Medicine Institute, Birmingham, Alabama

Preface

The idea of writing a comprehensive sports medicine board review book originated during a sports medicine board review course we participated in several years ago. At the time, there were a limited number of books available to assist physicians preparing for the sports medicine boards. To date, this deficiency has not been corrected and many of the books previously published for this purpose are no longer available. We recognized the need for a high quality, thorough but concise sports medicine board review book covering all of the major topics present on the sports medicine board examination. Therefore, we decided to undertake the task of creating a book to fill this education gap.

We began by reviewing the content of the sports medicine board examination and creating a list of chapters covering all of the subjects present on the examination. The length of each chapter was determined by the percentage of the board examination devoted to the subject. This ensured that the book weighted the importance of each subject appropriately.

After creating the initial outline, we decided to divide the book into three primary sections: (1) General Topics, (2) Health Promotion and Preventative Aspects of Sports Medicine, and (3) Diagnosis, Management and Treatment of Sports Injuries and Conditions. The third section is divided into the following 3 subsections: (1) Musculoskeletal, (2) Medical, Neurologic, Psychologic, and (3) Special Populations. Each section contains multiple chapters covering specific topics relevant to the section. Then we determined that the best way to convey important information in a concise manner is through an outline format. Thus, the chapters in the book use an outline format with tables and figures to supplement the text. For further study, a recommended reading list is also provided at the end of each chapter.

We are very proud of the final product and believe it provides the reader with an exceptional resource covering the entire breadth of sports medicine. The book is meant to be used as a study guide for primary care sports medicine physicians (e.g., family medicine, emergency medicine, internal medicine, pediatrics and physical medicine and rehabilitation) and orthopedic sports medicine physicians preparing to take the sports medicine board examination for initial certification or recertification. However, it also can serve as a sports medicine reference for other medical professionals such as athletic trainers, physical therapists, physicians in training (ie: interns, residents and fellows), and other physicians interested in sports medicine.

We would like to thank all of the authors who contributed to this book. Without their efforts, the book would not have come to pass. We would also like to thank our publisher, Beth Barry at Demos Medical Publishing for her belief in our vision and her guidance and assistance throughout the process.

Mark A. Harrast, MD

Jonathan T. Finnoff, DO

I

General Topics

1

Overview of the Examination

Mark A. Harrast and Jonathan T. Finnoff

Introduction

This chapter is aimed at those readers who are preparing for the Sports Medicine Certificate of Added Qualifications (CAQ) (or Subspecialty) Examination and the recertifying examination. The information presented in this section was collected in 2011 from the following American Board of Medical Specialties websites:

1. American Board of Emergency Medicine (ABEM) (www.abem.org)
2. American Board of Family Medicine (ABFM) (www.theabfm.org)
3. American Board of Internal Medicine (ABIM) (www.abim.org)
4. American Board of Pediatrics (ABP) (www.abp.org)
5. American Board of Physical Medicine and Rehabilitation (ABPMR) (www.abpmr.org)

The ABFM administers the examination; however, the subspecialty certificates are issued by the physician's primary Board.

Eligibility for the Sports Medicine CAQ Examination

Applicants must meet the following requirements to take the Sports Medicine CAQ examination:

1. Board certification in one of the primary fields that participates in this examination (listed above)
2. In good standing with the respective Board
3. Unrestricted medical license
4. Completion of 12 months of training in an ACGME-accredited Sports Medicine Fellowship program affiliated with an ACGME-accredited residency program in Emergency Medicine, Family Medicine, Internal Medicine, Pediatrics, or Physical Medicine and Rehabilitation

Special Circumstances for PM&R thru 2013

Since ABPMR diplomats were granted eligibility to sit for the subspecialty examination in 2007, additional examination eligibility criteria were established for physiatrists that will expire at the end of 2013.

These temporary criteria include fulfilling one of two pathways below:

1. Nonaccredited fellowship pathway:
   a. Completion of 12 months of nonaccredited Sports Medicine fellowship training in a fellowship program affiliated to an ACGME-accredited PM&R residency program. The fellowship program must meet the ACGME requirements for primary care Sports Medicine fellowship training.

2. Practice and Continuing Medical Education (CME) pathway:
   a. Participation in a Sports Medicine practice for a minimum of 5 years following residency completion. More than 20% of the time averaged over 5 years must have been devoted to Sports Medicine.

AND

   b. Completion of 30 CME credits relevant to Sports Medicine within the 5-year practice period.

For the July examination, practice requirements or training must be completed by July 31st of the examination year. If training is completed after July 31st, but before November 30th of the examination year, applicants will apply during the regular application period, but will take the examination in November/December.

Examination Format and Application Process

The examination is a computer-based test with 200 multiple-choice questions. Four hours are allotted for completion. The content of this review book is based on the "outline of examination content" for the Sports Medicine CAQ examination. A link to this outline can be found on the websites of each of the primary fields that participate in Sports Medicine subspecialty certification.

The examination is offered each year in July and November/December. Applicants must apply through their respective Boards. Applications can be found on their Board's websites. Application deadlines and fees vary according to the respective Board and thus, the appropriate Board's website should be reviewed for the most current information. Once you are approved to sit for the examination, you will be asked to select an examination date and location at one of the computer-based testing centers.

Other Resources

The ABFM offers an online tutorial to gain familiarity with the computer-based testing system used for this examination. It can be found on their website.

The American Medical Society of Sports Medicine (www.amssm.org) offers a computer-based self-assessment examination each February for current sports medicine fellows. Each June, this examination is also offered to practicing sports medicine physicians (who are planning to recertify). AMSSM also offers a Sports Medicine Fellowship "pre-test" computer-based examination each August for beginning fellows to help familiarize them with the typical content of the subspecialty examination and what they will be learning during their fellowship.

The American Academy of Physical Medicine and Rehabilitation (www.aapmr.org) also offers a downloadable written self-assessment examination in sports medicine. This is available for purchase anytime of the year.

Recertification

Subspecialty certification in Sports Medicine is time-limited. The certificate expires on December 31st of the 10th year after passing the examination. Sports Medicine subspecialty maintenance of certification (MOC) requirements currently include:

1. Maintaining primary Board certification
2. Holding an unrestricted medical license
3. Passing the recertifying examination (which is currently the same as the primary certifying Sports Medicine examination). The examination must be taken in July of years 9 or 10 of the MOC cycle. In case of failure, a candidate can re-take the examination in November/December.

MOC is an evolving process; so be certain to review your primary Board's requirements at least yearly. Currently, each of the primary care Boards that participates in Sports Medicine subspecialty certification has the above three requirements for recertification. However, ABIM has one other requirement and ABFM is developing one. Both are noted below.

Special Note for MOC from ABIM and ABFM

ABIM: the above three requirements plus diplomats must earn 100 points of self-evaluation.

ABFM: The ABFM is developing a Sports Medicine Self-Assessment Module (SAM) that will become a requirement for family physicians to maintain certification. This Sports Medicine SAM will also be applicable for credit toward the ABFM primary MOC program.

2

The Role of the Team Physician

Katherine Louise Dec and Larry Leone Benson

I. Role of the Team Physician

    A. A collaborative consensus statement developed by six medical organizations suggests the following requirements for team physicians:

        1. Provide the best medical care for athletes at all levels of participation.

        2. Be an MD or DO in good standing, with an unrestricted license to practice medicine.

        3. Possess a fundamental knowledge of emergency care regarding sport events.

        4. Be trained in cardiopulmonary resuscitation (CPR).

        5. Have a working knowledge of trauma, musculoskeletal injuries, and medical conditions in athletes.

II. Ethics: maintain professionalism and remember *primum non nocere*: above all, do no harm

    A. Patient Autonomy: defined as the ability of an athlete/patient to make their own decisions regarding medical or surgical options. For autonomy to occur, informed consent must be present.

        1. Informed Consent

            a. American Medical Association's (AMA) Code of Medical Ethics notes "The patient's right of self-decision can be effectively exercised only if the patient possesses enough information to enable an intelligent choice."

            b. Requires the disclosure of diagnosis, the nature and purpose of any proposed treatment, the risks and consequences of that treatment, any reasonably feasible treatment alternatives, the risk of return to play, and the prognosis if the proposed treatment is not performed.

        2. The necessary conditions for legitimate informed consent as it pertains to the sideline physician are as follows:

            a. *Disclosure:* all relevant information that a reasonable person in this player's position would want to know regarding the proposed treatment, nontreatment, and alternate treatments must be explained to the player in an appropriate fashion.

            b. *Capacity:* players must have the capacity to understand this information and appreciate how it applies to them. In the legal system this concept is known as *competency.*

            c. *Voluntariness:* in an environment without coercion, a player must voluntarily express their wishes regarding the proposed options.

    B. Patient Confidentiality

        1. Laws such as the Health Insurance Portability and Accountability Act of 1996 (HIPAA) and the Federal Educational Rights and Privacy Act (FERPA) play major roles in patient confidentiality.

            a. If an independent physician cares for a patient in his or her private office, HIPPA rules apply.

       i. Recommended to have an athlete's consent to release information to coaches and other members working with the team.

    b. However, a physician who is an employee of the team MAY disclose an athlete's health conditions with coaches and team owners because the information may be considered as part of the athlete's employment record and therefore would not fall under HIPAA regulations.

    c. FERPA permits team physicians employed by a college or university student health clinic to release health information without the patient's consent or authorization to other school officials who have an educational interest in the information.

    d. FERPA, however, does not allow disclosure of health information to the media or other outside entities without the athlete's signed authorization.

    e. On-field treatment and evaluations may not fall under HIPPA if they are considered emergencies.

III. Medical–Legal

A. Physician Responsibility

  1. Fiduciary obligation of the physician

    a. A physician focuses exclusively on a patient's health and what is best for the patient's health. Athlete–doctor relationship is a patient–physician relationship. Trust is an expected part of the relationship.

    b. Requires a physician to give an athlete full disclosure of medical condition and risks of participation.

  2. Remain an *objective* medical expert during treatment and return-to-play decisions.

  3. Ensure safety of other participants on the playing field. Example: officials are notified if contagious skin disease is detected in a wrestling match.

  4. Coverage of game or practice may involve team physician or other sports medicine health professional.

    a. Negligence related to oversight may be considered the responsibility of the team physician.

  5. Preparticipation physical examination clearance determination.

  6. Postinjury return to sports decisions.

    a. Has the athlete been evaluated by the appropriate physician? Has the athlete received adequate treatment? Were images of the injury documented (if necessary)? Has functional testing been applied before returning? Have the risks of returning been discussed with the athlete and documented?

  7. Communication with other health care professionals for athlete's health care needs.

  8. Knowledge of the pharmacology regarding medications their team members are prescribed. Must recognize banned drugs and follow appropriate governing bodies guidelines if therapeutic use exemption is required. NCAA (National Collegiate Athletic Association) and WADA (World Anti-Doping Agency) have policies and procedures in place outlined at www.ncaa.org and www.wada-ama.org, respectively.

B. Physician Liability

  1. Guided by tort law

    a. Tort = a wrong that involves a breach of civil duty owed to someone else.

    b. A person who suffers tortuous injury is entitled to receive "damages" from the person responsible.

    c. Medical malpractice is usually based on negligence torts, which require establishment of the following:

       i. The defendant had a duty to act

       ii. The defendant breached that duty

       iii. Harm to the plaintiff occurred due to this breach

       iv. The harm is measurable

2. Physicians protect themselves by practicing good medicine (i.e., use published guidelines and consensus statements when able) and placing the health care needs of the athlete over all competing interests.
    a. Clinical practice guidelines have been allowed in evidence to establish standard of care; however, they are not conclusive to the standard of care.
    b. Guidelines also allow reference for treatment decisions and return to play as they reduce uncertainty into the "customary practice."
3. Professional sports: Athlete–physician relationship on professional teams involves employment contracts. Physician may have a direct contract for salary payment or an indirect financial benefit from association, name/title as team physician, advertising and location to help the financial increase of their practice.
    a. If the physician is an "employee" of the professional team, those athletes on the professional team may be considered under worker's compensation and the physician is usually protected legally from being sued as they are "co-employees".
4. Educate the athlete regarding expected treatment outcomes and risks of returning to play.
5. Understand your state law regarding "first responder" and "Good Samaritan" statutes.
    a. When a patient consents to follow the care you have recommended, and you have assessed and rendered an opinion on their injury, a doctor–patient relationship has been established, regardless of free care/volunteer.

C. **Preparticipation Physical Examination (PPE)** (*specific medical conditions covered in other chapters)
1. Assess medical history, family history, and perform a physical examination.
2. Goals of PPE are:
    a. To detect conditions that may predispose athletes to injury, illness, or death.
    b. To detect conditions that may put other athletes at risk of illness or injury.
    c. To meet legal and insurance requirements.
    d. To determine *general* health, to counsel patients on health-related issues, and to assess fitness level for specific sport.
3. PPE content may vary based on age/level of competition
    a. Professional athlete
        i. Implications for contract and employment by athletes for a professional team.
        ii. Discuss with athlete confidentiality aspects regarding informing coaches or team management.
    b. College athlete
        i. After first-year PPE, subsequent assessments to update history and examination may be focused on any new medical conditions or injuries.
    c. Secondary schools or youth travel squads
        i. Confirm history information with parent/guardian or accompanying documents provided. Need parental consent.
        ii. Clearance also relates to psychological, cognitive, and physical readiness to participate in chosen sport.
        iii. Youth mature musculoskeletally and cognitively at different rates. This should be considered when clearing an athlete for a particular sport.
4. Follow clinical practice guidelines or consensus statements by expert panels if no standard of care for clearance to participate.
    a. Some clinical guidelines may concern certain age levels and/or level of competition; however, limited legal standards for preparticipation evaluation and clearance in professional athletes.

D. **Return to Play** (*specific conditions are covered in other chapters)
1. Physical Injury or Medical Condition

  a. Utilize clinical practice guidelines in treatment and return to play decisions.
  b. Understand an athlete's practice and competition environment to prevent further injury.
  c. Understand psychosocial aspects that may affect recovery and prevent injury in return-to-play decisions.
  d. Engage other members of medical management team for complex issues, that is, post-substance abuse with academic and physical function implications.

 E. Waiver of Liability
  1. Signed waivers (e.g., exculpatory agreements) do not absolve team physicians from liability.
  2. Little legal framework for waiver agreements and have been viewed as unenforceable.
   a. Assumption of risk: May be incorporated into informed consent form.
   b. Prospective release of risk: May not be unenforceable, but, will undergo scrutiny and may be considered in athletes requesting release against medical advice.

IV. Administrative Responsibilities

 A. Development of policies and procedures related to medical injuries and conditions that may affect athlete participation in sport.
  1. Understand intrinsic and extrinsic risks of sport. Identify athletes at risk. Establish prevention strategies, including athlete education, for injuries and medical conditions.
  2. Written policies outlining communication, testing, and outside consultant referral for certain conditions.
   a. Athletes sign a document outlining understanding of how information may be shared with team administration, coaches, and other health professionals if injury should occur. If athletes are minors, have parent or legal guardian also sign.
  3. Keep medical records documenting preparticipation physical injuries, treatments, risks of sports participation, and return-to-play decisions.
   a. Documents medical care and establishes athletes' awareness of injury/medical condition as well as risks of returning to sports.
  4. Review policies and procedures regularly. Follow state and federal guidelines and local standard of medical care when developing these policies.

 B. Communication between appropriate school officials and rest of medical team for care of athletes' health.
  1. The team physician should be the athlete's advocate in return-to-play decisions.
  2. The team physician should collaborate with outside specialists and other health care professionals, in addition to the athlete's family, coach, and administrators as appropriate.

 C. Policies and procedures for emergency management of athletes participating in school-sponsored sports
  1. Written emergency action plan that are understood by all members of athletic sports medicine team.
  2. Practice emergency procedures with members of athletic sports medicine team for catastrophic events and coordination with community medical systems.

 D. Coordination of care with other health care professionals for athletes' care.
  1. Meeting with community agencies to provide cohesive implementation of medical care policies, such as emergency transport for catastrophic injury.
  2. Collaborative efforts with community and legislature to increase safety in the sports venue, and, to develop universal policies to prevent injury.

Recommended Reading

1. American College of Sports Medicine. Sideline preparedness for the team physician: A consensus statement. *Med Sci Sports Exerc.* 2001;33:846–849.
2. *American Medical Association Council on Ethical and Judicial Affairs, Code of Medical Ethics: Current Opinions and Annotations, AMA, Opinion 8.08 on Informed Consent.* Chicago: AMA; 2004–2005.

3. Bernstein J, Perlis C, Bartolozzi AR. Ethics in sports medicine. *Clin Orthop Relat Res.* 2000;378:50–60.

4. Dunn WR, George MS, Churchill L, et al. Ethics in sports medicine. *Am J Sports Med.* 2007;35(5):840–844.

5. Furrow BR. The problem of the sports doctor: Serving two (or is it three or four?) masters. HeinOnline. *St. Louis University Law J.* 2005–2006;50:165–183.

6. Howe WB. Ethical considerations in sports medicine. In: Birrer RB, et al., eds. *Sports Medicine for the Primary Care Physician.* 2nd ed. Boca Raton, FL: CRC Press Inc; 1994:37–39.

7. Magee JT, Almekinders LC, Taft TN. HIPAA, the team physician. *Sports Med Update.* 2003;March–April:4–8.

8. Matheson GO, Shultz R, Bido J, et al. Return-to-play decisions: Are they the team physician's responsibility? *Clin J Sport Med.* 2011;21(1):25–30.

9. Mitten MJ. Team physicians as co-employees: A prescription that deprives professional athletes of an adequate remedy for sports medicine malpractice. *HeinOnline—St. Louis University Law J* 2005–2006;50:211.

10. Pearsall AW, Kovaleski JE. Medicolegal issues affecting sports medicine practitioners. *Clin Orthop Relat Res.* 2005;433:50–57.

11. Stovitz SD, Satin DJ. Professionalism and ethics of the sideline physician. *Curr Sports Med Rep.* 2006;5:120–124.

3

Exercise Physiology
Jonathan T. Finnoff

I. Muscles

A. Muscle Cells

  1. Muscle cells = myofibers or muscle fibers

    a. Long, cylindrical multinucleated cells

  2. Muscle cell membrane = sarcolemma

  3. Muscle cell cytoplasm = sarcoplasm

  4. Bundled groups of muscle cells = fascicles

B. Connective Tissue (Figure 3.1)

  1. Endomysium = surrounds each muscle cell

    a. Sarcolemma is continuous with the endomysium

  2. Perimysium = surrounds each fascicle

  3. Epimysium = surrounds the entire muscle

C. Tendons

  1. Connects muscle to bone periosteum

  2. Endomysium, perimysium, and epimysium all connect to the tendon

D. Innervation

  1. Each muscle cell is innervated by a single motor nerve, but a single nerve can innervate multiple muscle cells

  2. Motor unit = single motor nerve and all the muscle cells in it

    a. All the muscle cells in a motor unit contract when they are stimulated by their motor nerve

E. Myofibrils

  1. Contractile apparatus of muscles

  2. Composed of the myofilaments myosin (thick filament) and actin (thin filament)

    a. Myosin has a globular head which can form cross-bridges with actin

    b. Actin has a two-stranded double-helix structure

    c. Each actin is surrounded by three myosin

    d. Each myosin is surrounded by six actin

  3. Sarcomere (Figure 3.1)

    a. Smallest contractile unit in skeletal muscle

    b. Z-line = ends of the sarcomere

      i. Actin attaches to the Z-line

    c. M-line = center of the sarcomere

      i. Myosin attaches to the M-line

    d. A-band (dark)

      i. Contains myosin and actin

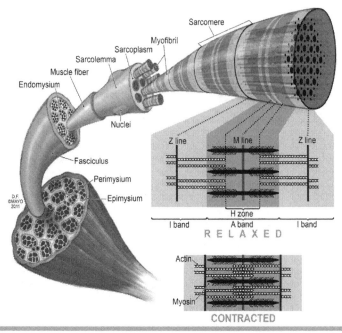

Figure 3.1   Muscle anatomy including the connective tissue layers (epimysium, perimysium, endomysium), muscle organization (fascicles, muscle fibers), and contractile units (sarcomere). During muscle contraction, the H zone and I band decrease in size due to increased overlap of actin and myosin.

    e. I-band (light)
       i. Contains only actin
    f. H-zone = in the middle of the A-band
       i. Contains only myosin
       ii. H-zone and I-band get smaller with muscle contraction

F. Muscle Contraction (Figure 3.1)
  1. At rest
    a. Minimal calcium in the sarcoplasm
    b. Few myosin heads bound to actin
    c. Troponin and tropomyosin cover the actin-binding sites on the myosin head
  2. Muscle contraction
    a. Acetylcholine released from the motor neuron binds to receptors on the muscle cell membrane
    b. Sarcolemma depolarizes
    c. Depolarization transmitted rapidly into the interior of the muscle cell via the transverse tubules (T-tubules)
    d. Intracellular calcium released from the sarcoplasmic reticulum
    e. Calcium binds to troponin, which causes a conformational change in tropomyosin and the myosin-binding sites on the actin filament are uncovered
    f. Myosin head forms a cross-bridge with the actin filament, flexes, then dissociates from the actin

      g. Myosin head re-cocks to its original position prior to beginning the process again

      h. Two adenosine triphosphate (ATP) converted into adenosine diphosphate (ADP) for muscle contraction

         i. One to form cross-bridge with actin and flex the myosin head

        ii. One for dissociation of myosin from actin and to re-cock the myosin head

  G. Muscle Fiber Types (Table 3.1)

    1. Type I (slow twitch—oxidative)

    2. Type II (fast twitch—glycolytic)

      a. Type IIa (fast twitch—oxidative glycolytic)

      b. Type IIb (fast twitch—glycolytic)

  H. Recruitment

    1. Henneman Size Principle

      a. Smaller, lower-threshold motor neurons (innervated by Type I muscle cells) recruited first

      b. Type II fibers recruited if more force is required

    2. Exception = high-velocity-type activities (i.e., plyometrics)

      a. Type II fibers recruited first.

II. Energy Systems

  A. Three energy systems

    1. ATP-phosphocreatine

      a. Phosphocreatine donates its phosphate to regenerate ATP from ADP in muscle

      b. Catalyzed by the enzyme creatine kinase

      c. Main energy source for maximal exercise lasting up to 30 s

      d. Most of the phosphocreatine can be regenerated after resting 3 min

    2. Anaerobic (glycolytic) (Figure 3.2)

      a. Metabolism of glucose to pyruvate via glycolysis

      b. No oxygen is required

      c. Produces two ATP if beginning with glucose, or three ATP if beginning with glycogen

      d. In the presence of oxygen, the end product of glycolysis (pyruvate) is metabolized via the aerobic energy system (see next section). When pyruvate is created faster than it can

Table 3.1   Characteristics of Muscle Fiber Types

Characteristic	Type I	Type IIa	Type IIb
Contraction speed	Slow	Fast	Fast
Force production	Low	Intermediate	High
Endurance	High	Intermediate/low	Low
Aerobic enzymes	High	Intermediate/low	Low
Anaerobic enzymes	Low	High	High
Fatigability	Low	Intermediate/high	High
Capillary density	High	Intermediate	Low
Fiber size	Small	Intermediate	Large
Mitochondria	High	Intermediate	Low
ATPase activity	Low	High	High
Myoglobin	High	Low	Low
Color	Red	White	White

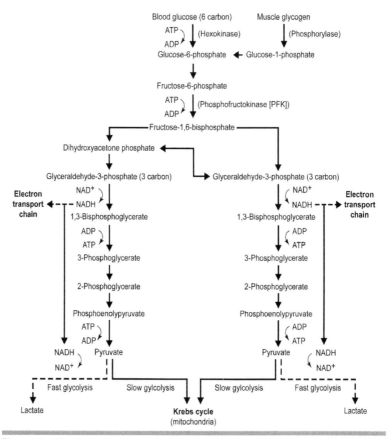

Figure 3.2 Glycolysis

be metabolized, it is reversibly converted into lactate. Pyruvate into lactate conversion is facilitated by a low-oxygen environment

  e. Glycolysis is the primary energy source for exercise lasting 1–3 min
  f. The rate-limiting step of glycolysis is catalyzed by the enzyme phosphofructokinase
3. Aerobic (oxidative)
  a. Occurs in the mitochondria via oxidative phosphorylation, which has two parts:
    i. Krebs cycle (Figure 3.3a)
      (A) By-product is CO_2
    ii. Electron transport chain (Figure 3.3b)
      (A) By-product is H_2O
  b. In the presence of oxygen, pyruvate is converted into acetyl coenzyme A, which is metabolized through the Krebs cycle and electron transport chain to produce 36 ATP per glucose molecule. Therefore, the net ATP produced from glycolysis and oxidative phosphorylation is 38 (beginning with glucose) or 39 (beginning with glycogen)
  c. Aerobic metabolism is the primary energy source for exercise lasting more than 3 min
  d. Fat is also metabolized in the mitochondria
    i. Triglycerides are broken down into glycerol and three free fatty acids by lipolysis

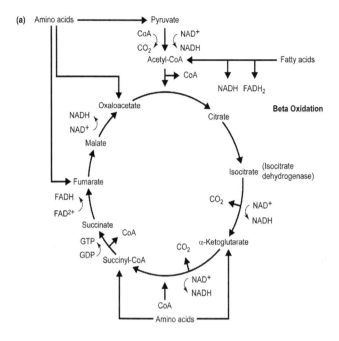

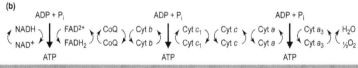

Figure 3.3   (a) Krebs cycle, (b) Electron transport chain.

    ii. Free fatty acids enter the mitochondria and are converted into acetyl coenzyme A through β-oxidation

    iii. Acetyl coenzyme A metabolized by the Krebs cycle and electron transport chain

    iv. Net ATP produced from free fatty acid metabolism is far greater than for glucose (e.g., 129 ATP for one palmitic acid molecule).

III. Adaptations to Exercise

A. Aerobic Exercise

  1. Results in an increase in:

    a. Muscular capillary density

    b. Size and number of mitochondria

    c. Oxidative enzymes

    d. Fatty acid transport across the sarcolemma

    e. Fat metabolism

    f. Arterial oxygen extraction

      i. Increased arterio-venous oxygen concentration difference

  2. Owing to the increase in fat utilization, there is a relative sparing of glycogen/glucose metabolism, which results in a reduction in lactate production

  3. There is no change in muscle cell lactate buffering capacity

    4. Pyruvate is metabolized faster due to the increase in oxidative enzymes

    5. After the first 2 weeks of aerobic exercise, many Type IIb fibers will convert into Type IIa fibers

B. Anaerobic Exercise

    1. Results in an increase in:

        a. Intramuscular anaerobic enzymes such as phosphofructokinase, phosphorylase, and lactate dehydrogenase

        b. Moderate increase in oxidative enzymes (Table 3.2)

    2. Improved muscle cell lactate buffering capacity

C. Resistance Exercise

    1. Causes muscle cell hypertrophy (increased muscle cell size)

        a. Due to an increased number of sarcomeres

        b. Occurs after 6–8 weeks of training

        c. Predominantly in Type II muscle cells

    2. Strength gains that occur prior to 6 weeks are due to neural factors including improved motor unit recruitment and repression of self-protection reflexes

    3. No substantial evidence supporting hyperplasia (increased number of muscle cells) in humans due to resistance exercise

    4. Fiber-type conversion from Type IIb to Type IIa begins after a few weeks

    5. Resistance exercises can lead to improved aerobic exercise as evidenced by the improved running economy of long-distance runners following maximal squat strength training three times weekly for 8 weeks

    6. Aerobic exercise does not appear to enhance the strength benefits of resistance training alone

    7. Resistance training increases

        a. Bone mineral density

        b. Ligament and tendon strength and collagen content

        c. Anaerobic energy stores (glycogen, phosphocreatine, ATP)

Table 3.2   Adaptations to Aerobic and Anaerobic Exercise

Anatomic/Physiologic Adaptation	Aerobic	Anaerobic
Muscular capillary density	↑↑	–
Mitochondrial number and size	↑↑	–
Oxidative (aerobic) enzymes	↑↑	↑
Glycolytic (anaerobic) enzymes	–	↑↑
Fatty acid transportation across sarcolemma	↑↑	–
Fat metabolism	↑↑	–
Glucose/glycogen metabolism	↓	–
Arterial oxygen extraction/arterio-venous oxygen difference	↑↑	–
Lactate production	↓	↓
Lactate buffering capacity	–	↑↑
Type IIb to Type IIa fiber-type conversion	↑↑	–
Muscle hypertrophy	–	–
Improved aerobic exercise performance	↑↑	↑

8. Capillary and mitochondrial density decrease due to larger degree of muscular hypertrophy compared to increase in capillarization
9. High-volume, low-load resistance exercises increase:
   a. Creatine phosphokinase
   b. Myokinase
   c. Phosphofructokinase
10. Low-volume, high-load resistance exercise:
    a. Decrease creatine phosphokinase
    b. No change in myokinase or phosphofructokinase
11. Lactate dehydrogenase concentrations do not change with either high-volume, low-load or low-volume, high-load resistance exercises

D. Flexibility
   1. Three main stretching techniques
      a. Static
         i. Hold muscle in stretched position for a sustained period of time, usually 30 s
         ii. Easy to perform
         iii. Minimal activation of the muscle spindles
      b. Ballistic
         i. Bouncing motion is utilized to stretch the muscle
         ii. Activates muscle spindles causing reflex contraction of the muscle being stretched
         iii. As effective as static stretching BUT more painful and has a higher potential for injury
      c. Proprioceptive neuromuscular facilitation (PNF)
         i. Muscle contraction, either the agonist or antagonist, is used to facilitate the stretch through reflexes (e.g., contracting the quadriceps muscle while stretching the hamstring muscle)
   2. Effectiveness of stretching techniques
      a. PNF > static = ballistic
   3. Factors that influence flexibility:
      a. Joint range of motion is limited by the joint's bony anatomy, as well as the muscles, fascia, tendons, and ligaments that cross the joint
      b. Muscle elasticity is reduced with age due to fibrocartilaginous replacement of degenerated muscle fibers, increased adhesions, and calcium deposits
      c. Females are more flexible than males, primarily due to pelvic structure and hormonal differences
      d. Physically active people tend to be more flexible than their sedentary counterparts
   4. Increased flexibility from stretching due to:
      a. Acute = musculotendinous viscoelastic properties
      b. Chronic = increased number of sarcomeres and increased stretching pain tolerance.

IV. Lactate Kinetics

A. At rest and during low-intensity exercise, blood lactate levels are low and remain relatively constant

B. As intensity increases, there comes a point above which lactate begins to accumulate

C. If exercise intensity continues to increase, a shift takes places where anaerobic metabolism becomes the predominant energy source rather than aerobic metabolism

D. This point is called the lactate or anaerobic threshold and usually occurs at 4 mmol/L of blood lactate

E. In untrained individuals, the lactate threshold may reside at 50–60% of their maximal oxygen uptake, while in trained individuals it may be closer to 80–90% of their maximal oxygen uptake

F. The lactate threshold is trainable

G. Lactate is an energy substrate for glycolysis and does not appear to cause the "muscle burn" associated with exercise.

V. Cardiovascular Response to Exercise

A. As exercise intensity increases, there is a linear increase in heart rate

B. Stroke volume increases initially, but then plateaus

C. Early increases in cardiac output associated with exercise are due to a combination of increased heart rate and stroke volume (CO = HR × SV), whereas the increased cardiac output associated with higher intensity exercise is nearly completely due to an increase in heart rate

D. There is a linear relationship between cardiac output and maximal oxygen consumption. Therefore, cardiac output is an important determinant of aerobic exercise capacity

E. During a prolonged aerobic exercise session, there is a gradual increase in heart rate and decrease in stroke volume at a given work load. This is referred to as cardiac drift and is likely due to a greater percentage of the blood being diverted to the skin for heat dissipation, and a reduction in blood volume due to sweating

F. Long-term aerobic exercise training causes:
  1. Increased:
     a. Stroke volume at rest and during maximal exercise
     b. Left ventricular wall thickness, internal diameter, and mass
     c. Blood volume
        i. Initial due to increased plasma volume likely due to increased antidiuretic hormone and aldosterone levels
        ii. Later due to increases in both plasma volume and red blood cell number
        iii. Since the increase in blood volume is greater than the increase in red blood cell volume, there is a net reduction in the hematocrit referred to as a "pseudoanemia"
  2. Decreased:
     a. Resting and submaximal exercise heart rate
     b. Systolic and diastolic blood pressures

G. Long-term resistance training causes:
  1. Increased left ventricular wall thickness and mass
  2. No change in internal left ventricular diameter.

VI. Respiratory Response to Exercise

A. Initial rapid increase in ventilation, followed by a brief plateau, and another gradual rise until a steady state is reached

B. During submaximal exercise, increased ventilation has a linear relationship with oxygen uptake

C. Initial increase in ventilation due to increase in tidal volume
  1. With increased exercise intensity, breathing rate becomes the predominant mechanism for increased ventilation.

VII. Endocrine Response to Exercise

A. Testosterone
  1. Temporarily increases after resistance exercise
     a. Increase enhanced by:
        i. Shorter rest periods (1 min rather than 3 min)
        ii. Less intensity but higher volume (10 repetition maximum (RM) rather than 5 RM)
        iii. Exercise lasting longer than 20 min

    2. Temporarily increases after anaerobic exercise

    3. Lower than normal resting testosterone levels in endurance athletes

  B. Growth hormone

    1. Increases after resistance exercise

      a. Increase enhanced by:

        i. Shorter rest periods (1 min rather than 3 min)

        ii. Less intensity but higher volume (10 repetition maximum (RM) rather than 5 RM)

        iii. Exercise lasting longer than 20 min

    2. Increases after aerobic exercise

  C. Insulin

    1. Decrease during exercise

    2. Insulin sensitivity increased by exercise

  D. Cortisol

    1. Increased after:

      a. Resistance training

      b. Prolonged aerobic exercise above 70% of maximal oxygen uptake.

VIII. Immune System Response to Exercise

  A. Exercise reduces:

    1. Mucosal IGA concentrations

    2. Leukocyte counts

    3. Natural killer cell numbers

    4. Infections in previously sedentary individuals

  B. Exercises increases:

    1. Upper-respiratory infections in endurance athletes.

IX. Delayed-Onset Muscle Soreness (DOMS)

  A. Occurs following high-force, unaccustomed eccentric (and occasionally isometric in an extended position) muscle contractions

  B. Reason for eccentric specificity of DOMS is unknown, but the following events occur following eccentric exercise:

    1. Disruption of the sarcomere's Z-lines called "Z-line streaming"

    2. Sarcolemma damaged

    3. Calcium is released within the cell

    4. Calcium-dependent proteolytic enzymes degrade the damaged sarcomere Z-lines

    5. Circulating neutrophil concentrations increase within a few hours of the injury

    6. Creatine kinase leaks from the muscle cell into the circulating plasma and attracts monocytes to the area within 6–12 h of the injury

    7. Monocytes transform into macrophages, which phagocytose damaged structures

    8. Macrophages release prostaglandin PGE2, and Type III and IV nerve endings are sensitized

    9. Mast cells are attracted to the area and release histamine causing tissue edema, hyperthermia, and further sensitization and mechanical compression of nociceptors

    10. Monocyte/macrophage concentrations peak at approximately 48 h postinjury

    11. Oxygen-free radicals are also produced throughout this process causing secondary tissue damage

  C. Pain typically begins 6–12 h after exercise, peaks 2–3 days postexercise, and resolves 5–7 days postexercise

  D. Symptoms treated with analgesics such as NSAIDS or acetaminophen, massage, electrical stimulation, cryotherapy, heat, and rest

E. The most effective prevention measure for DOMS is the "repeated bout effect"
   1. Single bout of eccentric exercise prevents the development of DOMS from the same exercise for approximately 6 weeks.

X. Children

A. Due to variable maturation rates, classify children by their biological rather than chronological age

B. Biological age can be determined by skeletal age, sexual maturation, or physical maturity (e.g., five Tanner stages)

C. Muscle mass increases during maturation with 25% of a baby's birth weight attributable to muscle versus 40% of an adult's weight
   1. Increase in muscle mass is due to hypertrophy not hyperplasia
   2. Prepuberty strength/muscle mass is similar between males and females
   3. Males have a larger increase in muscle mass than females during puberty due to higher testosterone levels
      a. Larger increases in male muscle mass mirrored by larger increases in strength

D. Females have increased estrogen levels during puberty, which causes fat deposition, secondary sex characteristic development, and widening of the hips.

XI. Elderly

A. Decrease in muscle:
   1. Strength
   2. Mass
   3. Function

B. Decreased muscle mass predisposes to:
   1. Osteoarthritis of the knee
   2. Falls
   3. Osteoporotic fractures

C. Endurance decreased due to:
   1. Decreased:
      a. Muscle mass
      b. Capillary blood flow
      c. Impaired oxygen uptake
      d. Nutritional status
   2. Increased presence of chronic diseases such as:
      a. Chronic obstructive pulmonary disease (COPD)
      b. Coronary artery disease (CAD)
      c. Congestive heart failure (CHF)

D. Balance decreased due to:
   1. Inactivity and deconditioning
   2. Chronic diseases that effect balance such as:
      a. Peripheral vascular disease (PVD)
      b. Diabetes mellitus (DM)
      c. Parkinson's disease
      d. Peripheral neuropathy
   3. Poor nutrition
   4. Alcoholism
   5. Medications

E. Flexibility decreased due to:
   1. Immobilization and/or a lack of regular joint movement through a full range of motion

F. Physiologic changes seen with aging (Table 3.3)

Table 3.3   Physiologic Changes with Aging

System	Type of Change	Effect/Amount of Change
Cardiovascular	↓ Maximum heart rate of	10 beats/min/decade
	↓ Blood vessel compliance	↑ blood pressure 10–40 mm Hg
	↓ Restring stroke volume	30% by 85 years of age
	↓ Maximum cardiac output	20–30% by age 65
	↓ Maximum cardiac output	
Respiratory	↑ Residual volume	30–50% by age 70
	↓ Vital capacity	40–50% by age 70
Metabolism	↓ VO$_{2max}$	9% per decade
Neurologic	↓ Nerve conduction velocity	1–15% by age 60
	↓ Proprioception	↑ falls 35–40% by age 60
Musculoskeletal	Bone loss when 35–55 years old	1% per year
	Bone loss when >55 years old	3–5% per year
	↓ Muscle strength	20% by age of 65
	↓ Flexibility	

G. Progressive resistance exercises:
   1. Increase:
      a. Strength
      b. Endurance
      c. Submaximal aerobic capacity
      d. Bone mineral density
   2. Decrease:
      a. Blood pressure
      b. Fall risk
      c. Osteoarthritic knee pain
      d. Disability
H. Aerobic exercise:
   1. Improves:
      a. Efficiency (i.e., reduced metabolic demands for a given activity)
      b. Endurance
      c. Oxygen uptake
      d. Multiple chronic diseases (see chronic disease section)
   2. Reduces
      a. Resting heart rate
      b. Disability
      c. Pain
 I. Balance training reduces:
   1. Falls
   2. Osteoporotic fractures
 J. Flexibility training improves:
   1. Joint range of motion
   2. Muscle flexibility.

XII. Patients with Chronic Disease

A. Regular exercise is a beneficial adjunctive treatment of chronic diseases such as:
   1. Hypertension

    a. Fifty percent greater risk of developing hypertension in sedentary than active people

    b. In people with hypertension (systolic blood pressure (SBP) ≥ 140 and/or diastolic blood pressure (DBP) ≥ 90), regular exercise reduces resting SBP by approximately 7.4 mm Hg, and DBP by 5.8 mm Hg

    c. Moderate-intensity aerobic exercise (40–70% of VO_{2max}) is as effective as high-intensity aerobic exercise at reducing blood pressure

    d. Some reductions in SBP and DBP from resistance training:

        i. Regular resistance training also blunts the acute elevations in blood pressure that occur in untrained individuals who perform resistance exercises

    e. Small reductions in blood pressure (2 mm Hg of SBP and DBP) result in significant reductions in stroke risk (14%) and coronary artery disease (9%)

    f. Decreased BP probably due to reduction in sympathetic tone

  2. PVD

  3. Osteoarthritis

  4. Claudication

  5. COPD

  6. Dementia

  7. Pain

  8. Congestive heart failure

  9. Syncope

  10. Cerebrovascular accident

  11. Deep-venous thromboembolism

  12. Back pain

  13. Constipation

  14. DM

    a. Increases GLUT4 production (a glucose-transporting protein), thus improves glucose transport in Type 2 DM

    b. Aerobic exercises performed for 30–60 min, 3–4 times per week at 50–80% of VO_{2max} reduces glycosylated hemoglobin levels (HbA_{1c}) by 10–20% in Type 2 diabetics

    c. Circuit-type resistance training or high-intensity progressive resistance training performed twice weekly for 3 months decreases HbA_{1c} 8.2–8.8% in Type 2 diabetics

    d. High exercise intensity is more predictive of improved glycemic control than high exercise volume

    e. Regular physical activity reduces the mortality in athletes with Type 1 or Type 2 DM

  15. Dyslipidemia

    a. Triglycerides reduced 18–24 h after an acute bout of high-intensity aerobic exercise

        i. Shorter duration and lower intensity blunts this response

    b. Total cholesterol and low-density lipoprotein (LDL) have small reductions following acute exercise

    c. High-density lipoprotein (HDL) levels frequently increase after an acute bout of aerobic exercise

    d. Consistent aerobic exercise for 3–12 months can reduce triglyceride levels by 10–20%

    e. Reductions in LDL are approximately 5% following ≥ 12 weeks of aerobic exercise

    f. Total cholesterol does not appear to decrease with regular exercise

    g. Regular exercise can increase HDL levels between 4% and 25%

  16. Depression

    a. Aerobic and resistance training decreases depressive symptoms in men and women

    b. Exercise appears to be as effective as psychotherapy for treating depression

    c. The American College of Sports Medicine (ACSM's) recommendations for exercise in the treatment of depression are 20–60 min of aerobic exercise 3–5 days per week

17. Osteoporosis
    a. Physically active youth have higher peak Bone Mineral Density (BMD) than their sedentary counterparts
    b. The ACSM's position stand on exercise in the treatment of osteoporosis recommends weight-bearing endurance activities (moderate-to-high intensity, 30–60 min, 3–5 times per week), activities that involve jumping, and resistance exercise (2–3 times per week)
18. Obesity
    a. Weight loss requires more caloric expenditure than intake (i.e., negative caloric balance)
    b. Dieting alone better for weight loss than exercise alone, BUT once an individual has lost weight, they are more likely to keep it off if they participate in regular physical activity
    c. Regular aerobic exercise modifies multiple cardiovascular disease risk factors in obese individuals.

Recommended Reading

1. American College of Sports Medicine Position Stand. Physical activity and bone health. *Med Sci Sports Exerc.* 2004;36(11):1985–1996.
2. Anish E, Klenck CA. Exercise as medicine: The role of exercise in treating chronic disease. In: McKeag D, Moeller JL, eds. *ACSM's Primary Care Sports Medicine.* 2nd ed. Philadelphia, PA: Lippincott, Williams & Wilkins; 2007: 107–131.
3. Baechle T, Earle RW. *Essentials of Strength Training and Conditioning.* 2nd ed. Champaign, IL: Human Kinetics; 2000.
4. Cheung K, Hume PA, Maxwell L. Delayed onset muscle soreness: Treatment strategies and performance factors. *Sports Med.* 2003;33(2):145–164.
5. Foster C, Faber MJ, Porcari JP. Exercise physiology and exercise testing. In: McKeag D, Moeller JL, eds. *ACSM's Primary Care Sports Medicine.* 2nd ed. Philadelphia, PA: Lippincott Williams & Wilkins; 2007: 29–34.
6. Frankel J, Bean JF, Frontera WR. Exercise in the elderly: Research and clinical practice. *Clin Geriatr Med.* 2006;22:239–256.
7. Hoffman J. *Physiological Aspects of Sport Training and Performance.* 1st ed. Champaign, IL: Human Kinetics; 2002.
8. Hough D, Barry HC, Eathorne SW. The mature athlete. In: Mellion MB, ed. *Sports Medicine Secrets.* 2nd ed. Philadelphia, PA: Hanley and Belfus, Inc; 1999: 47–52.
9. Howatson G, van Someren KA. The prevention and treatment of exercise-induced muscle damage. *Sports Med.* 2008;38(6):483–503.
10. Storen O, Helgerud J, Stoa ME, Hoff J. Maximal strength training improves running economy in distance runners. *Med Sci Sports Exerc.* 2008;40(6):1087–1092.
11. Thigpen L. Building strength. In: Mellion MB, ed. *Sports Medicine Secrets.* 2nd ed. Philadelphia, PA: Hanley & Belfus, Inc; 1999.

4

Sports Biomechanics

Mark A. Harrast

THROWING

I. Throwing as a kinetic chain of motion

A. Whole-body activity involving transfer of momentum from body to ball

B. Begins with drive from the large leg muscles and rotation of the hips progressing through segmental rotation of the trunk and shoulder girdle, transferring energy through elbow extension, next through the small forearm and hand muscles to the ball

C. When an initial segment of the body (e.g., trunk) accelerates, the next segment (e.g., arm) is physically left behind. The momentum from the accelerating trunk is transferred to the arm with an increased velocity of the arm that is accentuated by the forces acting on the shoulder/arm. Ultimately, this motion and the forces are transferred to the ball

D. The role of the trunk

  1. Approximately 50% of the velocity of the pitch results from the step and body rotation (i.e., from the large leg and trunk musculature)

  2. The other 50% comes from the shoulder, elbow, wrist, and fingers

  3. Peak velocity of a pitched ball dropped to

    a. Eighty-four percent when forward stride is not allowed

    b. Sixty-four percent when lower body is restricted

    c. Fifty-three percent when lower body and trunk are restricted

  4. Peak ball velocities in water polo are ~50% that of baseball due to the lack of ground reaction force.

II. Throwing: Six Phases of the Baseball Pitch (see Figure 4.1)

A. Wind-up

  1. Begins when pitcher initiates motion

  2. Ends when removing the ball from glove (at maximum knee lift with lead leg)

  3. Push off

    a. Stride leg (contralateral to pitching arm) pushes off from behind the pitcher

    b. Moves the center of gravity of the body forward

  4. As stride leg pushes off, three simultaneous motions occur:

    a. Both arms forward flex

    b. Body rotates 90°

    c. Stride leg is elevated and flexed in front of the body

    d. This positions the pitcher so that all body parts can contribute to propulsion forces of the ball

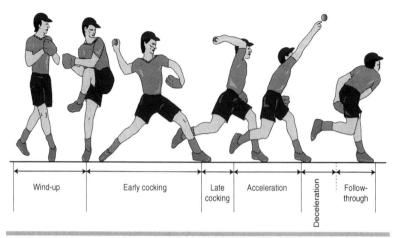

Figure 4.1 **Six phases of the baseball pitch.**

    B. Early cocking (Stride phase)
        1. As the stride leg extends toward the batter, the knee and hip of the pivot leg extend as well, propelling the body forward into the stride
        2. Hips rotate forward → forward rotation of trunk → throwing shoulder abducts, extends, and externally rotates, leaving the shoulder in a "semi-cocked" position
        3. Ends when the stride foot contacts the ground
    C. Late cocking
        1. Trunk rotates forward
        2. Shoulder maximally externally rotates
            a. From 50° of external rotation (ER) to ~175° at maximal ER
            b. To allow the greatest accelerating force to the ball over the greatest possible distance
            c. The amount of external rotation correlates with the speed of the pitched ball
    D. Acceleration
        1. Shoulder is powerfully internally rotated
            a. From 175° of ER to 90–100° of ER at ball release
        2. Very explosive phase
            a. Average peak angular velocity of shoulder internal rotation (IR) during the acceleration phase is approximately 7200°/s
        3. Shoulder abduction of 90° is relatively fixed in all throwers, regardless of style; trunk lateral flexion creates what position the arm is in relative to the vertical plane
            a. "Over the top" throwers
                i. Greater amount of contralateral lateral trunk flexion
            b. "Sidearm" throwers
                i. Less contralateral lateral trunk flexion
    E. Deceleration
        1. After ball release
        2. Decelerating internal rotation
        3. Ends when arm reached 0° of IR
    F. Follow-through
        1. A "passive phase" with the body merely catching up with the throwing arm
        2. Arm is adducted across pitcher's body, elbow is flexed.

III. Timing sequence of these phases

A. Preparation phase: Wind-up thru late cocking → 80%

B. Acceleration phase → 2%

C. Deceleration and follow-through → 18%.

IV. Pitching injuries and muscle activity according to the phase

A. Most injuries occur in the late cocking and deceleration phases, followed by the acceleration phase

B. Wind-up and early cocking
1. Few injuries occur in the early phases
2. Shoulder musculature is relatively inactive during wind-up
3. Most forces arise in the lower half of the body
4. Early cocking
   a. Trapezius and serratus anterior demonstrate moderate-to-high activity—to protract and upwardly rotate scapula
   b. Middle deltoid generates the abduction force
   c. Supraspinatus fine tunes humeral head positioning within the glenoid
   d. Static stabilizers are also active
      i. Inferior glenohumeral ligament limits anterior and posterior translation of the humeral head

C. Late cocking
1. Extreme degree of shoulder external rotation
   a. Subscapularis, pectoralis major, and latissimus dorsi stabilize the anterior glenohumeral joint during maximal ER
   b. Long head of the biceps limits anterior translation of the humeral head, restrains excessive ER, and alleviated strain on the inferior glenohumeral ligament
      i. Biceps is at its peak activity
2. Rotator cuff activity is highest here
   a. Infraspinatus and teres minor create the extreme ER
   b. Supraspinatus (less active) is at a mechanical disadvantage in extreme ER
3. Static stabilizers (glenohumeral ligaments, capsule, and labrum) are important in extremes of shoulder motion
   a. These ligaments increase in laxity due to the extreme ROM in overhead athletes
   b. This laxity is necessary for performance, however, overstretching of these ligaments (from throwing) enhances the work of the dynamic stabilizers (rotator cuff), thus with potential injury to them
4. Common injuries
   a. Anterior instability
      i. Results from repetitive microtrauma to the anterior static and dynamic stabilizers
         (A) Stretching the static ligaments
         (B) Eccentric contractions of the dynamic musculature
   b. Internal (posterior–superior) impingement
      i. Posterior–superior rotator cuff tendons (undersurface of the supraspinatus–infraspinatus junction) and posterior–superior labrum are pinched between the greater tuberosity of the humeral head and the posterosuperior glenoid rim
      ii. Two potential mechanisms:
         (A) Resulting from anterior instability
         (B) May be a normal phenomenon in all shoulders noted at 90° of abduction and external rotation; but becomes a clinical concern from repetitive motion.
      iii. Clinical exam
         (A) Posterior–superior shoulder pain in an apprehension position
         (B) May improve with scapular retraction and with the relocation test

    c. Type II superior labral antero-posterior (SLAP) lesion
        i. Instead of true anterior instability occurring with excessive ER at 90° of abduction, the arc of rotation is shifted such that ER is increased and IR is decreased
        ii. In symptomatic shoulders, this IR loss (glenohumeral internal rotation deficit, i.e., GIRD) greatly exceeds the ER gained
        iii. Loss of IR (i.e., GIRD) is caused by posterior–inferior capsule contracture
           (A) Side-to-side loss of IR > 20° is consistent with shoulder impingement
           (B) Side-to-side loss of IR < 20° is usually tolerated well
        iv. Anterior capsule stretching/laxity may or may not occur
        v. In order to get the extreme ER range, sheer forces increase at the biceps anchor and posterior superior labrum which eventually produces a posterior type II SLAP lesion
    d. Both internal impingement and posterior SLAP lesions can result in undersurface RC fraying/tears
    e. Bicipital tendonitis
        i. Results from repetitive trauma to the long head of the biceps tendon over the lesser tuberosity during abduction with external rotation
    f. Elbow
        i. Medial tension injuries due to high valgus forces
           (A) Little Leaguer's Elbow
              (1) Injury to the medial elbow in young throwing athletes
              (2) Includes:
                  (a) Medial epicondylitis
                  (b) Traction apophysitis
                  (c) Stress fracture of the medial epicondyle epiphysis
           (B) Ulnar collateral ligament (UCL) injury
              (1) During late cocking and early acceleration phases
              (2) "Dropped elbow" pitching increases the stress on the UCL and also creates less control of the ball (thus, pitchers should keep "elbow up")

D. Acceleration
    1. Latissimus dorsi and pectoralis major are the primary active internal rotators
    2. Subscapularis positions the humeral head in the glenoid and prevents its subluxation
    3. Teres minor provides a posterior restraint to limit humeral head translation during this forceful internal rotation
        a. Posterior rotator cuff (teres minor) tenderness is common in pitchers
    4. Injury
        a. Subacromial impingement in older pitchers as they internally rotate and adduct the abducted arm during acceleration
        b. Medial tension injuries such as Little Leaguer's Elbow and UCL injuries (see above) occur in the late cocking and early acceleration phases due to the high valgus forces (64 Nm) reached during these phases

E. Deceleration
    1. Muscle forces are eccentric, which generate the greatest tensile loads
    2. To decelerate rapid internal rotation, eccentric contraction of the posterior shoulder musculature is important
        a. Scapular muscle activity is highest
        b. Rotator cuff external rotators (esp teres minor)
        c. Posterior deltoid
    3. To decelerate rapid elbow extension, eccentric contraction of the biceps muscle occurs
    4. Common injuries
        a. Posterior instability
           i. Posterior structures are stressed as they resist glenohumeral distraction and horizontal adduction

    b. Isolated RC tears

    c. SLAP lesion

       i. Due to repetitive traction forces

       ii. Long head of the biceps eccentrically contracts to decelerate the rapidly extending elbow, which, in turn places significant stress on the biceps–labral complex (particularly the anterior superior labrum)

    d. Bennett lesion

       i. An extra-articular ossification of the posterior inferior capsule arising at the insertion of the capsule onto the posterior inferior glenoid

       ii. Peculiar to the baseball pitcher

       iii. Associated with rotator cuff syndrome and/or instability

       iv. Etiology unclear. Potential mechanisms:

          (A) Subluxation and impingement of the humeral head on the posterior capsule

          (B) From a traction injury to the posterior inferior capsule

    e. Valgus Extension Overload (VEO)

       i. Impingement of the posteromedial olecranon against the medial wall of the olecranon fossa from valgus elbow stress combined with elbow extension

       ii. Repetitive impingement can cause olecranon osteophytes, loose bodies, and scarring

       iii. Pain at posteromedial olecranon during passive elbow hyperextension with valgus stress

       iv. Accounts for ~65% of surgeries for medial elbow pain in professional baseball players

F. Follow-through

    1. Low-grade eccentric loading of the shoulder muscles

    2. A "passive phase" where the body is merely "catching up" with the throwing arm and thus, a rare potential for injury.

V. Adaptive changes with repeated throwing

A. Shoulder

    1. Increased ER range

    a. Full rotational ROM (IR → ER) is still the same as the contralateral shoulder, but ER is increased and IR is decreased (through various means: posterior capsule tightness, anterior instability, progressive retroversion of the humeral head, or all of the above)

       i. Total arc of shoulder rotation should be >=180°; that is, ER + IR >=180°

       ii. Pitchers at risk for impingement symptoms have a total arc <180° and/or a side-to-side GIRD of >20°.

       iii. Thus, be certain to measure the full arc of motion (with the scapula stabilized to isolate glenohumeral motion) before deciding if an internal rotation deficit is present

    b. May lead to anterior instability and impingement due to a shift in the glenohumeral rotation axis

    2. Imbalance in shoulder rotator strength

    a. Normal strength ratio of IR:ER → 3:2

    b. A common imbalance involves increased IR strength and decreased ER strength

B. Elbow

    1. Increased valgus stress at the elbow causes a breakdown of the medial stabilizing structures—particularly during the late cocking and early acceleration phases (see above)

    a. Ulnar collateral ligament

    b. Joint capsule

    c. Medial flexor muscles

2. Elbow flexion contracture sometimes develops from hypertrophy of soft tissues and osseous structures.

VI. Types of pitches

A. Determined by the spin imparted onto the ball by the hands and fingers at ball release

B. Normal follow through involves forearm pronation

C. "Breaking pitches"—forearm is relatively supinated at release and then pronates
   1. "Curve ball"—should not have much supination; the curve should come from the wrist

D. USA Baseball Guidelines
   1. Curve balls and sliders should not be pitched until puberty has been reached and bones are "more mature"
   2. Youth pitchers should not compete in baseball more than 9 months per year; during the three "off" months, they should not compete in other overhead arm sports (competitive swimming, javelin, etc.)
   3. Age-based pitch count guideline—see Table 4.1.

VII. Common biomechanical abnormalities in pitching

A. "Hanging" or "dropped elbow"
   1. A sign of fatigue
   2. Decreased shoulder abduction allows elbow to drop and thus a reduction in velocity
   3. Increased risk of injury to shoulder (rotator cuff injury) and elbow (UCL injury)

B. "Opening up too soon"
   1. Normally, once full external rotation is accomplished in late cocking, the body will begin to rotate forward into early acceleration
   2. If there is early forward body rotation, the arm lags behind and does not reach full ER
   3. Increases stress on the anterior shoulder, external rotators, and UCL (valgus stress at the elbow).

SWIMMING

I. Four competitive strokes

A. Freestyle (crawl)

B. Backstroke

C. Butterfly

D. Breaststroke.

II. Stroke phases for A–C (not breaststroke)

A. Entry/catch
   1. Hand entry into water to the beginning of it's backward movement

B. Pull
   1. Beginning of the hand's backward movement to the hand's arrival in the vertical plane of the shoulder

Table 4.1   Age-Based Pitch Counts

Age	Pitches Per Game	Per Week	Per Season	Per Year
9–10	50	75	1000	2000
11–12	75	100	1000	3000
13–14	75	125	1000	3000

Adapted from USA Baseball Medical and Safety Advisory Committee 2006.

C. Push

    1. Hand's movement from the vertical plane of the shoulder to its release from the water

D. Recovery

    1. Hand's release from the water to it's re-entry into the water for the next stroke (i.e., the aerial return of the hand).

III. Propulsive phase: pull and push

A. Pectoralis major and latissimus dorsi

    1. Move the arm through adduction and internal rotation starting from a stretched position of abduction and ER

B. Assistance is provided by the serratus anterior and the internal rotation function of the subscapularis and teres major.

IV. Recovery phase

A. Scapular retraction and external rotation

    1. Rhomboids and mid-trapezius retract scapula

    2. Posterior deltoid, teres minor, infraspinatus externally rotate the shoulder

B. Mid-recovery

    1. Hand entry preparation

        a. Serratus anterior and upper trapezius rotate the scapula upward for shoulder stabilization

C. Body roll

    1. Nearly 160°

    2. Paraspinals and abdominal musculature are important contributors to body roll

    3. Lack of body roll = lack of power

        a. Common in novice swimmers

    4. Decreases form drag (see below) as the cross sectional area of the body pushing through the water is decreased

    5. Helps with high elbow position during recovery and thus better placement of the hand/arm for the entry/catch.

V. Drag = water resistance

A. Form drag

    1. Dependent on body position

    2. The more horizontal the body is in the water, the less is the drag

B. Wave drag

    1. Turbulence at the water surface created by the moving swimmer

    2. Can rebound from the sides or bottom of pool

C. Frictional drag

    1. Contact of skin and hair with water

    2. Body suits (which have recently been banned from many competitions) are used to decrease frictional drag.

VI. Lift force

A. Perpendicular to the drag force

B. Bernoulli principle

    1. Water flows around the hand during the pull and meets on the back edge of the hand which creates a pressure known as the "lift force."

VII. "S" shaped pulling pattern

A. Designed to continually find still water that is not moving in order to propel the swimmer forward

    B. Over the last 10 years, there has been a change in coaching technique away from the "S" pull to more of a straight through pull and sometimes somewhere in between

    C. Other new techniques

        1. Earlier catch

        2. Earlier exit (at beltline instead of at the trochanter).

VIII. Kick patterns

    A. Knees should flex only 30–40° in the flutter kick of the freestyle stroke

    B. Hip flexion should be minimal

    C. Two-beat flutter kick

        1. One down beat and one up beat of each leg during the stroke cycle

    D. Six-beat flutter kick

        1. Three down and three up beats during one arm cycle

    E. Whip kick in breaststroke

        1. Creates a valgus stress at knee

        2. Predisposes to knee injuries (i.e., more knee injuries in breaststrokers)

          a. Medial collateral ligament sprain

          b. Medial plica/synovitis.

IX. Common stroke flaws

    A. Body position

        1. Head and shoulders are high in the water and hips/legs are lower

          a. Sometimes due to lack of kicking

          b. Decreases horizontal position

          c. Increases drag force

    B. Hand entry past midline

        1. Exacerbates impingement

        2. Creates side-to-side movement

          a. Increases form drag

    C. Poor body roll

        1. Increased form drag

        2. Predisposes to impingement

        3. Bilateral breathing increases body roll

        4. Ideally, swimmer should roll body 45°

    D. Excessively straight arm during recovery

        1. Predisposes to impingement

        2. Teach "high elbow" on recovery

    E. Striving for too much length in the stroke

        1. A long stroke improves propulsion

        2. But, the resultant prolonged shoulder adduction and internal rotation may lead to hypovascularity of the supraspinatus and risk of tendinopathy, which hand paddles can exacerbate.

X. General rehabilitation (and prehabilitation) principles for the swimmer

    A. Most shoulder pain (impingement and RC tendinopathy) in swimmers is due to dynamic muscle imbalances, weakness, and biomechanical faults (and not hard anatomical factors)

    B. Strengthen scapular stabilization

    C. Endurance training for serratus anterior and lower trap

        1. During swimming, the serratus anterior has been demonstrated to function at 75% of its maximum test ability (i.e., it is an overused muscle in swimming)

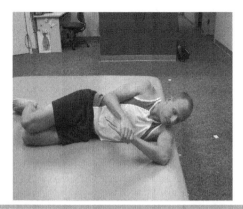

Figure 4.2   Posterior capsule shoulder stretching with a stabilized scapula ("Sleeper stretch").

    D. Stretch internal rotators and posterior capsule (Figure 4.2)
       1. Not the anterior capsule which is what many swimmers do regularly (Figure 4.3)
    E. Cervical and thoracic mobilization.

WALKING AND RUNNING

I. Walking gait (Figure 4.4)

    A. Two phases of gait
       1. Stance (60%)
         a. Loading response
         b. Midstance
         c. Terminal stance—propulsive portion of cycle until toe off and swing begins
         d. Pre-swing/toe off

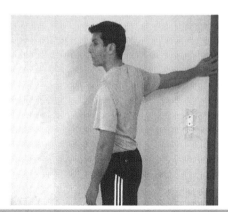

Figure 4.3   Anterior capsule shoulder stretching is commonly performed by swimmers, but rarely needed. They should focus their stretching routine on the posterior capsule and internal rotators (see Figure 4.2).

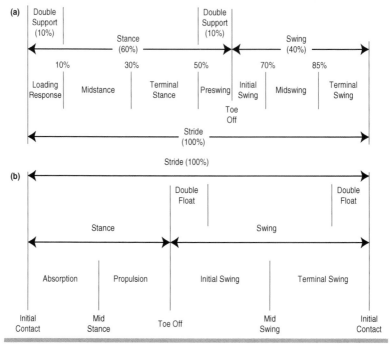

Figure 4.4 **Phases of gait. (Modified from Ounpuu, S. The biomechanics of walking and running.** *Clin Sports Med.* **1994;13(4):843–863. Permission Granted 02/11.)**

    2. Swing (40%)
        a. Initial swing
        b. Mid-swing
        c. Terminal swing
    3. Double limb support
        a. Occurs in the first and last 10% of stance phase
   B. Forward momentum for walking is provided by the stance leg.

II. Running gait
   A. Three phases
    1. Stance (decreased to 30% while running and 20% while sprinting (from 60% while walking))
        a. Initial contact
            i. Lateral foot contacts the ground with the foot slightly supinated
            ii. Energy absorption is key here
                (A) Vertical ground reaction force may reach $2.2 \times$ body weight in running (whereas in walking it is $1.1\times$)
                (B) Subtalar joint pronation, ankle dorsiflexion, knee and hip flexion help to dissipate forces
                (C) Eccentric contractions of the proximal muscles prevent excessive hip and knee flexion and falling to the ground
            iii. Hip adductors provide stability

      b. Midstance

        i. Dorsiflexion maximizes and results from forward progression of the tibia while foot is on the ground

        ii. Supination starts the propulsive phase as the heel begins to lift off the ground

      c. Toe off/propulsion

    2. Swing

      a. Initial swing

      b. Mid-swing

      c. Terminal swing

    3. Float

      a. Occurs at the beginning of initial swing and the end of terminal swing

      b. Neither foot contacts the ground

  B. Forward momentum needed for running is provided by the swinging leg and arms

  C. Most kinematic difference between walking and running occur in the sagittal plane of motion

    1. The body lowers its center of gravity by increasing

      a. Hip flexion

      b. Knee flexion

      c. Ankle dorsiflexion

  D. As speed increases, stance phase lessens

    1. This increases the velocity and range of lower limb motion

      a. Serves to minimize vertical displacement

    2. Energy costs increase

    3. Faster running changes foot contact

      a. Slower running and walking: heel to toe

      b. Faster running: foot strikes with forefoot and heel simultaneously or forefoot initially followed by heel lowering to the ground

      c. Sprinting: maintains weight-bearing on the forefoot from contact to toe-off.

  E. Angle of gait

    1. Angle between the longitudinal bisection of the foot and the line of progression

    2. Walking $= 10°$

    3. Running $=$ approaches $0°$ as footstrike is on the line of progression which allows more efficient locomotion by limiting lateral deviation of the center of gravity (i.e., decreased base of support).

III. Pronation

  A. Triplanar motion

    1. Ankle dorsiflexion

    2. Subtalar eversion

    3. Forefoot abduction

  B. Effect of pronation up the kinetic chain

    1. Tibial internal rotation

    2. Knee flexion and adduction (valgum)

    3. Femoral internal rotation

    4. Hip flexion and adduction

    5. Pelvis rotates anteriorly

    6. Lumbar spine extends and laterally flexes to the same side

  C. Pronation phase (first half of stance phase) of gait involves mostly eccentric muscular contractions to provide joint control and shock absorption.

IV. Supination

  A. Triplanar motion

    2. Subtalar inversion

    3. Forefoot adduction

  B. Effects of supination up the kinetic chain

    1. Tibial external rotation

    2. Knee extension and abduction (varum)

    3. Femoral external rotation

    4. Hip extension and abduction

    5. Pelvis rotates posteriorly

    6. Lumbar spine extends and laterally flexes to opposite side

  C. Supination phase (second half of stance phase) of gait involves mostly concentric muscular contractions (particularly gluteals) to provide acceleration and propulsion.

V. General rehabilitation (and prehabilitation) principles for the runner

  A. Core stabilization

  B. Pelvic girdle stabilization

    1. Hip abductor neuromuscular reeducation and strengthening and endurance training

  C. Hip flexibility

  D. Ankle and foot flexibility to better accommodate ground reaction forces.

JUMPING AND LANDING

I. Noncontact anterior cruciate ligament (ACL) injury prevention programs have attempted to influence a variety of noncontact ACL injury risk factors

  A. Balance

  B. Flexibility

  C. Strength

  D. Jumping and landing technique.

II. ACL injuries occur more frequently with the knee in less flexion

  A. Greater knee extensor loads

  B. Greater anterior tibial translation forces.

III. Gender differences which may predispose female athletes to noncontact ACL injuries

  A. Females

    1. Land more erect with less knee and hip flexion

    2. Land with less hip external rotation and abduction

    3. Increased quadriceps activation over hamstrings (less knee flexion/greater knee extension force).

IV. Teaching appropriate jumping/landing techniques is important in ACL injury prevention programs

  A. Increase knee and hip flexion during landing

  B. Balance quadriceps to hamstring activation ratio.

CYCLING

I. The key to assessing the injured cyclist is assessing their bike fit and how the rider interacts, statically and dynamically, with their bike. Static bike fits are still quite common; though many clinicians (who treat cyclists) and coaches (who train cyclists) are using modern bike fit technology to assess the rider dynamically and how the cyclist interacts with their bike (see section III) for injury prevention and performance enhancement.

II. Static bike fit

A. Saddle height
  1. Measured from a straight line taken from the saddle down the seat tube through the crank axis to the pedal at the bottom of downstroke
  2. Appropriate height
     a. Knee flexion angle of 20–30° when the pedal is at the bottom of downstroke and foot is neutral, or
     b. Riders inseam length × 0.883
  3. Should not have pelvic tilt when seat height is optimal
     a. Improves quadriceps power
     b. Improves core stability
  4. Saddle too high
     a. Power is diminished
     b. Excess stress on the posterior structures
        i. Hamstrings, gastrocs, posterior knee joint capsule
     c. Excessive hip extension
        i. Loss of pelvic and core stability
        ii. Pelvis rocks from side to side
        iii. Fatigues adductors, gluteals, spine/core, and upper body musculature
  5. Saddle too low
     a. Power is diminished—due to suboptimal length–tension relationships of lower limb musculature
     b. Increased knee flexion throughout the pedal cycle
        i. Patellofemoral pain
        ii. Suprapatellar bursa loading

B. Saddle fore/aft position
  1. Plumb line dropped from the inferior pole of the patella should fall over the front pedal spindle (or up to 2 cm behind) when the cranks are in the horizontal position (3:00)
  2. Check cleat positioning
     a. First metatarsal head should lie directly over the pedal axel
  3. Too far forward
     a. Knees are more flexed, hips more extended
     b. Increased patellofemoral loading
     c. More upright position
        i. Less aerodynamic
        ii. May need to raise the saddle height if the saddle needs to be so forward
  4. Too far back
     a. Hamstrings and gluteals will be overlengthened
        i. Inhibits force production

C. Saddle tilt
  1. Close to level or parallel to ground
  2. 10–15° of anterior tilt may reduce low back pain
  3. Aerobar users (time trialists/triathletes) prefer a slight downward/anterior tilt to decrease perineal pressure

D. Stem and handlebar height
  1. Affects "reach"
  2. Appropriate reach
     a. Pelvis is tilted forward so that the back is flat without kinks in the thoracolumbar and cervicothoracic junctions
     b. Shoulder girdle is not excessively protracted
     c. Slight elbow flexion with hand on brake hoods
  3. Different sized stems can optimize reach if the frame (top tube length) was properly fitted.

    4. Drop between saddle height and top of handlebars
      a. Usually 3–5 cm, but range is 0–8 cm
      b. Larger drop
        i. More aerodynamic
        ii. Only effective if the rider has the postural stability and flexibility to control the bike in this position
    5. Wrists held in neutral
      a. Prolonged weight-bearing on the ulnar aspect of an extended wrist can compress the ulnar nerve in Guyon's canal.

III. Dynamic fit

A. Video analysis

B. Wattage measure (power output)
    1. Once a fit change has been made, assess the power output; if the power output improves, the change made will likely improve performance

C. Heart rate
    1. Heart rate (similar to power output) can be used as a performance measure to determine if a static fit change is beneficial

D. Pedal torque measurement and spin analysis
    1. Can help even out the pedal stroke so the rider is pulling up during the upstroke as well as pushing down during the downstroke.

IV. Specific injuries

A. Anterior knee pain
    1. Saddle too low or far forward
    2. Excessive climbing/hilly rides
    3. Pushing too big of a gear/low RPMs
    4. Cranks too long

B. Medial knee pain
    1. Toes pointing out with cleats
    2. Too much pedal float
    3. Feet too far apart

C. Lateral knee pain
    1. Toes pointing in with cleats
    2. Too much pedal float
    3. Feet too close

D. Posterior knee pain
    1. Saddle too high or far back

E. Cervical or thoracic pain
    1. Reach too great
    2. Handlebars too low

F. Lumbar pain
    1. Overstretched riding position
    2. Poor pelvic and hip mobility causing pelvic rocking, commonly seen when saddle is too high

G. Perineal pain/numbness
    1. Saddle too high
    2. Saddle tilt excessive
    3. Saddle too narrow (not supporting the ischial tuberosities).

Recommended Reading

1. Agosta J, Biomechanics of common sporting injuries. In: Brukner P, Khan K, eds. *Clin Sports Med*. 2002:43–83. McGraw-Hill, Australia.
2. Burkhart SS, Morgan CD, Kibler WB. The disabled throwing shoulder: Spectrum of pathology Part 1: Patho-anatomy and biomechanics. *Arthroscopy*. 2003;19:404–420.
3. Chappell JD, Creighton A, Giuliani C, Yu B, Garrett WE. Kinematics and electromyography of landing preparation in vertical stop-jump risks for noncontact ACL injury. *Am J Sports Med*. 2007;35:235–241.
4. Dugan SA, Bhat KP. Biomechanics and analysis of running gait. *Phys Med Rehabil Clin N Am*. 2005;16:603–621.
5. Meister K. Injuries to the shoulder in the throwing athlete Part one. *Am J Sports Med*. 2000;28:265–275.
6. Park SS, Loebenberg ML, Rokito AS, Zuckerman JD. The shoulder in baseball pitching. Biomechanics and related injuries—Part 1. *Bull Hosp Joint Dis*. 2002;61:68–79.
7. Pollard H, Fernandez M. Spinal musculoskeletal injuries associated with swimming: A discussion of technique. *ACO*. 2004;12:72–80.
8. Silberman MR, Webner D, Collina S, Shiple BJ. Road bicycle fit. *Clin J Sport Med* 2005;15:271–276.
9. Yu B, Lin CF, Garrett WE. Lower extremity biomechanics during the landing of a stop-jump task. *Clin Biomech*. 2006;21:297–305.

5

Pharmacology

William J. Sullivan

I. Therapeutic Drugs

A. Analgesics
   1. Acetaminophen
      a. Mechanism of action:
         i. Exact mechanism unclear
         ii. May elevate pain threshold, may affect inhibition of the nitric oxide pathway mediated by a variety of neurotransmitter receptors including N-methyl-D-aspartate and substance P.
         iii. Fever reduction by inhibition of endogenous prostaglandins in the central nervous system
         iv. Little to no anti-inflammatory effects
      b. Indications
         i. Excellent safety profile
         ii. Good initial choice
            (A) First-line agent for mild-to-moderate osteoarthritis
               (1) American College of Rheumatology
               (2) American Academy of Orthopedic Surgery
               (3) American Pain Society
            (B) First-line agent for medically complex patients
               (1) American Geriatric Society: mild-to-moderate musculoskeletal (MSK) pain in those over 50
               (2) American Heart Association: for those with cardiac conditions or risk factors
               (3) National Kidney Foundation: for those with underlying renal conditions
         iii. Temporary relief of minor aches and pains associated with the common cold, headache, toothache, muscular aches, backache, for the minor pain of arthritis, for the pain of menstrual cramps, and for the reduction of fever
         iv. Superior gastrointestinal (GI) safety compared to nonsteroidal anti-inflammatory drugs (NSAIDs)
      c. Contraindications
         i. Chronic alcoholics may be at risk for liver disease, but conflicting reports
         ii. Reported safe in chronic, stable liver disease, but other evidence conflicting
         iii. Overdose in conjunction with taking anticonvulsants may increase risk of liver disease
         iv. High caffeine intake may elevate risk
         v. Recommended maximum daily dose 4000 mg/day, narrow safety window
         vi. Maximum daily recommended dose higher in some European countries, may lead to higher toxicity

2. Opioids
   a. Mechanism of action
      i. Various opioid receptors, primarily mu, kappa, and delta
      ii. CNS and peripheral effects
      iii. Codeine conversion into morphine in liver dependent on cytochrome P-450, may not be efficacious in some populations
      iv. Propoxyphene adds little analgesia to acetaminophen, has been withdrawn from market
   b. Indications
      i. Moderate–to-severe pain
      ii. Cough (e.g., codeine)
      iii. Diarrhea (e.g., loperamide)
   c. Contraindications
      i. Hypersensitivity/allergy
      ii. Concern regarding combination medications (acetominophen toxicity)
      iii. Dependency versus addiction
      iv. Increased scrutiny from Food and Drug Administration (FDA), also concern with combination medications and additional acetaminophen use leading to liver toxicity
      v. Drug testing may limit use (see below)
   d. Relative potency (Table 5.1)
3. Tramadol
   a. Mechanism of action
      i. Synthetic analog of codeine
      ii. Low affinity for opioid receptors, but primary metabolite has a high affinity for opioid receptors
      iii. Only partially inhibited by naloxone
      iv. Norepinepherine and Serotonin reuptake inhibition also part of the mechanism of action
      v. Available as combination medications
   b. Indications
      i. Moderate–to-severe pain
B. Antibiotics
   1. Penicillin and derivatives
      a. Mechanism of action
         i. Weaken bacterial cell wall by inhibiting formation of peptidoglycan cross-links
      b. Little research on athletic performance
      c. May be overprescribed for elite athletes for nonbacterial conditions

Table 5.1 Potency of opioid medications relative to morphine

Medication	Morphine equivalent
Dextropropoxyphene	0.025
Codeine	0.1
Demerol	0.36
Hydrocodone	0.6
Morphine	1.0
Oxycodone	1.5–2
Fentanyl	75–100

       d. Many athletes fear adverse effects

         i. GI side effects may impair performance

   2. Fluoroquinolones

       a. Mechanism of action

         i. Inhibit bacterial enzymes responsible for DNA replication and transcription

       b. Contraindications

         i. Known hypersensitivity

         ii. Central nervous system (CNS) conditions: epilepsy, stroke, meningitis

         iii. Prolonged QT syndrome

         iv. Children: risk of growth plate injury, tendon rupture

       c. Risks

         i. May cause tendinopathy or spontaneous tendon rupture (particularly in the elderly and in patients taking corticosteroids)

C. Antidiabetic agents

   1. Insulin and oral medication doses may need to be adjusted during periods of exercise

   2. Injection site not recommended to be at area of primary muscle use (e.g., thigh for cyclist) due to increased uptake during exercise which may lead to hypoglycemia

   3. May be used as performance enhancer: produces similar anabolic effects to insulin-like growth factor-I (IGF-I) when taken with glucose.

   4. Thiazolidinediones

       a. Mechanism of action

         i. Complete mechanism unclear

         ii. Lowers insulin resistance

         iii. Pioglitazone (Actos®) reduces triglycerides and increases high-density lipoprotein (HDL)

         iv. Rosiglitazone (Avandia®) increases HDL and slightly increases low-density lipoprotein (LDL), less interaction with oral contraceptives and erythromycin

         v. Generally not first-line agent

       b. Risks/side effects

         i. Upper respiratory infections and sinusitis

         ii. Headaches

         iii. Anemia

         iv. Fluid retention which may lead to congestive heart failure (CHF)

         v. Weight gain

         vi. Muscle pain

         vii. Increased risk of fracture in women

         viii. Possible risk of liver damage, as seen in older thiazolidinediones

   5. Sulfonylureas

       a. Mechanism of action

         i. Increased amount of insulin produced by the pancreas

         ii. Combination medications contain metformin, decreased amount of glucose produced by the liver

         iii. Long acting

         iv. Dose adjustment may be necessary to prevent hypoglycemia during competitive or training activity

         v. Chlorpropamide (Diabinese®)

         vi. Glipizide (Glucotrol®)

         vii. Glyburide (DiaBeta®)

         viii. Glimpiride (Amaryl®)

       b. Risks/side effects

         i. Sulfa allergy cross reactivity

         ii. Teratogenic, do not take while pregnant or if trying to become pregnant

        iii. Unsafe if liver or kidney problems, metabolized by liver, excreted via kidneys

        iv. Alcohol increases risk of low blood sugar

        v. Hyperinsulinemia may lead to increased cardiovascular disease

        vi. May cause weight gain

6. Meglitinides

    a. Mechanism of action

        i. Novel agents

        ii. Increase amount of insulin produced by pancreas, similar to sulfonylurea agents

        iii. Faster acting, shorter duration

        iv. Repaglinide (Prandin®)

        v. Nateglinide (Starlix®)

    b. Risks/side effects

        i. May not be safe in pregnancy

        ii. Similar side effects as sulfonylureas

        iii. May not be safe in liver or renal disease

7. Biguanides

    a. Mechanism of action

        i. Not completely understood

        ii. Decrease glucose production in liver

        iii. Increase glucose absorption in muscle

        iv. Decrease insulin resistance

        v. Metformin (Glucophage®)

            (A) Do not increase insulin production

            (B) Not associated with hypoglycemia

    b. Risks/side effects

        i. Nausea

        ii. Loss of appetite

        iii. Diarrhea

        iv. Increased abdominal gas

        v. Metallic taste

        vi. Rarely lactic acidosis during exercise, may limit use in athletes. Higher likelihood if liver or kidney problems exist, and associated with dehydration

        vii. Associated with menstrual irregularities in women with polycystic ovary syndrome, may lead to unplanned pregnancy

D. Antihypertensives: Diuretics and β-blockers often listed as first-line agents for treatment of hypertension (JNC 7), but banned by many organizations (see below)

    1. ACE inhibitors

        a. Mechanism of action

            i. Inhibit angiotensin-converting enzyme

            ii. Decreased production of angiotensin II

            iii. Dilation of blood vessels leads to lower blood pressure

        b. Indications

            i. Elevated blood pressure

            ii. CHF

            iii. Stroke prevention

            iv. Improves postmyocardial infarction survival

        c. Contraindications

            i. Not for use in pregnant individuals

            ii. Not for use if renal artery stenosis

            iii. Hypersensitivity

        d. Risks/side effects

            i. Cough

        iii. Hypotension, dizziness
        iv. Headache
        v. Weakness
        vi. Rash
        vii. Metallic taste
        viii. May increase lithium levels

2. Calcium channel blockers
   a. Mechanism of action
      i. Dilate blood vessels
      ii. Decreased resistance to blood flow
      iii. Decreased cardiac oxygen requirement
   b. Indications
      i. Hypertension
      ii. Angina
      iii. Abnormal cardiac rhythms
   c. Contraindications
      i. Verapamil and diltiazem reduce heart rate and strength of contraction, may not be best in those with CHF or in athletes
      ii. Amlodipine has little effect on heart rate, poor choice if arrhythmia, but good choice for athletes
   d. Risks/side effects
      i. Verapamil and diltiazem decrease elimination of many drugs by liver
      ii. Grapefruit juice may elevate concentrations of some calcium channel blockers
      iii. Common side effects include constipation, nausea, headache, rash, edema, hypotension

3. Angiotensin-II receptor blockers
   a. Mechanism of action
      i. Block action of angiotensin II, a potent blood vessel constrictor
      ii. Decreased blood pressure
      iii. Decreased cardiac work
   b. Indications
      i. Hypertension
      ii. Prevention of kidney failure in those with hypertension (HTN) or diabetes
      iii. May prevent recurrence of atrial fibrillation
      iv. Used when ACE inhibitors not tolerated, for example, due to cough
   c. Contraindications
      i. Pregnancy due to birth defects
      ii. Hypersensitivity
      iii. Renal artery stenosis
   d. Risks/side effects
      i. Couch
      ii. Hyperkalemia
      iii. Hypotension
      iv. Dizziness
      v. Headache
      vi. Rash
      vii. Diarrhea
      viii. Metalic taste

4. Diuretics
   a. Mechanism of action
      i. Increase sodium chloride excretion in urine
      ii. Distal tubule (hydrocholorthiazide) or loop segment (furosemide) as site of action

    b. Indications

        i. Hypertension, often initial choice in general population

        ii. Fluid retention

    c. Contraindications

        i. Pregnancy

        ii. Limited use in athletic population since it is a prohibited substance (used as a masking agent)

    d. Risks/side effects

        i. Volume depletion—may predispose to dehydration

        ii. Potassium imbalance

        iii. Decreased athletic performance

        iv. May contribute to cardiac events

  5. β-Blockers

    a. Mechanism of action

        i. Slows heart rate by decreasing response to sympathetic input

        ii. Decreases contraction of smooth muscle in peripheral arteries and airways

        iii. Slows resting heart rated

        iv. Decreases cardiac response to exercise

        v. Adverse affect on cardiovascular training

    b. Indications

        i. Hypertension

        ii. Tachycardia

        iii. Angina

        iv. Recent myocardial infarction

    c. Contraindications

        i. May increase asthma symptoms

        ii. Prohibited substance for participation in several sports (shooting, archer, powerboating) due to antianxiety effects

    d. Risks/side effects

        i. Depression

        ii. Fatigue

        iii. Male impotence

        iv. Increased wheezing

        v. Nightmares

        vi. Impaired athlete performance

E. Asthma medications

  1. Anti-inflammatories (glucocorticoids)

    a. Mechanism of action

        i. Inhaled glucocorticoid, upregulate gene expression of anti-inflammatory proteins, downregulate gene expression of pro-inflammatory proteins

    b. Indications

        i. Treatment of chronic asthma

    c. Contraindications

        i. Hypersensitivity to glucocorticoids

        ii. Should not be used as a rescue agent (i.e., takes 1–3 weeks for effect)

    d. Risks/side effects

        i. Chronic use may lead to osteopenia/osteoporosis

        ii. Thrush, especially in older population

        iii. Hoarseness

  2. Khellin derivatives—often used in children for mild symptoms

    a. Derived from plant *Amnivisnaga*

        i. Bronchodialator, inhibit histamine release from mast cells

      ii. Cromolyn sodium (Intal®)

      iii. Nedocromil sodium (Tilade®)

3. Antileukotrienes

  a. Mechanism of action

    i. Block leukotriene effect of potent bronchoconstriction

    ii. Block synthesis (zileuton) or receptors (zafirlukast/montelukast)

    iii. Decrease inflammation, rapid onset

  b. Indications

    i. Allergy and asthma symptoms

  c. Contraindications

    i. Hypersensitivity

    ii. Phenylketonurics should not be used, contains phenylalanine (aspartame)

  d. Risks/side effects

    i. Zileuton not approved for children, requires hepatic testing

    ii. Runny nose, headache, fever, stomach pain, diarrhea

4. Bronchodilators

  a. Mechanism of action

    i. Relax bronchial smooth muscle

    ii. Decrease mucus secretion

  b. Indications

    i. Short-acting B2-agonists

      (A) Main rescue medication

      (B) Oral forms not approved by NCAA

    ii. Long-acting B2-agonists such as salmeterol (Serevent®)

      (A) 12-h duration, not rescue/acute medication

  c. Risks/side effects

    i. Oral medication (clenbuterol) banned due to anabolic effects. However, not an ingredient in any FDA-approved drug in the United States

F. NSAIDs/cyclooxygenase-2 (COX-2) inhibitors

  1. No evidence to suggest individual superiority for pain

    a. May be individual patient preference

    b. Dose-dependent side effects

    c. Lower doses may provide analgesic effect

    d. Higher doses anti-inflammatory

  2. Conventional NSAIDS block cyclooxygenase

    a. Pain/inflammation

    b. Prostaglandins in GI tract

    c. Renal dysfunction

    d. Platelet inhibition

  3. Cox-2 specific (celecoxib)

    a. Decreased GI toxicity

    b. Increased cardiovascular risks

  4. Cox-2 selective (etodolac, meloxicam)

    a. Decreased GI side effects

    b. Unknown cardiovascular risks

    c. Etodolac with higher COX-2 selectivity

  5. General properties

    a. Mechanism of action

      i. Block cyclooxygenase, reduce prostaglandins

    b. Indications

      i. Pain

      ii. Fever

  iii. Inflammation
  iv. Arthritis
 c. Contraindications
    i. Hypersensitivity
   ii. Reye's syndrome risk with chicken pox or influenza in children
  iii. Avoid aspirin (ASA) and conventional NSAIDs if known or high risk of GI ulcers
 d. Risks/side effects
    i. Renal disease
   ii. GI bleeding, ulcers
  iii. Headache, rash, nausea, vomiting
  iv. GI protectivity of COX-2 agents mitigated by concomitant ASA use
   v. Animal studies suggest COX-2 may affect ligament strength, no clinically demonstrated difference in human muscle strength

G. Viscosupplementation
 1. Hyaluronic acid (HA) is an unbranched, high-molecular weight polysaccharide
 2. Distributed throughout the body, especially as a major component of the synovial fluid and of cartilage
 3. Primary role of the HA in synovial fluid and cartilage is to maintain the viscoelastic structural and functional characteristics of the articular matrix
  a. Mechanisms of action
     i. Rheological
       (A) Immediate restoration of synovial fluid rheologic properties (i.e., restoration of viscosity and elasticity)
       (B) Maintenance of increased rheological properties for 3–7 days after injection
       (C) Antinociceptive effect
       (D) Mechanical sponge or sieve (i.e., assist with removal from the joint of immune complexes and inflammatory cells)
    ii. Biological
       (A) Anti-inflammatory effect
       (B) Effect on immune cells
       (C) Restoration of hyaluronate synthesis; positive feedback for endogenous hyaluronate synthesis
       (D) Effects on cartilage: increased biosynthesis, decreased degradation
       (E) Effects on chondrocytes: decreased apoptosis, proliferation
       (F) Antioxidant effect
  b. Indications
     i. Multiple brands of viscosupplementation (Synvisc®, Hyalgan®, Supartz®, Orthovisc®, Euflexxa®)
    ii. Differences based on molecular weight and how they are produced (e.g., Euflexxa® bacterially derived, all of the rest are derived from rooster combs)
   iii. Strength gains demonstrated after viscosupplementation, due to pain relief?
  c. Contraindications
     i. Known allergy
    ii. Allergy to poultry/eggs (except Euflexxa®)
  d. Risks/side effects
     i. Local reaction, hypersensitivity
    ii. Injection site pain
   iii. Infection
   iv. Bleeding

H. Corticosteroids
 1. Various routes—oral, inhaled, injected, topical, ionto/phonophoresis
 2. Limited efficacy studies, both for acute and chronic condition

3. Injection complication
   a. Fat pad atrophy and hypopigmentation most common
   b. Injection into tendon not recommended, paratendon probably safe
   c. Use remains controversial
4. Systemic use is prohibited when administered orally, rectally, or by intravenous or intramuscular injection
5. Topical preparations for skin, ophthalmic (eye), otic (ear), nasal, buccal cavity (mouth), and iontophoresis or phonophoresis are permitted
6. Intraarticular and epidural injections are also permitted

I. General Athletic Concern: Photosensitivity reaction
   1. Diuretics, antipsychotics, older generation antidepressants, hypoglycemics, cardiovascular drugs, and antimalarials.
   2. NSAIDs, antimicrobials, antihistamines (diphenhydramine, loratidine), and estrogen/progesterone
      a. Most photoactive NSAIDs are the 2-arylpropionic acid derivatives (ibuprofen, naproxen, ketoprofen)
      b. Other NSAIDs include diclofenac, piroxicam, indomethacin, sulindac, and the COX-2-specific inhibitors
      c. Antibiotics include the tetracyclines (lower incidence with doxycycline and minocycline), the fluoroquinolones, and sulfamethoxazole.
      d. In female athletes, combined oral contraceptive use and topical medicines such as the retinoid creams for acne.

II. Performance-Enhancing (or Potentially Performance-Enhancing) Agents Drugs

A. History
   1. Long history of "doping"
      a. Chinese Emperor Shen-Nung depicted with *Ephedra*
      b. Ancient Olympians drank herbal teas and ate mushrooms
      c. Mixing sweat of athletes into drinks
      d. Late 1800s cycling death due to overdose
   2. Gradual process of fighting against performance-enhancing drugs
      a. First listed banned substances by International Olympic Committee Medical Commission in 1967
      b. Other medications added to the list, some as masking agents
   3. Doping
      a. Original use of term controversial
         i. South African dialect
         ii. Boers religious festivity infusion: the "doop"
         iii. Amsterdam canal workers: "doopen"
   4. Modern Olympics
      a. Amphetamines
      b. Later anabolic steroids
      c. Both had prior military applications

B. Definition
   1. Two of three affirmative to define doping
      a. Use of substances or methods that artificially increment performance
      b. Substances that are harmful to athletes
      c. Doping is against the spirit of the games

C. Structure
   1. Multiple organizations involved in determining banned substances, developing rules for testing, setting punishments

    a. IOC
        i. Anti-Doping Resolution passed 1962
        ii. Banned substance list 1967
        iii. First testing Mexico Olympics 1968
  2. World Anti-Doping Agency (WADA)
    a. Idea developed after 1998 Tour de France
        i. Due to difference between governments and International Cycling Federation
    b. Took over many aspects for IOC after Sydney 2000
    c. Now based in Montreal, Canada
    d. http://www.wada-ama.org/Documents/World_Anti-Doping_Program/ WADP-Prohibited-list/To_be_effective/WADA_Prohibited_List_2011_EN.pdf
  3. Other
    a. Various International Sport Federations
    b. NFL
    c. MLB
    d. NCAA
D. Categories of Performance-Enhancing Agents
  1. Any substance without approval by government health agency for human use
  2. Substances Prohibited at All Times (In- and Out-of-Competition)
    a. Anabolic steroids
        i. Initially developed post-World War II to treat emaciated Prisoners of War (POWs)
        ii. 1954 Soviet athletes began using steroids
        iii. Used for strength gains, speed, endurance, healing injury
            (A) Applicable to nearly all sports
        iv. Initial control in London, 1974
        v. Added to IOC banned list in 1975 (prior to Montreal Olympiad)
        vi. WADA list 2011 includes:
            (A) Endogenous: Androstenediol, androstenedione, DHEA, epitestosterone,
            (B) Exogenous: bolasterone, boldenone, danazol, desoxymethyltestosterone, drostanolone, methasterone, methyl-1-testosterone, methyltestosterone, prostanozol, nandrolone, norbolethone, oxandrolone, stanozolol, tetrahydrogestrinone (THG), trenbolone, and similar substances
            (C) Other: clenbuterol, selective androgen receptor modulators (SERMS), tibolone, zeranol, zilpaterol
        vii. Risks
            (A) Implicated in liver disease, however limited data
            (B) Psychiatric effects: mood swings, aggression
            (C) Overall limited data despite decades of use/abuse
    b. Peptide hormones, growth factors, related substances
        i. Erythropoiesis-stimulating agents
            (A) Erythropoietin EPO
            (B) Darbepoetin (dEPO)
            (C) Peginesatide (Hematide)
            (D) Continuous erythropoietin receptor activator (CERA)
            (E) Typical uses
                (1) Endurance events
                (2) Relatively high use in cyclists
            (F) Risks
                (1) Implicated in cyclist deaths due to hyperviscosity, thrombosis
        ii. Chorionic gonadotrophin and luteinizing hormone (males)
        iii. Insulins
        iv. Corticotrophins

    v. Growth hormones and growth factors
        (A) Including insulin-like growth factor, platelet-derived growth factor, vascular-endothelial growth factor
  c. β-2 Agonists
    i. All inhaled β-2 agonists allowed
    ii. Salbutemal (via inhalation) has a maximum allowable urine concentration
        (A) Max 1600 μg/24 h
        (B) Urine concentration >1000 ng/mL presumed to be adverse analytic finding, require proof that result due to intended therapeutic use
  d. Hormone antagonists and analogs
    i. Aromatase inhibitors
    ii. Selective estrogen receptor modulators
        (A) Tamoxifen
    iii. Antiestrogen substances
    iv. Myostatin inhibitors
  e. Diuretics
    i. Lasix
    ii. Hydrochlorothiazide (HCTZ)
    iii. Risks include dehydration and myriad of conditions associated
  f. Masking agents
    i. Diuretics
    ii. Plasma expanders
        (A) Glycerol
        (B) Dextrose
3. Prohibited methods in- and out-of-competition
  a. Enhancement of oxygen transfer
    i. Blood doping
        (A) Included autologous, homologous, or heterologous blood or blood products
        (B) Artificial enhancement of uptake, transport or delivery of oxygen
            (1) Perfluorochemicals
            (2) Efproxiral (RSR13)
            (3) Hemoglobin substitutes
            (4) Does not include supplemental oxygen
    ii. Chemical and physical manipulation
        (A) Tampering with samples
        (B) IV infusions, except those for legitimate medical reasons
        (C) Sequential withdrawal, manipulation, reinfusion of whole blood
    iii. Gene doping
        (A) Transfer of nucleic acids or nucleic acid sequences
        (B) Use of genetically modified cells
        (C) Use of agents that alter gene experession
            (1) Peroxisome proliferator activated receptor gamma
4. Substances prohibited in-competition
  a. Stimulants
    i. Initially developed in World War II for military use
    ii. 1940s football, 1950s other sports
    iii. Amphetamines: lack of evidence of performance enhancer
    iv. Demonstrated and perceived positive effects on self-confidence, mood, attention, aggression, and energy.
    v. Over-the-counter (OTC) stimulants such as phenylpropanolamine, ephedrine, and pseudoephedrine became substitutes in 1970s
    vi. Phenylpropanolamine and ephedra-containing supplements banned by DEA 2004

       vii. Modafinil/adrafinil

          (A) Developed in France, only modafinil legal in the United States

          (B) Not picked up on urine tests for stimulants

      viii. Bupropion, caffeine, phenylephrine, phenylpropanolamine, pipradol, synephrine are not considered prohibited

       ix. Adrenalin associated with local anesthetic injection not prohibited

        x. Ephedrine/methylephedrine/pseudoephedrine prohibited in competition

   b. Narcotics

      i. Prohibited: buprenorphine, morphine, hydromorphone, methadone, oxymorphone, fentanyl, oxycodone, others

      ii. Not prohibited: codeine

   c. Cannabinoids

      i. Natural

        (A) Cannabis, hashish, marijuana

      ii. Synthetic

        (A) Delta-9 tetrahydrocannabinol (THC)

      iii. Cannabimimetics

        (A) "Spice"

   d. Glucocorticosteroids

      i. Prohibited oral, IV, IM, rectal

5. Sport-specific prohibition

   a. Alcohol >0.10 g/L

      i. Archery, aeronautic, automobile, karate, motorcycling, powerboating, bowling

   b. β-Blockers

      i. Aeronautic, archery (also prohibited out-of-competition), billiards, Bobsleigh, boules, bridge, curling, darts, golf, motorcycling, pentathalon (shooting), bowling, powerboating, sailing, shooting (also prohibited out-of-competition), skiing, snowboarding, wrestling

6. Other agents

   a. Creatine

      i. Nitrogenous amino acid compound produced by the liver

      ii. Phosphocreatine, energy store for ATP in muscle

      iii. Discovered in 1830s, supplement since early 1900s

      iv. Mainly for short, high-intensity exercise

      v. Potential complications

        (A) Renal dysfunction

        (B) Liver dysfunction

        (C) Muscle cramping

        (D) Compartment syndrome

7. Supplements

   a. Supplies one or more nutrients purported to be missing from an athletes diet

   b. Many with unclear benefits/harm

   c. Rationale

      i. To maintain an adequate nutritional balance in terms of quality and correct quantities of specific nutrients (e.g., not less than minimal but not beyond the maximum safe daily macro- and micronutrient requirements)

      ii. To minimize any deterioration in physical or mental performance caused by possible daily-life or exercise-related reduction in the physiological quantity of essential nutrients in the body

      iii. To improve muscle protein balance when necessary for clinical purposes (e.g., aging, sarcopenia)

      iv. To reduce possible exercise-related, oxidative stress-linked damage (e.g., antioxidants: use of vitamin C, vitamin E, and β-carotene)

    d. Some have banned substances. Occasionally this is due to contamination at the manufacturing facilities

    e. NFL: multiple banned companies, including General Nutrition Centers, Met-Rx®, Metabolife®

    f. NCAA: "Ignorance is no excuse. What you don't know can hurt your eligibility"

    g. Belief in supplements/ergonomic aids driving force, without real consideration of effectiveness or risks

    h. Amino acids/Branched chain amino acids (BCAA)

E. Drug Testing

  1. NFL, New York, New York, USA

    a. Banned Substance List, Steroid Policy, and so on.

      i. http://www.nflpa.org/RulesAndRegs/RulesAndRegulations.aspx

  2. NCAA, Indianapolis, Indiana, USA

    a. Banned substances list

      i. http://www1.ncaa.org/membership/ed_outreach/health-safety/drug_testing/banned_drug_classes.pdf

  3. WADA, Montreal, Ottawa, Canada

    a. Banned substances list

      i. http://www.usantidoping.org/files/active/what/wallet_card.pdf

    b. Doping testing: urine, blood, or both

    c. Doping control

      i. In-competition: immediately after competition

    d. Out-of-competition: any time, more selective, including only anabolic agents, b2-agonists, agents with antiestrogenic activity, diuretic and masking agents, and all the banned methods. Stimulants, narcotics, and cannabis are not analyzed in this type of control.

    e. Control during Olympics to monitor level of red blood cells

      i. Nonstart determination

  4. WADA rulings accepted by all National Olympic committees, IOC, Paralympic committee, national governments, international sports federations

  5. Procedural issues

    a. WADA: The rights of the athlete are as follows:

      i. Check the credentials of the doping control officer to any type of control

      ii. Be notified in writing of a selection process

      iii. Be informed about the consequences of a refusal to cooperate

      iv. Be informed about the correct sequence of the control

      v. With the consent of the doping control officer, always accompanied by an escort, the athlete is entitled:

        (A) To receive a prize

        (B) To do a warm down (immediately after competition)

        (C) To receive medical attention (if necessary after competition)

        (D) To attend a press conference

        (E) Not to stay in the doping station, if you have other competitions that day

        (F) To select the equipment that will be used

        (G) To be observed in the passing of the urine by someone of the same gender

        (H) To receive a signed copy of all the documents

    b. The responsibilities of the athletes are as follows:

      i. To know the norms of the WADA, national antidoping organization (NADO), the national organizing committee (NOC), and the international and national federations of sports (IF)

      ii. To inform your personal physician and your pharmacologist that you are an athlete and may be submitted to doping controls

      iii. To consult your NADO, NOC, or IF with anticipation if you need to use any medical

      iv. Complete and submit TUE forms, when required (see below)
      v. To keep an actual list of all the medications, supplements, and herbal products that you are using, to declare it in the event of a doping control
      vi. To be careful in the ingestion of supplements or herbal products because they may contain banned substances
      vii. To bring always an identification with photograph with you to show to a doping control officer in the case of a doping control
      viii. In an in-competition or out-of-competition doping control, to remain at all times under the sight of an escort or doping control officer until the conclusion of the control
      ix. To hydrate with previously closed nonalcoholic beverages
      x. Be prepared to begin a doping control process as soon as notified and be in the doping control collection room until the sample is closed
      xi. Ensure that all documentation is correctly made and that you receive a copy of the documentation
    c. Testing procedures (e.g., NCAA: outlined in *NCAA Drug Testing Manual*)
      i. Athlete notified in writing by courier
      ii. Athlete remains in visual contact with courier, reports within 1 h
      iii. Sealed beverages without caffeine or other banned substances allowed
      iv. Athlete selects sealed beaker
      v. Specimen 85 mL, if less discarded
      vi. Specific gravity must be >1.005, pH between 4.5 and 7.5, otherwise discarded
      vii. Specimen A: 60 mL, Specimen B: 25 mL
      viii. Specimen prepared for shipping in the presence of athlete
      ix. Specimen A tested by approved laboratory
      x. Different lab personnel test B sample if necessary, considered final
      xi. Similar procedures for blood testing per WADA
    d. Therapeutic Use Exemption (TUE)
      i. Make possible, for therapeutic reasons, to prescribe to an athlete a restricted or prohibited substance
      ii. This information should be kept confidential by the Panel of Experts of the international sports federation responsible for granting permission
      iii. TUE should be submitted and approved at least 21 days before a competition
      iv. TUE should have a period of validity. After the expiration, it can be requested again by the athlete
      v. Some substances included in the List of Prohibited Substances are frequently used to treat medical conditions found in the athletic population
        (A) Insulin (long and short acting)
        (B) β-2 agonists (inhaled only)
        (C) Injected steroids
F. Future trends in doping
  1. Gene manipulation
    a. "the non-therapeutic use of cells, genes, genetic elements, or modulation of the gene expression, having the capacity to enhance athletic performance." (WADA Website [World Anti-Doping Agency]. www.wada-ama.org/.../2008_StPetersburg_Declaration_Dr.Rabin.pdf)
    b. Mentioned since 2000
    c. Site-specific sequence modification to affect disease versus gain-of-function expression of exogenous transgenes
    d. Risks
      i. Treatment-induced leukemia
      ii. Death

   e. Animal studies
      i. Peroxisomal proliferator-activated receptor delta
         (A) Lipid metabolism
         (B) Expression of slow twitch muscle fibers
   f. Gene transfer vectors
      i. Repoxygen
         (A) Expresses erythropoietin gene
   g. Testing
      i. WADA prohibited since 2004
      ii. Genetic markers may be used to identify perturbed physiological markers.

Recommended Reading

1. Ciocca M. Medication and supplement use by athletes. *Clin Sports Med*. 2005;24:719–738.
2. De Rose EH. Doping in athletes—An update. *Clin Sports Med*. 2008;27:107–130.
3. Gorsline RT, Caeding CC. The use of NSAIDs and nutritional supplements in athletes with osteoarthritis: Prevalence, benefits, and consequences. *Clin Sports Med*. 2005;24:71–82.
4. Kotevoglu et al. A prospective randomised controlled clinical trial comparing the efficacy of different molecular weight hyaluronan solutions in the treatment of knee osteoarthritis. *Rheumatol Int*. 2006;26:325–330.
5. McDuff DR, Baron D. Substance use in athletes: A sports psychiatry perspective. *Clin Sports Med*. 2005;24:885–897.
6. NCAA Drug Testing Program: Accessed February 15, 2008. http://www.ncaa.org/library/sports_sciences/drug_testing_program/2007-08/2007-08_drug_testing_program.pdf.
7. Sachs CJ. Oral analgesics for acute nonspecific pain. *Am Fam Phys*. 2005;71:913–918.
8. *United States Anti-Doping Agency Guide*. Accessed February 20, 2008. http://www.usantidoping.org/files/active/what/usada_guide.pdf.
9. World Anti-Doping Agency List of Banned Substances 2011.

6

Principles of Musculoskeletal Rehabilitation

Mederic M. Hall and Jay Smith

I. Tissue Injury and Repair Phases

A. Phase I: Injury and Inflammation
   1. Lasts days
   2. Bleeding and hemostasis
   3. Inflammation
      a. Characteristics:
         i. Edema
         ii. Pain
         iii. Warmth
         iv. Redness
         v. Dysfunction
   4. Essential for repair
   5. Short lived in most cases
      a. Too much/too long = bad
      b. Too little/too short = bad
         i. Inappropriate healing can lead to chronic tendinopathy
   6. Response influenced by:
      a. Injury site and severity
      b. Tissue type injured
      c. Patient factors

B. Phase II: Fibroplasia/Repair
   1. Lasts for 6–8 weeks
   2. Characterized by:
      a. Cell proliferation (e.g., fibroblasts)
      b. Growth factor release
      c. Fibroblast proliferation—Type III collagen deposition
      d. Formation of granulation tissue
      e. Neovascularization
   3. Tenuous time
      a. Many return to play (RTP) during this time
      b. Appearance > function; think they are better than they are
      c. Risk re-injury/regression
   4. Graded rehabilitation necessary
      a. Not based upon time, but based upon clinical examination and function
      b. Criterion based—every body and every injury different

    5. Education

        a. Patient, Parents, Coach

    6. Monitor for regression

  C. Phase III: Maturation/Remodeling

    1. Lasts for months

    2. Maturation of tissue

        a. Type III replaced by Type I collagen

        b. Fibers realign and remodel

           i. Dependent on force magnitude and direction across injured tissues

        c. Cellularity and vascularity decreases

    3. Injured tissue never returns to normal

        a. Prior injury is a major factor for reinjury

  D. Most athletes are able to RTP at some risk

    1. Many are not clinically "normal":

        a. Muscle imbalances

        b. Motion restrictions/imbalances

        c. Strength/endurance suboptimal/imbalanced

        d. Kinetic chain dysfunction

        e. Neuromuscular control deficits

        f. Technique alterations

        g. Often subtle

    2. Risk reinjury

  E. Rehabilitation

    1. Identify and treat deficits

    2. Monitor for trouble:

        a. Performance problems

        b. Prolonged recovery

        c. Pain

        d. Swelling

    3. Education

    4. If regress, treat accordingly.

II. Baseball Diamond Approach to Rehabilitation

  A. Cannot get to the next base without crossing the prior base

  B. Pain control → Motion → Strength → Neuromuscular control → RTP

  C. Control pain and inflammation

    1. PRICE:

        a. Protect (vs long immobilization)

        b. Relative rest

        c. Ice

        d. Compression (not too much)

        e. Elevation (above heart)

    2. Medications:

        a. Analgesics

        b. Acetaminophen

        c. Tramadol/opioids

        d. Antiinflammatories:

           i. Nonsteroidal antiinflammatory drugs (NSAIDs):

               (A) Analgesic benefit

          (B) Antiinflammatory benefit debatable
          (C) May impair healing
      ii. Not corticosteroids—detrimental
  3. Modalities:
      a. Heat—generally bad in phase I (inflammatory phase)
          i. Ultrasound = heat
      b. Ice—generally good in phase I (inflammatory phase)
      c. Electrical stimulation (e.g., "stim"):
          i. Possibly beneficial
          ii. Antiedema
          iii. Analgesic
          iv. Data mixed

D. Restore Range of Motion:
  1. Benefits:
      a. Antinociceptive
      b. Antiedema (at right dose)
          i. Provides neuromuscular training
          ii. Prerequisite for restoration of strength/endurance
          iii. Promotes tissue healing
          iv. Mentally gratifying (function)
      c. Types of motion:
          i. Passive (PROM)
          ii. Active assisted (AAROM)
          iii. Active (AROM)
          iv. Resisted (RROM)
      d. Range of motion prescription depends on:
          i. Healing phase
          ii. Injury specifics
          iii. Pain control
      e. Beware PROM in acute joint
          i. Increased pain
          ii. Increased inflammation
          iii. Potential damage
      f. General sequence of AAROM → AROM → RROM
      g. Control motion arc
      h. Control forces
      i. Begin in Phase II (Repair)
      j. Monitor for regression
      k. Types of stretching to improve ROM
          i. Static
          (A) 3–5 reps of 30–60 s
          ii. Splint—gentle, prolonged
          iii. Proprioceptive neuromuscular facilitation (PNF)
          (A) Common types
          (1) Contract–relax agonist
          (2) Contract–relax antagonist
          (B) Possibly more efficient acute gain in ROM, some evidence to suggest better maintenance of ROM gains
          (C) Usually requires another person
          iv. Ballistic—generally not recommended due to increased risk of injury

E. Strengthening
   1. Remember goal of restoring adequate functional strength and endurance
   2. Strength gains are specific for:
      a. Range of motion
      b. Contraction type
      c. Speed
      d. Energy system
      e. Movement pattern
   3. Isometric strengthening:
      a. No *intentional* joint motion (but joints may still move, especially with maximal contractions)
      b. Muscles co-contract
      c. For example, 5–10 reps of 6 s
      d. Can start early
         i. Even in splint/cast
      e. May reduce pain, edema, and atrophy
      f. Role in increasing strength and mass debatable, but should not be primary strengthening mode if hypertrophy is a priority
      g. Strength gains are angle specific $\pm 15°$. Would need to perform isometric contractions in about four to five different positions to isometrically strengthen the entire ROM arc of the elbow
   4. Isotonic strengthening:
      a. Muscles changing length against constant resistance. Speed can be varied
         i. Concentric—shortening
         ii. Eccentric—lengthening
         iii. Carryover better from eccentric to concentrate than from concentric to eccentric
      b. Need prerequisite motion
      c. Issue of elastic resistance:
         i. Nonphysiologic due to increased resistance provided by elastic band at a weak point in a muscle's length tension curve (i.e., end range of motion)
         ii. Can be partially mitigated by positioning
      d. During progression, consider % increase in load:
         i. Moving from 1 to 2 lb is not a large quantitative increase (e.g., 1 lb) but is a 100% increase in load to that muscle
         ii. Common mistake in rehab is too large of a jump in resistance
      e. Functional progressions/increased stress:
         i. Higher resistance
         ii. Eccentrics
         iii. Higher speeds
         iv. Terminal motion arcs
         v. More reps.
         vi. More joints
      f. Manipulate strength/end parameters as clinical condition (e.g., healing phase) dictates, with the ultimate goal in mind
   5. Isokinetic strengthening
      a. Variable resistance, constant speed:
         i. Move slow, resistance reduces
         ii. Move faster, resistance increases
      b. Training benefits unclear; may not translate into better performance.
      c. May exacerbate symptoms
      d. Can detect and monitor speed specific deficits in both eccentrics and concentrics:
         i. Research applications
         ii. Assist in detecting muscle imbalances, within limitations of test

F. Restore neuromuscular control/proprioception/return to sports
   1. Neuromuscular control (NMC):
      a. Afferent = proprioceptive
      b. Efferent = muscle contraction
      c. Coordination requires afferent input detection and processing to produce an appropriate efferent output
   2. Strength does not guarantee good NMC:
      a. Proprioceptive deficits may persist despite normal strength
      b. Poor movement patterns may persist despite normal strength
   3. Detect deficits:
      a. Assess balance
      b. Assess movement patterns
      c. Sport-specific scenarios
   4. Training Continuum for NMC:
      a. Early—AROM, Wobble boards, foam rollers
      b. Later—Rhythmic stabilization, body blades
      c. Even later—Plyometric training
         i. Jumps, hops, and so on.
      d. Throughout NMC training continuum, consider motion, speed, energy specificity
      e. Build movement patterns into sports-specific motions
      f. Graduated return to sports
      g. Appropriate monitoring
      h. Post-RTP rehabilitation.

III. Principles of Rehabilitation

A. A. During rehabilitation process, must constantly consider
   1. What is needed to RTP?
   2. Where are they in healing process?
   3. Is there regression?
   4. Can also simultaneously address pain, motion, strength/endurance, and NMC with appropriately prescribed exercises
   5. Importance of core:
      a. Component of all phases
      b. Integrate throughout
   6. Conditioning:
      a. Energy system specificity
      b. Integrate throughout
   7. Technique:
      a. Before vs after injury
      b. Do not wait until you are on your way home. Assess and treat technique at all phases of rehabilitation.

IV. Conclusions

A. Despite a paucity of data on specific rehabilitation for specific clinical problems, sufficient evidence exists to facilitate development and execution of rationale rehabilitation programs.
B. Clinicians should consider the healing stage of the injured tissue in the context of the "baseball diamond approach" to rehabilitation, realizing the ultimate goals of pain control, restoration of motion, restoration of functional strength and optimization of neuromuscular control.

Recommended Reading

1. Clover J, Wall J. Return-to-play criteria following sports injury. *Clin Sports Med.* 2010;29(1);169–175.
2. Dale RB, Harrelson GL, Leaver-Dunn D. Principles of rehabilitation. In: Andrews JR, Harrelson GL, Wilk KE, eds. *Physical Rehabilitation of the Injured Athlete.* 3rd ed. Philadelphia: Saunders, 2004:157–188.
3. Kinch M, Lambart A. Principles of rehabilitation. In: Brukner P, Khan K eds. *Clinical Sports Medicine Revised.* 3rd ed. Australia: McGraw-Hill, 2009:174–197.
4. Micheo WF. Concepts in sports medicine. In: Braddom RL ed. *Physical Medicine & Rehabilitation.* 3rd ed. Philadelphia: Saunders Elsevier, 2007:1021–1043.
5. Norris C. Healing. In: *Sports Injuries Diagnosis and Management.* 3rd ed. London: Butterworth-Heinemann, 2004:29–60.

Sports Medicine Procedures

Michael Henrie and Stuart Willick

BASIC PRINCIPLES

I. This chapter discusses common office-based procedures performed in most sports medicine clinics.

II. A thorough knowledge of joint and soft-tissue anatomy is essential to successfully performing the procedures discussed in this chapter.

III. Physicians performing these procedures should understand the indications, contra-indications, and complications of each procedure.

IV. Additionally, it is important to understand the different preparations and the side effects of the medications used.

JOINT INJECTION AND SOFT-TISSUE INJECTIONS

I. Basic Principles

A. Joint and soft-tissue injections have both a diagnostic and therapeutic role.

B. Although evidence-based reviews of the literature have found few studies to support or refute the efficacy of these procedures, there is substantial practice-based experience that supports their use.

C. Prior to performing a joint or soft-tissue injection the clinician must understand the rational for performing these procedures and should be able to identify those patients in whom they are most likely to be beneficial.

D. A variety of medication combinations can be used when performing joint and soft-tissue injections (see *Common Medications Used in Joint and Soft-Tissue Injections* below).

II. Indications

A. Indications generally fall into one of two categories: diagnostic or therapeutic.

B. Diagnostic indications:

  1. Aspiration of synovial fluid for laboratory analysis

    a. Gross examination

      i. Blood: hemarthrosis

      ii. Fat: violation of subchondral bone or fracture

    b. Polarized microscopy

      i. Monosodium urate crystals (negatively birefringent): gout

      ii. Calcium pyrophosphate crystals (weakly positive birefringent): calcium pyrophosphate disease (CPPD) or pseudogout

    c. Cell count

      i. See Table 7.1

Table 7.1   Synovial Fluid Analysis

	Normal	Hemorrhagic	Noninflammatory	Inflammatory	Septic
Appearance	Transparent	Bloody	Transparent	Mildly opaque	Opaque
WBC (per mm³)	<200	200–2,000	200–2,000	2,000–100,000	15,000– > 200,000
PMNs (%)	<25	50–75	<25	>50	>75
Total protein (g/dL)	1–2	4–6	1–3	3–5	3–5
Glucose difference vs. plasma	Nearly equal to blood	Nearly equal to blood	Nearly equal to blood	Lower than blood	Much lower than blood

2. Injection of contrast medium for arthrography
3. Injection of local anesthetic to confirm a presumptive diagnosis of a particular pain generator.

C. Therapeutic indications:
   1. General therapeutic indications include pain, swelling, and decreased mobility
   2. Indications for soft-tissue conditions include:
      a. Bursitis
      b. Tendonitis
      c. Trigger points
      d. Ganglion cysts
      e. Neuromas
      f. Nerve or tendon entrapment syndromes
   3. Indications for joint conditions include:
      a. Synovitis (commonly used in inflammatory arthritis)
      b. Crystalloid arthropathies
      c. Osteoarthritis
      d. Aspiration of a large joint effusion for relief of pain and stiffness.

D. Timing of injections:
   1. Generally, therapeutic injections are reserved for patients in whom physical therapy, physical modalities, NSAIDs, and other analgesics have failed.
   2. In some conditions such as calcific tendonitis, an early corticosteroid injection may augment therapy by reducing pain.
   3. The American College of Rheumatology Guidelines state: No more than four injections per year or a maximum of one injection every 3 months. These guidelines are based on expert opinion only.
   4. Patients who do not adequately respond to one or two injections should probably not have additional injections.

III. Contraindications

A. Absolute contraindications:
   1. Septic arthritis is a contraindication to corticosteroid injection into the involved joint, although diagnostic aspiration is allowed
   2. Skin or soft-tissue infection in the target area
   3. Bacteremia

4. Bacterial endocarditis
5. Joint prosthesis in the target joint with corticosteroid (diagnostic aspiration and injection allowed)
6. History of severe skin reaction or anaphylaxis with any of the medications being used
7. Fracture
8. Uncooperative patient.

B. Relative contra-indications:
1. Bleeding diathesis or coagulopathy
2. Anticoagulant therapy. (Note: There is no consensus on aspiration and injections in patients on anticoagulation therapy. Many practitioners safely perform soft-tissue and peripheral joint injections in these patients.)
3. Joint instability
4. Poorly controlled diabetes
5. Allergy to any of the medications being injected
6. Multiple failed injections.

IV. Risks and Complications

A. Bleeding

B. Local allergic reaction

C. Local infection

D. Iatrogenic septic arthritis
1. This is a rare (1/30,000–1/50,000) but serious complication.
2. Always use aseptic technique when performing joint injections.

E. Postinjection flare of pain.
1. This can occur within the first 24 or 36 h following a corticosteroid injection and is likely related to corticosteroid crystal formation within the joint and surrounding soft tissues
2. Occurs in 1–6% of injections
3. It typically manifests as increased joint pain, swelling, tenderness, and warmth
4. Symptoms are self-limited.
5. They can be treated with rest, application of ice, and antiinflammatory medications
6. When these symptoms occur the clinician should always consider the possibility of iatrogenic infection
7. If symptoms persist beyond 24 or 36 h the patient should be properly evaluated.

F. Fat necrosis and depigmentation of the overlying skin can occur with a corticosteroid injection.

G. Tendon rupture can occur with corticosteroid injections. Injection into a tendon should be avoided.

H. Traumatic injection can occur causing direct damage to articular cartilage, local nerves, or soft-tissue structures.

I. Pneumothorax has been reported with thoracic trigger point injections.

J. Systemic complications:
1. Generalized hypersensitivity reaction
2. Anaphylaxis
3. Systemic absorption of corticosteroids
   a. More common with water-soluble steroid preparations, higher injection dose, and injecting multiple joints.
   b. Systemic absorption of corticosteroids may cause a transient hyperglycemia, particularly in diabetics.
   c. Systemic absorption may cause a transient increase in the white blood cell count.

V. Sterile Technique

A. After identification of the target site, the area of skin overlying the target joint should be adequately cleansed with an appropriate antiseptic solution such as iodine-based or chlorohexidine-based soap.

B. Sterile technique should be used when performing these procedures.

C. Sterile gloves allow palpation of anatomic landmarks and the target area after skin preparation has been completed.

VI. Common Supplies Used for Joint and Soft-Tissue Injections

A. Providone-iodine or chlorohexidine-based swabs

B. Sterile gloves

C. Sterile drape

D. 25- to 30-gauge, 0.5–1 in. needle for local skin anesthesia

E. 22- to 25-gauge, 1–1.5 in. needle for injection

F. 18- to 20-gauge, 1–1.5 in. needle for aspiration

G. 1–5 mL syringe for local skin anesthesia

H. 1–10 mL syringe for medication

I. 30–60 mL syringe for aspiration (depending on the suspected size of the joint effusion)

J. Medications

K. Laboratory tubes for the aspirated fluid specimen

L. Bandage for puncture site.

VII. Postprocedure Instructions

A. There is a wide variety of clinician preference regarding postinjection care instructions, but often include the following:
1. Application of ice to the injection site
2. NSAIDs may be used for postinjection discomfort
3. Avoid strenuous exercise or strenuous activity for several days following the injection
4. The injection site should be cleaned and a Band-Aid should be placed over the area
5. Patients should be instructed about signs and symptoms of infection.

COMMON MEDICATIONS USED IN JOINT AND SOFT-TISSUE INJECTIONS

I. Corticosteroids

A. Corticosteroid preparations differ with respect to potency and solubility (see Table 7.2).
1. Less soluble preparations are likely to remain in the joint for a longer period of time.
2. Corticosteroid preparations differ by solubility, concentration, and duration. However, evidence is lacking that efficacy differs between preparations of different potency and duration of action.

B. Mechanism of action:
1. Suppression of inflammation occurs by several mechanisms:
   a. Increasing synovial fluid viscosity
   b. Limiting capillary dilation and altering synovial permeability
   c. Stabilizing lysosomal membranes
   d. Decreasing synovial fluid compliment proteins
   e. Preventing degranulation of granulocytes, mast cells, and macrophages
   f. Inhibiting the release of arachadonic acid from phospholipids, thus reducing the formation of leukotrienes, thromboxanes, prostaglandins, and prostacyclines.

Table 7.2 Common Corticosteroid Preparations Used for Intraarticular and Soft-Tissue Injection

Agent	Trade Name	Dose Equivalent	Potency	Duration
Hydrocortisone acetate	Hydrocortone	20 mg	Low	Short
Triamcinolone acetonide	Kenalog	4 mg	Intermediate	Intermediate
Methylprednisolone acetate	Depo-Medrol	4	Intermediate	Intermediate
Betamethasone sodium phosphate	Celestone	0.6 mg	High	Long
Dexamethasone sodium phosphate	Decadron	0.75 mg	High	Long
Betamethasone sodium phosphate– betamethasone acetate	Celestone Soluspan	0.6 mg	High	Long

C. Adverse reactions:
1. Systemic symptoms are related to the systemic uptake of the injected corticosteroid
   a. Systemic uptake is related to the solubility of the corticosteroid preparation
2. Systemic side effects, if present, are generally mild and include:
   a. Hyperglycemia
   b. Facial flushing and warmth
   c. Rash
   d. Headache
   e. Agitation and emotional lability
   f. Elevated blood pressure
   g. Transient increase in white blood cell count
3. Local side effects:
   a. Crystalline synovitis (postinjection flare)
   b. Tendon rupture.

II. Local Anesthetics

A. Different preparations of local anesthetics are available
1. They differ primarily in onset and duration of action (see Table 7.3)
2. Most commonly 1% lidocaine, 0.25–0.5% bupivacaine, or a combination of both is used. There have been recent reports of local anesthetic toxicity to chondrocytes and some studies have implicated all of the local anesthetics commonly used for joint injection procedures. The data are not definitive, however, and more studies are required to better understand the use of local anesthetics and their potentially harmful effects to articular cartilage.
B. Rarely patients exhibit signs of mild anesthetic toxicity:
1. Flushing
2. Hives

Table 7.3 Common Local Anesthetics Used for Intraarticular and Soft-Tissue Injection

Agent	Class	Concentration	Onset (min)	Duration (h)	Max Dose (adults)
Lidocaine	Amide	1 or 2%	1–2	1.5–2	5 mg per kg, up to 300 mg total
Prilocaine	Amide	1%	1–2	>1	700 mg per kg, up to 280 mg total
Bupivicaine	Amide	0.25 or 0.5%	5–30	2–8	2 mg per kg, up to 175 mg total
Mepivicaine	Amide	1%	3–5	1–1.5	4 mg per kg, up to 400 mg total

3. Tinnitus
4. Anxiety
5. Chest or abdominal discomfort.

C. Other serious adverse reactions include:
1. Seizures
2. Respiratory arrest
3. Worsening of arrhythmias
4. Heart block
5. Bradycardia.

III. Hyaluronic Acid Preparations

A. Several different formulations of hyaluronic acid are available and are under the following trade names:
1. Synvisc (hylan G-F 20)
2. Orthovisc (hyaluronan)
3. Hyalgan (sodium hyaluronate)
4. Supartz (sodium hyaluronate)
5. Euflexxa (sodium hyaluronate).

B. No serious reaction has been reported with use of hyaluronic acid.

C. Common reactions include:
1. Aseptic synovitis
   a. Occurs 24–72 h after injection at a rate of <3%
   b. Can potentially be reduced by also injecting corticosteroid into the joint with the first hyaluronate injection
2. Joint pain
3. Joint swelling
4. Joint effusion
5. Pruritis
6. Rash.

D. Clinical efficacy
1. Literature is conflicting with a known publication bias; most literature pertains to knee osteoarthritis
2. Meta-analyses suggest:
   a. Pain improvement over placebo
   b. Later onset with more slightly prolonged improvement over corticosteroids.

CASTING AND SPLINTING

I. Basic Principles of Splinting and Casting

A. Splints and casts are used to immobilize musculoskeletal injuries and serve to maintain alignment, decrease pain, and protect the injury.

B. An accurate assessment of the stage, severity and stability of the injury is necessary to determine what type of immobilization is appropriate.

C. A thorough evaluation of bone and soft-tissue anatomy, skin structure, and neurovascular status should also be performed.

D. Once the clinician determines that immobilization is required, a decision about the type of splint or cast should be made.

E. When deciding on immobilization in a splint or cast it is important for the clinician to understand the patient's functional requirements as well as the risks and complications associated with immobilization.

Improper application of a cast or splint can increase the risks associated with immobilization.

II. Indications

A. Splinting

1. Acute fracture management—splints allow for the natural swelling that occurs in the acute phase of the injury
2. Soft-tissue injuries
3. Definitive treatment for some fractures

B. Casting

1. Provides the most effective immobilization
2. Definitive management of many fractures
3. Some nonacute soft-tissue injuries not manageable by splinting.

III. Complications

A. Compartment syndrome

B. Skin breakdown

C. Ischemia

D. Nerve injury

E. Infection

F. Joint stiffness.

IV. Types of Splints

A. Hand and fingers:

1. Buddy taping: injured finger is taped to adjacent finger
2. Dorsal extension block splint
   a. Prevents extension, but allows flexion of the PIP joint
   b. Joint placed in progressively decreasing PIP flexion
3. Mallet finger splint
   a. Immobilizes the DIP joint
   b. DIP placed in hyperextension
4. Radial gutter splint
   a. Stabilizes the second and third metacarpals
   b. MCP joints placed in 70–90° of flexion and PIP and DIP joints in 5–10° of flexion
5. Ulnar gutter splint
   a. Stabilizes the fourth and fifth metacarpals
   b. MCP joints placed in 70–90° of flexion and PIP and DIP joints in 5–10° of flexion
6. Thumb spica splint (Figure 7.1)

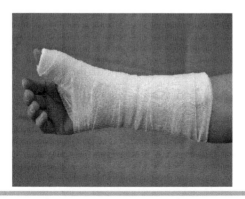

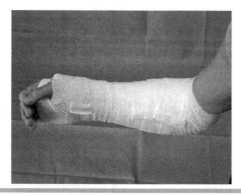

Figure 7.2   Single sugar-tong splint

      a. Stabilizes the thumb and radial wrist bones
      b. The forearm is placed in neutral with the wrist in about 25° of extension. The thumb is placed in position similar to "holding a soda can."
   B. Wrist, forearm, and arm
      1. Single sugar-tong splint (Figure 7.2)
         a. Stabilizes wrist and elbow flexion and extension and limits wrist supination and pronation
         b. The elbow is placed in 90° of flexion with the forearm in a neutral position
      2. Volar/dorsal forearm splint
         a. Stabilizes wrist flexion and extension but does not limit supination and pronation.
         b. The wrist is placed in slight extension
      3. Double sugar-tong splint
         a. Stabilizes wrist and elbow flexion and extension
         b. Offers more control of supination and pronation
      4. Long arm posterior splint
         a. Stabilization of injuries to the elbow, forearm, and wrist
         b. The elbow is placed in 90° of flexion and the wrist is slightly extended
      5. Coaptation splint
         a. Stabilizes humeral shaft fractures
         b. Elbow is placed in 90° of flexion and shoulder is neutral.
   C. Foot, ankle, and leg
      1. Posterior ankle splint and stirrup splints:
         a. Stabilizes the ankle
         b. Ankle placed in a neutral position
         c. If considerable swelling is anticipated, a bulky Jones splint can be created by adding additional padding and stabilizing with a stirrup splint.

V. Types of Casts

   A. Most of the splints mentioned above can be converted into a cast by the application of circumferential casting material.
   B. Wrist and hand (positioning is the same as when placing a splint)
      1. Ulnar gutter and radial gutter casts
      2. Thumb spica cast

Table 7.4 Criteria for Compartment Pressure Testing for the Leg

Compartment	Preexercise	1 min postexercise	5 min postexercise
Anterior, lateral, superficial posterior, and deep posterior	>15 mmHg	>30 mmHg	>20 mmHg

C. Wrist, forearm, and arm
   1. Short arm cast
     a. The wrist is slightly extended
     b. The MCP joints are free
   2. Long arm cast
     a. Stabilization of all elbow and wrist motion
     b. The elbow is flexed to 90° with the wrist slightly extended.
D. Foot, ankle, and leg
   1. Short leg cast
     a. Used for many foot and ankle fractures
     b. The foot is placed in a neutral position.

MUSCLE COMPARTMENT PRESSURE TESTING

I. Indications

A. Compartment pressure testing is typically used for diagnosing chronic exertional compartment syndrome.

B. It can also be used in the diagnosis of acute compartment syndrome when the history and physical examination findings are equivocal, or in anesthetized or comatose patients.

C. Some authors advocate using compartment testing anytime compartment syndrome is suspected.

II. Technique

A. This procedure is performed using sterile technique.

B. A large bore needle attached to a pressure monitor is inserted into the affected muscle compartment after infiltrating the area with local anesthesia.

C. Numerous commercial tonometers are available for measuring compartment pressures.
   1. Only a small amount of fluid (0.3 cm^3) is necessary to inject into the compartment.
   2. Once equilibrium is reached, the pressure should be recorded.

D. When evaluating for chronic exertional compartment syndrome both preexercise and postexercise pressure measurements should be obtained (Table 7.4).
   1. To obtain postexercise measurements, the athlete is instructed to perform the symptom-provoking exercise until significant symptom provocation, and then reevaluated 1 and 5 min postexercise.

III. Complications

A. Bleeding at the puncture site

B. Pain or discomfort at the puncture site

C. Local infection of the skin and underlying soft tissues.

Recommended Reading

1. Boyd AS, Benjamin HJ, Asplund C. Principles of casting and splinting. *American Family Physician.* 2009;79(1):L16–22.
2. Cardone DA, Tallia AF. Joint, soft tissue injection. *American Family Physician.* 2002;66(2):283–288.
3. Egol K, Koval KJ, Zuckerman JD. *Handbook of Fractures.* Philadelphia, PA: Lippincott Williams & Wilkins, 2010.
4. McNabb JW. *A Practical Guide to Joint & Soft Tissue Injection & Aspiration.* 2nd ed. Philadelphia, PA: Lippincott Williams & Wilkins, 2010.
5. Stephens MB, Beutler AI, O'Connor FG. Musculoskeletal injections: A review of the evidence. *American Family Physician.* 2008;78(8):972–976.

II

Health Promotion
and
Injury Prevention

8

Preparticipation Examination

D. Harrison Youmans and Tracy R. Ray

I. Administration

  A. Introduction

    1. Over 30 million children, adolescents, and college students are involved in organized sports in the United States.

    2. The development of the Preparticipation Physical Examination (PPE) was initially driven by American Heart Association (AHA) to decrease risk of sudden death.

    3. The PPE has become standard of care, although evidence of its effectiveness is conflicting. It fulfills legal and insurance requirements for participation in sports for many municipalities and organizations.

    4. Goals of the PPE include the following:

      a. Evaluate for the presence of medical conditions with life-threatening complications during participation

      b. Evaluate for conditions that require a treatment plan before or during participation

      c. Evaluate and rehabilitate old musculoskeletal injuries prior to participation

      d. Evaluate and treat conditions/diseases that interfere with performance

      e. Remove unnecessary restrictions on participation

      f. Advise athletes regarding appropriate sports in which to participate.

    5. Physician responsibilities during the PPE include:

      a. Identifying athletes with medical conditions that increase their risk of death or significant injury, and disqualify them until these risks can be controlled with treatment

      b. Ensuring that an athlete is not excluded from participation unless there is a compelling medical reason.

    6. The performing physician

      a. AHA recommends PPE be performed by a physician with background to reliably recognize heart disease

      b. Must be able to accurately evaluate the musculoskeletal system

      c. Majority of PPEs are performed by primary care physicians (PCP)

      d. Only a minority of PCP have received formal training in sports medicine or the musculoskeletal exam.

  B. Timing/frequency

    1. Frequency of the PPE is determined by individual governing bodies for its participants

    2. Thirty-five state high school athletic associations require annual exams

    3. AHA recommends a history and physical be performed every 2 years, with interim follow-up in the intervening year

    4. Others recommend PPE with each new level of participation (middle school, high school, college, etc.).

C. Mass vs. individual
   1. Most PPE occur either during individual office visits with a physician or in a station-based, mass examination setting
   2. Each of these methods has advantages and disadvantages (see Table 8.1).
D. Screening tests
   1. General medical history
      a. Chronic medical conditions
      b. Previous hospitalizations and surgeries
      c. Allergies
      d. Medications and supplements
      e. Previous exclusions from athletics
      f. Sports-related general medical history:
         i. Cardiovascular history
         ii. Musculoskeletal history
         iii. Seizure history
         iv. Respiratory symptoms or history of exercise-induced bronchospasm (EIB)
         v. Gastrointestinal symptoms
         vi. History of heat-related illness
         vii. Skin rashes (Tinea or MRSA)
         viii. Eating disorders
         ix. Sickle cell status
         x. Menstrual history
   2. Physical examination
      a. System-based examinations are detailed in the appropriate sections within this chapter. Examination should include the following:
      b. General appearance
      c. Vital signs (height, weight, BP, pulse)
      d. Cardiovascular examination
      e. Ocular examination
      f. Dermatologic examination: evaluate for infectious rashes or lesions
      g. Pulmonary examination
      h. Abdominal examination
      i. Genitourinary examination in males
      j. Musculoskeletal examination.

Table 8.1 **Advantages and disadvantages of individual vs. mass, station-based PPEs**

	Advantages	Disadvantages
Individual	More private	Less efficient
	Ability to build rapport	Increased cost
	Continuity of care	Lack of physician specialization
	Improved opportunity for counseling	
StationBased	More efficient	Less private
	Decreased cost	Decreased rapport with patient
	Increased specialization of physicians at stations	Decreased continuity of care
	Better communication between	Decreased opportunity for counseling
	ATCs, physicians, athletes, parents, coaches	

3. Laboratory testing
   a. General
      i. Lab testing, including complete blood count (CBC), basic metabolic panel (BMP), magnesium, phosphorous, liver function tests (LFTs), and fasting lipid panel (FLP), is not recommended as a part of routine screening PPE
      ii. May be ordered prior to clearing an athlete for activity if there is a compelling medical condition that requires laboratory testing for diagnosis or monitoring
   b. Sickle cell
      i. New NCAA guidelines mandate that the sickle cell trait status of student-athletes be known, either by history or new testing
      ii. Student-athletes may opt out of testing by signing a waiver
      iii. The U.S. military does not test recruits for sickle cell trait or disease, opting instead for universal prevention and treatment strategies
      iv. Not recommended as part of routine screening for non-NCAA athletes
   c. Ferritin
      i. Many advocate for screening ferritin tests, especially in female endurance athletes, to evaluate for iron deficiency
         (A) Controversy exists as to whether iron replacement in nonanemic iron-deficient patients may improve athletic performance
   d. Electrocardiogram (ECG)
      i. Evidence suggests that inclusion of ECG may increase sensitivity of the PPE for finding those at risk of sudden cardiac death (SCD)
      ii. The International Olympic Committee (IOC), European Society of Cardiology, and several governing bodies of sports within and outside the U.S. advocate screening ECG.
      iii. Not currently recommended by the AHA
   e. Echocardiogram
      i. Some propose its use as a screening tool for hypertrophic cardiomyopathy (HCM)
      ii. False-positive results may occur
      iii. Not recommended as part of routine screening PPE.

II. Cardiovascular (See Chapter 33 "Sports Cardiology" for More Details)

A. Introduction
   1. SCD in athletes can be caused by a diverse set of structural and electrical abnormalities of the heart.
   2. Cardiovascular events are the leading cause of sudden death in athletes.
   3. The purpose of preparticipation screening, which should include a well-performed cardiovascular history and physical exam, is to detect those athletes at increased risk of SCD.
   4. Cardiovascular history
      a. Question athlete regarding past history of any of the following:
         i. Heart murmur
         ii. Hypertension
         iii. Coronary artery disease
         iv. Syncope or near-syncope with exertion
         v. Dizziness with exertion
         vi. Angina
         vii. Palpitations
         viii. Disproportionate dyspnea
         ix. Exertional chest pain
         x. Kawasaki's disease (consider obtaining previous medical records or new echocardiogram to rule out coronary artery aneurysm)

  b. Chest pain red flags:
   i. Occurs during exertion
   ii. Occurs after recent viral illness and/or fever
    (A) Fever is a contraindication to participation due to association with carditis
   iii. Associated with new murmur
   iv. Lack of reproducible pain on palpation
  c. Family history of the following:
   i. CV disease
   ii. Sudden death
   iii. MI <50 years of age
   iv. HCM or dilated cardiomyopathy
   v. Long-QT syndrome, Brugada syndrome, or other arrhythmias
   vi. Marfan's syndrome
   vii. Unexplained seizures or drowning.
 5. Patients with a positive screening history should have a cardiac work-up prior to participation.
 6. Physical examination
  a. Vital signs (height, weight, BP, pulse)
  b. Auscultation of precordium to evaluate rate, rhythm, and presence of murmurs
  c. Palpation of radial and femoral pulses to exclude coarctation of the aorta
  d. Inspection for stigmata of Marfan's syndrome (see below).
 7. *36th Bethesda Conference*—report has recommendations from 2004 committee meeting in New Orleans regarding sports participation decisions for athletes with cardiovascular conditions.

B. Valvular disease
 1. Introduction
  a. Valvular abnormalities are typically discovered by detection of a murmur on exam or using echocardiography
  b. Insignificant valvular regurgitation is common in athletes, with greater than 90% of athletes demonstrating at least single valve regurgitation
  c. Symptomatic abnormalities will often preclude participation in sports and may be indications for medical treatment or surgical repair of the affected valve
  d. An athlete's history regarding associated symptoms may be unreliable. In these cases, echocardiography and exercise tolerance tests can be important diagnostic and risk stratification tools.
 2. Aortic stenosis (AS)
  a. Underlying etiology can be congenital, rheumatic, or degenerative/calcific
  b. The majority of athletes competing with AS have a congenital lesion
  c. Murmur associated with AS is a harsh systolic ejection murmur heard best at the right upper sternal border
  d. Risk of SCD increases with severity of AS, and onset of symptoms (dyspnea, syncope, chest pain, etc.) represents a severe increase in risk
   i. Severity is graded based on calculated aortic valve area as determined by echo-cardiogram and estimated mean aortic pressure gradient:
    (A) Mild: Greater than 1.5 cm^2 and less than 25 mmHg
    (B) Moderate: From 1.0 to 1.5 cm^2 and from 25 to 40 mmHg
    (C) Severe: Less than 1.0 cm^2 and greater than 40 mmHg
  e. Recommendations:
   i. Mild AS: Can participate in all sports, but should have annual examinations and echocardiogram to assess disease progression
   ii. Moderate AS: Can participate in low-intensity sports. Should be allowed to compete in low-to-moderate static or dynamic sports if exercise testing at the

level of competition does not elicit symptoms, ST-segment changes, ventricular tachyarrhythmia, or abnormal blood pressure response

iii. Severe AS or symptomatic moderate AS: Should not be allowed to participate in competitive sports.

3. Mitral valve prolapse (MVP)
   a. Sudden death is rare in athletes with MVP
   b. Usually able to compete in all competitive sports
   c. Five conditions that may be present with MVP should limit participation
      i. History of arrhythmogenic syncope
      ii. Family history of sudden death with MVP
      iii. Repetitive forms of supraventricular/ventricular arrhythmias
      iv. Moderate-to-severe mitral regurgitation
      v. Prior embolic event
   d. Patients with symptomatic MVP should be limited to low-intensity sports.
4. Other potentially disqualifying valvular abnormalities include aortic regurgitation (AR), mitral stenosis (MS), mitral regurgitation (MR), tricuspid stenosis (TS), and tricuspid regurgitation (TR)
   a. Current recommendations for athletes with these conditions can be found in the *36th Bethesda Report*
   b. Disqualification is generally based on presence of the following:
      i. Arrhythmia (e.g., atrial fibrillation)
      ii. Systolic dysfunction
      iii. Peak valvular gradients above recommended cut-offs
      iv. Increased chamber dimensions
      v. Symptoms during exercise.

C. Arteriosclerotic coronary artery disease (CAD)
   1. Most common cause of exercise-related SCD in adults >35 years of age
   2. Physical activity decreases cardiovascular mortality rates among healthy patients and those with diagnosed CAD
   3. Vigorous exercise transiently increases the risk of acute myocardial infarction and SCD, especially in sedentary individuals
      a. Likely secondary to plaque rupture and erosion during a period of increased myocardial oxygen demand.
   4. Assess LV function in patients with CAD diagnosed by any of the following:
      a. Coronary angiography
      b. Coronary artery risk score >100
      c. Evidence of inducible ischemia on stress testing
      d. History of prior coronary event
   5. Patients should have evaluation to assess exercise capacity and possible ischemia using treadmill or bicycle exercise testing.
   6. Risk stratification:
      a. Mildly increased risk: Must demonstrate *all* of the following:
         i. Preserved LV systolic function at rest (EF >50%)
         ii. Normal exercise tolerance for age on treadmill or bicycle exercise testing
         iii. Absence of exercise-induced ischemia or arrhythmia
         iv. Absence of hemodynamically significant coronary artery stenosis (50% or more luminal diameter narrowing)
         v. Successful myocardial revascularization if such procedure is performed
         vi. Recommendations: Can participate in low dynamic or low-to-moderate static sports. Should avoid intensely competitive situations.
      b. Substantially increased risk: Present if *any* of the following are demonstrated:
         i. Impaired LV systolic function at rest (EF < 50%)

        iii. Hemodynamically significant coronary artery stenosis (50% or more luminal diameter narrowing)

        iv. Recommendations: Should be restricted to low-intensity competitive sports.

    7. Patients with recent MI may benefit from cardiac rehabilitation in the weeks following the myocardial injury.

    8. Patients should refrain from vigorous activity for a period of 4 weeks following stent placement.

D. Athletic heart syndrome

    1. Term used to describe the physiologic adaptations of the heart to endurance training, which include increases in atrial and ventricular volume, LV wall and septal thickness, and overall cardiac mass in a heart with preserved systolic and diastolic function.

    2. Differentiation between athlete's heart and other cardiac abnormalities such as HCM or dilated cardiomyopathy can be difficult, especially in males. This is particularly true when LV thickness lies within the gray zone of 13–15 mm. However, "athlete's heart" shows increased wall thickness AND increased cardiac chamber volume, whereas HCM has an increased wall thickness with reduced chamber volume.

    3. Exercise may also increase LV wall thickness in athletes with the genetic disorders listed above, and a period of decreased training may partially reverse their cardiac remodeling.

    4. Proper differentiation from serious cardiac abnormalities is important to avoid unnecessary disqualification from sports. Tools that may be used include electrocardiography, echocardiography, genetic testing, and serial measurements of cardiac anatomy and function.

E. ECG

    1. Use of the ECG as a preparticipation screening tool is a highly debated topic in sports medicine currently.

    2. Proponents of screening ECGs cite cost effectiveness, ease of access, and higher sensitivity rates for detecting HCM with the combination of history, physical exam, and ECG compared to history and physical exam alone.

    3. Opponents of screening ECGs cite a high rate of false-positive exams (which can lead to needless testing and disqualification from sport), low positive predictive values, overall cost, need for a large number of physicians to interpret the studies, and low prevalence of disease.

    4. As of its 2007 recommendations, the AHA does not advocate universal ECG screening of athletes.

    5. The International Olympic Committee (IOC), European Society of Cardiology, and several governing bodies of sports within and outside of the U.S. advocate screening ECGs.

    6. Many athletes demonstrate ECG changes that correspond to the trained condition of the cardiovascular system. These are likely normal for the athlete and include the following:

        a. Sinus bradycardia

        b. Sinus arrhythmia

        c. Prolonged PR interval or 1st degree AV blocks

        d. Junctional rhythm

        e. Early repolarization abnormalities

        f. Incomplete right bundle branch block (RBBB) pattern

        g. Left ventricular hypertrophy (LVH) voltage criteria (sum of S wave in V1 and R wave in V5 greater than 35 mm) without ST segment or T-wave changes.

    7. ECG changes that may be associated with specific cardiac abnormalities:

        a. HCM: Left axis deviation with findings of LVH

        b. Prolonged-QT Syndrome: QTc (QT interval/square root of RR interval) >450 ms in men and >470 ms in women

        c. Brugada syndrome: RBBB pattern with ST elevation in precordial leads V1–V3

      d. ARVD: T-wave inversions in precordial leads V1–V3

      e. CAD: Pathologic Q waves, ST elevation, T-wave inversion

      f. Wolff–Parkinson–White (WPW): Presence of delta waves.

F. Hypertension

  1. Systemic hypertension is the most commonly encountered cardiovascular condition in athletes. It is present in nearly 30% of U.S. adults.

  2. Definition

    a. Adults: systolic blood pressure (SBP) >140 mmHg or diastolic blood pressure (DBP) >90 mmHg on at least two separate occasions

    b. Children: SBP or DBP greater than or equal to the 95th percentile for age, gender, and height.

  3. Aerobic exercise can be beneficial in both long- and short-term blood pressure control, decreasing risk of death from heart disease and stroke.

  4. Strenuous exercise can elevate blood pressure to dangerous levels in patients with hypertension, increasing risk of myocardial infarction, or stroke. Therefore, blood pressure measurement should be a routine part of the screening PPE.

  5. Recommendations:

    a. Prehypertension (120/80–139/89 mmHg): lifestyle modification without activity restriction. Echocardiography if LVH is suspected.

    b. Stage 1 hypertension (140/90–159/99 mmHg): Lifestyle modification without activity restriction if no evidence of end organ damage. Monitor BP every 2–4 months to evaluate effect of exercise.

    c. Stage 2 hypertension (>160/100 mmHg in adults; SBP or DBP >99th percentile + 5 mmHg in children): Patient should be restricted from activity until BP is controlled by lifestyle modification or drug therapy.

G. Hypertrophic cardiomyopathy (HCM)

  1. Most common cause of SCD in the United States, accounting for 25–33%

  2. Estimated to affect 1:500 Americans and 1:1,000–1,500 competitive athletes

  3. Diagnosis based on LV wall thickness >13–15 mm

  4. Genetic testing can also be useful for diagnosis

  5. Associated murmur is harsh, systolic, located at left or right sternal border. Murmur INCREASES in intensity with standing and during Valsalva maneuver, which decrease venous return, allowing for increased outflow tract obstruction.

  6. Murmur is only present in 25% of patients with HCM

  7. ECG is abnormal in 75–90% of patients with HCM. Abnormal findings can include:

    a. Prominent Q waves

    b. Deep negative T waves

    c. Increased QRS amplitude with associated ST changes

  8. Recommendations:

    a. Asymptomatic athletes with HCM phenotype should be excluded from all but low-intensity sports

    b. Asymptomatic athletes with HCM genotype who are phenotypically normal should not be excluded due to lack of evidence base

    c. Symptomatic athletes should be withheld from all sports. SCD is often the sentinel event, however.

    d. Asymptomatic athletes participating in sports should have ECG, echocardiogram, and Holter every 12–18 months.

H. Marfan's syndrome

  1. Inherited connective tissue disease associated with mutation of the gene for fibrillin-1 protein

  2. Affects two to three patients out of 10,000

3. Major cause of mortality is due to aortic rupture or dissection due to dilation and weakness of the aortic root caused by cystic medial necrosis
4. Patients should be questioned regarding family history, consider genetic testing if family history is positive
5. Ghent criteria have been developed to aid in diagnosis. See Figure 33.2, Chapter 33.
6. Diagnosis
   a. Patients with family history of Marfan's syndrome require one major and one minor criterion from different organ systems
   b. Patients without family history of Marfan's syndrome require two major criteria and one minor criterion from different organ systems
7. Recommendations:
   a. Patients may participate in low and moderate static/low dynamic sports if they are without the following conditions:
      i. Aortic root dilation
      ii. Moderate or severe mitral regurgitation
      iii. Family history of dissection or sudden death in a relative with Marfan's
      iv. Patients should have echocardiogram every 6 months to evaluate for worsening aortic root dilation
      v. Contact or collision sports should be avoided as these increase the risk or aortic dissection or rupture.

I. Murmurs
1. Precordial auscultation should be performed in supine and standing positions with and without Valsalva maneuver
2. Innocent murmurs are generally I–III/VI and systolic
3. Murmurs associated with outflow obstruction increase in intensity with maneuvers that decrease preload, such as Valsalva or moving from lying to standing
   a. These murmurs should prompt further evaluation with ECG and echocardiogram, and the athlete should be withheld from competition until the work-up is complete
4. Still's murmur
   a. Common benign murmur present in young children
   b. Vibratory in nature, located over apex, II–III/IV intensity
   c. Decreases in standing position
   d. Caused by blood flow into the aorta.

J. Syncope
1. Defined by AHA as "temporary loss of consciousness and posture ... usually related to temporary insufficient blood flow to the brain"
   a. The examiner should differentiate true syncope from other symptoms such as fatigue, dizziness, and light-headedness
2. History of syncope or presyncope without a defined cause may warrant a thorough evaluation, as it may be a manifestation of a dangerous cardiovascular condition
3. Potential causes can be cardiac (structural or electrical abnormalities), neurologic (TIA, CVA, seizure), vasovagal/orthostatic, or psychiatric in nature
4. History, physical examination, and clinical judgement should be used to guide further evaluation in patients who report a history of syncope
   a. Patients with a well-defined cause for syncope, such as vasovagal syncope during an injection or syncope occurring during an acute febrile illness, may not require further work-up
   b. Reassuring factors include postexertional timing; single episode; and negative family history, cardiac exam, ECG, echocardiogram, and stress testing
5. History should address stimulant use (cocaine, ephedra, etc.) as potential cause

    6. A thorough cardiac work-up is recommended for patients whose history and physical suggest a possible underlying cardiovascular cause. Testing to be considered includes:

      a. 12-lead ECG

      b. Echocardiogram

      c. Event monitor or Holter monitor

      d. Exercise stress test (consider performing test at the intensity of the athlete's sport, e.g., maximal intensity for a sprinter)

    7. Decisions regarding clearance for play should be made based on the diagnosis made during the history, physical, and subsequent work-up. In certain conditions, treatment of the underlying abnormality (e.g., accessory pathway ablation for WPW) may make participation safer for the athlete

    8. Certain cardiac arrhythmias that cause excessively fast or slow heart rates may place an athlete at increased risk for SCD or injury due to syncope/presyncope, as in diving or motorsports. These include:

      a. Ventricular tachycardias

      b. Atrial flutter/fibrillation with rapid ventricular response

      c. WPW syndrome

      d. AV blocks

      e. Sinus node disease

      f. Congenital long-QT syndrome

      g. Brugada syndrome

    9. In general, patients with arrhythmias may participate in all sports if they are without underlying structural heart disease and have been treated with medications or ablation that keep their ventricular rates within normal limits for their activity.

III. Neurologic

  A. Seizure

    1. Defined as uncontrolled electrical activity of the brain which may lead to physical convulsions, alterations in mental status, or a combination of both

    2. Well-controlled seizures are not a contraindication for participation in contact or collision sports

      a. The physician and athlete should be aware of individual governing body restrictions on the use of antiepileptic medications

    3. Poorly controlled seizures should be appropriately medically managed prior to beginning competition

      a. Consider referral to neurologist and/or electroencephalogram (EEG)

      b. Water sports (swimming, SCUBA, surfing, etc.), shooting sports (archery, riflery), and other sports during which an alteration in consciousness could be fatal (skydiving, auto racing, etc.) should be restricted in patients with poorly controlled seizures

    4. Patients with history of seizures should never train for or compete in water sports without supervision.

  B. Traumatic brain injury (see Chapter 45 "Sports Concussion and Traumatic Brain Injury" for more details)

    1. Preparticipation evaluation should include questioning regarding the following:

      a. History of concussion or injuries to the head, face, or cervical spine

      b. Quality and duration of symptoms and signs associated with these injuries

      c. Types of protective equipment used at the time of each injury and currently

    2. Controversy exists regarding the inclusion of neuropsychological testing as a part of the screening PPE

      a. Proponents site the ability to obtain objective measurements of neuropsychologic function and to compare these to preinjury baseline measurements

        i. May be useful for return-to-play decisions and research purposes

    b. Opponents site cost and availability of the tests and limitations in the reliability of serial measurements, including false-negative tests

      i. Test results may vary based on environmental factors (noise, lighting, etc.) and internal factors (athlete's hydration status, motivation, illness, etc.)

    c. These tools may be used as part of a comprehensive evaluation to aid in return to play and clearance decisions after a concussion

3. Decisions regarding clearance for play should be made on an individual basis for each athlete based on the history and physical exam as outlined above if the athlete is without symptoms and has completed a graduated return-to-play protocol

4. Consider withholding an athlete from further contact or competition for the following:

    a. The athlete remains symptomatic from most recent head trauma

    b. Severity or duration of symptoms after each head trauma are increasing

    c. Symptoms are occurring with increasingly mild trauma

5. The PPE should be used as an opportunity to educate athletes, parents, coaches, and athletic trainers about symptoms, treatment, and prevention of concussion.

C. Cervical stenosis

  1. Condition in which there is narrowing of the cervical canal, with or without encroachment upon the spinal cord

  2. Cervical stenosis may be defined as:

    a. Canal measurement less than 14 mm at level of C4 on cervical spine MRI

      i. Currently the most utilized method

    b. Torg ratio

      i. Measurement used historically to define stenosis, prior to routine use of MRI

      ii. Ratio of canal width to vertebral body width in saggital plane of less than 0.8

      iii. No longer recommended due to increased size of vertebral bodies in athletes, which causes variability of measurements and difficulty in interpretation of results

    c. Functional spinal stenosis

      i. Presence of symptoms, including pain, weakness, numbness, paresthesias, or bowel/bladder dysfunction with normal imaging studies

  3. Athletes with a history of bilateral paresthesias or transient quadriparesis should have a cervical spine MRI to evaluate the underlying cause of symptoms

    a. Causes of spinal stenosis may be acquired (degenerative changes, bulging disc, cervical instability) or congenital

  4. Return-to-play decisions should be made based on the degree of stenosis, presence or history of symptoms, and degree of contact associated with sports being considered.

IV. Musculoskeletal

A. Joint disorders

  1. Musculoskeletal complaints are the most common ailments seen by athletic trainers and sports medicine physicians

  2. Musculoskeletal history should include questions regarding the following:

    a. Previous fractures, sprains, strains, or dislocations

    b. Previous use of assistive devices, prosthetics, orthotics, or physical therapy

    c. Signs or symptoms consistent with inflammatory arthropathies

    d. Any current injuries or symptoms requiring rehabilitation

    e. Previous imaging studies including x-rays, CT scans, or MRI

  3. Musculoskeletal examination

    a. Introduction

      i. Begin with screening exam as described below

      ii. If the athlete has a history of prior injury, perform a more detailed exam for the injured body part

        iii. An accurate diagnosis must be established before making return-to-play decisions

        iv. Larger institutions may include functional movement assessments

    b. General inspection

        i. Patient standing, facing the examiner

        ii. Evaluate symmetry of trunk and limbs

    c. Cervical exam

        i. Observe range of motion in flexion, extension, rotation, and side bending

        ii. Important for athletes with previous history of neck injury and stingers

        iii. Consider exclusion from play if limited range of motion, weakness, pain with movement, or radicular symptoms are present

    d. Shoulder exam

        i. Observe range of motion and strength against resistance in abduction, forward flexion, internal rotation, and external rotation of the shoulders

        ii. Consider further evaluation if a significant side-to-side difference exists in strength or range of motion

    e. Elbow exam

        i. Observe range of motion and strength against resistance in flexion and extension, as well as pronation and supination of the forearm with the elbow flexed to $90°$

        ii. Consider further evaluation if a significant side-to-side difference exists in strength or range of motion

    f. Hand exam

        i. Evaluate for asymmetry and limited range of motion as the patient:

            (A) Spreads fingers in abduction

            (B) Makes a fist

            (C) Flexes fingers

            (D) Extends fingers

    g. Back exam

        i. Evaluate symmetry and range of motion during back flexion and extension

        ii. Also assess symmetry of trunk and extremities facing away from the examiner

        iii. Inspect for scoliosis (see section IV B)

        iv. Palpate for tenderness along entire spinal column

    h. Leg exam

        i. Assess symmetry of musculature and bony prominences

        ii. Assess range of motion:

            (A) Hip: Flexion, extension, internal and external rotation

            (B) Knee: Flexion and extension

            (C) Ankle: Plantar-flexion, dorsi-flexion, inversion, eversion

        iii. Inspect for edema or venous insufficiency

        iv. Duck walk

        v. Assess tibial tuberosities in adolescents (Osgood Schlatters)

        vi. Toe raise and heel walk

        vii. Five hops test

    i. If the athlete has a history of prior injury, perform a more detailed exam of the injured body part

    j. An accurate diagnosis must be established before making return-to-play decisions.

B. The PPE should be used as a time to communicate with athletic trainers and physical therapists regarding need for further treatment and evaluation for protective devices.

C. Scoliosis

    1. Defined as a lateral curvature of the spine greater than $10°$ accompanied by vertebral rotation

2. Present in 2–4% of children between 10 and 16 years of age
3. Of adolescents diagnosed with scoliosis, only 10% have curves that progress and require medical intervention
4. The three main determinants of progression are:
   a. Patient gender (more common in females)
   b. Future growth potential
   c. Curve magnitude at the time of diagnosis
5. Adam's test
   a. Evaluate the patient's back for a "rib hump" with patient flexed to 90° at the waist and arms extended forward
   b. Represents curves greater than 10° and should prompt radiographic evaluation
6. Surgery is considered for curves greater than 40–45° if the patient has potential for increased growth
7. Recommendations:
   a. Evidence is lacking regarding risks associated with sports participation in patients with scoliosis, and the decision regarding participation should be individualized for each patient
   b. General guidelines exist, and are as follows:
      i. Those with mild curves may participate without restriction
      ii. Those with larger curves should consider avoiding collision sports and activities that load the facet joints heavily (e.g., volleyball, swimming, diving, gymnastics, etc.)
      iii. Patients who use bracing should exercise in their brace
      iv. Postoperative patients should gradually increase activity in the 6 months following surgery assuming that there are no complications
         (A) Contact sports and activities that load the facets should be avoided
         (B) Noncontact endurance sports (running) should be encouraged.

V. Paired Organs

A. Eyes
   1. Eye injuries are common in sports and appropriate steps should be taken to minimize the risk of these injuries
   2. History should address the following:
      a. History of vision abnormalities
      b. Use of glasses or contacts for vision correction
      c. History of eye injuries, surgeries, or infections
      d. Use of protective eyewear
   3. Visual acuity testing should be a part of the screening PPE
   4. Athletes, parents, coaches, and athletic trainers should be familiar with protective eye equipment requirements for their sports
   5. High-risk sports for eye injuries include those that involve projectiles, balls, sticks, bats, rackets, close contact, or intentional facial injury
   6. A patient is considered functionally one-eyed if corrected visual acuity in an eye is less than 20/40
      a. These athletes should be withheld from sports involving intentional injury, including boxing, full-contact martial arts, and wrestling
      b. These athletes should be counseled regarding risks of injury to the eyes, as well as proper use of protective eye equipment, prior to being cleared for other high-risk sports
   7. Patients with history of eye injury, infection, surgery, retinal detachment, or severe myopia should be evaluated and cleared for participation by an ophthalmologist
   8. Patients with abnormal visual acuity at the time of the PPE should be referred to an eye-care professional for evaluation and vision correction.

B. Kidneys

1. Examination for abnormalities of the kidneys should be performed during the abdominal examination
2. Congenital or traumatic absence of a kidney does not preclude an athlete from participation
3. Individual assessment and counseling regarding risks of injury to the remaining kidney (including the potential needed for transplant or dialysis) should be performed during the PPE
4. Descriptions and limitations of protective equipment should be discussed
5. Some experts believe athletes should be withheld from contact sports if the solitary kidney is multicystic, pelvic or iliac in location, or hydronephrotic
6. Consultation with a urologist or nephrologist is recommended prior to clearance for participation in patients with a solitary functioning kidney
7. Functional assessment of renal function, including serum creatinine, glomerular filtration rate, and functional kidney scans may be considered to aid in decisions regarding participation in athletes with renal abnormalities
8. The decision regarding clearance for participation should be made on an individualized basis for each athlete based on the issues discussed above.

C. Testicles

1. Testicular examination should be performed on male athletes to assess size, shape, tenderness, and presence of both testicles
2. Evaluation of inguinal canal for hernias should be performed in patients with symptoms of a hernia, but is not necessary in asymptomatic patients
3. Single testicle
   a. Congenital or traumatic absence of a testicle does not preclude an athlete from participation
   b. Individual assessment regarding risks of participation (including infertility) and protective equipment should be performed before participation in collision or contact sports
   c. A protective cup should be used if the athlete plans to participate in contact, collision, or projectile sports.

D. Ovaries

1. Absence of an ovary does not preclude patients from participation as risk of injury to the solitary ovary is minimal.

VI. Abdominal and Pelvic

A. Introduction

1. Examination of the abdomen should be performed with the patient in the supine position, and should include auscultation of abdominal vessels as well as palpation of all four abdominal quadrants
   a. Should include evaluation for organomegaly, kidney abnormalities, gravid uterus, abdominal tenderness, and, in males, genital examination
   b. Pelvic examinations in females and Tanner staging are not recommended as a part of the routine PPE.

B. Conditions that may limit participation include:

1. Infectious diarrhea
   a. Athletes should be withheld from competition to avoid dehydration and heat illness unless symptoms are mild and athlete is well-hydrated
2. Organomegaly
   a. Hepatomegaly
      i. May be secondary to infection (hepatitis) or malignancy
      ii. Athletes should be withheld from competition until resolution

   iii. Athletes with chronic hepatomegaly should have individual evaluation regarding clearance to play based on sport, symptoms, and type and severity of underlying hepatic condition

  b. Splenomegaly

   i. Most commonly caused by infectious mononucleosis

    (A) Athletes should be withheld from competition for 28 days from onset of symptoms or date of diagnosis. See section VII F

   ii. Athletes should be withheld from competition until resolution due to risk of splenic rupture

 3. Malabsorption syndromes

  a. Athletes require individual assessment to determine ability to meet caloric needs to avoid nutritional deficits

  b. Presence of indwelling catheter or external devices for delivery of parenteral nutrition requires prevention strategy and emergency action plan in the event of damage to these devices

 4. Inguinal hernia

  a. Patients with inguinal hernia should not be precluded from participation, although symptoms may limit performance or ability to participate

  b. Symptoms may include inguinal heaviness, swelling, or pain

   i. Symptomatic patients will often require surgical correction

  c. Athletes should be advised to seek care if they develop severe pain, erythema, increased swelling, nausea, or vomiting, as these may represent strangulation of the hernia.

VII. Education/Prevention

 A. Asthma

  1. Introduction

   a. Pulmonary disease caused by bronchial hyperreactivity and airway inflammation leading to reversible obstruction of airflow

   b. Symptoms may include dyspnea, wheezing, cough, or chest tightness

   c. Exercise-induced asthma (EIA) is used to describe exercise-induced symptoms in patients with underlying asthma

   d. Exercise-induced bronchospasm (EIB) is used to describe symptoms in patients without underlying asthma, although undiagnosed asthma should be considered in athletes who show symptoms

   e. History questions should address the following:

    i. Past history of asthma, wheezing, dyspnea, or chronic cough

    ii. Previous and current use of bronchodilators or other asthma medications

    iii. Previous hospitalizations or intubations for asthma exacerbations

    iv. Current frequency and severity of symptoms

    v. Presence of tobacco abuse or second-hand smoke exposure

  2. Diagnosis

   a. Pulmonary function testing (PFTs) may be normal at rest, and are therefore unreliable in the diagnosis of EIA

   b. PFTs performed before and after exercise may be more reliable as a diagnostic test if there is a reversible decline in FEV1 after exercise

    i. Some patients may only develop symptoms under certain environmental conditions, and therefore portable spirometry may be required to adequately diagnose EIA

   c. Eucapnic voluntary hyperventilation (EVH) testing is the preferred method of testing identified by the IOC

    i. Requires specialized equipment, therefore often used only at higher levels of competition

        ii. Six-minute protocol of hyperventilation of gas containing 21% oxygen and 5% carbon dioxide at a prescribed ventilatory rate recreates exercise conditions

        iii. Considered diagnostic if FEV1 decreases by 10% or more

  3. Treatment

    a. Use of short-acting beta-agonist (SABA) bronchodilators prior to exercise may be useful in preventing symptoms

    b. Athletes who require bronchodilator use more than twice weekly may benefit from addition of inhaled corticosteroids, long-acting beta-agonists (LABA), mast cell stabilizers, or leukotriene inhibitors

  4. Recommendations

    a. Athletes with well-controlled asthma should not be restricted from activities

    b. Athletes with poorly controlled symptoms should be evaluated for need for additional treatment

    c. Patients with febrile respiratory illness or acute symptoms should be withheld from competition until they are well

    d. Athletes, coaches, athletic trainers, and covering physicians should have inhalers available during coverage and should work together to develop an emergency action plan in the event that this treatment is inadequate to reverse symptoms.

B. Diabetes mellitus

  1. Athletes with diabetes should be evaluated for potential complications of the disease in the same manner as any diabetic patient, including:

    a. Cardiovascular disease

    b. Retinopathy

    c. Neuropathy

    d. Nephropathy

    e. Gastroparesis

  2. Athletes with well-controlled blood glucose levels and without any other contraindications should be allowed to participate in sports

  3. High-risk sports for athletes with diabetes include rock climbing, skydiving, scuba, and auto sports

  4. Other sports such as swimming or endurance running require proper support for the athlete, including access to insulin and food or caloric drinks

  5. Athletes with retinopathy should avoid sports that are high impact or that acutely increase blood pressure

  6. Blood glucose should be monitored during exercise, and insulin dosing and caloric intake should be adjusted accordingly

  7. Patients with ketosis and preexercise blood glucose greater than 250 or preexercise blood glucose greater than 300 with or without ketosis should avoid exercise.

C. Drugs

  1. Introduction

    a. The PPE affords the physician an excellent opportunity for counseling patients, many of whom are in good health and may not seek healthcare frequently

    b. Adolescent athletes should be informed that discussions regarding drug and alcohol questions will be confidential

  2. Prescription medications

    a. Athletes participating in organized team sports should provide their team physician and athletic trainer with a list of current prescription medications and drug allergies prior to participation

      i. Some medications should be kept on the sideline for immediate use if needed (e.g., albuterol, insulin, epinephrine, etc.)

    b. Athletes participating in individual sports should discuss medication use with their physician at the time of the PPE

         i. Consider counseling athletes with medical problems to carry a list of medications and allergies or to use one of many commercially available accessories that provide emergency contact information

      c. Athletes, physicians, and athletic trainers should familiarize themselves with the list of medications that may be banned by their sport's governing bodies

  3. Alcohol

      a. Screening for use and abuse may be performed at the time of the PPE

      b. Athletes should be counseled regarding potential health problems from alcohol use, as well as associated dangers such as motor vehicle accidents

      c. Alcohol use is banned in some sports that require fine motor control, such as archery

  4. Tobacco

      a. Tobacco use is the chief cause of preventable deaths in the United States each year

      b. Cigarette smoking is associated with increased risk of many types of cancer, COPD, heart disease, and stroke

      c. Smokeless tobacco use is very common in young male athletes, and may lead to oral or laryngeal cancers

  5. Drugs of abuse

      a. Screening and counseling regarding abuse of prescription drugs and street drugs may be performed during the PPE as well

  6. Supplements

      a. Supplement use is extremely common in the athletic population

      b. Athletes should provide physicians and athletic trainers with a list of supplements being used, and should be counseled regarding possible adverse effects of their use

      c. Athletes should be counseled regarding the following information:

         i. Supplements are not regulated by the Food and Drug Administration

         ii. Ingredients present in supplements and their concentrations may vary

         iii. Claims made by the manufacturer may not have scientific evidence to support them

         iv. Listed or unlisted ingredients in supplements may cause them to have positive drug screens.

D. Female athlete triad (see Chapter 50 for more details)

  1. Introduction

      a. Female athletes have special concerns that should be addressed during the PPE, including increased risk relative to males for stress fractures, disordered eating, non-contact ACL injuries, and menstrual irregularities

      b. The female athlete triad is a constellation of symptoms caused by inadequate caloric intake that leads to decreased energy stores, causing decreased blood levels of estrogen. The triad includes the following:

         i. Disordered eating

         ii. Menstrual irregularities

         iii. Decreased bone mineral density

  2. Disordered eating

      a. History questions should address the following:

         i. History of disordered eating

         ii. Previous or current dietary restrictions

         iii. Previous or current use of diuretics, laxatives, stimulants, sweat suits, purging behavior, and so on.

         iv. Pressure from parents, coaches, athletic trainers, and so on to maintain or achieve a certain body weight

         v. Concerns of the athlete regarding current weight or body image

   b. Physical examination
   i. Exam should include height and weight measurements
      (A) An adult female athlete is considered underweight if her BMI is less than 18.5
      (B) A child or adolescent female athlete is considered underweight if her BMI is less than the 5th percentile for her age
   ii. Exam findings associated with anorexia nervosa may include bradycardia, hypotension, lanugo hair on the skin, abdominal distension as a result of constipation from hypomotility, pallor related to anemia, or musculoskeletal abnormalities associated with decreased bone density
   iii. Exam findings associated with bulimia nervosa may include parotid gland hypertrophy, wear of dental enamel, and calluses on the knuckles from repeated induced vomiting
3. Menstrual irregularities
   a. Caloric deficit created by overtraining or caloric restriction leads to decreased estrogen levels, which can cause menstrual irregularities
   b. Amenorrhea is common in active females, but should be viewed as a potential sign of a serious disorder
   i. Primary amenorrhea is the lack of menses by age 16
   ii. Secondary amenorrhea is the lack of three consecutive menstrual periods after menarche
      (A) Can have a number of causes, including pregnancy, some forms of contraception, or endocrine disorders
   iii. A thorough work-up should be performed to look for the cause of amenorrhea prior to attributing it to disordered eating or overtraining
   c. History should address the following:
   i. Length and frequency of menstrual periods
   ii. Current use of contraceptives
   iii. Age or presence of menarche
   d. Pelvic examination is not recommended as part of the PPE unless the PPE is part of a comprehensive health maintenance exam
   i. Patients with concerning history who may require a pelvic exam should have this scheduled with their PCP or Ob/Gyn at a later time
4. Decreased bone mineral density (BMD)
   a. Results from secondary amenorrhea and decreased estrogen levels, which simulates a postmenopausal state
   b. History should address the following:
   i. Presence or history of stress fractures or fractures
      (A) Details regarding the development of these injuries, including training regimen and diet at the time of injury, number and chronicity of injuries, and adequacy of treatment
   c. Physical exam should include the screening musculoskeletal exam and more thorough exam of sites of previous injuries
5. Further evaluation
   a. Athletes with menstrual irregularities should have a thorough work-up for underlying causes, which may include urine pregnancy test, CBC, BMP, thyroid function tests, and FSH and LH levels
   b. Athletes with disordered eating may require further work-up, including CBC, BMP, iron studies, magnesium and phosphorous levels, EKG to evaluate for heart blocks or prolonged QT intervals
   c. Athletes with decreased BMD may require testing of calcium and vitamin D levels, as well as monitoring with DEXA scanning

6. Treatment
   a. Treatment of the female athlete triad requires a multidisciplinary approach, which should include the physician, a nutritionist, a psychologist or psychiatrist, and if applicable, the patients parents, coaches, and athletic trainers to an appropriate extent
   b. Oral contraceptive pills have not been shown to be effective in restoring bone mineral density or preventing further decreases
   c. Decisions regarding clearance for sports participation should be made on an individualized basis
      i. Athletes should be withheld from sports if their participation puts them at risk for further injury
      ii. In many cases, athletes may require mental health treatment prior to returning to sport
      iii. Activity should be resumed gradually, with monitoring to ensure that overtraining does not occur
      iv. Parents, coaches, and athletic trainers should be counseled that behavior intended to restrict calories or weight is likely to be detrimental to the patient's health
      v. Contracts may be used with the athlete to encourage adherence with treatment recommendations and follow-up.

E. Injury prevention
   1. Introduction
      a. The PPE affords the physician an excellent opportunity for counseling patients, many of whom are in good health and may not seek healthcare frequently
      b. Athletes, parents, coaches, and athletic trainers should all be aware of options and requirements for protective athletic equipment, especially as this equipment pertains to specific medical conditions present in the athlete
      c. Young athletes and their parents should be counseled to avoid specialization in sports at a young age, as specialization may lead to an increased rate in overuse injuries and decrease the athlete's ability to develop balanced strength and flexibility
      d. Consider counseling of parents and coaches of young athletes to allow them adequate opportunity to rest, recover, and rehabilitate injuries between athletic seasons
   2. ACL prevention programs
      a. Many programs have been developed in recent years in attempt to decrease ACL injuries
         i. Females are up to four times more likely than males to have an ACL injury
         ii. The majority of these injuries occur in noncontact situations (i.e., pivoting, landing)
         iii. Emphasis is to place the athlete in a typical setting of injury in a controlled environment so that they may recognize proprioceptive cues and develop mechanisms to avoid injury
      b. Many authors have reported success in decreasing ACL injury rates after seasons incorporating these programs.

F. Infectious disease
   1. Human immunodeficiency virus (HIV) and Hepatitis B and C
      a. These viral infections can be transmitted through exposure to blood of infected bodily fluid though open wounds, mucous membranes, or parenteral administration, sexual contact, IV drug abuse, and perinatal transmission
      b. The risk of transmission through sport is minimal, and presence of these diseases alone should not preclude an athlete from sports participation
      c. The athlete should be evaluated for any complications from the diseases that may limit performance or place the participating athlete at risk
      d. Changes in the athlete's health status warrants reevaluation for participation clearance
   2. Infectious mononucleosis
      a. Viral infection caused by the Epstein–Barr virus (EBV)

    b. Diagnosed based on serology or rapid Monospot test

    c. Symptoms include fatigue, fever, myalgias, pharyngitis, cervical lymphadenopathy

    d. Symptoms may be severe enough to limit performance

    e. Splenomegaly occurs in the majority of patients with mononucleosis, and splenic rupture is a possible complication

      i. Splenic rupture is most common within the first 21 days of the illness, but rarely occurs after 28 days

      ii. Recommendations are to withhold an athlete from competition for 4 weeks after the onset of symptoms, or the time of diagnosis if the timing of symptoms is unclear

      iii. Serial ultrasound can be used to monitor for resolution of splenomegaly, but is limited by the lack of data and consistency among spleen sizes.

VIII. Special Populations

A. Disabled athletes

   1. "Disability" is defined by the Americans with Disabilities Act as "a physical or mental impairment that substantially limits one or more major life activities of such individual"

   2. The International Paralympic Committee (IPC), a division of the International Olympic Committee (IOC), is the governing body for athletic competitions for athletes with physical disabilities

    a. At the Beijing 2008 Paralympics, there were 3,951 athletes competing, representing 146 countries

   3. Disabled athletes are given a class score (one (severely impaired) to eight (minimally impaired)) based on testing of upper limb, lower limb, and trunk function

    a. This scoring system allows participants to compete against opponents with similar levels of functioning

   4. History and physical exams should be performed in a manner similar to the general PPE with some exceptions:

    a. Dermatologic considerations

      i. All wheelchair athletes should be evaluated for presence of ischial and sacral decubitus ulcers

        (A) Consider withholding athletes from competition if ulcers are present until they are completely healed

      ii. Skin should also be evaluated for callus or ulcer formation from wheelchair propulsion and bruising, abrasions, or lacerations from blunt trauma from equipment, other wheelchairs, and so on

    b. Urologic considerations

      i. Athletes with neurologic bladder dysfunction should have the normally recommended GU examination

      ii. In addition, any external collection systems (catheters, etc.) should be evaluated as these athletes are at increased risk for urinary tract infections

    c. Musculoskeletal considerations

      i. Wheelchair athletes should be evaluated for shoulder pain and impingement syndromes

      ii. Amputees should have prosthetics and orthotics evaluated for proper fit and mechanical function prior to using for athletic competition

    d. Neuroendocrine considerations

      i. Should be addressed in athletes with spinal cord injuries

      ii. Patients should be questioned regarding history of heat-related illness as they may have impaired thermoregulation mechanisms due to decreased ability to sweat below the level of injury

        iii. Questioning and education regarding autonomic dysreflexia should also be performed

           (A) Autonomic dysreflexia is a potentially life-threatening autonomic response of overstimulation from noxious stimuli

             (1) Occurs in patients with spinal cord injury at T6 level or above

             (2) Can lead to potentially fatal elevations in blood pressure

             (3) Other signs and symptoms include flushing, excessive sweating above level of spinal injury, headache, nausea, bradycardia, and piloerection below the level of spinal injury

             (4) Can be used by athletes to gain competitive advantage in a process known as "boosting"

               (a) Commonly achieved by mechanically obstructing urinary catheter, ingesting large quantities of fluid to cause bladder distension, wearing tight-fitting clothes, or sitting on sharp objects

               (b) May also be caused by infections or skin ulcers.

B. Special olympians

    1. Special Olympics is a charitable organization founded in the 1960s to promote "empowerment, competence, acceptance and joy" in individuals with intellectual disabilities through athletic competition.

    2. There are currently over 3 million Special Olympic athletes in 180 countries participating in over 30 sports.

    3. Due to the significant numbers of participants, sports medicine physicians and other PCPs are likely to encounter these athletes in practice, and should be aware of their specific needs for proper PPE.

    4. History and physical exams should be performed in a manner similar to the general PPE with some exceptions:

        a. A third party (parent, caregiver, etc.) may need to be present during the PPE to provide the most accurate history possible

        b. Emphasis should be placed on conditions common to intellectually disabled athletes, including congenital heart disease, vision and hearing limitations, ligamentous laxity leading to joint injuries, and seizure history

        c. Athletes with Trisomy 21 (Down Syndrome) should be evaluated for asymptomatic atlanto-axial instability (AAI) prior to competition using lateral cervical flexion and extension views

           i. In children, AAI is considered to be present when the distance between the posterior aspect of the anterior arch of the atlas and the anterior aspect of the odontoid is greater than 4.5 mm

           ii. This testing is required prior to competing in the following sports:

             (A) Judo, equestrian, high jump, alpine skiing, diving, snowboarding, squat lift, soccer, pentathlon, swimming (butterfly stroke or diving starts)

        d. Decisions regarding further evaluation (ECG, echocardiogram), specialist referrals (neurology for uncontrolled seizures, cardiology for congenital heart defects), and clearance for participation in different sports should be made in the same manner as for any other athlete.

C. Sickle cell trait

    1. Condition of inheriting one gene for sickle cell hemoglobin and one normal

    2. Present in one of 12 African Americans and one in 2,000 to 10,000 White Americans

    3. Intense exercise can lead to exertional sickling in those with sickle cell trait

    4. Exercise provides four conditions that can account for this in combination:

        a. Hypoxemia

        b. Metabolic acidosis

        c. Muscle hyperthermia

5. Clinical presentation can include fatigue, muscle cramps or weakness, shortness of breath, dizziness, inability to continue with exercise, or collapse in the setting of extreme exertion
6. While exertional sickling may lead to severe metabolic complications and even death, it is a self-limited event if symptoms are treated early with rest, oxygen, cooling if necessary, and monitoring of vital signs
7. Methods to prevent exertional sickling should include the following:
   a. Build training slowly
   b. Longer rest and recovery time between efforts
   c. Immediate cessation of activity with symptoms
   d. Avoidance of exercise during illness
   e. Adequate control of asthma if present
   f. Maintain adequate hydration
8. Education should be provided to athletes, athletic trainers, coaches, and medical staff regarding signs of deteriorating status in an athlete as well as an institutional emergency action plan
9. Screening for sickle cell trait has become mandatory for all NCAA athletes as of the 2010–2011 academic year
10. Concerns that exist regarding global screening include cost and the potential for discrimination against a sickle trait positive athlete (e.g., professional sports contracts, teammates' views of work ethic, personal view of training efficacy)
11. The U.S. military discontinued sickle cell screening after a 10-year prospective trial of modified training protocols, including enforced hydration and environmental monitoring, demonstrated no deaths in 40,000 recruits with sickle cell trait
    a. Military sites not participating in the study had mortality rates comparable to those of the participating sites prior to the training modifications
12. Presence of Sickle Cell Trait is not a contraindication to sports at any level.

D. Hematologic disorders
   1. Introduction
      a. Patients with hematologic disorders should have individualized evaluations to determine exercise capacity and effectiveness of oxygen utilization prior to clearance for participation in sports
      b. Testing to consider includes:
         i. Exercise stress test with oxygen saturation monitoring
         ii. Serial hematocrit assessments during the season
   2. Iron-deficiency anemia
      a. Can cause impaired performance in athletes
      b. Symptoms may include fatigue, dyspnea, tachycardia, or headache
         i. Consider CBC in patients reporting these symptoms at PPE
      c. Supplementation with iron should be initiated to correct anemia, and is recommended for a period of 6 months to correct residual depletion of total body iron stores
   3. Ferritin
      a. Laboratory marker representing total body iron stores
      b. Controversy exists as to whether a CBC and ferritin should be included as screening tests, and whether iron supplementation should be initiated in athletes with non-anemic iron deficiency
      c. Levels below 12 ng/dL represent decreased bone marrow iron stores
      d. Recommendations exist for iron supplementation for ferritin levels less than 30–35 ng/dL, to be continued for 6 months or until ferritin levels reach 50 ng/dL
      e. Ferrous iron products are recommended as they are better absorbed than ferric iron
   4. Hemophilia
      a. Inherited disorder caused by deficiency of factor VIII or IX in the clotting cascade
      b. Leads to spontaneous bleeding, which may be severe
         i. Frequent hemarthroses can lead to synovitis, joint degeneration, joint pain, limited

      c. Risk of bleeding with physical activity varies amongst patients, and may differ based on treatment, extent of disease, and amount of contact

      d. Recommendations

        i. Patients should be evaluated for joint injury and function prior to participation

        ii. Protective equipment, disease treatment, and injury rehabilitation should be maximized

        iii. Contact sports are not strictly contraindicated, but care should be taken in sport selection based on disease state and informed decisions by patients and parents

        iv. Emergency action plan should be in place to prevent and treat acute bleeds

    5. Anticoagulated athletes

      a. Evidence-based return-to-play guidelines for those receiving anticoagulant therapy have not been established

      b. Multiple case reports have demonstrated successful return to prior activity levels for patients receiving short-term anticoagulation for disorders such as deep-venous thrombosis (DVT) or Paget–Schroetter syndrome

      c. Risks must be discussed with patients regarding the dangers of contact or impact sports while on anticoagulant medications, including intracerebral hemorrhage, compartment syndrome, hemarthroses, hematomas, and so on.

        i. These activities should be discouraged due to the inherent risks.

E. Cystic fibrosis

    1. Disease process caused by mutation in the gene for the cystic fibrosis transmembrane conductance regulator (CFTR) protein

      a. Involved in the transport of chloride ions across cell membranes

      b. Mutation leads to fibrosis of the pancreases and abnormalities in sweat, digestive enzyme, and mucous secretions

    2. Hallmark symptoms include poor weight gain and growth, presence of thick mucous secretions, cough, dyspnea, and frequent lung infections

    3. Sports participation should be determined on an individual basis

      a. Exercise testing to determine oxygenation during exercise is recommended

      b. Patients should also be screened for effects of gastrointestinal malabsorption and ability to meet caloric needs for exercise

    4. Medical therapy, including bronchodilators, antibiotics, and so on, should be maximized prior to participation in sports

      a. Consider pulmonology referral in these patients.

Recommended Reading

1. Bernhardt DT, Roberts WO, eds. *Preparticipation Physical Evaluation.* 4th ed. Elk Grove Village, IL: American Academy of Pediatrics, 2010.
2. Maron BJ, Thompson PD, Puffer JC, McGrew CA, Strong WB, Douglas PS, Clark LT, Mitten MJ, Crawford MH, Atkins DL, Driscoll DJ, Epstein AE. Cardiovascular preparticipation screening of competitive athletes. A statement for health professionals from the Sudden Death Committee (clinical cardiology) and Congenital Cardiac Defects Committee (cardiovascular disease in the young), American Heart Association. *Circulation.* 1996;94(4):850–6.
3. Maron BJ, Zies DP. Bethesda Conference Report. *36th Bethesda Conference*: Eligibility Recommendations for Competitive Athletes With Cardiovascular Abnormalities. *J Am Coll Cardiol.* 2005;45(8):1313–1375.
4. McCrory P, Meeuwisse W, Johnston K, Dvorak J, Aubry M, Molloy M, Cantu R. Consensus statement on concussion in sport: The 3rd International Conference on Concussion in Sport held in Zurich, November 2008. *Br J Sports Med.* 2009;43:i76–i84.
5. Philpott JF, Houghton K, Luke A. Physical activity recommendations for children with specific chronic health conditions: Juvenile idiopathic arthritis, hemophilia, asthma, and cystic fibrosis. *Clin J Sport Med.* 2010;20(3):167–172.
6. Wingfield K, Matheson GO, Meeuwisse WH, Garrick JG, Beckerman J, Wang P, Hlatky M. The preparticipation evaluation: Thematic issue. *Clin J Sport Med.* 2004;14(3):107–187.

9

Conditioning and Training Techniques

Jacob L. Sellon and Jonathan T. Finnoff

I. Principles of Training

A. General adaptation syndrome (GAS) = response to new exercise-related stress
1. Shock phase
   a. Several days to a few weeks
   b. Performance drops
   c. Muscle soreness and stiffness
2. Resistance phase
   a. Body adapts and returns to supranormal performance level
      i. Initially neural adaptations
      ii. Later muscular, cardiovascular, and metabolic adaptations
3. Exhaustion phase = overtraining
   a. Result of excessive stress
   b. Performance declines

B. Sports specificity
1. Adaptations specific to type of exercise performed
   a. Neuromuscular specificity
      i. Motor learning due to repetition of specific movement pattern
         (A) Muscle action (e.g., concentric, eccentric, isometric)
         (B) Speed of movement
         (C) Range of motion
         (D) Muscle groups trained
   b. Metabolic specificity
      i. Energy systems (i.e., ATP/creatine phosphate, anaerobic lactic, aerobic) stressed during training should closely match metabolic demands of the specific sport

C. Overload
1. Physiologic adaptation occurs if exercise stimulus > normal
2. Key variables are intensity and volume
   a. Intensity = percent of maximal functional capacity of exercise mode
   b. Volume = total amount of exercise performed in a period of time

D. Progression
1. Volume and/or intensity must be periodically increased to continue improving

E. Recovery
1. Adaptations occur during recovery, not training
2. To maximize training adaptations, optimize recovery
   a. Rest days, appropriate nutrition, adequate sleep, restorative techniques (e.g., massage, relaxation)

F. Prioritization
   1. Not all elements of a conditioning program can be optimized simultaneously
   2. Develop training priorities based on athlete's abilities and sport-specific demands
G. Individuality
   1. Different individuals respond differently to same training stimulus
H. Diminishing returns
   1. The greatest improvements occur in individuals who are inexperienced
   2. Experienced individuals make much smaller gains
I. Reversibility
   1. If training not continued, benefits will be lost (e.g., VO_{2max} can decrease by 4–6% in just 2 weeks of inactivity).

II. Periodization

A. Periodization = planned variation in training in a given time period
   1. Developed in the 1960s by Russian physiologist Leo Matveyev
   2. Concept based on GAS
   3. Optimizes adaptations over long-term training while minimizing overtraining
   4. Typically general physical training → sport-specific physical training
B. Periodization cycles
   1. Macrocycle = a year or more (4 years for Olympics)
   2. Mesocycle = 2–6 weeks
   3. Microcycle: = 1 week
C. Periodization types
   1. Linear (classical) periodization
      a. Gradual variation of volume and intensity over mesocycles
      b. Volume (high → low)
      c. Intensity (low → high)
      d. Focus on one quality (e.g., endurance, strength, power, etc.) each mesocycle
      e. Preferable for sports with limited number of in-season competitions and well-defined off-season
   2. Nonlinear (undulating) periodization
      a. Acute variation of volume and intensity within microcycles
      b. Attempt to train various components of neuromuscular system (e.g., maximal strength, speed, endurance) simultaneously within microcycles
      c. Preferable for sports with long competitive seasons, multiple competitions, and year-round practice
D. Linear periodization macrocycle
   1. Preparatory period (2 major phases)
      a. First and longest mesocycle
      b. Develop general fitness base in preparation for future high-intensity, more specific training
      c. Higher volume, lower intensity
         i. High repetition resistance training
         ii. Low-intensity plyometrics
      d. Progressive microcycles increase resistance loads, aerobic exercise intensity, and sports technique training
      e. Often three resistance training microcycles
         i. Hypertrophy/endurance phase
            (A) Focus is increasing muscular strength endurance and lean body mass
            (B) High volume, high repetition
            (C) Light loading

    f. General preparation phase

       i. Develop anaerobic/aerobic work capacity in preparation for future high-intensity, sport-specific training

    g. Sport-specific preparation phase

       i. Develop physical capacity specific to the physiologic demands of the sport

       ii. Perfect sport technique

       iii. Transition to the competitive phase

    h. Progressive mesocycles may increase resistance loads, aerobic exercise intensity, and/ or sport technique training

    i. Classically three resistance training mesocycles in the preparatory period

       i. Hypertrophy/endurance phase

          (A) Focus is increasing muscular strength, endurance and lean body mass

          (B) High volume, high repetition

          (C) Light loading

          (D) Low-speed movements

          (E) Minimal sport-specific activities

       ii. Maximal strength phase

          (A) Focus is increasing maximal strength

          (B) High loading

          (C) Low repetition

          (D) Relatively low-speed movements

          (E) More emphasis on sport-specific movements

       iii. Strength/power phase

          (A) Focus is on power development

          (B) Moderate to high loading

          (C) Low repetition

          (D) High-speed, sport-specific movements

  2. Competition period = peaking

    a. Peak fitness difficult to maintain more than 2–3 weeks without overtraining

    b. Emphasis on maintaining high-intensity and sport-specific technique training

    c. Significantly reduced volume

  3. Active rest period

    a. Goal is physical and mental recovery from competitive season

    b. Injury rehab/prehab

    c. Low intensity and volume

    d. Unstructured, non-sports-specific recreational training.

III. Strength Training

A. Definitions

  1. Strength = ability to produce force

  2. Hypertrophy = increase in muscle cell size due to increases in intracellular fluid and contractile protein

  3. Power = ability to produce force quickly

B. Muscle strength factors

  1. Muscle fiber cross-sectional area positively correlated with maximal force production

  2. Expression of strength altered by muscle length, joint angle, pennation angle, and contraction velocity

  3. Enhanced neural function

    a. Motor unit recruitment (Henneman size principle)

    b. Rate coding (increased action potential frequency)

C. Strength programming variables

  1. Type of muscle action

      b. Eccentric (muscle lengthening)

         i. Greatest force per muscle fiber

         ii. Greatest stimulus for hypertrophy

      c. Isometric (no net change in muscle length)

2. Loading = resistance = weight lifted per repetition or set

      a. Intensity

         i. Percentage of one-repetition maximum (1-RM) load

         ii. Measurement of loading

      b. Loading (resistance) type

         i. Isotonic (e.g., free weights)

           (A) Resistance is constant and speed increases with force applied

         ii. Isokinetic (e.g., Cybex machine)

           (A) Speed is constant and resistance increases with force applied

         iii. Isometric (e.g., pushing against a wall)

           (A) Joint angle does not change

           (B) Resistance increases with force applied

         iv. Elastic (e.g., band, spring)

           (A) Both resistance and speed are variable

           (B) Allows resistance in multiple planes

3. Volume = total number of repetitions times load in a training session

4. Frequency = number of training sessions per week (or microcycle)

      a. Whole-body versus split routines

5. Exercise selection

      a. Multijoint versus single-joint exercises

         i. Multijoint (compound) exercises (e.g., squat, bench press)

           (A) Allow for more loading

           (B) Work more muscles with fewer exercises

           (C) Coactivation of muscles around joint promotes stability

         ii. Single-joint (isolation) exercises (e.g., leg extension, biceps curl)

           (A) Technically easier

           (B) Allow for focus on single joint movement

           (C) Less coactivation about joint → more shear force

      b. Closed kinetic chain (CKC) versus open kinetic chain (OKC) exercises

         i. CKC = distal aspect of limb is fixed (e.g., squat, push-up)

           (A) Require movement of proximal muscle segments resulting in coactivation of core musculature and larger muscle groups → arguably better transfer to sport (more functional)

           (B) Usually multijoint exercise → coactivation of muscles around joint promotes stability

         ii. OKC = distal aspect of limb is mobile (e.g., leg extension, bench press)

           (A) Less core and proximal muscle coactivation → arguably less transfer to sport

           (B) May be single-joint (e.g., leg extension) or multijoint (e.g., leg press) exercises

      c. Bilateral (two limb) versus unilateral (single limb) exercises

         i. Bilateral allow for more loading

         ii. Unilateral require more stabilization and allow correction of side-to-side imbalances

      d. Free weights versus machines

         i. Free weights train intra- and intermuscular coordination, allowing better movement specificity

         ii. Machines are technically easier to use

6. Exercise order

      a. More technically demanding exercises (e.g., Olympic lifts, CKC, multijoint) should be performed before simpler exercises

    b. Larger muscle groups should be trained before smaller muscle groups

    c. Muscle force and power are potentiated when antagonist movements paired

  7. Repetition speed

    a. Can be fast, moderate, or slow

      i. Unintentionally slow = due to loading or fatigue

      ii. Intentionally slow

        (A) Studies have shown decreased force production

  8. Rest periods = amount of rest taken between exercises, sets, or repetitions

    a. Affects metabolic, hormonal, and cardiovascular responses to exercise

    b. More rest is required for more complex exercises (e.g., Olympic lifts)

D. American College of Sports Medicine (ACSM) recommendations for muscular strength training

  1. Type of muscle action: should include exercises with concentric, eccentric, and isometric muscle contractions

  2. Loading

    a. Novice to intermediate: 60–70% one-repetition maximum (1-RM) for 8–12 repetitions

    b. Advanced: cycle loads of 80–100% 1-RM

    c. Progress loading no more than 2–10% between sessions

  3. Volume

    a. Novice: 1–3 sets per exercise

    b. Intermediate to advanced: multiple sets with systematic variation

  4. Frequency

    a. Novice: whole-body training 2–3 days per week

    b. Intermediate: 3 (whole body) or 4 (split routine) days per week

    c. Advanced: 4–6 days per week with option of twice per day

  5. Exercise selection

    a. Bilateral and unilateral exercises

    b. Emphasis on multijoint (vs. single-joint) exercises

    c. Free weights and machines with emphasis on free weights for advanced trainees

  6. Repetition speed

    a. Novice: slow to moderate speed

    b. Intermediate: moderate speed

    c. Advanced:

      i. Include continuum or speed (slow, moderate, fast)

      ii. Intent should be to maximize concentric speed

  7. Rest periods

    a. At least 2–3 min for main (heavy load) exercises

    b. 1–2 min for assistance (lighter load) exercises

E. ACSM recommendations for muscular hypertrophy training

  1. Type of muscle action: include concentric, eccentric, and isometric exercises

  2. Loading

    a. Novice to intermediate: 70–85% one-repetition maximum (1-RM) for 8–12 repetitions

    b. Advanced: cycle loads of 70–100% 1-RM for 1–12 repetitions (majority 6–12)

  3. Volume

    a. Novice to intermediate: 1–3 sets per exercise

    b. Advanced: 3–6 sets per exercise

  4. Frequency

    a. Novice: whole-body training 2–3 days per week

    b. Intermediate: 3 (whole body) or 4 (split routine) days per week

    c. Advanced: split routine training 4–6 days per week

5. Exercise selection
   a. Multi- and single-joint exercises
   b. Free weights and machines
6. Repetition speed
   a. Novice and intermediate: slow to moderate speed
   b. Advanced: slow, moderate, and fast speed
7. Rest periods
   a. Novice to intermediate: 1–2 min
   b. Advanced: variable

F. ACSM recommendations for muscular power training
   1. Power training should be incorporated with a concurrent strength training program as part of a periodized plan
   2. Loading
      a. Novice to intermediate
         i. Upper body: 30–60% 1-RM for 3–6 repetitions
         ii. Lower body: 0–60% 1-RM for 3–6 repetitions
      b. Advanced
         i. Upper body: 30–60% 1-RM for 1–6 repetitions
         ii. Lower body: 0–60% 1-RM for 1–6 repetitions
         iii. Integrate with 85–100% 1-RM for 1–6 repetitions
   3. Volume
      a. Novice to intermediate: 1–3 sets per exercise
      b. Advanced: 3–6 sets per exercise
   4. Frequency
      a. Novice: whole-body training 2–3 days per week
      b. Intermediate: 3 (whole body) or 4 (split routine) days per week
      c. Advanced: whole-body or split routine training 4–5 days per week
   5. Exercise selection:
      a. Multijoint exercises (e.g., jump squats, cleans, medicine ball throws)
      b. For vertical jump and long jump training:
         i. CKC are more effective than OKC resistance exercises
         ii. Plyometric training should be incorporated into routine
   6. Repetition speed: fast/explosive
   7. Rest periods
      a. At least 2–3 min for main exercises
      b. 1–2 min for assistance exercises

G. Plyometric training

   1. Trains the stretch-shortening cycle (SSC) → rapid eccentric contraction followed immediately by a powerful concentric contraction
   2. Developed by Russian and European coaches in the 1960s
   3. Physiologic basis
      a. Mechanical: stored elastic energy in musculotendinous unit
      b. Neurologic: stretch reflex of eccentrically stretched muscle
      c. Rate (not magnitude) of eccentric stretch is key to powerful concentric contraction → effort should be made to minimize ground contact time
   4. Exercise examples (easy → hard)
      a. Lower body
         i. Tuck jumps → hurdle jumps → bounding → depth jumps
      b. Upper body
         i. Medicine ball catch–throw → hand-clap push-up

5. National Strength and Conditioning Association (NSCA) position statement on plyometric exercises
   a. Plyometric training can improve performance in most sports
   b. Plyometric training should include sport-specific exercises
   c. Carefully applied plyometric training programs are no more harmful than other forms of sports activity and may be necessary for safe adaptation to the rigors of explosive sports
   d. Only athletes who have already achieved high levels of strength through standard resistance training should engage in plyometric drills
   e. Athletes weighing over 220 lbs should not depth jump from >18″
   f. Plyometric drills involving a particular muscle/joint complex should not be performed on consecutive days
   g. Plyometric drills should not be performed when an athlete is fatigued
   h. Time for complete recovery should be allowed between plyometric exercise sets
   i. Footwear and landing surfaces used in plyometric drills must have good shock-absorbing qualities
   j. Thorough warm-up should be performed before beginning a plyometric training session
   k. Less demanding drills should be mastered prior to attempting more complex and intense drills.

IV. Speed and Agility Training

A. Definitions
   1. Speed = distance traveled per unit time
   2. Linear speed = ability to move the body in one intended direction as fast as possible
   3. Multidirectional speed (MDS) = ability to produce speed in any direction or body orientation (e.g., forward, backward, lateral, diagonal)
   4. Agility = ability to change direction or body orientation based on rapid processing of internal or external information without significant loss of speed

B. Speed training concepts
   1. Speed and agility training should be done in a rested, nonfatigued state
      a. Beginning of training session
      b. After a rest day
   2. Other than speed technique training, speed drills should be done at high intensity (95–100%)
   3. Allow full recovery between sprint/drill repetitions
   4. Progression of training: technique mastery → speed → speed endurance
   5. Strength training for speed
      a. Untrained: speed may improve by strength training alone
      b. Strength trained: further improvement in speed requires addition of high speed or power training

C. Linear speed
   1. Reaction time
      a. Reaction time and starting technique can be trained with reactive drills
         i. Block starts
         ii. Sport-specific drills with a whistle or visual cue
   2. Acceleration = phase from static start to top speed
      a. Important component in short sprints (64% of 100 m sprint)
      b. Common methods of training acceleration
         i. Short sprints (e.g., 10–30 m)
         ii. Resisted sprints (e.g., uphill sprints, sled push/pull, bungee cord resisted)
         iii. Resistance training (e.g., power cleans, squats)

3. Top speed = stride length times stride rate
   a. Stride length and rate are interdependent → optimize combination
   b. Stride length = distance covered with each stride
      i. Largely depends on height and leg length
      ii. Optimal stride length is 2.3–2.5 times leg length
      iii. Overstriding creates deceleration force and may lead to injury
      iv. Directly related to force applied into the ground
      v. Resisted sprints improve stride length by increasing drive phase force production
         (A) Light resistance (<10% body weight) → maximizes sprint specificity by better replicating joint velocities
   c. Stride rate = amount of time needed to complete a stride cycle
      i. Most important determinant of maximum speed
      ii. Limited by stride length
      iii. Elite sprinters commonly run five strides per second
      iv. Overspeed drills effective for improving stride rate
         (A) Downhill running (5–6% grade)
         (B) Bungee cord-assisted sprints
4. Speed endurance = ability to maintain speed for a sustained period of time
   a. Strongly linked to athlete's conditioning of anaerobic and phosphocreatine metabolic systems
   b. Important in 100 m or longer sprints
   c. Common speed endurance training methods
      i. Sprint intervals
         (A) Choose distance (e.g., 100 m), then alternate sprinting and jogging that distance for specified time or repetitions
      ii. Repetition relays
         (A) Athletes run legs of a relay (e.g., 4 × 100 m) around a track for specified time or repetitions

D. Agility and MDS
   1. Key skills in athleticism
   2. Gambetta in 2006 described seven components of agility
      a. Body control and awareness
      b. Recognition and reaction time
      c. Starting and first step
      d. Acceleration
      e. Footwork
      f. Change of direction
      g. Stopping
   3. Agility/MDS training often resembles sporting activity
   4. Progression of training
      a. Beginner: master movement patterns
         i. Acceleration
         ii. Deceleration
         iii. Direction change
      b. Intermediate: develop speed of movement in above patterns
         i. Planned drills = predictable; athlete knows drill path (e.g., cone drills)
      c. Advanced: reactive drills
         i. Unpredictable environment simulating sport
         ii. Response to sound or visual cue (e.g., push-up sprints on whistle or ball movement)

E. ACSM recommendations for speed and agility training
   1. Sprinting, plyometric training, and explosive resistance training should be used in combination to maximize speed potential

    2. Agility-specific drills are most beneficial for enhancing agility performance
    3. While increasing maximal (absolute) strength is not highly related to reducing sprint times, increasing relative (to bodyweight) strength is highly correlated to speed and acceleration.

V. Endurance Training

  A. Definitions
    1. Endurance = ability to withstand prolonged physical stress
    2. Cardiorespiratory endurance = ability to perform prolonged, large-muscle, dynamic exercise at moderate to high levels of intensity
    3. Muscular endurance = ability to perform prolonged, repetitive, or sustained muscular contractions against resistance

  B. Endurance factors
    1. VO_{2max} = maximum oxygen uptake
      a. Indicator of aerobic capacity (potential)
      b. Limiting factors
        i. Cardiopulmonary transport of oxygen
        ii. Cellular utilization of oxygen
      c. May increase 10–30% in untrained individuals
      d. Upper limit can be reached within 8–18 months of training
    2. Lactate threshold = exercise intensity at which lactate production exceeds utilization; thus lactate begins to accumulate in the bloodstream
      a. Strong predictor of endurance performance
      b. Expressed as % of VO_{2max}
    3. Exercise economy
      a. Efficient technique requires less oxygen consumption
      b. Influences running speed at which lactate threshold and VO_{2max} occurs
    4. Substrate utilization
      a. With training, greater % of fat used at a given work rate → spares glycogen so higher intensity can be maintained for longer duration
    5. Muscle fiber composition
      a. Type 1 (slow twitch) fibers have more mitochondria and higher oxidative enzyme capacity, but endurance training to improve the oxidative capacity of both type 1 and type 2 fibers

  C. Cardiorespiratory endurance programming variables
    1. Mode = type of exercise
      a. Should be sport-specific for athletes
      b. Cross-training may decrease risk of overuse injury
    2. Intensity = expressed as a percentage of items a–d below:
      a. Maximum heart rate (HR_{max}) = 220 − age
      b. Heart rate reserve (HRR) = HR_{max} − HR_{rest}
      c. Maximum oxygen consumption (VO_{2max})
      d. Oxygen consumption reserve (VO_2R) = VO_{2max} − $VO_{2resting}$
      e. Rate of perceived exertion (RPE) = Borg scale
        i. 15 point scale ranging from 6 (no exertion) to 20 (maximal exertion)
        ii. RPE × 10 = heart rate (estimate)
        iii. Table 9.1 below equates intensity, RPE, HR_{max}, HRR, METs, and VO_2R
      f. MET = ratio of the rate of energy expended during an activity to the rate of energy expended at rest
    3. Duration = time performing exercise
      a. Continuous training
        i. High volume training (long, slow distance)

Table 9.1   Equating Exercise Intensity, RPE, %HRR, %VO$_2$R, HR$_{max}$, and METS

Intensity	RPE	%HRR or %VO$_2$R	HR$_{max}$	METS 20–39 y/o	40–64 y/o
Very light	<10	<20	<35	<2.4	<2.0
Light	10–11	20–39	35–54	2.4–4.7	2.0–3.9
Moderate	12–13	40–59	55–69	4.8–7.1	4.0–5.9
Hard	14–16	60–84	70–89	7.2–10.1	6.0–8.4
Very hard	17–19	85–99	90–99	10.2–11.9	8.5–9.9
Maximal	20	100	100	≥12	≥10

Adapted from Pollock ML, Gaesser GA, Butcher JD, Després JP, Dishman RK, Franklin BA, Garber CE. American College of Sports Medicine position stand: The recommended quantity and quality of exercise for developing and maintaining cardiorespiratory and muscular fitness, and flexibility in healthy adults. *Med Sci Sports Exerc.* 1998;30(6),975–991.

    (A) Low intensity (below lactate threshold)
    (B) Long distance, time
    (C) Gradually increase 10–20% per week
  ii. Maximal steady-state training (tempo runs)
    (A) Target intensity is lactate threshold
    (B) Estimate intensity with heart rate
      (1) Trained = 80–90% HR$_{max}$
      (2) Untrained = 50–60% HR$_{max}$
    (C) Estimate intensity with RPE = 13–15
    (D) Should make up no more than 10% weekly volume
  b. Interval training
    i. Alternating work/rest periods
    ii. High intensity (above lactate threshold)
    iii. Short duration
      (A) One example = Tabata method: 8 sets with work:rest = 20:10 s
      (B) Tabata et al. compared the above program to 1 hr/day or continuous exercise at 70% VO$_{2max}$
      (C) After 6 weeks of 5 days/week training, both groups had similar increases in VO$_{2max}$, but Tabata interval group also had 28% improvement in anaerobic capacity
  4. Frequency = number of training sessions per week
    a. 2 days per week is minimum for VO$_{2max}$ improvements
    b. >5 days not significantly better and much higher injury rate
D. ACSM recommendations for cardiorespiratory endurance
  1. Mode: any exercise that requires the continuous, rhythmic use of large muscle groups, such as walking, running, cycling, swimming, etc.
    a. Different modes have similar cardiorespiratory adaptations
    b. Recreational athletes should prioritize activities that are enjoyable and pose minimal risk
    c. Athletes should consider sport specificity, and training time should prioritize exercise modes that simulate the demands of their sport
    d. While circuit training has been shown to improve VO$_{2max}$ (6%), resistance training should not be utilized as the primary form of exercise when the goal is to improve cardiorespiratory fitness

2. Intensity
   a. For most adults:
      i. 65–90% of HR_{max}
      ii. 50–85% of VO_2R or HRR_{max}
   b. For severely unfit:
      i. 55–65% of HR_{max}
      ii. 40–49% of VO_2R
   c. Athletes may benefit from higher-intensity exercise, but these have higher cardiovascular and musculoskeletal risk and have been associated with poor adherence in the general population
3. Duration
   a. 20–60 min of continuous or intermittent (10 + min bouts) aerobic activity
   b. Short-duration, high-intensity exercise will result in a similar training effect as an isocaloric long-duration, low-intensity activity
4. Frequency: 3–5 days per week

E. ACSM recommendations for muscular endurance training
1. Muscular endurance = ability to perform repetitive or sustained muscular contractions against some resistance for an extended period of time
2. Loading/intensity
   a. Novice to intermediate: light loads for 10–15 repetitions
   b. Advanced: various loads for 10–25 + repetitions
3. Volume: multiple sets; progressing to higher volume over time
4. Frequency
   a. Novice: whole-body training 2–3 days per week
   b. Intermediate: 3 (whole body) or 4 (split routine) days per week
   c. Advanced: split routine training 4–6 days per week
5. Exercise selection
   a. Multi- and single-joint exercises
   b. Free weights and machines
6. Repetition speed
   a. Intentionally slow speed for moderate (10–15) repetition sets
   b. Moderate to fast speed for higher (15–25+) repetition sets
7. Rest periods
   a. 0–1 min for moderate (10–15) repetition sets
   b. 1–2 min for high (15–20+) repetition sets
   c. Circuit training: duration it takes to move from one station to the next.

VI. Altitude Training

A. Altitude training = hypoxic training = exercising in, living in, or otherwise breathing reduced-oxygen air for the purpose of improved athletic performance
B. Physiology of altitude training
1. Increased VO_{2max} correlated with increased serum erythropoietin (EPO)
   a. Increased erythrocyte volume (5%)
   b. Increased hemoglobin concentration (5–9%)
2. Serum EPO increase mediated by hypoxia-inducible factor 1α (HIF-1α) on chromosome 14
   a. HIF-1α upregulates EPO mRNA production
   b. EPO gene alleles vary in altitude training response
      i. D7S477 allele → 135% increased serum EPO after 24 hr high-altitude exposure
      ii. Other alleles → only 78% increase in serum EPO
      iii. Results in "responders" and "nonresponders" to altitude exposure
3. Improved mitochondrial efficiency → improved exercise economy (3–10%)

    4. Improved pH regulation and muscle buffer capacity → anaerobic adaptations

    5. Negative effects of altitude training

      a. Decreased cardiac output

      b. Dehydration

      c. Decreased muscle mass

      d. Decreased training intensity and power output

        i. Brosnan et al. showed athletes at 4,000 m elevation only able to exercise at 40% VO_{2max} compared to 80% VO_{2max} at sea level

      e. Longer recovery time from training

      f. May negate ergogenic effects of altitude training

C. Approaches to altitude training

    1. Live and train at high altitude (LHTH)

      a. Acclimatization phase: no high-intensity exercise first (7–10 days)

      b. Primary training phase: progressive intensity and volume (2–3 weeks)

      c. Peak performance generally 2–3 weeks after return to sea level

      d. Studies have shown increased VO_{2max} (~5%) but generally have not supported improved performance with LHTH

    2. Live at high altitude and train at low altitude (LHTL)

      a. Consistently most beneficial in studies

        i. Maintains sea-level training intensity

        ii. Minimizes detrimental effects of chronic hypoxia

      b. Peak performance generally 7–10 days after return to sea level

      c. Studies have shown increased VO_{2max} (~5%) and improved performance (1–1.5%)

    3. Artificial LHTL = intermittent hypoxic exposure during rest

      a. Artificial hypoxia exposure seconds to hours repeated over days to weeks

      b. Attempt to simulate LHTL when geographically not feasible

      c. Studies have been equivocal for performance effects

    4. Live at low altitude and train at high altitude (LLTH) = intermittent hypoxic training

      a. Artificial hypoxia during training only

      b. Attempt to minimize detrimental effects of chronic hypoxia

      c. Studies have been equivocal for performance effects

D. Optimal altitude

    1. Related to hypoxia exposure time

    2. ≥22 h per day: 2,000–2,500 m

    3. 12–16 h per day: 2,500–3,000 m

    4. >3,000 m: no additional benefits and increases overtraining risk

    5. <2,000 m: inadequate stimulus for physiologic adaptations

    6. Minimum 12 h per day required for physiologic adaptations

E. Optimal duration of altitude training

    1. Minimum 2 weeks to detect erythropoietic response

    2. 4 weeks for significant erythropoietic response.

VII. Flexibility Training

A. Flexibility = range of motion (ROM) of a joint or series of joints

    1. Stretching increases musculotendinous length by:

      a. Mechanoreceptor-mediated reflex inhibition

      b. Elastic (transient) and plastic (permanent) properties of musculotendinous unit that allow lengthening

      c. Possibly through addition of sarcomeres

B. Flexibility factors

    1. Gender: women are typically more flexible than men

2. Age: flexibility tends to decrease with age

3. Temperature: flexibility increases with heat and decreases with cold

4. Activity level: flexibility decreases with inactivity

5. Joint specific: flexibility may vary between joints

C. Flexibility programming variables

    1. Mode

        a. Static stretching

            i. Holds the muscle in a lengthened position

            ii. Avoids activation of stretch reflex

        b. Proprioceptive neuromuscular facilitation (PNF)

            i. Static stretching after isometric activation of stretched muscle

                (A) Stimulates Golgi tendon organs → reflexive muscle relaxation

            ii. May incorporate isometric activation of antagonist (stretched muscle) then agonist muscles (e.g., hamstring activation → quadriceps activation → hamstring stretch)

                (A) Contraction of agonist inhibits contraction of antagonist

            iii. Sequentially increased range with each repetition

            iv. More effective than static stretching alone

            v. May require assistance to perform properly

        c. Dynamic stretching

            i. Gently using momentum to propel body part in a controlled manner through full range of motion

            ii. Acutely improves muscle stiffness

        d. Ballistic stretching

            i. Similar to dynamic stretching, but uses rapid, repetitive, bouncing movements to exceed range of motion

            ii. Counterproductively activates the muscle spindles and stretch reflex

            iii. Associated with injury from overstretching muscle

            iv. May induce muscle soreness

D. ACSM recommendations for flexibility training

    1. Mode

        a. All major muscle groups should be stretched

        b. Include static and/or dynamic stretching techniques

        c. PNF is more effective than static stretching for improving flexibility

    2. Intensity: muscle stretched to point of mild discomfort

    3. Duration

        a. Static stretching: 10–30 s for 2–4 repetitions

        b. PNF: 3–6 s isometric activation (agonist or antagonist) followed by a 10–30 s static stretch for 3–5 repetitions

    4. Frequency

        a. Minimum: 2–3 days per week

        b. Ideal: 5–7 days per week

E. Warm-up

    1. Raises body temperature in preparation for vigorous exercise

        a. Warm muscles contract more forcefully and relax more quickly

        b. Warm blood facilitates transfer of oxygen to muscles

        c. Warm tendons and ligaments are less viscous

    2. Warm-up (to point of perspiration) should be done prior to flexibility training

    3. Methods

        a. Passive

            i. External heat (e.g., hot shower, heating pad, massage)

            ii. Usually do not achieve adequate temperatures

    b. Active

      i. Low- to moderate-intensity rhythmic movements of large muscle groups (e.g., jogging, cycling, jumping rope)

      ii. More effective than passive warm-up methods

    c. Specific

      i. Involve movements that are part of sport activity

      ii. Added advantage of technique rehearsal

      iii. Easily transitioned into dynamic stretching

F. Stretching and performance

  1. Growing evidence that preactivity static stretching acutely inhibits:

    a. Maximal force or torque production

    b. Running speed

    c. Vertical jump

    d. Muscle endurance

  2. However, regular static stretching (not preactivity) improves all of the above

  3. Some studies suggest that preactivity dynamic stretching acutely improves all of the above

G. Stretching and muscle soreness

  1. Stretching (pre- or postexercise) does not reduce delayed onset muscle soreness

H. Stretching and injury prevention

  1. Preactivity stretching does not appear to acutely reduce injury risk.

VIII. Overtraining

A. Overtraining is a syndrome characterized by a decline in performance that occurs when stress (training and nontraining) chronically exceeds recovery capacity

  1. Overreaching = early stages of overtraining

    a. Increased volume and/or intensity → fatigue and performance decline

    b. Easily reversible with 1–2 weeks relative rest → subsequent large improvement in performance (supercompensation)

    c. Often used by intermediate to advanced athletes as part of periodized training plan

  2. If excessive training continues, performance will continue to drop

    a. Frequently interpreted as sign of undertraining → intensity/volume further increased → further performance decrement with chronic fatigue

    b. Recovery may require 6+ months of rest

B. Overtraining factors

  1. Excess training stress (e.g., intensity, volume)

  2. Emotional stress (e.g., occupational, educational, family, social)

  3. Inadequate recovery (e.g., nutrition, sleep, alcohol)

    a. Inadequate dietary protein → muscles catabolized for amino acids

C. Autonomic dysfunction

  1. Sympathetic (early overtraining)

    a. Elevated resting heart rate and blood pressure, sleep disturbance, irritability, and weight loss

    b. Due to down-regulation of β-adrenergic receptors

    c. Catecholamines released during both rest and exercise to overcome poor receptor sensitivity

  2. Parasympathetic (late overtraining)

    a. Decreased resting and exercising heart rate

    b. Decreased resting blood pressure, blood glucose, and exercise-induced lactate accumulation

    c. Urinary catecholamines reduced 50–70%

D. Neuroendocrine dysfunction
1. Disturbance of both hypothalamic–pituitary–adrenal and hypothalamic–pituitary–gonadal axes
2. Decreased free testosterone to cortisol ratio of 30% or more (or absolute value of $<0.35 \times 10^{-3}$) suggests catabolism due to insufficient recovery (acutely) or overtraining (chronically)
   a. Not sensitive, so cannot be used as a sole measure of overtraining
3. Overtrained endurance athletes have blunted release of ACTH, growth hormone, and prolactin in response to insulin-induced hypoglycemia
4. Growth hormone and luteinizing hormone concentrations reduced
5. Menstrual and reproductive abnormalities in female athletes
6. Decreased sperm counts and libido in male athletes

E. Mood disturbance
1. Profile of mood states (POMS) = self-reported test of athlete's mood
   a. Normal athlete = "iceberg profile"
      i. Low tension, anxiety, anger, confusion, and fatigue scores
      ii. High vigor score
   b. Overtrained athlete
      i. High tension, anxiety, anger, confusion, and fatigue scores
      ii. Low vigor score
      iii. Less self-confidence in athletic ability

F. Immune deficiency
1. Reduced leukocytes, lymphocytes, neutrophil activity, and immunoglobulin concentrations
2. Increased susceptibility to upper respiratory infections

G. Biochemical alterations
1. Increased creatine kinase and uric acid levels
2. Decreased glycogen, glutamine, and lactate levels
3. These findings may be present acutely in normal athletes following a high-intensity training period → adequate rest required prior to using these studies as indicators of overtraining

H. Performance decrement
1. Careful monitoring of performance can assist in early identification of overtrained (or overreaching) athlete
2. Use sport-specific performance tests relevant to athlete's sport

I. Medical evaluation of overtraining
1. Look for other etiologies of declining performance, mood, and energy level
   a. Pulmonary (e.g., exercise-induced bronchospasm)
   b. Cardiac (e.g., cardiomyopathy)
   c. Endocrine (e.g., hypothyroidism, adrenal insufficiency)
   d. Hematologic (e.g., iron deficiency anemia)
   e. Infectious (e.g., mononucleosis, Epstein–Barr, Lyme)
   f. Malignancy (e.g., leukemia)
   g. Nutritional (e.g., bulimia nervosa, magnesium deficiency)
   h. Toxic exposure (e.g., anticholinergic medications)
   i. Neuromuscular (e.g., myopathy)
   j. Psychological (e.g., depression, substance abuse)
   k. Pregnancy

J. Treatment of overtraining
1. Key treatment is REST

    2. Since early identification is difficult, prevention is best treatment
      a. Structured (periodized) training program
      b. Regular monitoring of performance parameters
    3. If athlete begins to exhibit signs of overtraining:
      a. Several days of rest should be instituted immediately
      b. Training error should be identified and addressed
      c. Athlete should resume training at slightly decreased level
    4. If athlete develops overtraining syndrome:
      a. Prolonged period of rest from training/competition (often 6+ months)
      b. Consider prescribing counseling to assist in identifying and treating the psychological aspects of overtraining
      c. If concomitant psychological disorder identified, this should be addressed by a sports psychologist with or without an antidepressant medication.

Recommended Reading

1. Baechle TR, Earle RW. *Essentials of Strength Training and Conditioning*. 3rd ed. Champaign, IL: Human Kinetics; 2008.
2. Bompa TO, Haff GG. *Periodization: Theory and Methodology of Training*. 5th ed. Champaign, IL: Human Kinetics; 2009.
3. Bonetti DL, Hopkins WG. Sea-level exercise performance following adaptation to hypoxia: A meta-analysis. *Sports Med*. 2009;39(2):107–127.
4. Gambetta V. *Athletic Development: The Art & Science of Functional Sports Conditioning*. Champaign, IL: Human Kinetics; 2006.
5. Garber CE, Blissmer B, Deschenes MR, et al. American College of Sports Medicine position stand: Quantity and Quality of Exercise for Developing and Maintaining Cardiorespiratory, Musculoskeletal, and Neuromotor Fitness in Apparently Healthy Adults- Guidance for Prescribing Exercise - MSSE 2011. *Med Sci Sports Exerc*. 2011;43(7):1334–1359.
6. Herring SA, Bergfeld JA, Boyd JL, et al. The team physician and conditioning of athletes for sports: A consensus statement. *Med Sci Sports Exerc*. 2007;39(11):2058–2068.
7. Hoffman J. Anaerobic conditioning and the development of speed and agility. In: J Hoffman. ed. *Physiological Aspects of Sport Training and Performance*. Champaign, IL: Human Kinetics; 2002:93–108.
8. Hoffman J. Overtraining. In: Hoffman J, ed. *Physiological Aspects of Sport Training and Performance*. Champaign, IL: Human Kinetics; 2002:261–272.
9. Millet GP, Roels B, Schmitt L, Woorons X, Richalet JP. Combining hypoxic methods for peak performance. *Sports Med*. 2010;40(1):1–25.
10. Purvis D, Gonsalves S, Deuster PA. Physiological and psychological fatigue in extreme conditions: Overtraining and elite athletes. *PM&R*. 2010;2(5):442–450.
11. Ratamess NA, Alvar BA, Evetoch TK, et al.. American college of sports medicine position stand: Progression models in resistance training for healthy adults. *Med Sci Sports Exerc*. 2009;41(3):687–708.
12. Shrier I. Does stretching improve performance? A systematic and critical review of the literature. *Clin J Sport Med*. 2004;14(5):267–273.
13. Tabata I, Nishimura K, Kouzaki M, et al. Effects of moderate-intensity endurance and high-intensity intermittent training on anaerobic capacity and VO_{2max}. *Med Sci Sports Exerc*. 1996;28(10):1327–1330.
14. Winchester JB, Nelson AG, Landin D, Young MA, Schexnayder IC. Static stretching impairs sprint performance in collegiate track and field athletes. *J Strength Cond Res*. 2008;22(1):13–19.
15. Zatsiorsky VM, Kraemer WJ. *The Science and Practice of Strength Training*. 2nd ed. Champaign, IL: Human Kinetics, 2006.

10

Nutrition

Susan M. Kleiner, Abbie E. Smith and
Cassandra Forsythe-Pribanic

I. General Principles of Nutrition

A. Sports nutrition paradigm for mind and body performance:
   1. Eat more → gain energy → train hard → build muscle → burn fat

B. Hydration
   1. Greatest impact on training, performance, and recovery

C. Energy consumption/metabolism/weight control
   1. Set goals for a balance between performance enhancement and body composition/body weight maintenance

D. Carbohydrates, protein, and high-performance fats
   1. Timing and combining
   2. Recovery nutrition
      a. Pre-, during, and postexercise

E. Vitamins/minerals/antioxidants/anti-inflammatory compounds
   1. Whole, unrefined foods
   2. Variety among and within food groups
   3. Vegetables, fruits, fish, plant fats, whole grains, nuts, seeds, dairy, animal and plant proteins

F. Supplements
   1. Important for dietary support and convenience.

II. Fluid Replacement

A. Overview
   1. Five to ten percent of total body water is turned over daily through obligatory losses (respiratory, urine, and sweat)
   2. The Institute of Medicine (IOM) recommends in general that men aged 19 to 70+ consume 3.7 L/day and women aged 19 to 70+ ingest 2.7 L/day of total fluids
   3. Physically active adults in warmer climates have daily water needs of 6 L with highly active populations needing even more to remain euhydrated
   4. Elite marathoners tend to sweat at a rate of 2 L/h

B. Dehydration
   1. A 1% or greater loss of body weight due to fluid losses
   2. Severe dehydration: 3% or greater losses of body weight in fluid

Table 10.1 Symptoms of Dehydration

Early Signs	Severe Signs
Fatigue	Difficulty swallowing
Loss of appetite	Stumbling
Flushed skin	Clumsiness
Burning in stomach	Shriveled skin
Light-headedness	Sunken eyes and dim vision
Headache	Painful urination
Dry mouth	Numb skin
Dry cough	Muscle spasm
Heat intolerance	Delirium
Dark urine with a strong odor	

3. Adverse effect on muscle strength, endurance, coordination, mental acuity, and thermo-regulatory processes
4. Early and severe signs: Table 10.1
5. Losses as small as 1–2% of body weight stimulate thirst, but the athlete is already dehydrated
6. Greater than 3% loss of total body fluids may require oral rehydration solutions and food for complete rehydration, and may require 18–24 h

C. Fluid replacement
   1. Volume recommendation:
      a. 480–600 cc fluid: 1–2 h preexercise
      b. 300–480 cc fluid: 15 min preexercise
      c. 120–180 cc fluid: every 10–15 min during exercise
      d. In general start fluid intake 24 h prior to exercise event
      e. Continue fluid and food consumption for 24–48 h postevent
   2. Beverage
      a. 6–8% typical glucose–electrolyte solution or a carbohydrate–protein mixture
      b. For exercise lasting less than an hour, water or noncaloric fluid is recommended
      c. Taste acceptance is very important for compliance
   3. Hyperhydration
      a. Beverages that contain >100 mmol/L sodium chloride (NaCl) can temporarily induce hyperhydration, thus aiding in rehydration
      b. Adding glycerol to a typical sports drink at a concentration of 1.0 to 1.5 g/kg/BW can induce hyperhydration
      c. Benefit includes protection against dehydration and enhanced performance in hot environments
      d. Risks include headaches, blurred vision, and GI distress
   4. Hyponatremia (see Chapter 30 for more details)
      a. Risk factors
         i. Overconsumption of hypotonic fluids
         ii. Cooler than predicted environmental conditions
         iii. Slower pace in running events
      b. Prevention
         i. During endurance races, it is safe for slower athletes to drink according to thirst.

III. Carbohydrates

A. Not all carbohydrates in the diet are equally beneficial
1. Carbohydrates from whole, minimally processed plant sources are preferable to processed carbohydrate-rich foods
2. Refined carbohydrates in sports drinks and energy gels may not be more advantageous before, during, or after exercise, than whole food
   a. 1 g/kg carbohydrate from raisins or energy gel given to endurance athletes before a 1-h cycling time trial had similar performance effects but caused less of an insulin response, and generated more free fatty acids, indicating a sparing of muscle glycogen
   b. Simple or easily digested carbohydrates taken 30–60 min before exercise may result in rebound hypoglycemia and decreased performance
      i. Consuming slower-digesting, unrefined carbohydrate along with protein and/or fat is preferable
   c. 1.0–1.5 g carbohydrate/kg/h of rapid-digesting carbohydrates are ideal 1–4 h following exercise
   d. A high-glycemic, very high-molecular-weight starch supplement (e.g., Vitargo S2) following glycogen-depleting exercise appears to stimulate greater glycogen resynthesis and improved performance in a subsequent exercise bout compared to a typical low-molecular-weight sports drink
B. Athletes in events >1 h will benefit from carbohydrate ingestion during activity
1. Most researched is a 6–8% carbohydrate–electrolyte solution consumed every 15 min during prolonged endurance exercise for improved performance
   a. However, carbohydrates taken in solid form during exercise produce similar mean and peak oxidation rates as a liquid or gel source
   b. Sports gels, drinks, and solid foods containing glucose + fructose lead to higher carbohydrate oxidation rates during exercise compared to glucose alone
2. An oral carbohydrate rinse (without ingestion) in a fasted state boosts performance during short-duration (≤1 h), high-intensity endurance events, which may have important implications for those with sensitive gastrointestinal systems
   a. Little to no advantage in a fed state
   b. No benefits noted for maximum strength or strength endurance performance
C. A high-carbohydrate daily diet is typically recommended for athletes because of its role in maintaining adequate muscle glycogen, but it should not be so high that it greatly displaces protein or essential fats
1. Recommend 5–10 g carbohydrate/kg body weight (bw) for anaerobic and aerobic sports, with women and strength athletes consuming near the lower end
   a. During extreme training, intake can be as high as 10–12 g/kg/day
2. Although most athletes tolerate high carbohydrate intakes, some do not respond well and do better with more dietary fats and protein
D. Endurance athletes versus strength athletes
1. Less muscle carbohydrate/glycogen used during strength exercise
2. Long-distance endurance athletes often benefit from carbohydrate intake before, during, and after exercise and overall higher carbohydrate intakes/day
   a. Protein and carbohydrate together promote greater muscle glycogen, protein repair, and synthesis than carbohydrate alone
E. Men versus women
1. Women use less glycogen and more stored fat than men during both endurance and strength exercise
   a. Women have greater muscle protein content of major enzymes involved in long- and medium-chain fatty oxidation
   b. Women do not require as much dietary carbohydrate as men.

Table 10.2   Protein Requirements

Sedentary	0.8 g/kg
Recreationally active	1.0–1.4 g/kg
Resistance trained	1.2–1.8 g/kg
Endurance trained	1.2–1.4 g/kg
High-intensity sprints	1.2–1.8 g/kg
Weight-restricted sports	1.4–2.0 g/kg

IV. Protein

  A. Necessary protein consumption (Table 10.2)
   1. Athletes have increased protein needs
   2. Excessive consumption of protein may lead to mild effects of dehydration
      a. Adequate water consumption can minimize these effects
   3. Individuals with previous liver and/or kidney damage, should refrain from excessive amounts of protein (>2.8 g/kg per day)
  B. Protein quality
   1. High-quality protein
      a. Proteins containing all essential amino acids (EAA) and branched chain amino acids (BCAA) (Table 10.3)
         i. Typically animal proteins, including meats, eggs, and milk
         ii. Soy protein is also categorized as high quality

Table 10.3   Essential, Conditionally Essential, and Nonessential Amino Acids

Essential Amino Acids

Isoleucine[a]	Phenylalanine
Leucine[a]	Threonine
Lysine	Tryptophan
Methionine	Valine[a]

Conditionally Essential Amino Acids

Arginine	Proline
Cysteine (cystine)	Taurine
Glutamine	Tyrosine
Histidine	

Nonessential Amino Acids

Alanine	Glutamic acid
Asparagine	Glycine
Aspartic acid	Serine
Citrulline	

[a]Branched-chain amino acid.

Adapted from Di Pasquale, 2000.

2. Lower-quality proteins
   a. Plant proteins lacking one of the essential amino acids
3. Consumption of high-quality proteins leads to positive nitrogen balance and greater gains in lean body mass and strength compared to plant proteins
   a. BCAA in high-quality proteins directly stimulate muscle protein synthesis

C. Nitrogen balance

1. When amino acid contribution equals excretion rates, this is referred to as nitrogen balance
2. Preventing a negative nitrogen balance in athletes is key
   a. Negative nitrogen periods are stimulated by overtraining and fasting
   b. It reflects muscle protein breakdown and prevents muscle growth
3. A positive nitrogen balance is the ideal environment for building lean body mass and fostering performance gains
   a. Consume optimal amounts of high-quality protein
4. Ideal timing of protein consumption, pre- and postexercise, helps maintain nitrogen balance
   a. Consume at least 20 g of protein (with a mix of carbohydrate) within 30 min postexercise for muscle recovery and gains in strength and lean body mass. This is stimulated by the 3 g of leucine found in roughly 20 g of protein
   b. Recent research suggests integrating protein preexercise carries the same importance as post-workout consumption for gains in lean body mass.

V. Fat

A. Fats from natural, minimally processed sources preferable to manufactured foods
1. Animal and plant fats should be included in a successful athletic diet
2. Land-based animal fats (meats, poultry, dairy) should be balanced with marine-based animal fats (salmon, seafood, krill) and omega-3 essential fatty acid-rich plant oils

B. Diets high in fat and moderate to low in carbohydrate consumed for more than 7 days increase fat oxidation
1. Also lengthens time to exhaustion, but conversely may make physical exercise feel harder, which may depend on the duration of fat adaptation

C. Women athletes benefit from at least 30% of calories as dietary fat to ensure rapid replenishment of stored muscular fat, which is used more readily
1. This is critical for continued performance benefits

D. Beneficial high-performance fats that can help reduce cortisol and inflammatory markers while enhancing recovery include:
1. Oleic acid from olive and canola oils
2. Long-chain omega-3, eicosapentanoic acid (EPA) and docosahexanoic acid (DHA) from marine oils
3. Short-chain omega-3 linoleic acid from flax, walnut, hemp and pumpkin
4. Conjugated linoleic acid (CLA) from dairy products
5. Medium-chain triacylglycerols (MCT) from coconut oil

E. Other athletic benefits of adequate and beneficial dietary fats:
1. Osteoarthritis and tendonitis improvement (reduced inflammation and breakdown of soft tissues)
2. Maintained sex hormone concentrations
3. Bone preservation
4. Resistance to overtraining-induced mental depression
5. Provision of fat-soluble vitamins (A, D, E, K).

VI. Metabolism

A. Energy currency for specific activities
  1. Adenosine triphosphate (ATP)
     a. Immediate energy
  2. Creatine phosphate (CP)
     a. ATP can be regenerated anaerobically by adding a phosphate group back to ADP, most often donated from the degradation of CP
     b. Muscle contains enough CP energy to support a maximal effort activity for 3–15 s
  3. Carbohydrate
     a. The breakdown of carbohydrate to glucose for energy is referred to as glycolysis
        i. ATP derived from glycolysis is enough for activities lasting 30 s to 3 min, and is anaerobic
        ii. Exercise lasting longer than 3 min requires aerobic metabolism in the form of oxidative phosphorylation to resynthesize ATP
        iii. Aerobic metabolism of glucose supplies energy for activities lasting from 3 min to 4 h
     b. Stored sources of glucose, known as glycogen, are the primary source of energy during exercise
        i. Individuals can store a limited amount of glycogen
        ii. With training, one can store more glycogen, and spare glycogen from use due to an enhanced reliance upon fat for fuel
  4. Fat
     a. Has the capability to supply an immense amount of energy
     b. Stored in muscle as triglycerides (TG; glycerol + 3 fatty acids)
        i. Can be a significant source of energy when an athlete consumes adequate fat in the diet for a significant period of time
     c. Disadvantage: slower metabolic energy-producing process
        i. Primary fuel for low-intensity, long-duration events
     d. Athletes can train their bodies to use more fat as fuel than carbohydrate and have similar or better exercise performance
     e. With resistance exercise, significant stores of intramuscular TG are depleted
  5. Protein
     a. Amino acids not used as a major source of energy during exercise
     b. Amino acids can undergo gluconeogenesis
     c. Depending on the intensity and duration of the activity, as well as the nutritional status of the individual, amino acids can contribute up to 6% of the required energy
        i. If an athlete is lacking available carbohydrate (as glycogen) for fuel, the use of amino acids for fuel is elevated
     d. Protein metabolism is particularly important for the repair and recovery of the muscle with exercise

B. Fuel for specific activities
  1. Short sprint activities, lasting 10–12 s, use an equal amount of ATP/CP (50%) and carbohydrate (50%)
  2. Intense events, lasting 4–6 min, rely primarily upon carbohydrate (~94%) and small amounts of ATP/CP (6%)
  3. Moderate events, such as a 10 km run (32–45 min), still use carbohydrate as the primary source of fuel (60%), with the addition of fat (40%)
  4. A marathon event uses ~75% carbohydrate, ~20% fat, and ~5% protein
  5. Longer low-intensity activities (e.g., walking 5–8 h) use fat as the primary fuel source (65%) and carbohydrate at ~35%.

VII. Vitamins/Minerals—Micronutrients

A. Regular exercise may cause greater needs due to increased losses and turnover
   1. Poor nutritional status and low energy intake may cause chronic insufficiency

B. Vitamins and minerals as antioxidants that prevent oxidative damage
   1. Minimizes production of free radicals that can accelerate recovery, reduce inflammation, and improve immune function

C. B vitamins
   1. Thiamin, riboflavin, vitamin B6, niacin, pantothenic acid, and biotin
   2. Act as cofactors in the metabolism of fats, proteins, and carbohydrates
      a. As energy needs and intake increase with exercise, the need for additional consumption of specific B vitamins may also increase
   3. Thiamin (B1)
      a. Acts as a coenzyme for the metabolism of carbohydrates
         i. Catalyzes the conversion of pyruvate to acetyl-CoA to enter into the tricarboxylic acid cycle (TCA)
      b. Is heavily involved in the metabolism of lipids and BCAA
      c. Current (1998) recommendations are as follows:
         i. Men: 1.2 mg/day; women: 1.0 mg/day
         ii. If greater carbohydrate and protein consumption, needs may increase
   4. Riboflavin (B2)
      a. Essential for the synthesis of the coenzymes: flavin mononucleotide (FMN) and flavin adenine dinucleotide (FAD), which are important for the metabolism of glucose, fatty acids, glycerol, and amino acids
      b. Involved in the conversion of B6 and folate to their active forms
      c. Current recommendations:
         i. Men: 1.3 mg/day; women: 1.1 mg/day
      d. Active individuals may need additional consumption of B2 above the current recommended dietary allowance (RDA)
   5. Pyridoxine (B6)
      a. Directly linked to energy production during exercise:
         i. Used for transamination of amino acids, the liberation of glucose from glycogen, as well as gluconeogenic processes
      b. Current recommendations are 1.3 mg/day for both men and women
         i. Recent evidence suggests this recommendation is too low, and higher amounts may be necessary
   6. Niacin (B3; nicotinic acid)
      a. Serves as the precursor for nicotinamide adenine dinucleotide (NAD) and NAD phosphate (NADP)
         i. Coenzymes that drive energy production through glycolysis, TCA cycle, and the electron transport chain
         ii. Also an influence on β-oxidation and amino acid synthesis
      b. Can be consumed through the diet or made endogenously with adequate amounts of tryptophan (an essential amino acid)
      c. Recommendations are reported in niacin equivalents (NE)
         i. 16 NE/day for men; 14 NE/day for women
   7. Pantothenic acid
      a. Involved in various metabolic processes
         i. Plays a role in gluconeogenesis
         ii. Synthesis of steroid hormones, acetyl choline, fatty acids, amino acids, and membrane phospholipids
         iii. Protein degradation
      b. No RDA set due to adequate consumption through food

8. Biotin
 a. Metabolic roles:
  i. Gluconeogenesis and fatty acid synthesis
  ii. Degradation of glucose and amino acids are influenced by biotin availability
 b. No published RDA, due to its wide distribution in food

D. Miscellaneous vitamins and minerals in sport
 1. Vitamin E
  a. Comprised of active antioxidant compounds
   i. Alpha-tocopherol and tocotrienols
  b. One of the most biologically active antioxidants, and plays a strong role in minimizing lipid peroxidation
   i. In turn, this helps stabilize the cell membrane and protect cellular structures from oxidative damage
  c. Deficiencies are rare; however, vitamin E requirements may be higher for active individuals
   i. A diet consisting of 25–35% fat should be adequate to maintain vitamin E levels. Lower-fat diets may be deficient
   ii. High doses (>400 IU/day) have been linked to adverse effects
 2. Vitamin C (ascorbic acid)
  a. Functions in exercise and an important antioxidant
   i. Influences collagen synthesis
   ii. Has a strong potential influence in maintaining the immune system under conditions of high stress (excessive training)
    (A) Reduces symptoms of upper respiratory infections
   iii. Influences amino acid metabolism
   iv. Enhances iron absorption
 3. Beta-carotene and vitamin A
  a. Beta-carotene is a precursor to vitamin A
  b. Both have strong antioxidant potential
   i. Primary influence is maintaining lipid integrity, by reducing lipid peroxidation
  c. High doses of vitamin A, via supplementation, may be toxic
  d. Consuming high doses of beta-carotene have not been reported to yield adverse effects
  e. RDA levels for beta-carotene are 3–6 mg/day
   i. Minimal research to suggest active individuals need enhanced amounts
 4. Vitamin D
  a. New data has linked vitamin D to several physiological roles
  b. Vitamin D_3 activates receptors within the skeletal muscle, stimulating contraction
  c. Sufficient amounts are related to an increase in size and number of fast-twitch muscle fibers
  d. Recent evidence suggests most individuals are vitamin D deficient
  e. There is a greater risk for deficiency in individuals that experience all four seasons due to lack of sun exposure
  f. Athletes that train indoors, live at higher latitudes, wear sunscreen, and have darker skin are at a greater risk for deficiency
  g. The vitamin D intake recommendations are 600 IU daily
   i. Recent evidence promotes the intake of higher levels: 1,000–2,000 IU, especially in active individuals
 5. Iron
  a. Primary function is to transport oxygen in red blood cells
  b. Also plays a role in exercise energy metabolism
  c. Exercise increases the need for iron consumption

    d. Current recommendations: 18 mg/day for premenopausal women and 8 mg/day for men, postmenopausal women and sedentary individuals

    e. Highly active individuals, especially female athletes, endurance runners, and vegetarian athletes are at risk for iron deficiencies.

VIII. Supplements

  A. The following are the few that are strongly supported by human data:

    1. Beta-alanine (BA)

      a. A naturally occurring, nonessential amino acid that is typically found in a carnivorous diet (i.e., chicken and turkey)

      b. Beta-alanine is the rate-limiting substrate necessary for the synthesis of a dipeptide protein called carnosine

      c. Supplementing with 4–6 g per day of BA for four weeks increases muscle carnosine concentration by 64%

      d. Muscle carnosine acts as a physiochemical hydrogen ion buffer, delaying the drop in pH associated with anaerobic metabolism

      e. BA supplementation alone has been shown to enhance performance by:

        i. Improving times to exhaustion during cycling and running

        ii. Delaying neuromuscular fatigue

        iii. Increasing ventilatory threshold

    2. β-Hydroxy-β-methylbutyrate (HMB)

      a. HMB is a metabolite of the essential amino acid leucine

      b. Chronic supplementation with HMB has demonstrated anticatabolic characteristics

      c. Consumption of 3 g HMB daily has consistently demonstrated a reduction in protein catabolism when combined with a resistance training program

      d. These results are most consistent in untrained individuals

      e. Supplementation in resistance-trained individuals has shown no improvements in protein synthesis, maximal strength, or body composition

      f. Positive influences on lean body mass for older athletes

    3. Caffeine

      a. Caffeine stimulates the central nervous system and augments metabolism

      b. Multiple research studies demonstrate reduced feelings of exertion during exercise following caffeine intake

      c. Supplementation prior to exercise has been shown to increase fat oxidation and spare muscle glycogen

      d. Can improve time to exhaustion and recovery time

      e. Primarily for improving aerobic performance

      f. No evidence to directly improve anaerobic/strength performance

      g. Indirectly, ingestion of caffeine prior to any type of exercise may be beneficial

      h. Most common effective dosing recommendation is to supplement with 3–6 mg per kg (1.4–2.7 mg/lb bw) 30–60 min preexercise

    4. Creatine (Cr)

      a. Small amounts of creatine are synthesized endogenously in the liver, pancreas, and the kidneys from the amino acids arginine, methionine, and glycine

      b. Also obtained from high-quality protein, such as fish and beef

      c. Over 500 studies have demonstrated an increase in intramuscular Cr with supplementation

      d. Cr supplementation of 20 g (4 × 5 g) daily for 5 days significantly increase muscle phosphocreatine (PCr) levels

      e. Increasing the initial amount of PCr can provide a greater source of immediate energy for exercise and enhance the rate of PCr regeneration

     f. Demonstrated to increase muscle cross-sectional area (Type I, IIA, IIB) and augment myosin heavy-chain expression

     g. Ergogenic effects lead to increases in muscle growth and strength and improvements in lean body mass, as a result of an increase in training volume

     h. There is no scientific evidence of detrimental short- or long-term effects of Cr supplementation

     i. Some research has noted an increase in body weight for men only, following a loading dose (5 days of supplementation), but this is not equivocal across studies, with some demonstrating no change in weight

     j. The quickest method to increase muscle Cr stores is to consume 0.3 g per kg of body weight per day of Cr monohydrate for at least three days followed by 3–5 g per day thereafter

     k. Ingesting a lower dose of Cr monohydrate (e.g., 2–3 g per day) will increase muscle Cr stores over a 3–4-week period

5. Whey protein

     a. Is a rich source of high-quality protein and the branched-chain amino acid, leucine, which has been shown to optimally stimulate protein synthesis

     b. Ideal for pre- and post-workout recovery, along with carbohydrate

     c. As a powdered protein supplement, is useful to help athletes incorporate inexpensive, high-quality protein into more daily meals

     d. Convenient and very palatable

6. Essential amino acids (EAAs)

     a. Research has demonstrated that consuming EAAs pre- and postexercise augments amino acid uptake and availability for protein synthesis

     b. Combining EAAs with carbohydrates before exercise has consistently demonstrated anticatabolic effects, attenuating myofibrillar protein degradation

     c. There may be a threshold of 20 g EAA intake, above which greater doses may not further improve protein synthesis

     d. To enhance the effects of training and to improve recovery, 3–20 g/day is recommended 30 min prior to exercise and within 1 h postexercise

     e. These effects can be augmented when consumed with a 6% carbohydrate solution.

IX. Weight Management

A. It is important for athletes to decide whether performance or a specific body composition is more important

     1. Athletes can beneficially change their body composition while maintaining excellent performance, but dietary factors are key

     2. Poor dietary choices of either inadequate or excessive energy intake along with less-than-ideal macronutrient composition will hinder these goals

B. Weight and fat loss

     1. The prevalence of overweight and obesity has increased substantially in the general population, and athletes are not immune to this phenomenon

     2. A society of excessive calories and processed foods has contributed to these issues

     3. Large energy-deficit diets often will impair athletic performance

     4. Athletes who struggle with excess, unhealthy body fat, should first examine their diet and remove manufactured food products and replace them with unprocessed whole foods like meats, fish, dairy (low-sugar, moderate-fat), eggs, vegetables, fruits, whole grains, legumes, nuts, seeds, and plant oils

          a. A higher-protein, moderate-fat, lower-carbohydrate diet compared to typical athlete diets is shown to enhance fat and weight loss

               i. Athletes who have kidney dysfunction should avoid excessive protein and instead reduce simple carbohydrates and incorporate plenty of beneficial, high-performance fats

5. If calorie-counting and estimations of energy expenditure are desired, two equations have been shown to have good accuracy with indirect calorimetry for calculation resting metabolic rate (RMR):

    a. Mifflin–St Jeor equation

        i. For men: RMR (kcal/day) = 10 (wt in kg) + 6.25 (ht in cm) − 5 (age in years) + 5

        ii. For women: RMR (kcal/day) = 10 (wt in kg) + 6.25 (ht in cm) − 5 (age in years) − 161

    b. Owen equation

        i. For men: RMR (kcal/day) = 879 + 10.2 (wt in kg)

        ii. For women: RMR (kcal/day) = 795 + 7.2 (wt in kg)

    c. To this RMR, activity factors must be multiplied to calculate total energy expenditure:

        i. 1.3 for very light; 1.5 for light; 1.6 for moderate; 1.9 for heavy

6. For very active athletes, can also multiply current body weight by 14–16 to determine calorie intake necessary for weight loss

    a. For moderately active exercisers, multiply body weight by 12–14

C. Weight gain

  1. Athletes looking to gain muscle mass and body weight must first ensure they are eating plenty of quality food

    a. Their total energy intake must exceed their energy output

    b. They must ensure they are eating regularly at all hours of the day and avoid fasted exercise or prolonged periods (greater than 4 h) between feedings

    c. To facilitate enough calories, liquid meals may be necessary, such as whey protein smoothies with fruits, nut butters, and/or yogurt

    d. Some simple carbohydrates, such as sugar-containing meal replacements and powdered protein supplements may be necessary to help athletes ingest enough energy at regular hours or at inconvenient times

    e. If athletes have a hard time gaining body weight and muscle, and have significant gastrointestinal distress that hinders food intake or impairs nutrient absorption, rule out food allergies or intolerances

        i. Common issues: gluten, wheat, lactose, and milk proteins.

Recommended Reading

1. Antonio J, Kalman DS, Stout JR, et al. *Essentials of Sports Nutrition and Supplements.* New Jersey: Humana Press; 2008.

2. Brooks GA, Fahey TD, Baldwin KM. *Exercise Physiology: Human Bioenergetics and Its Applications.* 4th ed. New York, NY: McGraw Hill; 2005:31–41;59–92.

3. Driskell JA, Wolinsky I. *Nutritional Concerns in Recreation, Exercise and Sport.* Boca Raton, FL: CRC Press; 2009:91–114;145–161;235–265.

4. Frankenfield DC, Rowe WA, Smith JS, Cooney RN. Validation of several established equations for resting metabolic rate in obese and nonobese people. *J Am Diet Assoc.* 2003;103(9):1152–1159. Erratum in: *J Am Diet Assoc.* 2003.

5. Jeukendrup AE. Carbohydrate and exercise performance: The role of multiple transportable carbohydrates. *Curr Opin Clin Nutr Metab Care.* 2010;13(4):452–457.

6. Johnson WR, Buskirk ER. *Structural and Physiological Aspects of Exercise and Sport.* Princeton, NJ: Princeton Book Co; 1980.

7. McArdle WD, Katch FI, Katch VL. *Sports & Exercise Nutrition.* Philadelphia, PA: Lippincott Williams & Wilkens; 1999:275–276.

8. Stephens FB, Roig M, Armstrong G, Greenhaff PL. Post-exercise ingestion of a unique, high molecular weight glucose polymer solution improves performance during a subsequent bout of cycling exercise. *J Sports Sci.* 2008;26(2):149–154.

9. Tipton KD. Efficacy, consequences of very-high-protein diets for athletes exercisers. *Proc Nutr Soc.* 2011;70(2):205–214.

10. Yeo WK, Carey AL, Burke L, Spriet LL, Hawley JA. Fat adaptation in well-trained athletes: Effects on cell

Exercise Prescription, Exercise Testing, and Exercise Screening

Kenneth R. Mautner and Jerome T. Nichols

I. Principles of Exercise Prescription

A. Regular participation in activity at 3–6 metabolic equivalents (METs) confers health benefits, even without changing aerobic fitness. See Table 11.1 for examples of activities and associated approximate METs.

   1. One MET is equal to ~3.5 mL of oxygen uptake per kg of body mass per minute for an average adult (1.2 kcal/min for a 70 kg person)

   2. For healthy adults under 65 years, the American Heart Association (AHA) and American College of Sports Medicine (ACSM) recommend:

      a. moderately intense cardiovascular exercise 30 min/day, 5 days/week

OR

      b. vigorously intense cardiovascular exercise 20 min/day, 3 days/week WITH 8–10 strength training exercises, 8–12 repetitions of each, twice/week

B. Individualized prescriptions targeted at achieving desired outcomes for each patient

   1. Prescription should address the FITT components (regardless of age, fitness level, or presence/absence of comorbidity):

      a. Frequency: most or all days of the week

      b. Intensity: several ways of specifying this

         i. Karvonen formula:

$$\text{Heart rate (HR)}_{target} = (HR_{reserve} \times \text{training intensity}) + HR_{resting}$$

[Goal training intensity is 40–80% of HR_{max} (220−age)]

         ii. Talk test: able to converse comfortably

         iii. Moderate intensity rate of perceived exertion (RPE) on Borg scale (see C.3. below)

      c. Type of exercise/mode (e.g., running, swimming, cycling)

      d. Time/duration: 30–60 min

   2. ACSM guidelines also address progression as an additional component

      a. Increasing duration, intensity, frequency, varying activity type as conditioning improves

C. Optimal exercise prescription written only after evaluating the individual's response to exercise, including:

   1. Heart rate (HR)

   2. Blood pressure (BP)

3. RPE utilizing a tool such as the Borg scale or ACSM RPE scale, wherein patients rate how hard they perceive they are working
   a. Borg scale: Ranges from 6–20, with a rating of 6–11 being "very, very light" exertion, 12–14 considered moderate effort, and 16–20 being "hard" to "very hard" effort
   b. ACSM RPE scale: Ranges from 0–10, with 0 being "nothing," and 10 being "very, very heavy—almost max"
4. Subjective response to exercise
5. Electrocardiogram (ECG) when appropriate
6. VO_{2max}.

Table 11.1 Examples of Activities and Associated Approximate METs

Physical Activity	METs
Light Activity	**<3**
Sleeping	0.9
Sitting quietly (e.g., watching TV)	1.0
Whirlpool sitting	1.0
Standing in line	1.2
Sitting-studying, reading, and/or writing	1.8
Walking 2.0 mph, firm, level surface	2.5
Moderate Activity	**3–6**
Walking 2.5 mph firm, level surface	3.0
Food shopping, with grocery cart	3.5
Walking 3.5 mph firm, level surface	4.0
Hand washing/waxing car	4.5
Skateboarding	5.0
Scrubbing floor on hands and knees	5.5
Tennis, doubles	6.0
Vigorous Activity	**>6**
Chopping wood/splitting logs	6.0
Softball, pitching	6.0
Wheelchair basketball	6.5
Running, 5ph (12 min/mile)	8.0
Calisthenics (e.g., push-ups, sit-ups, pull-ups) heavy, vigorous effort	8.0
Shoveling, digging ditches	8.5
Jumping rope	10.0
Bicycling 16–19 mph not drafting (>19 mph drafting)	12.0
Rock climbing, ascending rock	11.0
Running, 8.6 mph (7 min/mile)	14.0
Running upstairs	15.0

Adapted from Ainsworth BE, Haskell WL, Leon AS, et al. Compendium of physical activities: Classification of energy costs of human physical activities. *Med Sci Sports Exerc.* 1993; 25(1):71–80.

II. Medical Clearance/Screening

  A. Initial screening should evaluate for likelihood of adverse outcomes related to cardiovascular and pulmonary disease
  1. Assess for risk factors of coronary artery disease (CAD). ACSM has a useful tool for risk factor assessment of CAD. See Table 11.2.
  2. Patients can then be risk stratified into ACSM's low-, moderate-, or high-risk categories
    a. Low-risk patients:
      i. Men, <45 years of age, with no more than one positive risk factor (from the list above)
      ii. Women, <55 years of age, with no more than one positive risk factor
    b. Moderate-risk patients:
      i. Men ≥45 years of age or women ≥55 years of age
      ii. Individuals with two or more positive risk factors
    c. High-risk patients:
      i. Presence of known cardiac, peripheral vascular, or cerebrovascular disease
      ii. Presence of certain pulmonary conditions (chronic COPD, asthma, interstitial lung disease, or cystic fibrosis)
      iii. Presence of additional signs and symptoms associated with cardiac or pulmonary disease (angina, dyspnea at rest or with mild exertion, dizziness or syncope, ankle edema, palpitations or tachycardia, intermittent claudication, orthopnea or paroxysmal nocturnal dyspnea, unusual fatigue or dyspnea with usual activities, known heart murmur)
  3. Physicians can utilize the above risk stratification to make recommendations for exercise testing prior to engaging in an exercise program
    a. Low-risk patients: No exercise testing necessary
    b. Moderate-risk patients: Should undergo exercise testing if planning to engage in a vigorous-intensity exercise program
    c. High-risk patients: Exercise testing recommended prior to engaging in a moderate (40–60% VO_{2max}) or vigorous-intensity program (>60% VO_{2max})
    d. Additionally, physician supervision is recommended for submaximal testing in high-risk patients, and maximal testing in moderate- or high-risk patients
  4. Depending on results of risk stratification, exercise testing and thorough pretesting history and examination should be performed

Table 11.2   Risk Factors for Coronary Artery Disease

Family history	Male relative <55yo OR female relatives <65yo with MI, sudden death, or coronary revascularization
Smoking history	Current OR quit within the last 6 months
Hypertension	SBP ≥ 140 OR DBP ≥ 90 OR antihypertensive use
Dyslipidemia	LDL > 130, HDL < 40 OR total cholesterol > 200 if LDL not available; High HDL ≥ 60 is protective
Blood glucose	Fasting level > 100 on two occasions
Obesity	BMI > 30 OR waist size > 40 inches in men, 35 inches in women OR waist to hip ratio ≥0.95 in men, ≥0.86 women
Sedentary lifestyle	Not partaking in 30 min per day of moderate activities most days of the week

Adapted from Balady G, Ber K, Golding L, et al. Health screening and risk stratification. In: Barry F, ed. *ACSM's Guidelines for Exercise Testing and Prescription*. 6th ed. Philadelphia: Lippincott Williams & Wilkins; 2000:22–32.

B. Contraindications to exercise testing
 1. Absolute contraindications
   a. Recent significant change in resting ECG concerning for significant ischemia, acute cardiac event, or recent infarction
   b. Recent complicated myocardial infarction (MI)
   c. Unstable angina
   d. Uncontrolled symptomatic dysrhythmia
   e. Severe aortic stenosis
   f. Uncontrolled, symptomatic heart failure
   g. Recent, acute pulmonary embolism or infarction
   h. Myo- or pericarditis
   i. Dissecting aneurysm
   j. Acute infection
 2. Relative contraindications
   a. Left main coronary artery stenosis
   b. Moderate valvular stenosis
   c. Electrolyte abnormalities (e.g., disorders of potassium, magnesium)
   d. Systolic blood pressure (SBP) of >200 mm Hg and/or diastolic blood pressure (DBP) of >110 mm Hg at rest
   e. Tachyarrhythmia or bradyarrhythmia
   f. Hypertrophic cardiomyopathy or other outflow obstruction
   g. Neuromuscular, musculoskeletal, or rheumatoid conditions exacerbated by exercise
   h. Mental or physical impairment resulting in inability to exercise adequately
   i. High-degree atrioventricular (AV) block
   j. Ventricular aneurysm
   k. Uncontrolled metabolic disorder (e.g., diabetes mellitus, thyrotoxicosis, myxedema)
   l. Chronic infectious disease (e.g., mononucleosis, hepatitis, AIDS).

III. Exercise Testing for Performance
 A. Maximal oxygen uptake (VO_{2max}): accepted criterion measure for cardiorespiratory fitness
  1. Product of maximal cardiac output (L/min) and arterial–venous oxygen difference (mL O_2/L)
  2. Two- to threefold difference in VO_{2max} (L/min) across populations primarily due to difference in maximal cardiac output
  3. Open-circuit spirometry used to measure VO_{2max}
    a. Athlete breathes through low-resistance valve (nose-occluded)
    b. Pulmonary ventilation, expired fractions O_2 and CO_2 measured
    c. If direct VO_{2max} measurement not possible, submaximal and maximal exercise tests can be performed to determine estimated VO_{2max}
  4. Maximal testing more sensitive for diagnosing coronary artery disease in asymptomatic athletes
  5. Submaximal testing frequently more feasible for most practitioners to perform
    a. The aim of submaximal testing is to determine the HR response to a submaximal work rate and, using any of multiple available protocols and associated equations, use results to determine predicted VO_{2max}
    b. Tests should ideally be performed with electrocardiography (ECG), heart rate monitor, or stethoscope to determine HR
      i. When possible, use test mode most consistent with athlete's primary activity (e.g., treadmill, cycle ergometer, step)
  6. Field tests
    a. Field tests are always presumptively maximal tests

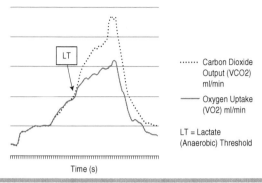

Figure 11.1   VCO2 versus VO2 for lactate (anaerobic) threshold

   i. subjects walk/run specified distance in a given time (i.e., 12-min run test, Cooper 1.5-mile run test, Rockport 1-mile walk test)

   ii. Able to test a large number of subjects simultaneously

   iii. Individual motivation and pacing ability can significantly impact test results, as some patients may not give true maximal effort

   iv. Unmonitored nature of test can increase risk of cardiovascular and musculoskeletal complications

B. Lactate (anaerobic) threshold is the level at which exercise intensity increases to the point where anaerobic metabolism, rather than aerobic metabolism, becomes the predominant energy source

   1. Typically occurs at 4 mmol/L of blood lactate

   2. May be as low as 40% of VO_{2max} uptake in the untrained, or as high as 80–90% VO_{2max} in trained endurance athletes

   3. Exercise below lactate threshold can be performed continuously for prolonged periods without discomfort or fatigue; exercise above this level is associated with systemic metabolic acidosis and augmented ventilatory demand (respiratory alkalosis), leading to fatigue and inability to continue activity above threshold

   4. Determined graphically by plotting VCO2 against VO2 (mL/min or a percentage of VO_{2max}). See Figure 11.1.

IV. The Pediatric Athlete

A. Important to tailor exercise prescription and testing with consideration of normal growth and development of young athletes

B. Fitness testing

   1. Common in school-based physical education

   2. Typically, a battery of 4–6 simple field tests are performed

     a. Fitnessgram and President's Challenge test are commonly utilized tools

     b. Measurements include:

       i. Aerobic capacity (e.g., 1-mile walk/run)

       ii. Muscular strength and endurance (e.g., curl-ups, pull-ups, push-ups)

       iii. Flexibility (e.g., sit-reach, V-sit reach)

       iv. Agility (e.g., shuttle run)

       v. Body composition (e.g., body mass index, skinfolds)

C. Clinical exercise testing
  1. The American College of Cardiology (ACC) and the AHA have published common reasons to recommend pediatric stress testing:
     a. Evaluate specific signs or symptoms that are induced or aggravated by exercise
     b. Assess or identify abnormal responses in children with cardiac, pulmonary, or other organ disorders, including the presence of myocardial ischemia and arrhythmias
     c. Assess efficacy of specific medical or surgical treatments
     d. Assess functional capacity for recreational, athletic, and vocational activities
     e. Evaluate prognosis, including both baseline and serial testing measurements
D. Exercise prescription
  1. Those greater than 6 years old should participate in 30 min or more of moderate-intensity physical activity most to all days of the week
     a. Focus on active play for very young children
     b. 20–30 min of vigorous exercise at least three times per week recommended for older children
  2. Typically, no need for HR prescriptions as children are able to self-adjust RPE
  3. Resistance training programs for children are safe if properly designed and supervised
  4. Prescriptions for strength training should specify intensity, duration, and frequency
     a. Intensity
        i. Avoid repetitive use of maximal weight until Tanner stage 5
        ii. Weight should be low enough to allow eight or more repetitions per set
        iii. Resistance exercises should not be performed to the point of severe muscle fatigue
        iv. First, achieve overload with increasing repetitions, then increase resistance
     b. Duration
        i. 1–2 sets (8–12 repetitions per set) of 8–10 exercises, training all major muscle groups
        ii. Rest 1–2 min between exercises; intersperse rest days between training days
     c. Frequency: Limit strength training sessions to twice per week; encourage other forms of physical activity
E. Considerations for pediatric athletes with specific diseases
  1. Bronchial asthma
     a. Program should focus on conditioning, reduction in exercise-induced bronchospasm, and confidence building
     b. Activities should be varied, with emphasis on lower-energy demand activities
        i. Aquatic activities and intermittent activities with long warm-up periods are recommended
  2. Cerebral palsy
     a. Focus of program should include increasing aerobic power, range of motion (ROM), and body mass control
     b. Activity recommendations are dependent on residual ability
  3. Cystic fibrosis (CF)
     a. Goal of training respiratory muscles, improving mucus clearance
     b. Jogging, swimming, walking, other selected games all recommended
  4. Diabetes mellitus
     a. Goal of activity is to help with metabolic control and BMI control
     b. Recommend a variety of activities with emphasis on equal daily energy output
  5. Hemophilia
     a. Activity recommended to prevent muscle atrophy and possible hemarthrosis
     b. Avoid contact sports—recommend cycling, swimming, etc.

6. Mental retardation
   a. Goal of exercise program should emphasize socialization, improve self-esteem, and prevent deconditioning
   b. Recommend a variety of activities that are recreational and intermittent
7. Muscular dystrophy
   a. Design a program to increase muscle strength and endurance, prolong the ambulatory phase
   b. Activity recommendations should include swimming, calisthenics, and wheelchair sports
8. Obesity
   a. Focus on reduction of BMI and body fat, conditioning, socialization, and self-esteem improvement
   b. Recommend activities high in caloric expenditure but feasible for a child (e.g., walking, swimming, recreational games)
9. Rheumatoid arthritis
   a. Propose a program focused on preventing contractures and muscle atrophy, increasing daily function
   b. Include activities such as swimming, cycling, calisthenics
10. Spina bifida
    a. Activity recommendations should be designed to increase upper body strength, control body fat and BMI, and increase maximal aerobic capacity
    b. Training should consist of arm–shoulder training, wheelchair sports.

V. The Geriatric Athlete

A. Higher rate of CAD makes exercise testing even more relevant than in the adult population at large
B. Medical clearance advised prior to maximal exercise testing or participation of geriatric athletes in vigorous activity
C. Exercise testing considerations
   1. If work capacity expected to be low, start with low workload, such as 2–3 METs
      a. Increase in small increments, 0.5–1.0 METs
   2. Be mindful of increased rate of exercise-induced arrhythmias in the elderly
   3. Medications that might interfere with hemodynamic responses and ECGs are commonly prescribed in this population
   4. Criteria for termination of exercise testing are the same in all adult populations, regardless of age, as are the general principles regarding exercise prescription
D. Exercise prescription
   1. Cardiovascular
      a. Recommended that the elderly participate in a cumulative 30 min of moderate-intensity exercise on most (preferably all) days of the week
      b. A conservative approach to increasing intensity is advised
      c. A measured peak heart rate is preferred in the elderly (vs. age-predicted value) given high variability in peak heart rates in patients over age 65
      d. May be safer initially increasing exercise duration rather than intensity
   2. Resistance/strength training
      a. At least one set of 8–10 exercises that involve all major muscle groups, at least twice weekly (48 h between sessions)
         i. Each set to include 10–15 repetitions with an RPE of 12–13 (somewhat hard)
      b. Initially, preferable to increase number of repetitions to achieve overload rather than resistance

    c. If a period of time-off from training has occurred, advise elderly patients to resume at 50% or less of previous training intensity with a gradual increase

    d. Initial close supervision of training sessions for the first 8 weeks with minimal resistance to allow connective tissue to adapt.

VI. Athletes with Cardiovascular/Cerebrovascular Disease

A. Athletes with cardiovascular disease

  1. Clinical indications for cardiac rehabilitation

    a. Medically stable post-MI

    b. Stable angina

    c. Coronary artery bypass graft (CABG) surgery

    d. Percutaneous transluminal coronary angioplasty (PTCA)

    e. Compensated congestive heart failure (CHF)

    f. Cardiomyopathy

    g. Heart or other organ transplantation

    h. Other cardiac surgery (e.g., valvular, pacemaker insertion)

    i. Peripheral vascular disease (PVD)

    j. High-risk cardiovascular disease in patients otherwise ineligible for surgical intervention

    k. End-stage renal disease (ESRD)

    l. At-risk for CAD, with concurrent diagnoses of diabetes mellitus, hyperlipidemia, hypertension, etc.

  2. Clinical contraindications for cardiac rehabilitation

    a. Recent EKG change or myocardial infarction

    b. Unstable angina

    c. Resting SBP of >200 mm Hg or resting DBP >110 mm Hg requires case-by-case evaluation

    d. Symptomatic orthostatic hypotension with >20 mm Hg drop (supine-to-stand)

    e. Critical aortic stenosis

    f. Acute systemic illness or fever

    g. Uncontrolled atrial or ventricular arrhythmias

    h. Uncontrolled sinus tachycardia (>120 beats/min)

    i. Uncompensated CHF

    j. Unpaced, high-degree AV block

    k. Active peri- or myocarditis

    l. Recent embolism

    m. Thrombophlebitis

    n. Resting ST segment displacement of >2 mm

    o. Uncontrolled diabetes (resting blood glucose >400 mg/dL)

    p. Orthopedic conditions that would preclude exercise

    q. Certain other metabolic conditions (e.g., acute thyroiditis, hypokalemia, hyperkalemia, hypovolemia)

  3. Relative contraindications to participation in cardiac rehabilitation

    a. Tachyarrhythmias

    b. Bradyarrhythmias

    c. Moderate valvular disease

    d. Hypertrophic cardiomyopathy

    e. Left main CAD

  4. Indications for cardiac stress testing prior to beginning an exercise program

    a. Asymptomatic persons with two or more risk factors of CAD (see Table 11.2)

    b. Men >45 years and women >55 years who plan to exercise >60% VO_{2max}

    c. Known cardiac symptoms to assess severity and prognosis

    d. Postmyocardial infarction for prognostic assessment

    e. Those involved in occupations in which cardiovascular events may affect public safety

  5. When preliminary exercise testing is not feasible, pharmacologic stress testing can be beneficial

    a. Highest heart rate obtained with dobutamine testing may be used to guide prescribed target heart rate (THR)

    b. Other complementary methods (symptoms, Holter monitoring, ECG-telemetry, heart rate monitors) may be useful in determining exercise intensity

  6. Exercise prescriptions in cardiovascular disease

    a. Frequency, duration, type, and time follow basic AHA guidelines (30–60 min, 5–7 days weekly of repetitive movements involving large muscle groups)

    b. Intensity parameters

       i. 40–85% maximal functional capacity (VO_{2max})

      ii. 40–85% of maximal heart rate reserve (HRR_{max})

     iii. 50–90% of maximal heart rate (HR_{max})

     iv. Moderate-intensity (12–13) RPE on Borg scale

      v. Exercise at more vigorous intensity is associated with a 10-fold increased risk of major cardiovascular event in patients with underlying CAD

  7. Progression should be over a 3–6 month period

B. Exercise prescriptions in patients with cerebrovascular disease

  1. Considerations:

    a. Assess strength, tone, ROM

    b. Emphasis on exercises that do not significantly increase BP in patients with hypertensive CVA

    c. Incorporate adaptive equipment (AFOs, etc.) and ensure adequate skin care

  2. Benefits of exercise include:

    a. Improved mood

    b. Improved cardiovascular fitness

    c. Modification of risk factors associated with stroke (BP, hyperlipidemia).

VII. Diabetes Mellitus

A. In some individuals with type 2 diabetes, adequate glycemic control can be achieved with exercise and weight reduction

B. In diabetics taking insulin, response to exercise is variable in regard to glycemic control

C. If under appropriate control or only slightly hyperglycemic without ketosis, exercise decreases blood glucose concentration, and a lower insulin dose may be required

D. Lack of sufficient insulin prior to exercise impairs glucose transport into muscles, may lead to ketosis and worsen the hyperglycemic state

  1. Adequate control prior to exercise is imperative

    a. Blood glucose concentration >300 mg/dL or >240 mg/dL with positive urine ketones is a relative contraindication to exercise

E. Exercise-induced hypoglycemia is common

  1. Hypoglycemia can result if too much insulin is present and with accelerated glucose absorption from the injection site—both can occur with exercise

    a. Can result during exercise or up to 4–6 h after completing exercise

  2. Decreasing insulin dose or increasing carbohydrate load prior to exercise can both compensate for this response

  3. Insulin-dependent diabetics should consider intake of 20–30 g of additional carbohydrates with preexercise blood glucose of <100 mg/dL

  4. Reduce risk of hypoglycemic events with basic precautions

    a. Measure glucose before, during, and after exercise

      b. Avoid exercise in periods of peak insulin activity

      c. Precede unplanned exercise with 20–30 g carbohydrates/ 30 min of exercise; if needed, decrease insulin dose after unplanned exercise periods

      d. Insulin doses prior to and following planned exercise should be decreased, dependent on exercise intensity, duration, and the personal experiences

      e. Instruct athletes to keep easily absorbable carbohydrates on hand for consumption during exercise

      f. Carbohydrate-rich snacks following exercise may be necessary

      g. Ensure athletes are knowledgeable about signs and symptoms of hypoglycemia

      h. Recommend exercise with a partner

  F. Exercise prescription in diabetics

    1. Be cautious for autonomic neuropathy that may be associated with silent ischemia, postural hypotension, and/or blunted heart response to activity

    2. Frequency: 4–6 days/week

    3. Duration: 20–60 min/session

    4. Intensity: 50–85% VO_{2max}

      a. RPE may be an excellent adjunct to heart rate when monitoring intensity

    5. In obese type 2 diabetics, maximize caloric expenditure.

VIII. The Disabled Athlete

  A. Benefits of physical activity in disabled athletes

    1. Usual benefits known to accompany regular physical activity (improved cardiovascular capacity, strength, VO_{2max})

    2. Reduced disability-associated health care costs in disabled individuals who participate in regular exercise

      a. Fewer visits to physicians and hospitalizations than inactive counterparts

  B. Difficult for some disabled individuals to exercise at sufficient intensity to optimize health benefits.

    1. Use of alternate modes of exercise (e.g., hand-cycles for wheelchair users) may enable disabled athletes to better achieve optimal health benefits of exercise

    2. While many exercise prescription recommendations will remain similar between disabled athletes and nondisabled athletes, it is important to understand different risks, capacities, and needs of athletes in different disability groups.

IX. Athletes With Fibromyalgia

  A. Aerobic exercise has most consistently demonstrated benefit in fibromyalgia (FM), with some benefits also noted with strengthening

    1. Mixed results with flexibility exercises (including yoga)

    2. Walking as well as activities performed in warm water have both shown positive results demonstrated in studies and endorsed by patients with FM

  B. Benefits of exercise in FM

    a. Studies demonstrate improvements in multiple areas including pain score, tender-point count, and symptom severity

    b. Some evidence that regular exercise may result in improved cognitive function in patients with FM (cognitive dysfunction often rated as FM patients' most distressing symptom)

    c. Improved anaerobic function, power, cardiac parasympathetic tone, and strength

  C. Strategies for optimizing exercise compliance in individuals with FM

    1. Obtain a focused medical history with emphasis on pain, sleep, fatigue, stiffness, mood disorders, and cognition

2. Identify potential pain generators—for example, osteoarthritis, spine pathologies, bursitis, and tendonitis, and modify exercises to minimize aggravation
3. Minimize eccentric muscle work to reduce muscle strain
4. A low-intensity, varied-exercise program is key to reduce symptom exacerbation
5. Screen for and treat autonomic dysfunction (severe fatigue, near-syncopal episodes, orthostatic hypotension, chronic low blood pressure)
6. Evaluate for fall risk, as patients with FM often have poor balance.

X. Athletes With HIV

A. Benefits of exercise in HIV
   1. Multiple studies demonstrate improvements in aerobic capacity, upper and lower limb strength, and VO_{2max}
   2. Reduction in symptoms of anxiety and depression
   3. Multiple studies demonstrate improvements in body composition
   4. Conflicting data indicate some sero-positive exercisers may demonstrate an improved CD4 count
   5. Effective exercise regimens include:
      a. Constant or interval aerobic exercise OR a combination of constant aerobic exercise and progressive resistive exercise for 20 min per session, three times per week, performed for at least 5 weeks prior to progressing intensity and duration.

XI. Athletes With Cancer

A. Systematic reviews indicate that exercise is safe and well tolerated in patients with curative disease during and after adjuvant therapy

B. Incorporating formalized preexercise screening into standard practice enables oncologists to provide safe and accurate exercise guidance to patients

C. Benefits associated with exercise in cancer patients and survivors
   1. Effective as part of treatment program for cancer-related fatigue (CRF)
   2. A few cohort studies demonstrate significant improvement in survival related to increased levels of physical activity after cancer diagnosis
   3. Studies demonstrate improvement in perceived quality of life (QOL), anxiety, and depression

D. Cancer-related fatigue
   1. Combined cytotoxic treatments and reduction in physical activity lead to decreased capacity for physical performance; ordinary activities become fatiguing
   2. Regular exercise can maintain and increase functional capacity, leading to greater exercise tolerance and cardiac output, reduced resting heart rate, and less fatigue

E. Exercise prescription
   1. Most studies demonstrate a positive effect from aerobic exercise of moderate intensity as well as strength training in treating CRF
   2. Should be prescribed in consultation with the patient's oncologist and an exercise physiologist
   3. Individualized based on patient's needs, age, comorbid conditions, physical condition, and planned cancer therapy
   4. ACSM guidelines recommend:
      a. 150 min per week of moderate exercise (e.g., brisk walking, light swimming) or 75 min per week of vigorous exercise (e.g., jogging, running, hard swimming)
      b. These guidelines serve as a long-term goal
   5. Sedentary patients not able to meet ACSM guidelines should start with a moderate-intensity exercise, 20 min per session, three times per week

      a. Reassessment every 2–3 weeks, and progression as appropriate should follow the initial prescription

    6. Resistance training should also be added

      a. Upper and lower multijoint exercises, two sets of 12–15 repetitions, 20 min per session, twice per week.

XII. Athletes With Osteoarthritis

  A. Deficits in muscle function associated with osteoarthritis (OA)

    1. Muscle function helps absorb limb loading, providing dynamic joint stability

      a. Muscle weakness potential risk factor for disease development due to increased joint loading

      b. Studies indicate patients with knee OA have 20–40% relative quadriceps weakness in comparison with healthy controls

      c. Loss of measurable strength likely related to multiple factors, including pain, anxiety, motivation, effusion, muscle atrophy, and aberrant joint mechanics

      d. Determining source of weakness is important in directing therapy—that is, if weakness due to atrophy, pure strengthening may suffice; if a deficit of activation is the main causative factor, removal of inhibitory source should be the primary initial goal

    2. Proprioception

      a. Deficits in knee-joint proprioception noted in individuals with knee OA compared to age-matched normals

  B. Requisite testing prior to prescribing exercise: none

  C. Exercise prescription in OA

    1. Mode: A low-impact program (e.g., stationary bike, water-based exercises, strength training) focused on strengthening, flexibility, and function

    2. Intensity: Likely need to be individualized to the patient. High-intensity, low-impact exercise may yield greater strength gains and take less time to perform the same overall work load, but may not be well tolerated by all individuals

      a. High intensity in one study of patients with knee OA defined as three sets of eight repetitions of a weight at 60% maximum

    3. Duration/frequency: 30 cumulative minutes daily, 3 or more days per week.

XIII. Athletes With Osteoporosis

  A. Trials suggest that regular physical exercise can reduce the risk of osteoporosis and delay the physiologic decrease of BMD

  B. Some trials demonstrate that use of resistance or mixed endurance–resistance exercise lead to gains in bone mass in older men and women, with other studies demonstrating only decreased bone loss compared to controls

  C. Exercise also demonstrated to reduce incidence of falls in the elderly

  D. An inclusive exercise program should include balance, postural, resistance, and weight-bearing exercises

  E. Severely osteoporotic patients should be on appropriate medication therapy for a minimum of 3 months before engaging in exercise to minimize fracture risks.

XIV. Athletes With Pulmonary Disease

  A. Exercise training in patients with respiratory disease provides benefit by increasing endurance, increasing functional status, decreasing severity of dyspnea, and improving quality of life

B. Exercise prescription
  1. Mode: Any aerobic exercise involving large muscle groups is appropriate for pulmonary patients
     a. Walking is often recommended, but other exercises such as cycle ergometry and rowing are also reasonable
  2. Frequency: 3–5 days/week
     a. For those with lower functional capacity, daily exercise may be recommended
  3. Intensity: Consensus on appropriate intensity for pulmonary patients is lacking
  4. Two approaches frequently utilized
     a. Exercise at 50% of peak oxygen uptake—allows pulmonary patients to perform exercise at the minimal intensity recommended for healthy adults and may improve adherence to training while still improving endurance and reducing dyspnea
     b. Maximal limits as tolerated by symptoms—patients with moderate-to-severe COPD are able to sustain ventilation at a high percentage of maximal minute ventilatory volume for a few minutes, and may be able to interval train in this fashion, increasing duration over time
  5. Duration: As most patients are unable to tolerate 20–30 min of continuous exercise when beginning a training program, specify intensity for a period of a few minutes, followed by a rest period.

XV. Exercise for Weight Control

  A. Obesity increases multiple health risks (e.g., cardiovascular disease, diabetes, some cancers)
  B. Assessment of patient to include weight, height, waist circumference, BMI, risk factors for chronic diseases
  1. Important to consider weight history, diet, exercise level, prior weight loss attempts
  C. Initial target goal of weight loss therapy for overweight patients: decrease body weight by ~10%
  D. Some advocate 60–90 min of moderate-intensity activity daily at a minimum of 6 days per week, in order to attain or maintain weight loss goals
  E. Strategies to overcome common barriers and pitfalls
  1. For patients who complain of a lack of adequate time for exercise, physical activity for shorter durations per session may be of benefit
  2. Important for patients to identify opportunities in normal daily activities to increase physical activity
     a. Use of a pedometer or step-counter may promote physical activity awareness
     b. 10,000 steps each day may improve cardiovascular fitness and overall health
        i. Average number of steps taken daily is 6,000 to 7,000
  3. As patients often grow discouraged at the absence of rapid changes in weight, it is important for physicians to educate patients on additional health benefits of physical activity independent of weight loss (blood pressure, insulin, lipids, etc.)
  4. Important to discourage weight cycling to avoid potential negative consequences
     a. Emphasize concept of "realistic" lifetime weight loss goals
  5. Encouraging patients to participate in any activities they find enjoyment in will increase the likelihood they will maintain long-term physical activity.

Recommended Reading

1. Balady G, Ber K, Golding L, et al. Health screening and risk stratification. In: Barry F, ed. *ACSM's Guidelines for Exercise Testing and Prescription*. 6th ed. Philadelphia: Lippincott Williams & Wilkins; 2000:22–32.
2. Coral DM, Klaege K. Exercise and weight management. *Prim Care Clin Office Pract.* 2007;34:109–116.

3. Evans WJ. Exercise for successful aging In: Garrett WE, Kirkendall DT. eds. *Exercise and Sport Science.* Philadelphia: Lippincott Williams & Wilkins; 2000:276–284.

4. Kannus P, Liu-Ambrose T. Exercise prescription for health. In: Brukner P, Khan K. eds. *Clinical Sports Medicine.* Revised 3rd ed. Australia: McGraw Hill Australia Pty Ltd.; 2009:912–934.

5. Mock V. Fatigue. In: MD Abeloff, JO Armitage, JE Niederhuber, et al. eds. *Abeloff: Abeloff's Clinical Oncology.* 4th ed. Philadelphia: Churchill Livingstone, an imprint of Elsevier Inc.; 2008:657–662.

6. O'Brien K, Nixon S, Glazier R, Tynan AM. Progressive resistive exercise interventions for adults living with HIV/AIDS. *Cochrane Database Sys Rev.* 2004;(4). Art. No.: CD004248. DOI: 10.1002/14651858.CD004248.pub2.

7. Paridon SM, Alpert BS, Boas SR, et al. Clinical stress testing in the pediatric age group a statement from the American Heart Association Council on Cardiovascular Disease in The Young, Committee on Athersclerosis, Hypertension, and Obesity in Youth. *Circulation.* 2006;*113*(15):1905–1920.

8. Plotnikoff GA. Osteoporosis. In: Rakel D, ed. *Rakel: Integrative Medicine.* 2nd ed. Philadelphia: Saunders, an imprint of Elsevier Inc.; 2007:417–426.

9. Sietsema KE. In: Mason RJ, Broaddus CV, Martin TR, et al. eds. *Mason: Murray and Nadel's Textbook of Respiratory Medicine.* 5th ed. Philadelphia: Saunders, an imprint of Elsevier Inc.; 2010:554–557.

10. Webbon N. The disabled athlete. In: Brukner P, Khan K, eds. *Clinical Sports Medicine.* Revised 3rd ed. Australia: McGraw Hill Australia Pty Ltd.; 2009:778–786.

11. Wolfe F, Johannes JR. Fibromyalgia. In: Firestein GS, Budd RC, Harris ED, et al. eds. *Firestein: Kelley's Textbook of Rheumatology.* 8th ed. Philadelphia: W.B. Saunders Company; 2008:555–566.

12

Event Administration

John C. Cianca

I. Personnel

    A. Medical Director (MD): The MD leads the medical team and delegates tasks and responsibilities to team members in order to create a team that works cohesively. The MD organizes the team, develops the medical plan and the budget for medical coverage, serves as an advisor to the race director, procures necessary equipment, and educates participants during the lead up to the event. The MD may be a caregiver, particularly in smaller events that have few team members. However, the most important role of the MD on race day is crisis management. Associate medical directors are useful to oversee large areas such as the course and the medical tent, allowing the MD to be free to trouble shoot.

    B. Team Members: The medical team is often made up of individuals from various medical disciplines, including physicians, nurses, emergency medical technicians, athletic trainers, physical therapists, and massage therapists.

II. The Medical Plan

Depending on resources, manpower, and community emergency service capacity the medical plan may involve a triage and transport methodology or it may be designed to treat on site and transport only emergency cases to local hospitals. The triage and transport model involves much less medical personnel but depends heavily on the community emergency response system to cover medical issues other than simple first aid cases. A medical plan that is designed to treat on site may be considerably more sophisticated and have many more medical personnel.

    A. Organization: The MD designates captains that serve as leaders of various aspects of the medical plan. These areas include the course and the finish line of the main medical tent. The course caregivers may include aid stations, cyclist medics, and finish line medics. The main medical tent is generally divided into the triage area, minor medical care, major medical care, and perhaps even an intensive care area. There is also an area for equipment disbursement.

    B. Planning: The process of planning begins weeks if not months in advance of the event. During this time meetings are held with the MD and lead personnel to identify and delegate tasks such as recruitment of medical volunteers, procurement of equipment, and the design of the medical area. One of the most important aspect of planning is the development of treatment protocols by the medical team.

    C. Implementation: The medical tent is built and stocked with the resources to implement the medical plan. Once the event is underway the plan is put into action. This will most often include deploying personnel and resources to the course. Ambulances or other types of transport vehicles are employed to bring injured participants back to the main tent. The majority of affected participants come to the medical area after they have finished the event; but it may be necessary to patrol the finish area for participants who become ill after completing the event.

Care inside the main medical tent is dispensed according to the protocols developed in the planning stage. This may include skin care for blisters, abrasions, and chafing. Simple supportive measures are frequently utilized for participants that are tired, concerned about aches and pains, and suffering from cramps and muscular fatigue. More extensive care for hydration and temperature-related illnesses and other medical conditions is also dispensed. It is important that contingencies be made for cardiovascular or other medical emergencies that may arise.

D. Wrap up and Evaluation: Once the event has concluded; the medical area is broken down and reusable supplies are stored or returned to donors. A postevent meeting to evaluate the medical operation is useful to identify and correct inefficiencies or breakdowns in the medical plan. An after-action report should be created to refer to for subsequent events.

III. Venue

A. Finish line: The finish line medical tent is the site where most medical care is rendered. It is also most often the command center for medical services.

1. *Areas:* Within the medical tent areas are designated for various aspects of medical care including triage, minor medical, and major medical. The communications center for all medical services may be based here or in a unified command center.

2. *Equipment:* Standard equipment for the medical tent includes cots, chairs, wheelchairs, leg bolsters (to elevate the legs when supine), and blankets. Additionally, instrumentation to obtain vital signs, automated electronic defibrillators (AEDs), and materials to cool or warm ill participants are necessities. More sophisticated instrumentation such as blood analyzers, advanced cardiac monitors, fluids for intravenous resuscitation, and a full code cart are often part of the medical tent.

B. Field

1. *Areas:* Field aid stations are frequently used in races from 5k to ultra-marathons. These stations serve mainly as first aid stations but may become very important in the event of an on course emergency. Additional bike teams of medical personnel provide mobile medical care that can respond rapidly to participants who fall ill or injured on the course. Ambulance backup for more intensive care or transport are employed after an initial assessment determines response needs.

2. *Equipment:* A 10′ × 10′ pop up tent is a very practical way to create an aid station on the course (Figure 12.1). Basic first aid equipment and two to three medical personnel are deployed to each aid station. Bike medics usually circulate in teams of two. Having AEDs available on the course is recommended, preferably spaced to have access within 3–5 min of a collapsed athlete.

C. Asset management: If equipment is owned by the medical team or the event, having a storage facility is a practical way to inventory and maintain equipment. Once deployed to the event, it should be housed in a central supply area and deployed as needed to the course or the main medical area.

IV. Communication

Communication must be optimized at several levels to ensure a safe event and allow efficient medical care. A unified central command center is the best way for all parties involved in event management and emergency response to maintain effective communication and response.

A. Team: The medical team may use cell phones, two-way radios, or HAM radio operators to maintain open lines of communication between the course personnel and the main medical tent. A central dispatcher is a vital intermediary to ensure rapid and accurate response.

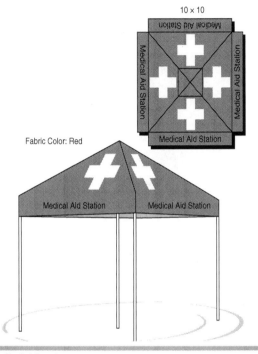

10 × 10

Fabric Color: Red

Figure 12.1   **Medical aid station**

B. **Event:** The MD will need to maintain communication with other race officials through any of the methods mentioned above.

C. **Participants:** Electronic message boards, electronic megaphones, or a system of warning signs (see Figure 12.2) is used to communicate with event participants about weather changes or other important information about course conditions.

V. Environmental Factors

Weather conditions are the most influential variable in predicting medical encounters in an event. Warm weather, particularly with humid conditions will result in more encounters than cooler conditions. The wet bulb globe temperature (WBGT) is used to calculate heat stress. The formula for calculating it is:

$$WBGT = 0.7T_{wb} + 0.2T_{bg} + 0.1T_{db} \text{ (with direct solar exposure)}$$
$$WBGT = 0.7T_{wb} + 0.3T_{bg} \text{ (without direct solar exposure)}$$

where:

T_{wb} = wet bulb temperature (humidity)
T_{bg} = black globe temperature (solar radiation)
T_{db} = dry bulb temperature (air temperature)

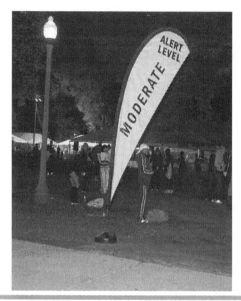

Figure 12.2   Warning flag

A. **Event timing:** Scheduling an event for a time of the year when conditions are moderate and less variable is preferred. Furthermore, the event should be staged at a time of the day, usually mornings, when conditions are cooler and the sun lower in the sky.

B. **Temperature:** Cool-to-moderate temperatures are preferred for most endurance events.

C. **Humidity:** As seen above in the WBGT formula humidity is the most heavily weighted variable in determining event heat stress. Humidity impairs cooling by reducing the efficiency of evaporative heat loss resulting in greater fluid and electrolyte losses via sweating. This may directly impact hydration status.

D. **Exposure:** Sun exposure is also a factor in heat stress so a shadier course on warm days is advantageous. However, during cooler conditions, an exposed course may be an advantage. Rain and wind accentuate heat loss and may make a day with moderate or low temperature an increased risk for hypothermia, particularly for endurance events.

VI. Emergency Planning

Unusual or unsafe conditions may arise during an event, which make it necessary to have a plan to handle such situations. Weather is the most likely for creating an emergency situation; but other scenarios have occurred in recent years.

A. **Event contingencies:** A plan to alter or cancel the event should be in place and stated on the event's web page or informational literature. Such a plan would outline under what circumstances the event would be cancelled. It would also describe how the event might be altered to accommodate an unsafe condition such as extreme heat. These contingencies would be enacted with input from the MD.

B. **Response:** Understanding the threat that may be in place is essential to making a reasonable and correct response. In the face of an emergency situation, the response of the event organizers and the medical team must be exact and well planned. Roles of team members should be clearly defined whether this is through rehearsed situational planning or a specific operational manual. An example of this would be an evacuation plan for the course that would allow the participants to be safely moved from the course to a more safe location.

C. **Preparation:** This is the essential ingredient to successful medical coverage of an event and in particular for an emergency situation. Thinking of possible scenarios in advance allows the team to make preparations for these situations. This should include unusual or extreme weather conditions, on course obstructions, or terrorist threats.

D. **Community interaction:** Communication is a vital link to enacting a contingency plan. Team members need to be in close communication within the team and also with community-based resources such as fire and police departments, local transportation agencies, and the community hospital system.

A unified command center ensures that this can happen effectively. Furthermore, the participants need to be able to receive clear communication from event officials. This can be done using messaging systems along the course and by having an event alert system (EAS) in place. Such a system would utilize simple messaging to communicate risk levels and appropriate responses (Figure 12.3).

CURRENT RISK LEVEL DUE TO WEATHER OR OTHER CONDITIONS

ALERT LEVEL	EVENT CONDITIONS	RECOMMENDED ACTIONS	POTENTIAL RISKS
EXTREME	EVENT CANCELLED/ EXTREME OR DANGEROUS CONDITIONS	STOP PARTICIPATION/ FOLLOW EVENT OFFICIAL INSTRUCTIONS	HYPERTHERMIA
HIGH	DANGEROUS CONDITIONS	SLOW DOWN/ OBSERVE COURSE CHANGES/FOLLOW EVENT OFFICIAL INSTRUCTION/ CONSIDER STOPPING	HYPERTHERMIA IN ALL INDIVIDUALS
MODERATE	POTENTIALLY DANGEROUS CONDITIONS	SLOW DOWN/BE PREPARED FOR WORSENING CONDITIONS	HYPERTHERMIA PARTICULARLY IN HEAT SENSITIVE INDIVIDUALS
LOW	GOOD CONDITIONS	ENJOY THE EVENT/ BE ALERT	HYPERTHERMIA RISK WITH INTENSE EFFORTS
< 50 F COLD WEATHER ALERT	COLD WEATHER CONDITIONS	COVER HANDS, FEET AND TOP OF HEAD	HYPOTHERMIA INCREASES AS TEMPERATURE DROPS AND WINDS AND DAMPNESS INCREASE

Figure 12.3 **Event alert system**

VII. Participants

Mass participation events have grown rapidly and expansively in the last three decades. There is a broad range of participants that present differing levels of experience and risks for injury.

   A. **Elite:** This group of participants is usually few in number and a low risk for injury. They are typically superbly trained and very experienced. Nonetheless, illness and injury do occur in this population but in far fewer numbers than in other participation groups. Medical care for these individuals is usually minimal but the medical team must remain alert to the possibility of sudden cardiac emergencies and heat-related illness.

   B. **Recreational:** This group is varied in their levels of preparation and experience; but usually makes up the largest contingent of event participants. This alone would make the occurrence of casualties higher than in other groups. In addition this group while highly motivated to perform well may be vulnerable to exceeding their capabilities and thus becoming more likely to become ill. Hydration-related illness, muscle cramps, and blisters are prevalent in this group.

   C. **Charity:** This group is increasing rapidly in numbers of participants and may include recreational participants and even elite level participants. It may also include poorly trained and often inexperienced participants. In addition to the maladies that occur in the recreational population these participants may be more prone to fatigue-related problems and gastrointestinal problems due to insufficient training and lack of experience with eating and drinking while exercising intensely.

   D. **Education:** Pre-race education is part of the role of the MD. This may include seminars to local clubs. It will likely include presentations at preevent expositions. Education can also be through e-mail blasts to race participants in advance of the event. Any of these forums can impart valuable and practical information to participants about injury and illness that may occur. Furthermore, using these opportunities allows the MD to communicate with participants about how information will be relayed to them during the event and how they should respond to it.

Recommended Reading

1. American Coll. Sports Med. Position stand: Exercise and fluid replacement. *Med. Sci. Sports Exerc.* 2007;*39*(2):377–390.
2. Armstrong LE, Casa DJ, Millard-Stafford M, Moran D, Pyne SW, Roberts WO. ACSM position stand: Exertional heat illness during training and competition. *Med. Sci. Sports Exerc.* 2007;*39*(3):556–572.
3. Chiampas G, Troyanos C. Best practices for providing cardiac emergency care at marathons. *J. Emer. Med. Ser.* 2010;(9) suppl:14–15.
4. Cianca JC, Roberts WO, Horn D. Distance running: Organization of the medical team. In: O'Connor FG, Wilder RP, eds. *Textbook of Running Medicine.* NY: McGraw-Hill; 2001:489–504.
5. Grollman LJ. Organization and administration of medical coverage for road races. In: Fu FH. ed. *Sports Injuries, Running: Mechanisms, Prevention and Treatment.* Baltimore: Williams & Wilkins; 1994.
6. McCann D.J., Adams W.C. Wet bulb globe temperature index and performance in competitive distance runners. *Med. Sci. Sports Exerc.* 1997;*29*(7):955–961.
7. Nicholl J, Williams B. Popular marathons: Forecasting casualties. *BMJ.* 1982;*285*:1464–1465.
8. Noble B, Bachman D. Medical aspects of distance race plan. *Phys. Sportsmed.* 1979;*6*:78–84.
9. Roberts WO. Assessing core temperature in collapsed athletes. *Phys. Sportsmed.* 1994;*22*(8):49–55.
10. Roberts WO. Medical management of athletic events. In: Kibler WB, ed. *ACSM: Handbook for the Team Physician.* Baltimore: Williams & Wilkins; 1996.
11. Roberts WO. Medical management and administration for long distance road racing. In: Brown CH, Gudjonsson B, eds. *IAAF Medical Manual for Athletics and Road Racing Competitions: A Practical Guide.* Monaco: International Amateur Athletic Federation; 1998.
12. Roberts WO. A twelve year profile of medical injury and illness for the twin cities marathon. *Med Sci Sports Exerc.* 2000;*32*(9):1549–1555.

13. Roberts WO. Determinig a "Do not start" temperature for a marathon on the basis of adverse outcomes. *Med. Sci. Sports Exerc.* 2010;42(20):226–232.

14. Robert WO, Maron BJ. Evidence for decreasing occurrence of sudden cardiac death associated with the marathon. *J. Am. Coll. Cardiol.* 2005;46(7):1373–1374.

15. Ronneberg K, Roberts WO, McBean AD, Center BA. Temporal artery and rectal temperature measurements in collapsed marathon runners. *Med Sci Sports Exerc.* 2008;40(8):1373–1375.

16. www.runningusa.org/statistics.

13

Braces and Protective Equipment

Kelli M. Kyle and Jonathan T. Finnoff

I. Braces

A. Knee—Four types of braces
1. Rehabilitative
a. Control motion following injury
2. Prophylactic
a. Reduce incidence of knee injuries
b. Evidence does not currently support their routine use
3. Functional
a. Support unstable knees (e.g., anterior cruciate ligament (ACL) brace)
4. Patellofemoral
a. Utilized for patellofemoral pain syndrome, patellar tendinopathy, and patellar instability

B. Ankle
1. Lace-up
a. Functional ankle brace
b. Typically made of a sturdy fabric such as muslin or leather
2. Lace-up with straps
a. Functional ankle brace
b. Same as the lace-up ankle brace with figure-8 straps that simulate the heel lock of taping an ankle, therefore providing superior stability
3. Stirrup
a. Hard plastic sides with foam or air-filled pads to stabilize the ankle
b. Good for immediate postinjury protection
4. Stirrup with hinges
a. Functional ankle brace
b. Hard plastic sides with foam padding and hinges at the ankle joint
c. Best combination of mobility and stability

C. Wrist
1. Neutral wrist splints with plastic or metal stays protect the wrist from hyperextension and hyperflexion injuries.

II. Eye Protection

A. Face shields
1. Polycarbonate shields utilized primarily in football and hockey; can fit between the helmet and facemask (e.g., football), or partially or fully cover the athlete's face independent of a facemask (e.g., hockey)

B. Goggles/glasses
  1. Worn for eye protection in multiple sports: lacrosse, swimming, tennis, basketball, racquetball, and so on
  2. Lenses made from polycarbonate.

III. Helmets

A. Certification
  1. Certified by one of the following certification bodies: the National Operating Committee on Standards for Athletic Equipment (NOCSAE), Hockey Equipment Certification Council, Inc. (HECC), or Canadian Standard Association (CSA), depending on the sport
  2. Certifying body determines testing methods, but all helmets must undergo impact testing
  3. Once a helmet passes the tests, the certification body's seal and warning label are placed on the helmet

B. Fitting
  1. Football Helmets:
    a. Depends on the manufacturer and style. Some feature inflatable jaw pads, whereas others use snap-in jaw pads in different sizes
    b. All helmets have either a hard polycarbonate or acrylonitrile butadiene styrene shell, and inner foam or air-filled chambers for energy absorption
    c. Helmets must be fit with facemask and chinstrap in place and tightened
    d. The front pad of the helmet should be approximately 1-in. above the athlete's eyebrows
    e. The jaw pads should be snug against the athlete's cheeks to prevent side-to-side rocking. You should be able to insert an index card without difficulty between the athlete's cheek and jaw pads
    f. The helmet's top and side padding should be inflated until the helmet fits the athlete's head snugly
    g. The helmet should cover the occiput posteriorly but should not impinge on the cervical spine during neck extension
    h. When properly fitted, minimal head rotation should occur when the helmet is held and the athlete tries to turn their head inside the helmet
    i. Facemasks:
      i. Lineman = full cage with a middle bar to minimize risk of eye injury
      ii. Quarterbacks, running backs, and wide receivers = less obtrusive facemask in order to improve their field of view
      iii. Players may wear untinted polycarbonate shields. The NCAA prohibits tinted eye shields without a letter of medical necessity
  2. Hockey Helmets
    a. Fit helmet with facemask attached. Facemasks may be wire cage, face shield, or combination.
      i. Facemasks:
        (A) Wire cage
          (1) Metal or composite shield that covers the entire face
          (2) Does not fog up like face shields
        (B) Face shield
          (1) High impact-resistant plastic
          (2) Better overall vision with no wires
          (3) Can be made with fog-resistant coating
        (C) Combination:
          (1) Plastic face shield upper half, wire cage lower half to offer better vision and ventilation
    b. Chinstrap should be snug without binding or pinching

    c. Helmet ear holes should align with the athlete's ears

    d. The posterior helmet should cover the occiput, but allow full cervical range of motion (ROM)

    e. There should be 1 in. between helmet's front pad and athlete's brow

    f. The helmet should have limited side-to-side and up and down motion when the chinstrap is secured

    g. Apply downward pressure to the anterior and superior aspects of the helmet to ensure that the athlete feels no head or neck discomfort

    h. The same steps are completed for fitting the goalkeeper's helmet with the addition of:

        i. A cage that extends down to protect the throat, anterior aspect of the cheek and jaw

        ii. Helmet should cover the entire crown, frontal, temporal, and posterior aspects of the head

        iii. An attached throat guard, typically made of a polycarbonate

  3. Lacrosse helmets

    a. Fit similarly to hockey helmets

  4. Concussions and helmets

    a. Several helmet manufacturers have designed helmets to "prevent" concussions. There is insufficient evidence to validate this claim.

IV. Padding

A. Shoulder

  1. Football

    a. Cantilevered

        i. Larger, disburse impact forces over a larger surface area via their cantilever strap.

        ii. Most commonly used by linemen

    b. Flat

        i. Less obstructive of shoulder range of motion

        ii. Preferred by quarterbacks and wide receivers

    c. All football padding has a hard plastic cover over foam padding to improve protection against a direct blow

  2. Hockey

    a. Lighter than football padding to allow freedom of movement

    b. No hard plastic covering over the padding

    c. Protective padding covers the shoulders, chest, and upper back. Padding extensions are available to cover more of the back

    d. Defensemen have thicker pads to protect from flying pucks

  3. Lacrosse

    a. Similar to hockey

  4. Special shoulder pads/braces:

    a. Acromioclavicular (AC) joint injury pad = extra pad underneath shoulder pads to protect the AC joint

    b. Shoulder dislocation brace = limit shoulder abduction and external rotation

B. Chest protectors

  1. Utilized in sports where impact to the chest can occur: baseball, softball, field hockey, and motor-cross motorcycle racing

  2. Some baseball leagues have made chest protectors mandatory to protect against commotio cordis, but research indicates that chest protectors do not prevent commotio cordis

  3. Chest protectors are not currently required in the United States

C. Elbow pads

  1. Utilized in sports such as in-line skating and skateboarding

  2. Protects the ulnar nerve and olecranon process from direct trauma

D. Wrist guards
   1. Neutral wrist pads protect the wrist from sprains and fractures due to wrist hyperflexion or hyperextension
E. Knee pads
   1. Utilized in sports such as softball, volleyball, baseball, hockey, and lacrosse where direct trauma may occur to the knee.

V. Gloves

A. Football
   1. Used by wide receivers to improve grip on the football
   2. Keep hands warm
B. Hockey
   1. Protect the hand and wrist from direct blows
   2. Goalkeeper's gloves are larger. On the stick hand, the glove has a large deflector pad. On the opposite hand, the glove is similar to a baseball glove to facilitate catching the puck
C. Lacrosse
   1. Protect the hand and wrist from direct trauma
D. Boxing
   1. Protect the opponent from trauma.

VI. Breakaway Bases

A. The majority of softball injuries occur due to sliding. Breakaway bases reduce the incidence of sliding-related injuries by up to 98%
B. Use suction cups to adhere the base to the base plate
C. The base will dissociate from the base plate if sufficient shear forces are applied to the base.

Recommended Reading

1. Chang C. Protective equipment: football. In: MB Mellion. ed. *Sports Medicine Secrets*. 3rd ed. Philadelphia: Hanley and Belfus; 2003: 131–42.
2. Dunn L, Jones BJE. Bracing in athletics. In: Mellion MB, ed. *Sports Medicine Secrets*. 3rd ed. Philadelphia: Hanley and Belfus; 2003: 428–33.
3. Hockey protective equipment buyer's guide (n.d.). Retrieved from http://shop.nhl.com/info/index.jsp?categoryId=222795.
4. Jeffers J. Sports related eye injuries. In: Mellion MB, ed. *Sports Medicine Secrets*. 3rd ed. Philadelphia: Hanley and Belfus; 2003: 294–9.
5. Naftulin S, Sherbondy P, McKeag DB. Protective equipment: baseball, softball, hockey, wrestling, and lacrosse. In: Mellion MB, ed. *Sports Medicine Secrets*. 3rd ed. Philadelphia: Hanley and Belfus; 2003: 143–50.
6. Pietrosimone B, Grindstaff TL, Linens SW, Uczekaj E, Hertel J. A systematic review of prophylactic braces in the prevention of knee ligament injuries in collegiat football players. *J Athletic Training* 2008;43(4):409–15.

III

Diagnosis and Treatment of Sports Injuries and Conditions

14

General Concepts of Muscle and Tendon Injuries and Conditions

Paul Gerrard and Joanne Borg-Stein

I. Muscle Strains: Stretching or Tearing of Muscle Fibers

A. Epidemiology
  1. Muscles affected
    a. Can occur in any muscle, but more common in:
      i. Muscles that cross two joints (rectus femoris, biceps femoris)
      ii. Muscles with a high proportion of fast twitch (Type II) fibers
  2. Risk factors
    a. Increased age
    b. Poor flexibility in the affected muscle
    c. Muscle weakness relative to its antagonist (e.g., hamstring strain occurring in a quadriceps-dominant athlete)
    d. Deconditioning or relative deconditioning with return to vigorous activity
      i. More commonly seen in preseason or early season workouts

B. Pathology and classification
  1. Generally occurs during an eccentric contraction with stretch of the muscle past its resting length with secondary biomechanical failure at the weak point in the muscle
  2. Can occur at one of three locations
    a. Muscle attachment site (tendon tear)
      i. In young athletes, a bony avulsion at the apophysis typically occurs instead of a tendon rupture due to the elasticity and tensile strength of tendons relative to the more vulnerable unfused apophysis
    b. Myotendinous junction
    c. Muscle belly
  3. Three grade classification system:
    a. Grade 1 (mild)—Stretching of the muscle or tendon with tearing of very few muscle fibers (<5%)
    b. Grade 2 (moderate)—Partial thickness tear or detachment from aponeurosis or surrounding fascia
    c. Grade 3 (severe)—Full thickness tear

C. Clinical features—The diagnosis can usually be made by history and physical examination alone, but ultrasound or MRI may be useful in unclear cases or to help guide prognosis and return-to-play decisions

1. History
   a. Generally presents as an acute injury, which occurs during activity involving contraction of the affected muscle
   b. Typically there is a sudden onset of pain in the middle of physical activity that is initially quite sharp and then may progress to a dull ache
   c. Athlete may hear a "pop"
2. Physical Examination
   a. Grades 1 and 2
      i. Swelling in the affected muscle
      ii. Tenderness to palpation over the affected muscle
      iii. Ecchymosis that may track distally
      iv. Pain with passive stretch
      v. Pain with resisted contraction
   b. Grade 3: In addition to the same findings as grade 1 and 2 strains
      i. Palpable mass (i.e., the retracted muscle belly)
3. Ultrasound findings—Compare both limbs to detect subtle findings
   a. Grade 1 strain
      i. Diffuse hyperechogenicity may be seen in up to 50% of mild strains
      ii. May see no evidence of abnormality
   b. Grade 2 strain
      i. Disruption of perimysial striae
      ii. Active muscle contraction enhances visibility and size of the tear
      iii. Hematoma
         (A) May be visible within the cavity of the torn muscle fibers
         (B) Appearance varies with time from the injury as granulation tissue develops
   c. Grade 3 strain
      i. Large hematoma or fluid collection almost always present acutely
      ii. "Clapper in Bell" sign—retracted tendon surrounded by hypoechoic hematoma
      iii. Hyperechoic muscle stump
4. MRI findings
   a. Grade 1 strain
      i. Edema present in the affected muscle appears as an area of diffuse or focal hyperintensity on fluid-sensitive sequences (STIR and T2)
      ii. No distortion of the overall muscle architecture, though muscle may appear slightly enlarged
   b. Grade 2 strain
      i. Edema appears as hyperintense areas on T2 in the acute phase
      ii. Retraction of the muscle fibers visible on T1 and T2 seen as a disruption in muscle fibers that appears to be in a plane parallel to fiber orientation
      iii. Hemorrhagic fluid in area of muscle fiber interruption
   c. Grade 3 strain
      i. Retraction of the affected muscle seen as a complete disruption in the muscle fibers in a plane that appears perpendicular to the fiber orientation
      ii. Pseudomass—rounded stump of retracted muscle
      iii. Edema may be seen in the retracted muscle stump

D. Treatment and return to play
   1. Treatment timeline
      a. Inflammatory phase (Immediately—1 week)
         i. Protection
         ii. Rest, ice, compression, elevation
         iii. Minimize stretching and strengthening
         iv. Assistive device for ambulation if needed

      b. Proliferative and remodeling phase (1 week–6 months)—Active exercise to restore normal strength and function; conditioning to maintain aerobic fitness

         i. Stretching: progressive as tolerated to restore flexibility

         ii. Strengthening: gentle isometrics first, followed by concentric and later eccentric strengthening

         iii. Excessively quick increases in exercise intensity can lead to repeat injury

      c. Return-to-play phase (3 weeks–6 months)—No good evidence base or consensus to support any particular return-to-play guidelines

         i. Superficial or small injuries usually require less than 5 weeks

         ii. Patients should be able to perform daily functional activities without pain

         iii. General return-to-play guidelines include: normal range of motion, 90% strength restoration compared to the contralateral limb, appropriate aerobic conditioning for the sport, and progressing appropriately through sport-specific drills and training.

    2. Medications—There is no good evidence to support or dispute the use of any particular medications in muscle strain injuries. Generally pharmacologic therapy is aimed at analgesia (most commonly with NSAIDs). Objections to the use of NSAIDs regard the role of inflammation in the repair process (see section IV. C) as the inflammatory cascade facilitates the recruitment of myogenic precursor cells for regeneration. Research shows mixed outcomes.

  E. Prognosis and outcomes

    1. Grade 1 and 2 strains usually have good outcomes and full recovery within 6–18 weeks with conservative management. However, some strains may take up to 6 months to fully recover. Additionally, repeated strains of the same muscle may lead to changes in muscle architecture and chronic injury.

    2. Grade 3 strains tend to have a poorer prognosis and may require surgery. Generally early surgery is the treatment of choice in young athletes, while rehabilitation is the treatment of choice in the older population.

  F. Prevention: After an initial strain, a primary focus should be on future prevention. However, there is no definitive strain prevention program. The most common guidelines include:

    1. Stretch to maintain flexibility and muscle elasticity, after a basic warm-up. However, research on stretching to prevent injury shows mixed results

    2. Allow adequate time for recovery from prior injury as well as appropriate rehabilitation prior to return to play

    3. Warm up prior to engaging in vigorous physical activity

    4. Tailor the exercise intensity to the level of current conditioning; thus, avoid forceful exercise if possible (Table 14.1).

II. Muscle Contusions

  A. Epidemiology

    1. Documented contusions account for one-third of all sports injuries

    2. Most commonly seen in lower limb muscles, including quadriceps and gastrocnemius

  B. Pathology

    1. Caused by rupture of blood vessels within the muscle

    2. Excessive damage/bleeding can cause compartment syndrome

    3. Graded in some cases by range of motion in the joint controlled by the affected muscle

    4. Acute injury may result in chronic myositis ossificans (see section III)

  C. Clinical findings

    1. History

      a. Blunt trauma to the affected area prior to the onset of symptoms is pathognomonic

      b. Onset of pain may be immediate or delayed by hours

Table 14.1   Characteristics of Muscle Strains

Muscle Strains	Grade I	Grade II	Grade III
Definition	Stretching of muscle with <5% fibers torn	Partial thickness tear or fascial detachment	Complete muscle tear
Exam	Swelling Tenderness to palpation Ecchymoses Pain with passive extension Pain with resisted flexion	Same as Grade I	In addition to the same findings as Grades I and II: Palpable mass off retracted muscle belly
Ultrasound	Diffuse hypoechogenicity	Disruption of perimysial striae	Clapper in bell sign—retracted tendon surrounded by hypoechoic hematoma
MRI	Edema No muscle architecture disruption	Disruption of muscle fibers Small hematoma	Pseudomass—Retracted muscle belly Large fluid collection
Treatment	Rest, ice, compression, elevation PT—advance activity as tolerated without pain	Same as Grade I	Possibly surgery PT—strengthen affected muscle
Outcome	Good	Good if given adequate recovery time	Retracted muscle unlikely to heal. Outcome based on surgery or ability to compensate with other muscles

    c. May have pain with active or passive range of motion

    d. Residual function should be present (even with pain)

  2. Physical examination

    a. Hallmark findings are tenderness to palpation and pain with active and passive range of motion.

    b. Swelling and ecchymosis in affected limb

    c. Document vascular status of the affected limb. If compromised, consider compartment syndrome.

    d. Decreased range of motion

  3. MRI

    a. Acute: Intermediate signal on T1 and T2

    b. Subacute: Hyperintense on T1 similar to fat

    c. Chronic: Hypointense T1 and T2

D. Treatment: Protection and rehabilitation are mainstays of therapy

  1. Immediate treatment

    a. Rest, ice, compression, and elevation for the first 24–48 h after injury.

    b. Monitor for evidence of compartment syndrome or vascular compromise, which requires surgical intervention

    c. An epinephrine injection may be considered acutely to limit bleeding

  2. Recovery phase

    a. Early mobilization has been shown to decrease recovery time, after a brief period (24–48 h) of immobilization

    b. Increase range of motion gradually so as not to cause pain

    c. Excessive stretching of previously immobile limb thought to increase risk of myositis ossificans

  3. Return to play: No good evidence to guide decisions

    a. Probably not all players need to be kept from play for any longer than it takes to adequately assess the injury

    b. The larger the muscle group involved and the greater the functional limitations caused, the more likely a player will need to be removed from the game and the more time that will likely be needed for recovery

  4. Medications: Therapy is aimed at pain relief, but there is no good evidence to support any particular treatment. Acetaminophen or NSAIDs are usually the treatments of choice. See section I.D.2

  5. No role for surgery except in the case of vascular compromise

E. Prognosis

  1. Single injury allowed adequate healing time usually has good prognosis without residual injury

  2. Chronic or repeat injuries may lead to myositis ossificans (see section III).

III. Myositis Ossificans Traumatica

A. Introduction

  1. A form of heterotopic ossification that results from traumatic insult to a muscle

  2. Frequently seen with repeated contusions to a particular muscle

B. Clinical findings

  1. Firm, nontender mass that develops in muscle at the site of prior trauma, usually multiple prior traumas.

  2. May slowly enlarge until the bone center matures

  3. Bone scan is the gold standard to detect but not very specific

  4. CT (better than MRI): Peripheral calcification that is distinct from nearby bone

5. MRI
  a. Young lesion is isointense to muscle on T1 and heterogenous on T2.
  b. Mature lesion: Central area is isointense to fat on T1 and T2 (bone marrow)
C. Treatment
  1. If symptomatic, surgical resection is considered once bone has matured at 6–12 months (to minimize recurrence risk)
  2. NSAIDs (usually indomethacin) immediately in the postoperative period for a limited course.

IV. Tendon Injury

A. Anatomy and histology of normal tendons
  1. Tendon
    a. Composed of parallel fibers of type I collagen, which provide tensile strength, embedded within a proteoglycan matrix, which maintains tendon shape
    b. Not a contractile structure
    c. Contains Golgi tendon organs, which provide the afferent component of the reflex arc
  2. Fibrous sheaths
    a. Dense fibrous canal though which long tendons move
    b. Provides structural support to maintain tendon in proper anatomical location
  3. Reflection pulleys: reinforce the fibrous sheaths where the tendon course curves. The most clinically significant pulleys are located in the fingers
    a. Numbered A1–A5 from proximal to distal in the fingers
    b. A1 pulley is responsible for trigger finger and can be surgically released
    c. A2 and A4 pulleys are biomechanically the most important for finger flexion
  4. Synovial sheath
    a. Composed of two thin serous sheets with lubricating fluid between them
    b. Parietal layer adheres to fibrous sheath, and the visceral layer adheres to the tendon.
    c. The two sheets glide along each other so as to minimize friction on the tendon
  5. Paratenon
    a. Present in tendons where there is no true synovial sheath (e.g., Achilles tendon)
    b. Composed of elastic alveolar tissue to minimize frictional resistance to tendon movement
B. Nomenclature
  1. Tendonitis: Strictly speaking refers to inflammation of the tendon but frequently used erroneously to describe noninflammatory tendon degeneration or overuse conditions
  2. Tenosynovitis: Inflammation of the synovial sheath. May be related to infection
  3. Tendinosis: Noninflammatory degeneration of the tendon (see section C for further details)
  4. Tendinopathy: A term which refers to any ailment of the tendon, but it is normally used in reference to chronic tendon injury. It is thought that tendinosis is primarily responsible for most chronic tendinopathy.
C. Histology and pathophysiology of tendon injury
  1. Normal tendon
    a. Composed of large amounts of type 1 collagen to provide tensile strength with little type 2 collagen
    b. Type 1 collagen organized from small to large into fibrils, fibers, and fiber bundles
    c. Fibrils embedded within proteoglycan matrix, which provides compressive strength and maintains tendon shape (Figure 14.1)
  2. Tendon responses to activity, stress, and injury
    a. Compressive force → increased production of proteoglycan matrix rather than collagen
    b. Inactivity → decreased type 1 collagen → decreased tensile strength
      Moderate tension   increased type 1 collagen   increased tensile strength

    d. Excessive tension → microtearing → collagen repair and turnover → immature cross-linking → mature cross-linking

3. Tendinosis

    a. Disruption of normal tendon architecture caused by repeated excessive tendon stress without adequate healing time

    b. Inadequate tendon recovery leads to a tendon with less tensile strength because of immature cross-linking and/or an abundance of proteoglycan compared with collagen

    c. Tendon may enlarge and show neovascularization

4. Tendonitis (inflammation)

    a. Local injury → acute inflammatory response → inflammation → tissue repair and regeneration → normal or altered tissue architecture

    b. Altered tissue architecture may include changes consistent with tendinosis or calcification and fibrosis

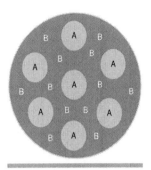

Figure 14.1 Collagen fiber containing collagen fibrils, A, surrounded by proteoglycan matrix, B.

D. Epidemiology

  1. Older athletes at higher risk, though may occur in all age groups

  2. Increased risk with diabetes

  3. Increased risk with history of quinolone use

E. Clinical features

  1. History

    a. Recent changes in activity level, terrain, or footwear

    b. Pain

      i. Progressive increase in pain over days to months without an identifiable origin suggests chronic tendinopathy

      ii. Sharp, burning, or aching pain present in both tendonitis and tendinosis

      iii. Usually well localizable

      iv. Acute onset of pain suggests tendonitis or strain

    c. Onset of pain relative to exercise in chronic tendinopathy

      i. Onset after exercise early in disease course

      ii. Onset of pain during activity or with even minor activity indicates more severe tendinopathy

    d. History of quinolone use or steroid use may predispose one to tendinosis

  2. Physical examination

    a. Normal neurovascular examination

    b. Tests for tendon integrity to rule out rupture (e.g., Thomson's Test of Achilles tendon)

    c. Normal stability and range of motion in nearby joints

    d. Enlarged tendon may be appreciated

    e. Point tenderness over affected tendon or pain with sonopalpation may help distinguish from age-related changes

    f. Exam to rule out biomechanical abnormalities

    g. Warmth, while rarely present, suggests tendonitis

  3. Imaging studies

    a. Plain films rarely useful but may show calcification of the affected tendon

    b. Ultrasound is the best imaging modality to diagnose tendinopathy.

    c. MRI has lower resolution and does not offer the dynamic testing of ultrasound but better for ruling out pathology in neighboring structures. Shows increased signal on T1 and fat

    d. Tendinosis

       i. Increased echogenicity on ultrasound compared with the contralateral tendon

       ii. No hematoma or masses

       iii. Neovascularization appreciated on Doppler imaging

       iv. Progression: Tendon thickening unchanged by dorsiflexion or plantarflexion → development of cystic collections → development of calcifications

    e. Tendonitis

       i. Fluid in tendon sheath and synovial thickening or paratenon irregularity (in Achilles tendon) on MRI and US

       ii. Hyperemia on MRI and US

F. Treatment—General principles of treatment are based upon tendon histology and reaction to injury (see section C for details). The goal is to encourage appropriate healing and relieve pain.

  1. Rest and ice, which allow for tissue regeneration and reduced inflammation

  2. Eccentric strengthening exercises, which promote increased synthesis of type 1 collagen

  3. Stretching of affected tendon, which increases flexibility and decreases risk of tearing

  4. Nonsteroidal antiinflammatory medications may be prescribed for pain relief, especially in the presence of acute pain, where inflammation is likely present. Chronic use of NSAIDs in the treatment of noninflammatory tendinopathy is controversial

  5. Return to full activity may take weeks or months. This decision is guided by the patient's symptoms; the pain should be improving

  6. Nitroglycerin transdermal administration (1–2 mg over 24 h) is used to increase nitric oxide in the tendon. This is believed to improve tendon strength by alleviating hypoxia, which plays a role in inadequate tendon healing and consequent degeneration

  7. Extracorporeal shockwave therapy may be used to help treat calcific tendinosis

  8. Recent injection therapies including sclerotherapy, autologous platelet-rich plasma or autologous whole blood are used (frequently in refractory cases) in chronic tendinopathy, where it is believed that restoration of normal tissue architecture has failed to occur. The goal of these therapies is to initiate an inflammatory response to promote tissue remodeling.

  9. Tendon rupture

    a. Treatment should be based upon functional deficits rather than anatomy (e.g., biceps long head rupture rarely requires repair)

    b. Complete ruptures (only those that impose functional deficits) will likely require surgical repair

    c. For incomplete rupture, the tendon should be protected from stress or weight bearing, frequently with a cast or splint. It should be given daily range of motion exercise within a protected range

    d. For operated tendons, a period of 1–2 weeks of rest is usually given followed by range of motion exercises with slow advancement

    e. Failure to provide range of motion may lead to contractures and also to weakened tendons

G. Prognosis and Outcomes

  1. Tendinopathy

    a. Early stage or mild tendinopathy usually carries a good prognosis if given an adequate chance to recover

    b. Continued overuse may lead to tendon rupture with a poor prognosis for return to competitive sports

    c. Sport-specific training

    d. Stretching and strengthening to correct muscle imbalances or biomechanical abnormalities

  2. Tendonitis

    a. Inflammation is typically quick to resolve

      b. Prognosis usually good if appropriate recovery opportunity is given to tendon

      c. Exercising or performing "through the pain" of acute tendonitis can lead to chronic tendinopathy and tendon damage.

V. Tendon and Tendon Sheath Tumors

  A. Ganglion cyst—Not a true tumor

    1. Epidemiology

      a. Typically seen in patients aged 20–40 years

      b. Three times more common in women

    2. Clinical Findings

      a. Uniloculated or multiloculated fluid-filled cysts adherent to tendon or to joint capsule

      b. Generally nontender

      c. Has potential to grow in size slowly over time

      d. MRI—Low signal intensity on T1 and high signal intensity on T2

    3. Treatment

      a. Aspiration—Will drain fluid within, but fibrous tissue remains with risk or recurrence

      b. Surgery is definitive treatment

    4. Prognosis and outcome

      a. Benign tumor without local invasion

      b. Surgery usually curative

  B. Giant cell tumor of tendon sheath—Benign

    1. Epidemiology

      a. Generally seen in individuals aged 30–50 but can occur in anyone

    2. Clinical findings

      a. Gelatinous-filled round nodule

      b. Small and firm nodule adherent to the tendon

      c. Most commonly seen in hand, but may be seen in lower extremities

    3. Treatment

      a. Surgical removal is the treatment of choice

    4. Prognosis and outcome

      a. Recurrence rate is high

      b. Injury in nearby joint increases recurrence risk

      c. Tumor otherwise benign.

VI. Muscle Tumors

  A. Rhabdomyosarcoma—Malignant tumor

    1. Epidemiology

      a. Incidence about six per 1 million per year

      b. Most common soft-tissue sarcoma in young children.

      c. Teenage onset tumor associated with PAX3-FKHR and PAX7-FKHR fusions

      d. Very rarely found in adults

    2. Clinical findings

      a. Rapidly growing soft-tissue mass

      b. In some cases may cause local pain and be tender to palpation

      c. Metastatic disease may present with bone pain or systemic symptoms

      d. MRI or CT is likely to show aggressive tumor along fascial plains

      e. PET scan indicated to look for metastases

    3. Treatment

      a. Surgery: Wide margin excision with limb sparing technique if possible. In metastatic disease, known metastases are also excised

      b. Adjuvant radiation and chemotherapy

4. Prognosis and outcome
   a. Moderate-to-well-differentiated tumors without deep fascial involvement have 98.8% 5-year survival rate.
   b. Metastatic disease has <20% 5-year survival

B. Desmoid tumor—Benign but very locally aggressive tumor
   1. Epidemiology and pathology—Rare in the general population
      a. 0.03% of all neoplasms
      b. Prevalence as high as 13% in patients with familial adenomatous polyposis
      c. More common in women after childbirth
      d. Usual age of diagnosis is 10–40
      e. Overgrowth of fibroblasts in the muscle
   2. Clinical findings
      a. Most commonly a seen in the shoulder, back, chest wall, or the thigh
      b. Usually no precipitating event, but sometimes local trauma is described prior to mass developing
      c. Very firm, mobile, nontender mass that does not affect the overlying skin
      d. MRI/CT—Contrast-enhancing mass with local invasion of surrounding tissues
      e. MRI—T1 and T2 low signal intensity fibrous bands
   3. Treatment
      a. MRI is the test of choice to identify the extent of invasion and plan for surgery
      b. Generally surgical excision with wide margins is the treatment of choice
      c. Adjuvant chemotherapy may also be used
   4. Prognosis and Outcome
      a. Morbidity related to disruption of local structures from tumor growth
      b. Tends to regress in menopause
      c. Low risk of recurrence if surgical margins are clear.

Recommended Reading

1. Brotz S, Wilk K, eds. *Clinical Orthopedic Rehabilitation*. 2nd ed. Philadelphia, PA: Mosby; 2003.
2. Frontera W, Silver J, Rizzo T, eds. *Essentials of Physical Medicine and Rehabilitation: Musculoskeletal Disorders, Pain, and Rehabilitation*. 2nd ed. Philadelphia, PA: Saunders/Elsevier; 2008.
3. Greene W, ed. *Essentials of Musculoskeletal Care*. 2nd ed. Rosemont, IL: American Academy of Orthopaedic Surgeons; 2001.
4. Józska L, Kannus P. *Human Tendons: Anatomy, Physiology, and Pathology*. Champagne, IL: Human Kinetics; 1997.
5. Maffuli N, Renström P, Leadbetter W, eds. *Tendon Injuries: Basic Science and Clinical Medicine*. London, UK: Springer-Verlag; 2005.
6. Stoller D, ed. *Magnetic Resonance Imaging in Orthopedics and Sports Medicine*. 3rd ed. Baltimore, MD: Lippincott, Williams, and Wilkins; 2007.
7. Weinstein S, Buckwalter J, eds. *Turek's Orthopedics: Principles and Their Application*. 6th ed. Philadelphia, PA: Lippincott, Williams, and Wilkins; 2005.

15

Bone Injuries and Conditions

Megan L. Noon, Anne Z. Hoch, and Omar Bhatti

I. Bone Matrix

A. Organic components (35% of bone weight)
1. Type I collagen fibers (90%) = tensile strength of bone
2. Ground substance—proteoglycans
   a. Glycosaminoglycan—protein complexes
   b. Promote mineralization and bone formation
   c. Compressive strength of bone

B. Inorganic components (60% of bone weight)
1. Bone salts:
   a. Calcium hydroxyapatite—primary mineral in bone
      i. Responsible for matrix mineralization
      ii. Compressive strength of bone
   b. Osteocalcium phosphate

C. Water (5% of bone weight, varies with age/location).

II. Types of Bone

A. Cortical bone (compact bone)—80% of skeleton mass
1. Basic structural unit: osteon
   a. Stress oriented: highly organized, tightly packed osteons—concentration of osteons determines the mechanical strength
   b. Concentrically arranged lamellae surround longitudinally oriented Haversian canals containing blood vessels
   c. Volkmann canals—horizontally oriented canals connecting osteons
2. Porosity: 5–10%
3. Found in the shaft of long bones; outer shell around trabecular bone at the ends of joints and the vertebrae
4. Woven bone
   a. Immature or pathologic bone—formed during embryonic development, fracture healing, and pathologic states (hyperparathyroidism, Paget's Disease)
   b. Poorly organized—composed of randomly arranged collagen bundles and irregularly shaped vascular spaces; does not contain osteons
   c. Not stress oriented; can become highly mineralized and brittle

B. Trabecular bone (cancellous bone)—20% of skeleton mass
1. Basic structural unit: trabeculae
2. Lamellae arranged longitudinally along the trabeculae
3. Porosity: 50–95%

    4. More compliant than cortical bone—distribute and dissipate energy from articular contact loads

    5. Found filling the ends of long bones; comprises the majority of vertebral bodies.

III. Cellular Biology

  A. Osteocytes

    1. Osteoblast encased in bone matrix

    2. Less bone deposition capability than active osteoblasts

    3. Play role in controlling extracellular calcium and phosphorus concentrations—directly stimulated by calcitonin, inhibited by parathyroid hormone (PTH)

  B. Osteoblasts

    1. Single nucleated cells derived from mesenchymal stem cell lineage

    2. Line the bone surfaces—disruption of cell layer activates osteoblasts

    3. Responsible for bone formation—synthesis and deposit bone matrix

  C. Osteoclasts

    1. Multinucleated giant cells derived from macrophage lineage

    2. Responsible for bone resorption—secrete acids and enzymes (collagenase) to break down bone matrix

    3. Resorption occurs in depressions, Howship's lacunae, and is more rapid than bone formation.

IV. Bone Remodeling

  A. Wolff's law—formation of bone takes place wherever stresses of pressure and tension occur in bone

  B. Bone mineral metabolism

    1. Bone—reservoir for 99% of the body's calcium, 85% of the body's phosphate

    2. Parathyroid hormone—PTH

      a. Regulates plasma calcium—PTH release is stimulated by decreased serum calcium concentrations

      b. Stimulates the kidney to increase fractional resorption of filtered calcium; promotes urinary excretion of phosphate; stimulates vitamin D conversion to its active form

      c. Net effect: increased serum calcium, decreased serum phosphate

    3. Vitamin D—1,25 active form

      a. Vitamin D from skin (UV light) or diet is hydroxylated twice (1-liver, 25-kidney)

      b. Factors promoting production: elevated PTH, decreased serum calcium, decreased serum phosphate

      c. Stimulates intestinal absorption of calcium and phosphate

      d. Net effect: increased serum calcium and phosphate

      e. Ideal serum level in athletes: 30—50

      f. Common replacement recommendations if low

        i. 50,000 IU per week × 6—8 weeks, followed by 600—800 IU daily

    4. Calcitonin

      a. Elevated serum calcium concentration increases calcitonin secretion

      b. Directly inhibits osteoclastic resorption of bone

      c. Net effect: decreased serum calcium

    5. Estrogens—prevents bone loss by inhibiting bone resorption

    6. Corticosteroids—increase bone loss by decreasing gut absorption of calcium and decreasing bone formation through inhibition of collagen synthesis

    7. Thyroid hormone—increases bone turnover, bone resorption exceeding formation.

V. Acute Fractures

  A. Location in bone

    1. Epiphyseal—end of bone, forming part of adjacent joint

   2. Metaphyseal—flared portion of the bone at ends of the shaft

   3. Diaphyseal—shaft of a long bone

B. Orientation/Extent of the fracture line(s)

   1. Transverse—fracture that is perpendicular to the shaft

   2. Oblique—angulated fracture line

   3. Spiral—multiplanar and complex fracture

   4. Comminuted—more than two fracture fragments

   5. Segmental—completely separate segment of bone bordered by fracture lines

   6. Intraarticular—fracture line crosses the articular cartilage and enters the joint

   7. Torus—buckle fracture of one cortex (often seen in children)

   8. Compression—impaction of bone

   9. Greenstick—incomplete fracture with angular deformity (seen in children)

  10. Pathologic—fracture through bone weakened by disease or tumor

C. Amount of displacement of the fracture fragments

   1. Nondisplaced—fracture fragments are in anatomic alignment

   2. Displaced—fracture fragments are no longer in their usual alignment

   3. Angulated—fracture fragments are malaligned

   4. Bayonet—distal fragment longitudinally overlaps the proximal fragment

   5. Distracted—distal fragment is separated from the proximal fragment by a gap

D. Integrity of skin and soft tissue

   1. Closed fracture—skin over and near fracture is intact

   2. Open fracture—skin over and near fracture is lacerated or abraded by injury.

VI. Fracture Healing

Primary fracture healing—cortex attempts to bridge the fracture gap, results from rigid stabilization (i.e., plate immobilization)

Secondary fracture healing—callus formation bridges the fracture gap, results from less rigid treatment methods (i.e., fracture bracing)

A. Inflammatory stage

   1. Hematoma formation: Bleeding from the fracture site provides a source of hematopoietic cells which secrete growth factors

     a. Transforming growth factor (TFG)-b, platelet-derived growth factor (PDGF)

   2. Inflammatory cells and fibroblasts infiltrate the bone under prostaglandin mediation

   3. Fibrovascular tissue forms around the fracture ends from fibroblasts, mesenchymal cells, and osteoprogenitor cells

   4. Anti-inflammatory or cytotoxic medications during the first week are detrimental (via inhibition of the cyclo-oxygenase pathway)

B. Repair stage

   1. Primary callus response occurs within 2 weeks

   2. Bridging (soft) callus can occur if bone ends are not in continuity

     a. Fibrocartilage develops, stabilizes bone ends—this soft callus is later replaced (via endochondral ossification) by woven bone (hard callus)

     b. Soft callus is weak in the first 4–6 weeks, requires adequate protection

   3. Medullary callus supplements the bridging callus

     a. Forms slowly and occurs later

   4. Amount and type of callus formation are dependent on the method of treatment (i.e., operative management, bracing, etc.)

     a. Rigid immobilization and anatomic reduction—primary cortical healing occurs, resembles normal remodeling

   b. Rigidly fixed fractures (i.e., compression plate)—direct osteonal or primary bone healing occurs without visible callus formation
   c. Closed treatment—endochondral healing with periosteal bridging callus formation occurs
C. Remodeling stage
   1. Begins during the middle of the repair phase, continues after the fracture has clinically healed (up to 7 years)
   2. Bone assumes its normal configuration and shape based on the stresses it is exposed to—Wolff's law
   3. Woven bone formed during the repair phase is replaced with lamellar bone
   4. Repopulation of marrow space completes the fracture healing
   5. Adequate strength is typically achieved in 3–6 months.

VII. Factors Affecting Fracture Healing (Table 15.1)

A. Nutrition
   1. A proper diet including all food groups in proper amounts is essential—diets deficient in calcium and protein may negatively affect fracture healing
B. Factors promoting fracture healing
   1. Vitamins A and B, thyroid hormone, growth hormone, calcitonin, insulin, anabolic steroids
   2. Weight-bearing, exercise and certain types of electric currents
C. Factors negatively affecting fracture healing
   1. Smoking, nonsteroidal antiinflammatories, diabetes, corticosteroids, denervation, irradiation.

Table 15.1   Biological and mechanical factors influencing fracture healing

Biological factors	Mechanical factors
Patient age	Soft-tissue attachments to bone
Comorbid medical conditions	Stability (extent of immobilization)
Functional level	Anatomic location
Nutritional status	Level of energy imparted
Nerve function	Extent of bone loss
Vascular injury	
Hormones	
Growth factors	
Health of the soft-tissue envelope	
Sterility (in open fractures)	
Cigarette smoking	
Local pathological conditions	
Level of energy imparted	
Type of bone affected	
Extent of bone loss	

From Brinker MR. Basic science. In: Miller MD, Brinker MR, eds. *Review of Orthopaedics.* 3rd ed. Philadelphia: WB Saunders; 2000:18.

VIII. Stress Fracture

A. Common overuse injury, partial or complete bone fracture that results from repeated application of a stress lower than the stress required to fracture the bone in a single loading

B. Incidence—0.7–20% of all injuries presenting to sports medicine clinics; less than 1% in general population

   1. Incidence varies with type of athlete—13–52% among runners

C. Etiology

   1. Sudden increase in duration, intensity, or frequency of activity without adequate periods of rest

   2. Bone remodels in response to a mechanical stress—rate and amount of remodeling depends on the number and frequency of loading cycles (Wolff's law)

   3. Imbalance between bone resorption and formation renders the bone susceptible to microfractures

   4. Under continued loading, microfractures may propagate into stress fracture

D. Risk factors

   1. Decreased bone mineral density (BMD)

   2. History of prior stress fracture

   3. Training patterns

      a. Intensity—Higher training volume, abrupt or rapid increase, higher weekly running mileage correlates with increased incidence

      b. Surface—uneven surfaces could increase risk by causing increased muscle fatigue and redistributing load to the bone. Less complaint surfaces (cement) could increase risk through higher mechanical forces being transmitted to bone during impact

      c. Footwear—athletes with old shoes (>6 months) have a higher incidence of stress fractures

   4. Female gender/Hormonal

      a. Amenorrhea/oligomenorrhea—decreased estrogen levels—increased osteoclastic activity—increased risk for fracture

   5. Leg length discrepancy noted in 70% of patients with lower extremity stress fractures

   6. Nutrition—weight <75% of ideal body weight increases risk of stress fracture

      a. Decreased calcium correlates with low BMD, not stress fractures

   7. Poor biomechanics—excessive pronation or supination

   8. Muscle mass—decreased strength and endurance is associated with increased incidence

E. Presentation

   1. Onset of localized pain initially related to activity, increasing in severity with increased activity

   2. Eventually pain with less strenuous activity and ultimately during normal ambulation (with lower limb injuries) and rest

F. Physical examination

   1. Point tenderness over affected bone, usually focal—limited to the site of injury

   2. May have soft-tissue swelling over stress fracture site in superficial areas; occasionally mild erythema or bony callus in chronic cases

   3. Maneuvers of stress to the bone at the area of pain may aid in diagnosis (Fulcrum test)

   4. Single leg hopping, hop test, may reproduce pain at fracture site

G. Location

   1. More common in lower limb weight-bearing bones

   2. Different sites depending on athlete

      a. Runners—tibia, metatarsals

      b. Throwing athletes—humerus

      c. Gymnasts—spine, foot

      d. Golfers, rowers—ribs

3. Bilateral stress fractures in 16% of cases
4. Common sites
   a. Tibia (49%)
   b. Metatarsals (19%)
   c. Fibula (12%)
5. High-risk sites—pose a problem, can progress to nonunion occasionally requiring surgical intervention
   a. Pars interarticularis of the lumbar spine
   b. Femoral neck
      i. Superior side of the femoral neck (tension side)
   c. Tibia—anterior cortex, middle third of tibia
      i. "dreaded black line" seen on plain radiographs
   d. Medial malleolus
   e. Talus
   f. Tarsal navicular
   g. Proximal 5th metatarsal
   h. Base of the 2nd metatarsal

H. Imaging
   1. Plain film radiography
      a. Poor sensitivity
      b. Typically normal for the first 2–3 weeks
      c. Periosteal elevation, cortical thickening, sclerosis, or a true fracture line are positive findings
   2. MRI (Figure 15.1)
      a. Study of choice for confirmation and definitive diagnosis
      b. Helpful in distinguishing between shin splints and stress fractures of the tibia
      c. Early in the stress fracture process MRI may show increased signal intensity secondary to edema surrounding the fracture
      d. MRI grading of stress fractures (Table 15.2)
   3. Three-phase bone scan
      a. Highly sensitive but nonspecific
   4. CT scan
      a. Preferred if extensive bony injury
   5. Single photon emission computed tomography (SPECT)
      a. Eliminates surrounding soft tissue resulting in improved detection and localization
      b. Provides axial views
      c. Commonly used for stress fractures of the spine and pelvis

I. Management
   1. Early intervention is essential to prevent further damage
   2. Conservative management for low-risk sites
      a. Protection of fracture site with reduced weight bearing and/or splinting, modification of activities
      b. Rehabilitation—ROM, proprioception, strengthening, gradual resumption of activities
      c. Risk factor reduction—evaluate for female athlete triad

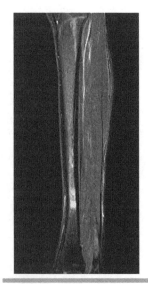

Figure 15.1 Tibia: Positive STIR image

Table 15.2   Radiological grading of stress fractures

	X-ray	Bone scan	MR image	Treatment
Normal	Normal	Normal	Normal	None
Grade 1	Normal	Poorly defined area of increased activity	Positive STIR image	3 weeks rest
Grade 2	Normal	More intense but still poorly defined	Positive STIR plus positive T2	3–6 weeks rest
Grade 3	Discrete line; discrete periosteal reaction	Sharply marginated area of increased activity focal or fusiform	Positive T1 and T2, but without definite cortical break	12–16 weeks rest
Grade 4	Fracture or periosteal reaction	More intense transcortical localized uptake	Positive T1 and T2 fracture line	16+ weeks rest

From Arendt E, Grifths H. The use of MR imaging in the assessment and clinical management of stress reactions of bone in high-performance athletes. *Clin Sports Med.* 1997;16(2):291–306.

3. Orthopedic consultation for possible surgical intervention for high-risk sites of nonunion or complete fracture.

IX. Osteochondrosis

A. Overuse syndromes associated with the development of secondary ossification or apophyseal centers or accessory ossification centers

1. Affect actively growing epiphyses, may be localized to one or more epiphysis

2. Thought to be due to lack of vascularity—result from trauma, infection, or congenital malformation

B. Common sites of osteochondrosis in children

1. Little leaguer's elbow—medial epicondyle of the humerus

  a. Repetitive throwing—medial traction and lateral compressive forces—leads to medial epicondyle fragmentation

2. Osgood–Schlatter disease—tibial tubercle

  a. Repetitive stress at the patellar tendon due to repetitive quadriceps contraction—patellar tendon traction leads to microscopic avulsion fractures at the tibial tuberosity

  b. Activity-related pain, swelling along tibial tubercle

  c. More common in males active in sports, early adolescence

3. Sever's disease—calcaneus

  a. Tenderness at the insertion of the Achilles tendon onto the calcaneus

4. Freiberg infraction—2nd > 3rd metatarsal head

  a. Localized tenderness, pain with weight-bearing

  b. Acute stage—6 months to 2 years

5. Iselin disease—5th metatarsal base

  a. Lateral foot pain with weight-bearing in early adolescence—girls 10+ years old, boys 12+ years old

  b. Prominent proximal 5th metatarsal is tender to palpation at peroneal brevis insertion, localized soft-tissue edema and erythema may be present, inversion stresses on forefoot increases pain, resisted eversion and dorsiflexion increases pain

  c. Oblique radiograph may reveal enlargement, often fragmentation of epiphysis

C. Treatment—activity modification (rest), short-term immobilization for severe symptoms, followed by functional rehabilitation of involved muscle group.

X. Bone Tumors

A. Presentation

1. Pain may be activity related, may have progressive pain at rest and at night

B. Cancers that present as musculoskeletal pain

1. Primary osteosarcoma

   a. Adolescents, male predominance

   b. Present with pain, swelling, and tenderness, eventual decrease in range of motion

      i. Seventy percent arise from the knee—(should be included in differential for non-traumatic knee pain), 15% from the hip or pelvis, 10% from the shoulder

   c. Most common primary malignant bone tumor

2. Chondrosarcoma

   a. Peak incidence: age 30–60

   b. Present with ill-defined, dull-achy pain and mass

      i. Proximal femur, pelvis, proximal humerus, scapula

3. Ewing's sarcoma

   a. Age range 5–25, peak incidence: age 10–20, male predominance (2:1)

   b. Present with pain, swelling and tenderness of affected site, dilated veins

      i. Pelvis, femur, tibia, humerus, scapula

   c. Elevated temperatures, elevated sedimentation rate—may be confused with osteomyelitis

   d. Onion-skin layering is classic appearance on plain radiographs

4. Giant cell tumors

   a. Age range 20–40, slight female predominance

   b. Present with nonspecific local pain, tenderness, and functional disability

Table 15.3   Bone tumor differential based on location

Epiphyseal lesions	Lesions of the spine
Chondroblastoma (age 10–25)	Older than 40 years of age
Giant cell tumor (age 20–40)	– Metastasis, multiple myeloma, hemangioma, chordoma
Clear cell chondrosarcoma (rare)	Younger than 30 years of age
	– Vertebral body—histiocytosis, hemangioma
	– Posterior elements—osteiod osteoma, osteoblastoma, aneurismal bone cyst
Diaphyseal lesions	**Multiple lesions**
Ewing sarcoma (age 5–25)	Histiocytosis
Lymphoma (adult)	Enchondroma
Fibrous dysplasia (age 5–30)	Osteoenchondroma
Histiocytosis (age 5–30)	Fibrous dysplasia
	Multiple myeloma
	Metastasis
	Hemangioma
	Infection
	Hyperparathyroidism

Combined tables from Heck RK. Tumors. In: *Canale & Beaty: Campbell's Operative Orthopaedics.* 11th ed. 2007.

      c. Distal femur, proximal tibia, distal radius

      d. Tumor can grow large, becoming palpable mass

C. Differential based on location (Table 15.3)

D. Imaging

    1. Plain radiograph—determine site of lesion

    2. CT scan

      a. Assess ossification and calcification; evaluate integrity of cortex

    3. MRI

      a. Replacing CT as the study of choice

      b. Able to determine size, extent, anatomical relationships—bone/soft tissue

      c. May yield specific diagnosis of characteristic tumors—lipoma, hemangioma, hematoma, pigmented villonodular synovitis

    4. Bone scan

      a. Determine activity of a lesion, presence of single/multiple lesions

      b. False negative may occur due to bone destruction without bone repair.

Recommended Reading

1. Arendt E, Griffiths H. The use of MR imaging in the assessment and clinical management of stress reactions of bone in high-performance athletes. *Clin Sports Med.* 1997;16(2):291–306.
2. Bennell KL, Brukner PD. Epidemiology and site specificity of stress fractures. *Clin Sports Med.* 1997;16:179–196.
3. Brinker MD, O'Connor DP, Almekinders LC, et al. Physiology of injury to musculoskeletal structures: 5. Bone injury. In: DeLee JC, Drez D, Miller MD, eds. *DeLee and Drez's Orthopaedic Sports Medicine*; 2009.
4. Miller MD, Kaeding CC, eds. Stress fractures. *Clin Sports Med.* 2006;25(1):1–174.
5. Wood GW. Fractures and dislocation. In: Canale ST, Beaty J, eds. *Campbell's Operative Orthopaedics*; 2007. Philadelphia, PA: Mosby/Elsevier.

Cartilage and Joint Injuries and Conditions
Brandee Waite

OSTEOARTHRITIS

I. Definition/Pathology

A. Degenerative loss of articular cartilage
   1. Excessive loads cause degeneration in an otherwise normal joint
      a. Predisposing factors: abnormal anatomy, prior trauma, or injury
   2. Begins in superficial cartilage zone, progresses to transitional zone, and finally to sub-chondral bone
   3. Additional cartilage changes: decline in chondrocyte replication, reduction in proteogly-can content, reduced size of type II collagen fibers, shortened glycosaminoglycan chains, decreased keratin sulfate concentration, and increase in proportion of chondroitin-4-sulfate (indicating immature cartilage is being produced in an attempt to regenerate lost cartilage)
   4. Cartilage matrix becomes more permeable and less stiff

B. Osteophytes (fibrous, cartilaginous, and osseous prominences)
   1. Occur around the periphery of the joints (marginal osteophytes), along joint capsule insertions (capsular osteophytes), or protrude from degenerative joint surfaces (central osteophytes)

C. Cyst-like bone cavities may form

D. Synovial fluid changes occur, causing decreased viscosity and elasticity
   1. Decreased concentration of normal molecular weight hyaluronate
   2. Increased water content
   3. Increased concentration of inflammatory mediators

E. Periarticular muscle atrophy in advanced cases due to disuse.

II. Epidemiology

A. Osteoarthritis (OA) is the most common form of arthritis in the United States

B. Affects 33% of adults, making it the most widespread disease in America

C. Risk factors: (1) age, (2) obesity, (3) prior trauma, (4) family history of OA, and (5) occupation with repetitive joint loads or high physical demands

D. Primary cause of disability, impairment, and job loss in U.S. adults

E. Prevalence higher in whites, men >45 years, women >55 years, overweight, sedentary, and persons with <8 years of education

F. Nearly 60% of people with OA are >65 years, and the incidence is increasing

G. Estimated annual cost = $65–$215 billion, including medical care, peripheral losses due to job limitations/time off, ADL limitations/care giver needs, and biopsychological issues including depression, anxiety, etc.

III. Clinical Symptoms/Diagnosis

A. Subjective: joint pain, stiffness

B. Objective: limited range of motion, deformity (e.g., genu valgum or genu varum at the knee), effusion

C. Table 16.1: American College of Rheumatology (ACR) knee OA clinical criteria.

IV. Physical Exam Findings/Tests

A. Inspection: check for malalignment, deformity, bony enlargement, asymmetry, atrophy, effusion (inflammation, if present, is usually mild and localized to the affected joint, unlike rheumatoid arthritis)

B. Palpation: tenderness to palpation at the joint lines, may also be tender over local ligaments/tendons

C. Range of motion (ROM): crepitus on motion, limitation of joint motion, sensation of pain or stiffness with ROM

D. Strength: may or may not be impaired

E. Sensation/reflexes: should be normal unless there is a history of prior surgery, which may have caused impairment

F. Special tests: compression of articular surfaces against each other/axial load with or without applied grind may cause pain.

V. Imaging Studies/Lab Tests

A. Radiographs: anterioposterior (AP) (weight bearing if examining the knee) and nonweight bearing lateral views are standard, with additional specific views by joint (Merchant's view in the knee, frog leg view in the hip, etc.), which may show decreased joint space, irregular articular surface, osteophytes, cystic change, subchondral sclerosis (see Figure 16.1)

B. Advanced imaging is not needed unless there is concern for ligament, tendon, or nonarticular cartilage (meniscus, labrum) pathology

C. Synovial fluid analysis is not crucial, but if conducted should show: viscosity—high; clarity—clear; color—straw/yellow; WBC/mm^3—200–2000, %PMN— <25; Gram stain—negative; crystals—none.

Table 16.1 **American College of Rheumatology Clinical Criteria Diagnosis of Knee OA**

Age older than 50 years
Morning stiffness for less than 30 min
Crepitus with knee motion
Bony tenderness
Bony enlargement
Lack of palpable rheumatoid nodules

At least three of these characteristics are required.

VI. Medical Management

A. There is no known cure for OA, nonsurgical treatment is aimed at symptom management, improved quality of life slowing progression of the disease

B. Nonpharmacologic management

1. Weight loss (if overweight): The Framingham study showed an increased risk of knee OA development in patients with high body mass index (i.e., 25 kg/m^2 or greater)

2. Aerobic and strengthening exercise programs

a. Aquatic exercise has been shown to benefit patients with severe arthritis or patients who are unaccustomed to exercise

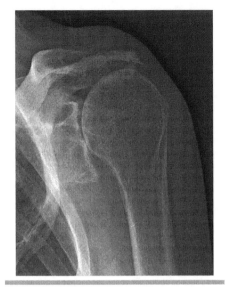

Figure 16.1   Radiograph showing osteoarthritis of the shoulder

3. Physical/occupational therapy: range-of-motion and muscle strengthening exercises

4. Assistive devices for ambulation (e.g., cane)

5. Table 16.2: additional nonpharmacologic management strategies

C. Pharmacologic management

1. Acetaminophen is first-line medication

a. Pain relief with acetaminophen similar to nonsteroidal anti-inflammatory drugs (NSAIDS) in patients with mild to moderate joint pain from OA. Has less risk of adverse gastrointestinal (GI) issues

Table 16.2   Nonpharmacologic Treatments for OA

1. Patient education: Explaining natural course and standard treatments/interventions

2. Self-management programs (e.g., Arthritis Foundation Self-Management Program)

3. Weight loss (if overweight)

4. Aerobic and strengthening exercise programs, including aquatic exercise

5. Physical/occupational therapy

6. Assistive devices for ambulation and activities of daily living

7. Patellar taping

8. Appropriate footwear/medial or lateral heel wedges

9. Bracing for comfort and subjective support (e.g., functional unloader brace, neoprene knee sleeve)

10. Joint protection and energy conservation (avoiding aggravating activities)

2. If symptoms not adequately improved with acetaminophen, trial of NSAIDS advisable. Consider adding gastroprotective agent (e.g., misoprostol) to NSAID therapy to reduce risk of GI events

3. COX-2 inhibitors have less GI side effects, but increased risk of nonfatal stroke and nonfatal myocardial infarction with chronic use

4. Other pure analgesic oral medication options: tramadol (synthetic opioid agonist that also inhibits reuptake of norepinephrine and serotonin), opioids

5. Topical medications: capsaicin, NSAID topical creams/ointments

6. Intra-articular therapy options: corticosteroids for acute/chronic OA pain, hyaluronic acid (viscosupplementation) for chronic OA pain.

VII. Surgical Management

A. Surgical indications = failed medical management, severe pain and progressive limitation in activities of daily living (ADLs)

B. Arthroscopic debridement for knee OA is unproven

C. In appropriately selected patients who are not candidates for total joint arthroplasty, osteotomy may relieve pain and prevent OA progression

D. Total joint arthroplasty reduces pain, improves function, and is a cost-effective treatment for OA in appropriately selected patients.

CHONDRAL LESIONS

I. Definition/Pathology

A. Injury or pathology affecting cartilage structure

B. Cartilage has poor blood supply, derives nutrition from diffusion

C. Term "chondral lesion" usually indicates articular cartilage lesion, though it may be considered to include meniscal or labral tears

D. Pathology can be degenerative (from repetitive overuse) or acute (from trauma)

E. Rotational forces are the most common cause of acute injury

F. Injury occurs generally in weight-bearing regions of articular cartilage, and is four times more common in medial than lateral knee compartment

G. In adults, the tidemark zone is the weak link between the overlying cartilage and subchondral bone and therefore shearing injuries most often produce a chondral injury rather than an osteochondral injury

H. Can occur in any joint, but most prominent in the knee, hip, ankle, and shoulder

I. Table 16.3: Outerbridge classification scheme.

Table 16.3   Outerbridge Classification of Chondral Lesions

Grade 0: normal cartilage

Grade I: cartilage with softening and swelling

Grade II: a partial-thickness defect with fissures on the surface that do not reach subchondral bone or exceed 1.5 cm in diameter

Grade III: fissuring to the level of subchondral bone in an area with a diameter more than 1.5 cm

Grade IV: exposed subchondral bone

II. Epidemiology

A. 60% of patients undergoing arthroscopy have chondral or osteochondral lesions
1. 30% are isolated lesions
2. Patellar articular surface (36%) and the medial femoral condyle (34%) are the most frequent location of cartilage lesions
3. Most lesions are Outerbridge Grade II (42%)
4. Most common associated lesions are the medial meniscus tear (37%) and anterior crucial ligament injury (36%).

III. Clinical Signs and Symptoms

A. Intermittent locking, recurrent effusions, crepitus, and persistent pain.

IV. Physical Exam Findings/Tests

A. Inspection: normal or with effusion

B. Palpation: tenderness over articular surface or joint line

C. ROM: may be impaired if loose body or free flap of cartilage blocks movement

D. Strength: may or may not be impaired

E. Sensation/reflexes: normal

F. Special tests: (+) McMurray's test = meniscal tear in the knee; other load and shift or load and pivot type maneuvers, which produce a "clunk" or sensation of instability at the joint may suggest cartilage injury.

V. Imaging Studies/Lab Tests

A. Plain radiographs = normal in low-grade lesions, may show defect in high-grade lesions, osteochondral lesions, or if there is a loose body

B. MRI = 30–85% sensitive and 85–99% specific for chondral lesions

C. Athroscopy is currently the gold standard for detecting chondral lesions.

VI. Medical Management

A. Oral analgesics or NSAIDS for pain management

B. Intra-articular corticosteroid injection for pain management

C. Bracing for joint unloading (i.e., valgus unloading knee brace).

VII. Surgical Management

A. Mosaicplasty/osteochondral autologous transplantation (OATs) procedure:
1. Harvest small circular (4–8 mm) autologous grafts from nonweight-bearing regions of the knee, and transplanting the grafts in a mosaic pattern in the lesion until the osteochondral defect is filled
2. Indications = age <45 years, chondral/osteochondral defects <2 cm

B. Arthroscopic debridement or microfracture

C. Allograft
1. Indications = age <30 years, chondral/osteochondral defects >2 cm
2. Graft needs to be harvested within 24 h of death.

OSTEOCHONDRAL LESIONS

I. Definition/Pathology

A. Osteochondral defect: complete or incomplete separation of the joint cartilage and subchondral bone

B. Osteochondritis dissecans (OCD): unknown etiology, characterized by degeneration and recalcification of articular cartilage and underlying bone
   1. Subchondral bone undergoes necrosis while overlying cartilage remains intact to variable degrees
C. Osteochondral defect: usually a traumatic injury in skeletally mature people, but may be undiagnosed "persistent" OCD
D. OCD: a condition of adolescents caused by an interaction between repetitive trauma and a genetic predisposition to the problem
E. Most common location in the knee for both conditions is the lateral aspect of the medial femoral condyle, but is also common in the talar dome and humeral capitellum (capitellar lesions seen in baseball players and gymnasts).

II. Epidemiology

A. OCD incidence: 15–30 cases per 100,000 persons, more common in males between 10 and 20 years of age
B. OCD incidence appears to be increasing in women and in younger children, perhaps because of increasing involvement in organized sports
C. 20–30% of cases are bilateral.

III. Clinical Signs and Symptoms

A. Pain and swelling
B. Intermittent locking or catching if a loose body is present.

IV. Physical Exam Findings/Tests

A. Same as in chondral lesions
B. Special tests: Patients with knee OCD may walk with affected limb in tibial external rotation or have a positive Wilson's sign (pain provoked by extending the knee from 90° to 0° of flexion with the tibia internally rotated).

V. Imaging Studies/Lab Tests

A. Plain radiographs may demonstrate the osteochondral lesion or a loose body (see Figure 16.2)
   1. Knee = AP, posteroanterior (PA) tunnel, lateral, and Merchant's views
      a. OCD usually located on the lateral aspect of the medial femoral condyle and are seen on the PA tunnel view
   2. Ankle = AP, mortise view, lateral
      a. May require ankle plantar or dorsiflexion with mortise view films to identify OCD lesions on the posterior or anterior talar dome, respectively
B. Table 16.4: Berndt and Harty OCD Scale
C. If radiographs are negative, consider repeat radiographs in 2–4 weeks
D. OCD lesions evident on radiographs should be staged for stability with MRI
   1. MRI has 97% sensitivity for detecting unstable lesions

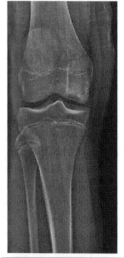

Figure 16.2 **Radiograph showing OCD of the knee**

Table 16.4   Berndt and Harty Scale: Radiographic Classification of
Osteochondral Lesions

I: Small area of compression

II: Partially detached osteochondral lesion

III: Completely detached, nondisplaced fragment

IV: Detached and displaced fragment

E. Bone scan or MRI may be ordered if symptoms persist 8–12 weeks with negative radiographs.

VI. Medical Management

A. Modified weight bearing can be used in stable cases

B. Approximately one half of lesions resolve in 10–18 months with conservative measures

C. Prognosis of OCD worsens with age and physeal closure.

VII. Surgical Management

A. Indicated for unstable lesions or persistent symptoms

B. Berndt and Harty Scale III and IV lesions

C. Arthroscopic debridement, microfracture, allograft, or removal of loose body.

CHONDROCALCINOSIS

I. Definition/Pathology

A. Acute arthritis (usually monoarthritis) caused by crystal deposition
1. Gout—monosodium urate crystals, associated with elevated uric acid
2. Pseudogout (aka calcium pyrophosphate dihydrate [CPPD])—calcium pyrophosphate dihydrate crystals; may occur in up to 72% of cases of hemochromatosis
3. Gout and CPPD are most common, but other acute crystal induced monoarthritis include calcium oxalate (especially in patients who are receiving renal dialysis) and calcium hydroxyapatite

B. Crystals activate the humoral and cellular inflammatory processes.

II. Epidemiology

A. Pseudogout is most common in the knee and wrist, while gout is most common in the great toe and knee.

III. Clinical Signs and Symptoms

A. Rapid onset of pain, edema and erythema over hours to days (without trauma) usually indicates an infection or a crystal-induced process.

IV. Physical Exam Findings/Tests for Acute Chondrocalcinosis

A. Inspection: effusion

B. Palpation: exquisitely tender, may be warm or hot

C. ROM: limited by pain and effusion

D. Strength: may or may not be impaired due to pain

E. Sensation/reflexes: normal

F. Special tests: none specific for chondrocalcinosis

G. Chronic cases present similarly to OA (see section on osteoarthritis).

V. Imaging Studies/Lab Tests

A. Arthrocentesis: synovial fluid collection/analysis is mandatory for diagnosis
 1. >2,000 WBC per mm^3
 2. Gout—polymorphonuclear leukocytes and intracellular monosodium urate crystals
  a. Monosodium urate crystals observed using polarized light microscopy are needle shaped and negatively birefringent
  b. If fluid analysis is negative and gout is highly suspected, repeat arthrocentesis and synovial fluid analysis 5 h to 1 day later
 3. Pseudogout/CPPD—calcification of cartilage or meniscus on plain radiographs is pathognomonic for diagnosis of pseudogout
  a. CPPD crystals observed using polarized light microscopy are rhomboid or rod shaped and positively birefringent.

VI. Medical Management

A. Acute treatment
 1. NSAIDs: most favored treatment for acute attacks
  a. Indomethacin (Indocin) is generally the drug of choice, but other NSAIDs can be used
 2. Corticosteroids: by intra-articular injection
  a. Systemic corticosteroids used only when NSAIDs are contraindicated or not effective

B. Chronic management of pseudogout/CPPD is similar to management of OA, with added screening for certain comorbidities (see "Prevention" below).

VII. Surgical Management

A. Synovectomy or joint replacement indicated in advanced disease.

VIII. Prevention

A. Pseudogout/CPPD: Screen for hemochromatosis, hyperparathyroidism, hypomagnesemia, hypophosphatasia, hypothyroidism, and familial hypercalcemia.

AVASCULAR NECROSIS

I. Definition/Pathology

A. Also known as AVN, osteonecrosis, or aseptic necrosis

B. Caused by impairment of blood supply to bone, causing bony death/necrosis

C. Initial osteocyte death followed by bony structural collapse

D. Occurs primarily in areas where vascular supply is precarious: femoral head, body of talus, scaphoid, lunate, and head of second metatarsal

E. May occur as sequelae of chronic corticosteroid exposure, trauma (femoral neck fracture, hip dislocation surgery), disease (coagulopathy, gout, diabetes, sickle cell, Gaucher's disease, decompression sickness, slipped capital femoral epiphysis [SCFE], Legg–Calve–Perthes disease, posttransplant, HIV), pregnancy, radiation treatment or chronic alcohol use/abuse.

II. Epidemiology

A. Hip AVN incidence: 10,000–20,000 per year in the United States
 1. Most common in third through fifth decade of life or in childhood/adolescence if associated with SCFE or Legg–Calve–Perthes
 2. Patients with confirmed AVN have a 70–80% chance of collapse after 3 years
 3. AVN of hips is often bilateral

   B. Freiberg's disease (AVN of metatarsal head) is most common in second metatarsal, followed by third and fourth

     1. Adolescent female:male ratio is 3–4:1

     2. More common if 1st metatarsal is shorter than 2nd metatarsal

   C. Kienbock's disease (AVN of the lunate) typically affects gymnasts, men with labor jobs, age between 20 and 40, ulnar negative variance, 20% incidence following lunate fractures.

III. Clinical Signs and Symptoms

   A. Hip: pain with weight bearing, antalgic gait, stiffness in hip

   B. Freiberg's: pain, tenderness, swelling, and stiffness in MTP joint; pain wearing high-heeled shoes

   C. Kienbock's: wrist pain/stiffness, may radiate to forearm, reduced grip strength.

IV. Physical Exam Findings/Tests

   A. Inspection: likely normal

   B. Palpation: hip provocative maneuvers positive, tender over affected bone in foot or wrist

   C. ROM: limited in affected joint (especially internal rotation of hip and extension of wrist)

   D. Strength: may or may not be impaired

   E. Sensation/reflexes: should be normal

   F. Special tests:

     1. Hip: hip/groin pain with FADIR (flexion, adduction, internal rotation), pain with FABER (flexion, abduction, external rotation), pain with resisted straight leg raise, Trendelenburg gait

     2. Foot: pain with palpation, forefoot squeeze, toe walking/toe raises

     3. Wrist: pain with palpation, passive wrist extension, passive middle finger extension.

Table 16.5   Ficat Stages of AVN in the Femoral Head

Stage 0: preclinical	X-ray: normal MRI: normal Clinical symptoms: none
Stage I: preradiographic	X-ray: normal or minor osteopenia MRI: edema Bone scan: increased uptake Clinical symptoms: pain typically in the groin
Stage II: precollapse (diffuse osteoporosis, sclerosis, cysts)	X-ray: mixed osteopenia and/or sclerosis MRI: geographic defect Bone scan: increased uptake Clinical symptoms: pain and stiffness
Stage III: collapse (abnormal contour of head)	X-ray: crescent sign and eventual cortical collapse MRI: same as X-ray Clinical symptoms: pain and stiffness $\pm$ radiation to knee and limp
Stage IV: osteoarthritis (flattened contour, decreased joint space)	X-ray: end stage with evidence of secondary degenerative change MRI: same as X-ray Clinical symptoms: pain and limp

V. Imaging Studies/Lab Tests

A. Radiographs may show bony deformity depending on site of AVN

1. Hip: AP view may show flattening and sclerosis of femoral head; frog leg views may show crescent sign/Caffey's sign (represents collapse of subcortical/medullary bone)

   a. Table 16.5: Ficat stages of femoral head AVN

2. Freiberg's: increased density and flattening of the metatarsal head, collapse, cystic changes, and widening of the MTP joint

3. Kienbock's: ulnar negative variance, lunate sclerosis

B. MRI is the preferred method for diagnosis of occult AVN, since it is more sensitive than bone scan or plain films (see Figure 16.3)

1. High incidence of bilateral AVN in nontraumatic etiologies, MRI may pick up AVN in opposite asymptomatic hip.

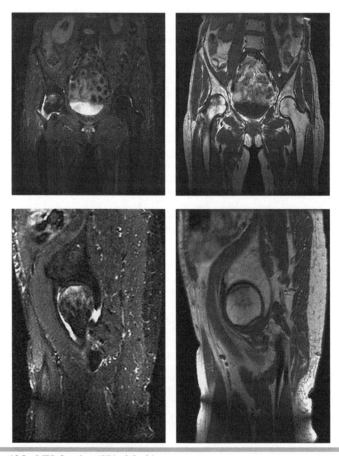

Figure 16.3   MRI showing AVN of the hip

VI. Medical Management

A. Hip: may be considered in Ficat stages I, II, and III
   1. Anticoagulants (enoxaparin) and bisphosphanates (alendronate)

B. Freiberg's: initial management includes proper foot wear w/ metatarsal bar or pad placed beneath the involved bone; limit activity for 4–6 weeks
   1. For severe symptoms consider immobilizing foot in short leg walking cast or boot until symptoms subside, usually in 3–4 weeks

C. Kienbock's: initial treatment consists of immobilization of the wrist for up to 12 weeks and analgesic medication.

VII. Surgical Management

A. Hip: Core decompression and bone grafting, arthroplasty (total vs. resurfacing)

B. Freiberg's: surgical intervention (removal of the metatarsal head) is rare, reserved for failure of conservative treatment with severe persistent pain

C. Kienbock's: if collapse is noted, then radiocarpal fusion or replacement of the lunate with a prosthesis.

ACUTE LIGAMENT INJURIES

I. Definition/Pathology

A. Traumatic sprain or tear of ligament, causing edema or disruption of ligament fibers

B. Can occur to any ligament when forces transmitted are beyond tensile strength of ligament, causing either mid-substance or avulsion injury

C. Table 16.6: Ligament injury grading scale.

II. Epidemiology

A. Varies depending on site of lesion, but common in adolescents and adults

B. If joint has been subluxed or dislocated, potential for acute ligamentous injury is high; however, ligament injuries may occur with shearing or twisting forces that do not cause dislocation.

III. Clinical Signs and Symptoms

A. Acute pain, swelling, and sensation of instability may have bruising

B. Urgent evaluation is recommended for patients with a high level of pain, rapid onset of swelling, coldness or numbness in the injured limb, inability to bear weight, or a complicating medical condition.

Table 16.6   Grading of Acute Ligament Injuries

Sign/Symptom	Grade I	Grade II	Grade III
Pain	Minimal	Moderate	Severe
Swelling	Minimal	Moderate	Severe
Ecchymosis[a]	Uncommon	Common	Frequent/all
Difficulty WB	None	Common	Frequent/all
Ligament tear	Minimal	Moderate	Complete

[a]Ecchymosis may not be seen with deep ligament injuries.

IV. Physical Exam Findings/Tests

A. Inspection: normal or may have swelling, deformity, or ecchymosis

B. Palpation: tender in region of injured ligament

C. ROM: may be limited due to pain, swelling, or subluxation/dislocation

D. Strength: likely impaired due to pain

E. Sensation/reflexes: should be normal

F. Special tests: vary depending on site of lesion; laxity noted when ligament is stressed. Examples:
1. Valgus and varus stress tests for collateral ligaments of elbow or knee
2. Lachman's or anterior drawer for anterior cruciate ligament (ACL)
3. Watson's test for scapholunate instability.

V. Imaging Studies/Lab Tests

A. Plain radiographs may be normal or show abnormal alignment

B. MRI is the gold standard imaging study for many ligament injuries.

VI. Medical Management

A. Conservative treatment for partial tears or certain complete tears (covered in individual chapters)

B. Protection, rest, ice, compression, and elevation (PRICE)

C. Active ROM and isometrics should usually begin within 48–72 h of injury

D. As pain subsides, patient begins targeted strengthening, physical therapy, endurance training, sport-specific drills, and training to improve functional stability

E. Supportive orthotics/bracing for stability can be used throughout medical management, weaning out of these devices as tolerated.

VII. Surgical Management

A. Early referral to an orthopedic surgeon in cases of bony avulsion, multiple ligament tears in one joint, gross instability, and any complete or partial tears that fail medical/conservative management.

VIII. Prevention

A. Appropriate strength training, alignment, technique, and protective equipment.

CHRONIC LIGAMENT INJURIES

I. Definition/Pathology

A. Nontraumatic, overuse ligament injury, causing edema or disruption.

II. Epidemiology

A. Seen in patients with chronic repetitive ligament loading/stressing

B. Incidence may be increased in patients with diabetes due to impaired healing.

III. Clinical Signs and Symptoms

A. Buckling, "clunking," or sensation of mechanical instability in affected joint

B. Pain associated with movements that stress the affected ligament.

IV. Physical Exam Findings/Tests

A. Inspection: usually normal, may have mild swelling

B. Palpation: tender over the affected ligament

C. ROM: full, possibly hypermobile

D. Strength: may or may not be impaired

E. Sensation/reflexes: normal

F. Special tests: same as in acute ligament injuries.

V. Imaging Studies/Lab Tests

A. Same as in acute ligament injuries.

VI. Medical Management

A. Oral analgesics

B. Activity modification, ensure normal movement patterns/technique

C. Closed kinetic chain and proprioceptive exercises

D. Supportive orthotics/bracing.

VII. Surgical Management

A. Surgical intervention may be warranted in cases when medical management fails to adequately resolve symptoms in an active patient.

Recommended Reading

1. Brophy RH, Silvers HJ, Mandelbaum BR. Anterior cruciate ligament injuries: Etiology and prevention. *Sports Med Arthrosc.* 2010;*18*(1):2–11.

2. Crosby J. Osteoarthritis: Managing without surgery. *J Fam Prac.* 2009;*58*(7):354–361.

3. Daniels JM, Dorsey JK. Arthritis update. FP essentials™, Edition No. 371, Leawood, Kansas. American Academy of Family Physicians; April 2010.

4. Eggebeen AT. Gout update. *Am Fam Physician.* 2007;15:76(6):801–808.

5. Ivins D. Acute ankle sprain: An update. *Am Fam Physician.* 2006;15;74(10):1714–1720.

6. McCauley TR. MR imaging of chondral and osteochondral injuries of the knee. *Radiol Clin North Am.* 2002;*40*(5):1095–1107.

7. Peck D. Pelvis, hip and upperleg. In: McKeag D, Moeller JL, eds. *ACSM's Primary Care Sports Medicine.* 2nd ed. Philadelphia, PA: Lippincott, Williams & Wilkins; 2007:447–460.

8. Pittman J, Bross M. Diagnosis and management of gout. *Am Fam Physician.* 1999;*59*(7):1799–1806.

9. Sitik T, Foye PM, Stiskal D, Nadler R. Osteoarthritis. In DeLisa J, Gans B, Walsh N, eds. *Physical Medicine & Rehabilitation Principles and Practice.* 4th ed. Philadelphia: Lippincott Williams & Wilkins; 2005:765–786.

10. Watson RM, Roach NA, Dalinka MK. Avascular necrosis and bone marrow edema syndrome. *Radiol Clin North Am.* 2004;*42*(1):207–219.

17

Fracture and Dislocation Management
Christopher A. Gee and Stuart Willick

FRACTURE MANAGEMENT

I. Principles of Fracture Management

A. Introduction
   1. Approximately 70% of primary care providers are involved in nonoperative fracture management
   2. Up to 70% of all fractures can be treated nonoperatively
   3. Fractures and dislocations make up 1.6% of all visits and rank 14th of the top 20 diagnoses seen in primary care
   4. Most common adverse outcome is missed diagnosis with resulting delay in treatment and referral
   5. Accurate fracture identification is the first step in deciding whether to treat a fracture nonoperatively or to refer

B. Bone composition (see Chapter 15 for more details)
   1. Consists of cells embedded in extracellular matrix of minerals and organic elements
   2. Primarily type I collagen
   3. Periosteum invests outside of bone in layer of strong fibrous tissue

C. Fracture healing—three continuous phases
   1. Phase one—Inflammation: Shortest phase; consists of release of inflammatory mediators and vasoactive substances that attract inflammatory cells. Bleeding from the ends of the fractured bones leads to formation of a hematoma
   2. Phase two—Repair: Hematoma serves as the scaffolding with various chemotactic factors that attract fibroblasts to begin the formation of a soft callous around the fracture site. After 2–3 weeks the soft callous begins mineralization as osteoblasts begin to lay down new bone. This process creates the hard callous that further stabilizes the fracture
   3. Phase three—Remodeling: Final phase, begins approximately 5–6 weeks after injury. Consists of replacement of irregular woven bone by lamellar or mature bone. Osteoclasts remove unnecessary bone and replace with bone that is more appropriately laid down along lines of physical stress and strain

D. Factors that influence healing
   1. Age: Younger patients tend to lay bone more quickly and heal faster
   2. Fracture issues: Contamination (open fractures), extensive soft tissue damage, vascular injuries, inadequate blood supply, soft tissue interposed between fracture fragments can all lead to impaired or delayed healing
   3. Nutritional status: Fracture healing requires adequate intake of protein, vitamins (C, D), and minerals (calcium)

4. Patient comorbidities: Diseases affecting vasculature (diabetes, atherosclerosis), osteoporosis, smoking, and chronic steroid use can all negatively impair bone healing
5. Proper stabilization through splinting and casting can lead to improved healing. Nonunion occurs when fragments fail to form solid osseous bridge. Delayed union occurs when fragments take an excessively long time to heal. Malunion is when a fracture has healed in an incorrect position.

II. Radiologic Description of Fractures

A. Description is key
   1. Describe findings anatomically—use landmarks for positioning (styloids, tuberosities, joints, malleoli, condyles, etc.)
   2. Describe location as distal versus proximal, lateral versus medial, dorsal versus volar/plantar, long bone location (midshaft, distal, proximal, thirds, etc.)
   3. Keys to describe: location, angulation, displacement, orientation, simple versus comminuted, open versus closed
B. Long bone anatomy (see Figure 17.1)
   1. Diaphysis = shaft of bone
   2. Epiphysis = one end of a long bone
   3. Metaphysis = growth plate region
   4. Medullary cavity = marrow cavity
   5. Cortex = compact outer part of bone that surrounds the medullary cavity
   6. Endosteum = lining of marrow cavity
   7. Periosteum = tough membrane covering bone but not cartilage
C. Alignment (angulation)
   1. Relationship of fragments along the long axis of the bone
   2. Degree of angulation of the distal fragment in relation to the proximal fragment. Can also describe as apex of angle volar or dorsal
D. Position (displacement)
   1. Defined as the relative surface of contact between the fracture surfaces
   2. Amount of displacement is partial or complete. Describe percentage of surface (or mm or cm) displaced (compare cortices)
E. Orientation
   1. Transverse—The fracture line runs 90° to the long axis of the bone. Usually produced by a bending force applied directly to the fracture site
   2. Oblique—The fracture line runs at an angle less than 90° to the long axis of the bone. Caused by torsional force applied at angle to fracture site
   3. Spiral—Produced by twisting or rotational forces. Fracture line "spirals" along long axis of bone
F. Rotation
   1. Described clinically by looking at the fractured limb and radiographs
   2. Defined as rotation around the long axis of the bone

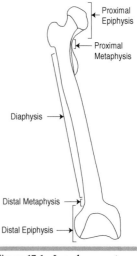

Figure 17.1   **Long bone anatomy**

G. Shortening/distraction
  1. Fragments overriding each other
  2. Impaction—two fracture fragments or two bones compressed into one another
  3. Separation—fragments have been pulled away from one another and a gap is interposed between fracture fragments

H. Other fracture types
  1. Open versus closed—Open fractures (compound) have contacted the external environment. Most commonly seen in high-impact trauma. High risk for infection and thus need emergent wash out in operating room and antibiotics
  2. Torus (buckle)—Caused by a compression force along the long axis of a child's bone that essentially creates a buckle of the cortex. Named after the small semicircular convexity near the ends of classical Roman columns
  3. Stress—Caused by repetitive overuse and stress of a bone leading to microfracture. Risk factors include acute change in training routine, footwear or fitness level, as well as overall body composition, bone density, and hormonal/nutritional factors. (see Chapter 15 for details)
  4. Greenstick—An incomplete long bone fracture seen in children due to increased bone elasticity. Only one cortex of the bone actually fractures
  5. Pathologic—This type of fracture occurs at the site of a bone that has been weakened by osteoporosis, tumor, or infection. Also called an "insufficiency fracture" or "osteoporotic fracture."

III. Fracture Reduction Techniques

A. Many different techniques exist; yet they often follow the same principles. The type of reduction technique used depends on a number of factors
  1. Training and level of comfort of the individual provider
  2. Clinical policies and resources (including availability of portable fluoroscopy, nursing support for patient monitoring, and on-site orthopedist)
  3. Presence of neurovascular emergencies
  4. Integrity of soft tissues. Closed fractures can be managed with manual reduction after anesthesia. Open fractures require surgical irrigation, stabilization, and closure

B. Anesthesia
  1. Patient comfort is an important part of a successful fracture reduction. Not only does anesthesia provide much needed pain relief to a suffering patient, but also helps to relax the patient's spasming muscles, which allows for an easier reduction
  2. Techniques:
     a. Local nerve blocks: Depending on the location of the fracture, a small amount of anesthetic injected proximally around the nerve providing innervation to the area can provide adequate relief during a reduction
     b. Hematoma block: This is when a small amount of anesthetic is injected into the fracture site itself using sterile technique. The syringe plunger is pulled back when entering the fracture to aspirate a small amount of the hematoma and thereby confirm proper placement. Especially useful in forearm fractures
     c. Bier block: Technique named after August Bier where the blood is squeezed out of an injured extremity, then a tourniquet is placed. Anesthetic is injected into a vein distal to the tourniquet. This provides anesthesia to the affected limb and allows for fracture reduction
     d. Procedural sedation: While this requires intensive resources and monitoring, it can provide maximal pain and anxiety control when a difficult and prolonged reduction is necessary. This is usually performed in the hospital setting where resources are available. A wide variety of medications can be used, including fentanyl, midazolam, propofol, or ketamine

C. Reduction
   1. Patient positioning: Provider should ensure that the patient is in the best position to perform the reduction properly. Usually this is recumbent on a bed so that if the patient does lose consciousness, they do not fall to the ground. It is important to ensure proper bed height to maximize leverage
   2. Casting/splinting: Make sure to obtain all necessary casting or splinting supplies prior to the reduction. The unaffected opposite limb can be measured for proper splint size. Usually, splinting is performed acutely so that subsequent swelling of the limb can occur without restriction
   3. Prereduction in-line traction: As much as is possible, weights (5–15 lbs) should be placed on the limb (after anesthesia) for 15 min in line with the fracture. This can lead to improved alignment of fracture fragments, and less movement required by provider
   4. Traction/countertraction: Once ready to reduce, the provider should have an assistant provider countertraction at the joint proximal to the fracture. The provider then firmly grasps the distal end of the fracture and "accentuates the deformity." By recreating the injury pattern, the provider unlocks any overlapped bone fragments and frees them to be reduced. After this the provider gives axial in-line traction to "pull the fracture" back out to the anatomic length. This may require several attempts and a good amount of feel and experience is required to know when a bone is properly aligned. It is important to limit the attempts to one with the most experienced provider attempting when the fracture involves an open growth plate
   5. Position check: While visual inspection is an important method of assessing proper alignment, other modalities can be particularly useful. Performing a quick fluoroscopic check in two planes with a portable C-arm can verify anatomic reduction. In some instances, bedside ultrasound may be useful in assessing cortical regularity after a reduction. It is important for the provider to maintain the reduction with firm pressure across the fracture site during these position checks
   6. Splinting:
      a. Fiberglass or plaster can be used, but any splint should do the following:
         i. Completely cover the length of the fractured bone
         ii. Cover the joint above and below to ensure maximal immobilization (for unstable fractures)
         iii. Adequately pad bony prominences
         iv. Immobilize the extremity in a position of function (i.e., the hand should be grasping, the elbow and ankle at 90°)
      b. Once an adequate splint has been applied, postreduction x-rays should further evaluate for adequacy of reduction. Near anatomic alignment is often necessary
   7. Neurovascular exam should be performed before and after any reduction.

IV. Indications for Referral

A. While the majority of fractures can be managed without specialty consultation or referral, it is important to know when and what to refer for orthopedic evaluation
B. Principles of referral
   1. Avoid managing any fracture outside of your comfort zone. If you feel unsure of how to manage the fracture, you should likely get some help
   2. Any open fracture should be referred to an orthopedist for surgical wash out and repair
   3. Any fracture with neurovascular compromise should be evaluated urgently by an orthopedist
   4. Significantly comminuted fractures often need orthopedic referral
   5. Complex intra-articular fractures often need open repair to adequately reduce and stabilize the fracture fragments. Unless the provider is comfortable managing such injuries, referral should be considered

6. Any fracture that cannot be adequately reduced; these often have intervening soft tissue and need operative reduction. This may include more than minor displacement of fractures that involve a joint surface. Even a few millimeters can lead to significant joint arthritis

7. Patient considerations: Any patient who will likely have difficulty complying with treatment should likely be referred. This may include those patients who are high-level athletes since even a week or two of decreased rehab time after a surgical repair relative to nonoperative treatment may be beneficial to their profession.

V. Fracture Emergencies

These fracture patterns require emergent evaluation and stabilization in a center experienced in the management of these injury patterns

A. Open fractures

1. A fracture is considered to be open if there is a skin laceration overlying or near the fracture site. During the injury, bone fragments can penetrate the skin then retract prior to evaluation. These can be subtle and skin integrity should be closely evaluated

2. Open fractures are at high risk for osteomyelitis and should be aggressively managed. This includes irrigation and debridement, which occurs in the operating room for long bone fractures, but can occur in the emergency room or clinic for open fractures of the phalanges

3. Antibiotics should be administered to patients with open fractures. Earlier administration has shown improved response to treatment. Tetanus prophylaxis should also be provided

4. While a bone sticking out of the skin can be distracting, it is critical for providers to perform a thorough evaluation of each patient to ensure no other injury is present. Providers should have a low threshold for sending the patient to a higher level of care for a full trauma evaluation

5. Splinting the extremity can go a long way in comforting the patient. Oftentimes, the simple movement of the fracture causes exquisite pain and limiting this movement helps reduce pain

B. Vascular compromise

1. Each bone has numerous associated blood vessels that can be lacerated from the sharp edges of the fracture

2. Venous bleeding will be slow, but can be significant (i.e., venous plexus tearing associated with pelvic fractures can lead to massive hemorrhage)

3. Significant hemorrhage can occur into the soft tissues after a long bone fracture. Femur fractures have been known to have 2 L of blood within the fracture hematoma and surrounding areas. This can cause any patient to be hemodynamically unstable

4. Arterial injury is an orthopedic emergency. The injured artery needs to be identified and repaired prior to onset of limb ischemia

    a. Pulses distal to the injury should always be evaluated with palpation and Doppler vascular tones (if available). Any discrepancy between limbs warrants emergent referral to an orthopedic or vascular surgeon

    b. Extremity will be cool, pale, or cyanotic with delayed capillary refill

    c. If vascular injury is suspected in a deformed fracture, reduction should be immediately attempted. The bony fragments may simply impinge the vessel and proper alignment may relieve the obstruction. Full evaluation should be performed in a trauma center after reduction

    d. An evaluation of arterial pulses should be performed and documented before and after any reduction is performed

C. Nerve injury can often occur with orthopedic trauma

1. Local mild paresthesia can occur due to tissue edema or temporary stretching of the nerve during the injury

2. Most neuropraxias resolve spontaneously
3. Nerve injuries associated with penetrating or open injuries should be emergently referred. In addition, complete loss of nerve function is often serious in nature, and needs orthopedic evaluation
4. Proximal humeral fractures can often have an associated nerve injury
5. Distal nerve function should be evaluated and documented before and after reduction attempts

D. Compartment syndrome
1. Occurs when pressures within fascial compartments exceed the arterial pressures leading to impaired muscle perfusion. Myonecrosis and ischemic nerve injury occur, eventually leading to ischemic limb contracture or limb loss
2. Most commonly occurs in the lower leg or forearm where numerous separate compartments exist. However, can occur anywhere a fracture occurs within a compartment
3. Symptoms are commonly described as the six Ps
   a. Pain, pallor, pulselessness, paralysis, poikilothermia (cool), and paresthesia. Unfortunately, many of these are late findings and often patients only complain of significant pain that is usually out of proportion to exam findings
4. Compartment pressure testing should occur as soon as possible. The offending compartment can feel hard, but deep compartments are often difficult to palpate. Simple bedside compartment testing devices exist, but a clinical suspicion is needed to be aware of this diagnosis
5. Patients with compartment syndrome require an emergent fasciotomy to open the compartment and restore muscle/nerve perfusion

E. Skin tenting
1. Significant skin tenting can be identified as fracture fragments displace the skin enough to be easily visible. This causes the overlying skin to be blanched or pale and is at high risk of becoming an open fracture
2. Urgent reduction should be performed to reduce fragments to their anatomic positions

F. Significant soft tissue damage
1. When significant soft tissue damage is present, adequate bony reduction may not be achieved. These injuries are at high risk of infection, compartment syndrome, or skin breakdown. In addition, other neurovascular structures may also be involved
2. Orthopedic referral should be considered

G. Associated life-threatening conditions
1. An acute fracture not only causes pain and disability, but potentially other associated injuries can occur. These include fat embolus, pulmonary embolus, gas gangrene, or hemorrhage. Any time these entities are associated with a fracture, specialty consultation and inpatient care should be sought.

DISLOCATION MANAGEMENT

VI. Principles of joint dislocation management

A. Introduction
1. A joint is dislocated when the congruity between the two (or more) articular surfaces is disrupted
2. Dislocation involves complete separation of these surfaces while subluxation involves only partial separation
3. Usually occurs due to a large traumatic force applied across the joint proper. However, due to prior joint damage, subsequent dislocations may occur with minimal force
4. Recognition, reduction, and proper rehabilitation of the affected joint are key to long-term joint stability. Recurrent instability causes pain and functional limitations

5. Although any joint can potentially dislocate, the most common dislocated joints are shoulders (45% of all dislocations), fingers, knees, wrists, and elbows
6. Description: When describing the position of a joint dislocation, convention is to note the distal bone's position to the proximal bone (i.e., anterior hip dislocation: femur dislocates anteriorly to the acetabulum)

B. Joint composition
1. Cartilage—Articular surfaces are covered with hyaline cartilage that provides a smooth articulating surface. Synovial membranes cover joint internally and secrete the lubricating synovial fluid contained within the joint. Cartilage is avascular
2. Joint capsule—A strong capsule encases the joint providing stability throughout the range of motion. Dislocations disrupt and stretch this capsule leading to recurrent instability. Associated ligaments (i.e., MCL or LCL in knee) often lie within or near the joint capsule and provide additional joint stability
3. Static restraints—These are the finite structures that provide consistent limitation to motion through each joint's range. They include:
   a. Bony joint configuration (extensive in hip, limited in shoulder)
   b. Joint capsule—has a finite joint volume
   c. Associated ligaments that stabilize particular facets of joint movement
   d. Adhesions or cohesions from prior injuries can also provide static restraints
4. Dynamic restraints—These are the muscles surrounding the joint that provide motion restriction when contracting through the range of motion of the joint
   a. Each muscle has an axis of force that is exerted across the joint depending on its insertion and origin
   b. Muscle activity can be inhibited due to prior injury and may need rehabilitation to improve its dynamic restraint capacity

C. Factors that affect recurrence
1. Congenital factors not only lead to increased joint laxity, but may actually increase athletic performance. Since some athletes have extreme joint ranges of motion in certain positions, they may have an advantage in their chosen sport. However, these joint positions often put them at risk for dislocations. This is especially common in swimmers, volleyball players, and baseball pitchers
2. Other congenital factors like collagen laxity (Marfan's syndrome), age, or bony configuration can also put patients at risk of recurrent instability.

VII. Reduction Techniques

A. Many different techniques exist; yet they often follow the same principles. The type of reduction technique used depends on a number of factors
1. Training and level of comfort of the individual provider
2. Clinical policies and resources (including availability of portable fluoroscopy, nursing support for patient monitoring, and on-site orthopedist)
3. Presence of neurovascular emergencies

B. Anesthesia
1. Patient comfort is an important part of a successful joint reduction. Not only does anesthesia provide the much-needed pain relief to a suffering patient, but also helps to decrease muscle spasm, which allows for an easier reduction
2. Techniques
   a. Local nerve block: Depending on the location of the dislocation, a small amount of anesthetic injected proximally around the nerve providing innervation to the area can provide adequate relief during a reduction
   b. Joint injection: Injection of anesthetic (i.e., lidocaine) into a joint space can provide for adequate pain relief and allow for reduction. This is commonly performed with shoulder dislocations because the large open joint space is easy to access

      c. Procedural sedation: While this requires intensive resources and monitoring, it can provide maximal pain and anxiety control when a difficult and prolonged reduction is necessary. This is usually performed in the hospital setting where resources are available. A wide variety of medications can be used, including fentanyl, midazolam, propofol, or ketamine

C. Reduction

    1. Patient positioning: Provider should ensure that the patient is in the best position to perform the reduction properly. Usually this is recumbent on a bed so that if the patient does lose consciousness, they do not fall to the ground. It is important to ensure proper bed height to maximize leverage.

    2. Sling/brace: Make sure to obtain all necessary bracing or sling supplies prior to the reduction. Usually, the unaffected opposite limb can be measured for proper sling size. It is important to tell patients to limit the motion of the joint after reduction to prevent acute dislocation recurrence.

    3. Prereduction in-line traction: As much as is possible, weights (5–15 lbs) should be placed on the limb (after anesthesia) for 15 min in line with the dislocation. This is particularly useful for shoulder reductions in patients that cannot be sedated. Patient is placed prone on the bed with weights on the affected limb's wrist.

    4. Traction/countertraction: Once ready to reduce, the provider should have an assistant provider countertraction at the joint proximal to the dislocation. The provider gives axial in-line traction to fatigue the muscles around the joint. Usually, after traction is applied, the joint is moved in such a way as to "unhook" the bony prominence that is preventing reduction. The provider and patient will often feel or hear a clunk as the joint is reduced. Patients often have significant relief of pain.

    5. Once an adequate reduction is attained, a sling or brace is applied and postreduction x-rays should be performed to further evaluate for adequacy of reduction.

    6. Neurovascular exam should be performed before and after any reduction.

VIII. Indications for Referral

A. While the majority of dislocations can be managed without specialty consultation or referral, it is important to know when and what to refer for orthopedic evaluation

B. Principles of referral

    1. Avoid managing any dislocation outside of your comfort zone. If you feel unsure of how to manage a dislocation, you should likely get some help

    2. Most dislocations associated with a fracture should be referred to an orthopedist for evaluation

    3. Any dislocation with persistent neurovascular compromise should be evaluated by an orthopedist, usually emergently

    4. Any dislocation that cannot be adequately reduced. These often have intervening soft tissue and need operative reduction or deep sedation to reduce

    5. Patient considerations: Any patient who will likely have difficulty complying with treatment should likely be referred.

IX. Dislocation Emergencies

A. Most dislocations can be reduced urgently and managed with careful rehabilitation and activity modification. However, certain conditions increase the urgency of the injury, and emergent orthopedic evaluation is recommended

    1. Arterial compromise is a surgical emergency. The injured artery needs to be identified and repaired prior to development of limb ischemia

        a. Pulses distal to the injury should always be evaluated with palpation and Doppler vascular tones (if available). Any discrepancy between limbs warrants emergent referral to an orthopedic or vascular surgeon

    b. Extremity will be cool, pale, or cyanotic with delayed capillary refill

    c. If vascular injury is suspected, a reduction should be immediately attempted. The dislocated joint may simply be kinking the vessel and proper alignment may relieve the obstruction. Full evaluation should be performed in a trauma center after reduction

    d. An evaluation of arterial pulses should be performed and documented before and after any reduction is performed

B. Nerve injury can often occur with dislocations

    1. Local mild paresthesia can occur due to tissue edema or temporary stretching of the nerve during the injury

    2. Most neuropraxias resolve spontaneously

    3. Nerve injuries associated with penetrating or open injuries should be emergently referred. In addition, complete loss of nerve function is serious in nature, and needs orthopedic evaluation

    4. Shoulder dislocations often have associated axillary nerve injury as evidenced by subjective numbness over the lateral deltoid

    5. Distal nerve function should be evaluated and documented before and after reduction attempts

C. Knee dislocations

    1. Dislocations of the knee joint proper are rare and require significant force. Patients may refer to a patellar dislocation as a knee dislocation, and it is important to distinguish between these entities.

    2. Have a high incidence of popliteal artery injury (up to 1/3 of patients)

    3. Requires close observation and angiography to evaluate for arterial injury in a confirmed knee dislocation

    4. Can be suspected in the patient with a multiple ligament injured knee that suffered significant force to the knee

    5. Evaluate patient closely for neurovascular integrity before and after reduction.

Recommended Reading

1. Bucholz RW, Heckman JD, Court-Brown CM, Tornetta P, eds. *Rockwood and Green's Fractures in Adults (Vol. 1).* Philadelphia, PA: Lippincott Williams & Wilkins; 2010.
2. Eiff MP, Hatch RL, Calmbach WL. *Fracture Management for Primary Care.* 2nd ed. Philadelphia, PA: Elsevier Science (USA); 2003.
3. Koval KJ, Zuckerman JD. *Handbook of Fractures.* 2nd ed. Philadelphia, PA: Lippincott Williams & Wilkins; 2002.
4. National Ambulatory Medical Care Survey 1989–1990.

18

Cervical Spine Injuries and Conditions

Christopher T. Plastaras and Somnang Pang

I. Cervical Spine Injuries and Conditions: Overview

A. Anatomy: 7 cervical vertebrae (C1–C7), 8 pairs of exiting spinal nerves; lordotic curve
   1. Occiput
   2. C1—Atlas
   3. C2—Axis, transverse process can be palpated posterior to angle of mandible
      a. Odontoid process = dens—articulates with anterior arch of atlas to restrain forward translation of atlas
   4. C3—surface landmark is hyoid bone
   5. C4, C5—directly posterior to thyroid cartilage
   6. C6—landmark includes first cricoid ring and carotid tubercle

B. Spinal canal
   1. Individual variance in size
   2. Lower cervical canal diameter: 14–23 mm on lateral radiograph
   3. Methods of evaluating central stenosis
      a. Lateral radiograph: sagittal canal dimension <13 mm
      b. Torg/Pavlov ratio = ratio of the posterior vertebral body to spinolaminar line over the AP diameter of the corresponding vertebral body (see Figure 18.1)
         i. Ratio <0.8 = "significant" stenosis
         ii. Low positive predictive value; not useful in screening
         iii. This is of historical use only given one can directly assess canal size and show the source of stenosis with an MRI
      c. Functional reserve (see Figures 18.1 and 18.2a and b)
         i. T2 images on MRI used to detect the extent of protective cushioning of cerebral spinal fluid around the spinal cord

C. Motion
   1. Flexion and extension greatest at C4–C5 and C5–C6
   2. Side bending greatest at C3–C4 and C4–C5
   3. Occipital–atlantal joint and C1–C2 contribute to 30–40% of all cervical flexion and extension
   4. C1–C2 accounts for about 55% of total cervical rotation

D. Static stabilizers (Figure 18.3)
   1. Ligaments
      a. Anterior longitudinal—limits hyperextension and forward movement
      b. Posterior longitudinal—prevents hyperflexion
      c. Intertransverse and capsular—limits lateral bending
      d. Interspinal—prevents excessive rotation

    e. Supraspinal—resists spinal separation and flexion

    f. Ligamentum flavum—maintains constant disk tension, elongates with flexion and shortens with extension

2. Other structures

    a. Intervertebral disk

        i. Annulus fibrosis—outer fibrous ring that encases nucleus pulposus

        ii. Nucleus pulposus (consistency of a bar of soap)—inner gelatinous material

    b. Zygapophyseal (facet) joint capsules

        i. Synovial joints in the coronal plane (cervical spine) that restrain forward translation

    c. Uncovertebral joints (of Luschka)

        i. Not true synovial joints; arise from the posterolateral margins of the vertebral bodies C3–C7

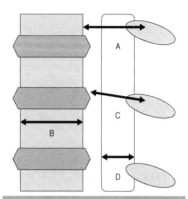

Figure 18.1   **Sagittal section through cervical canal. A = canal diameter; B = vertebral body width; C = disk level canal diameter; D = spinal cord diameter; Torg ratio = A/B; functional reserve = C–D**

3. Dynamic stabilizers/muscles

    a. Splenius capitis and cervicis: main action is extension of the head and neck; also laterally flex and rotate the head and neck to the same side with unilateral contraction

    b. Semispinalis capitis, semispinalis cervicis, and spinalis cervicis: main actions are extension and lateral flexion of the head and neck and rotation to opposite side of contraction

    c. Trapezius: arises from the external occipital protuberance, nuchal ligament, and spinous process of seventh cervical vertebrae as well as spinous process of thoracic vertebrae, to insert into lateral 1/3 clavicle, acromion process, and spine of scapula. Its main action is adduction and rotation of the scapula. It is also involved in extension of the head and neck, lateral flexion of head and neck to side of contraction and rotates head and neck away from side of contraction

    d. Sternocleidomastoid: two heads—sternal and clavicular. They act in a coordinated fashion to rotate the head opposite the side of contraction and flex the neck on the same side of contraction

    e. Anterior, middle, and posterior scalenes: The anterior and middle scalenes are involved in elevation of first rib and lateral flexion of the neck. The posterior scalene elevates the second rib

E. Testing and diagnostics

  1. Radiography

    a. Plain radiographs of cervical spine to evaluate for fractures, dislocation, instability, or foraminal stenosis (seen on oblique films)

    b. AP, lateral, obliques, odontoid (open mouth), and flexion/extension views

  2. MRI

    a. Evaluate soft tissues, including intervertebral disks, central spinal canal, foramina, functional reserve volume (cerebrospinal fluid around spinal cord), and spinal cord (see Figure 18.2)

  3. Electrodiagnostics

    a. Nerve conduction studies (NCS) and needle electromyography (EMG) are used to assess peripheral nerve conduction as well as nerve and muscle function, respectively

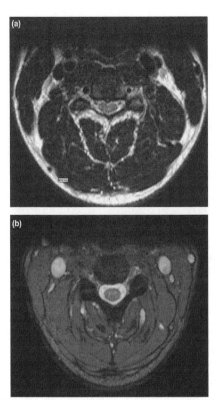

Figure 18.2   a) MRI T2-weighted axial image of C3–C4–decreased functional reserve or space available for cord. (b) MRI T2-weighted axial image of C3–C4–normal functional reserve or space available for cord.

    b. Timeline of findings in a nerve injury:
        i. 1 week—abnormal spontaneous activity detectable in paraspinals
        ii. 3 weeks—abnormal spontaneous activity present in the paraspinals and limbs
        iii. 5–6 weeks—reinnervation can occur
        iv. >6 months—increased motor unit action potential amplitude from reinnervation.

II. Diagnosis and treatment of cervical spine disorders

  A. Stingers/burners
    1. A transient neurological event lasting seconds to minutes characterized by pain, burning, or parasthesias in a single upper limb. Sometimes accompanied with weakness
    2. Precise incidence is unknown, but it is estimated that >50% of collegiate football players sustain a stinger each year
    3. A traction type trauma to the brachial plexus or nerve roots when the head is forcibly laterally tilted and extended as the contralateral shoulder is depressed
    4. May also occur from compression of nerve roots in their foramina during forced lateral neck bending or a direct blow to the brachial plexus at Erb's point

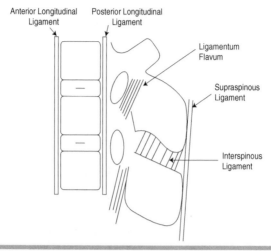

Figure 18.3   Spine ligaments: Static stabilizers

5. Upper trunk of brachial plexus (C5 and C6) most commonly involved (weakness of deltoid, biceps, infraspinatus)
6. Diagnostics
   a. Radiological studies indicated in an athlete with persistent symptoms or signs and recurrent stingers
      i. Plain films: relative value is limited but may reveal clues to pathoanatomy contributing to symptoms
      ii. MRI: most definitive study to evaluate neurologic symptoms
         (A) C-spine MRI most helpful to evaluate for foraminal stenosis or disk herniation as a source of the stinger
         (B) Brachial plexus MRI rarely needed but can evaluate for a compressing lesion of the plexus
   b. Electrodiagnostics (EMG/NCS) highest diagnostic yield ≥2 weeks after injury. Positive sharp waves and fibrillations indicate axonal injury and would prolong return to play. Sensory nerve action potential preservation, especially in the upper trunk, including lateral antebrachial cutaneous, median sensory to index finger and superficial radial sensory, are all better prognostic findings
      i. EMG testing can also help localize the lesion to the cervical spine (nerve root) versus brachial plexus
7. Treatment
   a. Remove from sport. Supportive treatment including oral anti-inflammatory medications and analgesics; ice followed by heat
   b. Return to play: full cervical range of motion, full upper extremity strength, absence of neurological symptoms
   c. Relative contraindication to return to play: symptoms lasting more than 24 h, three or more previous stingers/burners
   d. Absolute contraindication for return to play: continued neck discomfort with impaired range of motion or any evidence of neurological deficit, evidence of instability

B. Cervical cord neurapraxia (CCN)/transient quadriparesis (TQ)
   1. Definition
      a. Transient paresis (loss of motor function) and/or dysethesias in more than one limb
      b. A self-limited phenomenon with symptoms lasting typically <24 h
      c. "Burning hands syndrome"—a typical initial presentation of CCN, consistent with central cord syndrome
   2. Epidemiology
      a. Incidence in NCAA football: 7.3 per 10,000
      b. The overall recurrence rate after return to play is 56%
   3. Mechanism of injury: two
      a. Cervical hyperextension
         i. Creates functional spinal stenosis
         ii. Preexisting spinal stenosis is a significant risk factor for permanent spinal cord injury
      b. Axial loading
         i. Occurs with a slightly flexed cervical spine or spine with loss of the typical lordosis (spear tackler's spine)
            (A) Fracture–dislocation can occur
            (B) Transient compression of the anterior cord and anterior spinal artery can result in the setting of a central disk herniation
   4. Diagnostics
      a. Cervical spine radiographs—Used to assess any acute changes such as fractures, dislocations, instability. Lateral radiographs may suggest spinal stenosis using the Torg ratio (see Section I.B.3 above and Figure 18.1)
      b. MRI cervical spine—mandatory to assess stenosis and any spinal cord injury/sequelae
   5. Return to play—guidelines not uniformly accepted
      a. Absolute contraindications: more than one episode, persistent symptoms or neurologic deficit, MRI finding of cord edema, ligamentous instability, severe central stenosis
      b. Relative contraindications: one prior episode, history of mild to moderate central stenosis
C. Intervertebral disk injuries and cervical radiculitis/radiculopathy
   1. Cervical radiculitis:
      a. Process affecting the spinal nerve root, most commonly from disk herniation or foraminal stenosis
         i. Characterized as *radiculopathy* if strength deficit, reflex deficit, or if abnormal EMG
         ii. Radiating pain from neck into the arm, but can sometimes be present with pain into periscapular/shoulder area only
      b. Clinical presentation based on root level includes: see Table 18.1 and Figure 18.4

Table 18.1

Root Level	Muscle Weakness	Sensory Complaints
C5	Deltoid, biceps, infraspinatus	Lateral arm in the lateral brachial cutaneous nerve and axillary nerve distribution
C6	Deltoid, biceps, infraspinatus	Lateral forearm in lateral antebrachial cutaneous nerve distribution including thumb and index finger
C7	Triceps, wrist flexion/extension weakness	Index, middle, and long fingers
C8	Finger flexion, hand intrinsic weakness	Medial forearm in medial antebrachial cutaneous nerve and ulnar nerve distribution including little finger

2. Diagnostics
   a. Plain radiographs may demonstrate disk space narrowing and marginal osteophytes
   b. MRI may demonstrate a disk bulge or herniation and evaluate for foraminal or central stenosis
   c. EMG/NCS can be helpful in localizing a specific nerve root that is affected or to rule out other sources of limb pain and paresthesias (e.g., peripheral nerve entrapment)
3. Treatment
   a. Analgesics: NSAIDs, consider oral corticosteroids, neuromodulating agents, short course of opiates
   b. Physical therapy may include postural correction, cervical traction, and the McKenzie method (mechanical diagnosis and treatment). The McKenzie method consists of sustained postures or repeated movements and exercise for pain that is classified into one of three syndromes: derangement, dysfunction, or postural syndrome
   c. Fluoroscopically guided cervical epidural steroid injection if pain limits progress in rehabilitation
   d. Surgery indicated if progressive neurologic loss, signs of spinal cord dysfunction/myelopathy (bowel/bladder, loss of balance) or if the athlete has persistent disability due to pain
   e. Return to play once the athlete is asymptomatic with full painless range of motion of the cervical spine and no neurologic deficit

D. Cervical fractures
   1. Upper cervical spine fractures (C1–C2)
      a. Rare in sports
      b. Atlas (C1) fracture
         i. Jefferson fracture: burst fracture disrupting both the anterior and posterior arches of the atlas due to axial load
            (A) Treatment: unstable with transverse ligament rupture requires surgery

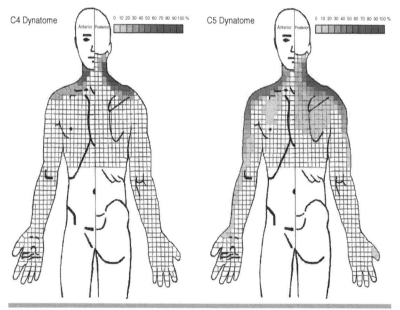

Figure 18.4 **Distribution of C4–C8 spinal nerve sensory complaints with fluoroscopically guided mechanical stimulation (dynatome).**

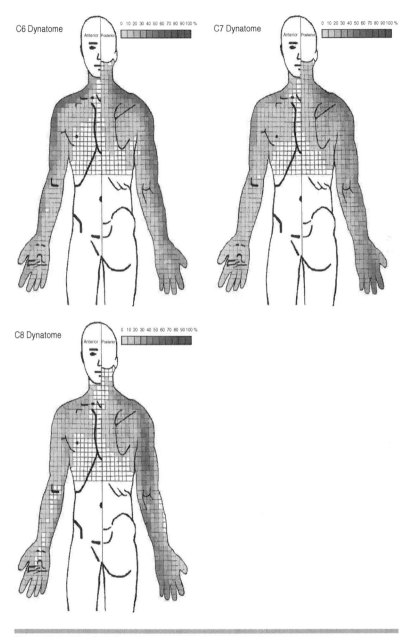

Figure 18.4 (Continued)

       ii. Posterior arch fracture alone

         (A) Treatment: brace without surgery

    c. Axis (C2) fractures

       i. Hangman's fracture: through the neural arch of C2

         (A) Hyperextension injury with a spondylolisthesis

       ii. Odontoid fractures

         (A) Type I : avulsion of the superior tip of odontoid; rare; stable

         (B) Type II : through the base; typically requires early surgical stabilization

         (C) Type III : through the body of C2

    d. Open mouth view on plain radiographs to visualize odontoid

  2. Middle cervical spine fractures (C3–C4)

    a. Rare injury; dislocation more common than fracture

  3. Lower cervical spine fractures (C4–C7)

    a. Most common cervical fractures in athletes

    b. Vertebral body compression fractures (from axial loading)

       i. Type I: simple wedge or endplate fracture

         (A) No neuro involvement

         (B) Nonsurgical management

       ii. Type II: isolated anterior-inferior body or teardrop fracture

         (A) No neuro involvement

         (B) Nonsurgical management

       iii. Type III: comminuted burst fracture

         (A) Displaced bony elements into spinal canal

         (B) Surgical stabilization

       iv. Type IV: three part fracture—fractures through anterior-inferior body, sagittal body, posterior neural arch

         (A) Associated with tetraplegia

         (B) Surgical stabilization

       v. Type V: Type IV with posterior element disruption of adjacent vertebrae

         (A) Extremely unstable

E. Ligamentous injury and instability

  1. Radiographic diagnosis

    a. Flexion–extension plain radiographs

       i. Passive: dangerous and should not be performed

       ii. Active: difficult as pain and muscle spasm may limit ROM

         (A) 30–70% of films show inadequate gross motion to determine instability

    b. CT scan if confirmation is needed

  2. Instability criteria

    a. Sagittal plane translation >3.5 mm or 20%

    b. Sagittal plane rotation >20°

F. Strains/sprains

  1. Strain: a muscular stretch injury—a diagnosis of exclusion in neck pain, as disk and zygapophyseal joint injuries can present as "muscular" pain

    a. Mostly occurs at musculotendinous junction

    b. Commonly affects trapezius, sternocleidomastoids, erector spine, scalenes, levator scapulae, and rhomboids. Results in local pain, tenderness, and weakness in the neck

    c. Imaging:

       i. Plain radiographs appropriate if there is a history of trauma, point tenderness, limited motion, or prior cervical surgery

       ii. Flexion/extension when able (after acute symptoms subside)

  2. Sprain: a ligamentous stretch injury that results from distraction to the spinal ligaments and capsular structures (zygapophyseal joints)

3. Treatment:
   a. Anti-inflammatory medications and modalities for pain
   b. Brief period of immobilizaton in a soft foam collar for severe injuries can be considered; limit to 48 h to prevent paraspinal atrophy
   c. Return to play when asymptomatic, regained neck muscle strength, and full cervical range of motion

G. Congenital anomalies
   1. Down syndrome (Trisomy 21): Atlantoaxial instability
      a. Epidemiology
         i. Affects 10–20% of individuals with Down syndrome
         ii. Symptomatic in 1–2%
      b. Athletes are screened with lateral neck radiographs in flexion and extension. The presence of an abnormally large anterior atlanto-odontoid distance (upper limit of normal is 3–4 mm) raises concern for instability
      c. Transverse atlantal ligament laxity contributes to instability
      d. Symptomatic athletes should be restricted from sports participation and are recommended for surgical stabilization
      e. Asymptomatic athletes may participate in sports on a case-by-case basis. However, the Special Olympics does restrict athletes with cervical spine instability from certain sports including diving, gymnastics, pentathlon, squat lift in power lifting, high jump, soccer, alpine skiing, swimming using flip turns, butterfly stroke, diving starts, or any competitive event or warm-up exercise that places undue stress on head and neck
   2. Klippel–Feil syndrome
      a. A congenital disorder of segmentation defects or fusion of the cervical spine, termed synostosis. There is a spectrum of phenotypic findings with more severely affected individuals having a short webbed neck with decreased range of motion and short hairline. These athletes are at risk of damage to cervical spinal cord or medulla from minor trauma due to hypermobility and instability at unfused levels
      b. Incidence is 1:40,000 with a female predilection
      c. Three types:
         i. Type 1—single fused segment
         ii. Type II—multiple fused segments, noncontiguous
         iii. Type III—multiple fused segments, contiguous
      d. Associated renal anomalies: In one study, 16 out of 41 patients (Hesinger's series) were found to have renal anomalies (hydronephrosis, solitary kidney). Renal ultrasound is an appropriate screening test.
      e. Evaluation includes cervical spine radiograph with flexion and extension to rule out instability and note location and number of fused segments
      f. Avoidance of contact sports in asymptomatic athletes. Obtain periodic flexion extension radiographs to monitor for instability
      g. Absolute contraindication to contact sports in symptomatic individuals
      h. Symptomatic treatment includes modification of activities, bracing, and surgical evaluation for progressive instability or neurologic compromise.

Recommended Reading

1. Ali FE, Al-Bustan MA, Al-Busairi WA, Al-Mulla FA, Esbaita EY. Cervical spine abnormalities associated with Down syndrome. *Int Orthop.* 2006;30:284–289.
2. Bransford R, Falicov A, Nguyen Q, Chapman J. Unilateral C-1 lateral mass sagittal split fracture: An unstable Jefferson fracture variant. *J Neurosurg Spine.* 2009;10:466–473.
3. Castro FP, Jr, Ricciardi J, Brunet ME, Busch MT, Whitecloud TS, 3rd. Stingers, the Torg ratio, and the cervical spine. *Am J Sports Med.* 1997;25:603–608.

4. Gill SS, Boden BP. The epidemiology of catastrophic spine injuries in high school and college football. *Sports Med Arthrosc.* 2008;16:2–6.
5. Herzog RJ, Wiens JJ, Dilingham MF, Sontag MJ. Normal cervical spine morphometry and cervical spine stenosis in asymptomatic professional football players: Plain film radiography, multiplanar computed tomography, and magnetic resonance imaging. *Spine.* 1991;16(Suppl):178–186.
6. Kjellman K, Oberg B. A randomized clinical trial comparing general exercise, McKenzie treatment and a control group in patients with neck pain. *J Rehabil Med.* 2002;34(4):183.
7. Oda T, Yonenobu K, Fujimura Y, et al. Diagnostic validity of space available for the spinal cord at C1 level for cervical myelopathy in patients with rheumatoid arthritis. *Spine.* 2009;34(13):1395–1398.
8. Pavlov H, Torg JS, Robie B, Jabre C. Cervical spinal stenosis: determination with vertebral body ratio method. *Radiology.* 1987;164:771–775.
9. Samartzis DD, Herman J, Lubicky JP, Shen FH. Classification of congenitally fused cervical patterns in Klippel-Feil patients: Epidemiology and role in the development of cervical spine-related symptoms. *Spine.* 2006;31(21):798–804.
10. Slipman CW, Plastaras CT, Palmitier RA, Huston CW, Sterenfeld EB. Symptom provocation of fluoroscopically guided cervical nerve root stimulation: Are dynatomal maps identical to dermatomal maps? *Spine.* 1998;23(20):2235–2242.
11. Tassone JC, Duey-Holtz A. Spine concerns in the special Olympian with Down syndrome. *Sports Med Arthrosc.* 2008;16:55–60.
12. Torg JS, Naranja RJ, Pavlov H, Talinat BJ, Warren R, Stine RA. The relationship of developmental narrowing of the cervical spinal canal to reversible and irreversible injury of the cervical spinal cord in football players. *J Bone Joint Surg Am.* 1996;78:1308–1314.
13. White A, Punjabi M. *Clinical Biomechanics of the Spine.* 2nd ed. Philadelphia, PA: JB Lippincott; 1990;67–71:184–186.

Emergency Evaluation and Management of Cervical Spine Injuries

Leah G. Concannon and Mark A. Harrast

I. Introduction

A. In all, 7–10% of spinal cord injuries occur during sports participation
1. Sporting accidents are the fourth most common overall cause of spinal cord injuries behind motor vehicle accidents, violent crime, and falls
2. In those under 30 years of age, sporting accidents are the second most common cause of spinal cord injury. The vast majority of these results in tetraplegia and approximately 60% are classified as complete injuries.

B. High-risk sports
1. Contact sports: American football, ice hockey, rugby, lacrosse
2. High-energy sports: skiing, gymnastics, diving
3. Highest total number occurs in recreational diving accidents, with the highest number in supervised sports occurring in American football
4. Incidence is higher in lacrosse, gymnastics, and ice hockey than in football
5. In American football, the total number of spinal cord injuries is highest in high school athletes, but the incidence increases with the level of the player
   a. 0.52 per 100,000 at the high school level
   b. 1.55 per 100,000 at the college level
   c. 14 per 100,000 in professional football

C. Mechanism of injury
1. In American football spinal cord injury most often results from a forced hyperflexion, such as with spear tackling. Since rule changes in 1976 that banned spear tackling, the incidence of permanent spinal cord injuries has declined.
2. Hyperextension and axial loading have both also been implicated as a cause
3. In ice hockey, checking from behind is a risk factor and is currently illegal

D. Pre-event planning for sporting events is necessary to deliver safe and efficient care
1. Formulation and practice of a standardized protocol for pre-hospital care that includes the following:
   a. Establishment of a clear chain of command
   b. Head and neck stabilization techniques
   c. Transfer of the injured player to a spine board
   d. Organization of all necessary equipment for on-field management
      i. The minimum equipment needed includes a spine board, tools for facemask removal, airway and cardiopulmonary resuscitation equipment

       e. Management of sports equipment, including when and how it should be removed

       f. Airway management

   2. Selection of a hospital for transfer of care

       a. Open channels of communication between team physician/trainer and emergency medical services as well as emergency department personnel should be established before the season starts

       b. Preseason in service training for emergency department personnel in equipment removal techniques

       c. The chosen hospital should be able to care for the critically injured athlete and provide access to spine surgeons.

II. On Field Evaluation of the Contact Sport Athlete With Altered Consciousness

  A. See Chapter 33 (Sports Cardiology) for specific details of cardiopulmonary resuscitation and care of the athlete with potential cardiogenic collapse and Chapter 30 (Exercise-Associated Collapse) for other medical causes of collapse in the unconscious athlete.

  B. All unconscious athletes should be presumed to have a cervical spine injury until proven otherwise

  C. Those athletes with altered consciousness, or significant distracting injury, and a probable mechanism should also be presumed to have a cervical spine injury

   1. Potential cervical spine injury is considered with the following:

       a. Mechanism consistent with potential for injury

          i. Spear tackle, axial load of cervical spine, hyperflexion or extension

       b. Midline cervical pain or tenderness on palpation

       c. Bilateral symptoms or signs, including paresthesias or weakness

       d. Obvious spinal deformity

  D. Early management should include cervical spine immobilization

  E. Acute management of the underlying condition should be undertaken. This may include CPR and airway management.

III. Initial Assessment of the Injured Contact Sport Athlete

  A. ABCDE of trauma care

   1. Airway

       a. Mouth guard and facemask should be removed as quickly as possible

       b. See section VI below for further description of airway management techniques

   2. Breathing

       a. High cervical injuries may inhibit phrenic nerve output and may require advanced airway management and ventilation

   3. Circulation

       a. Newer guidelines emphasize circulation as the primary goal for CPR, but without a primary cardiac event, inadequate perfusion is rare

       b. Neurogenic shock can occur with spinal cord injury

          i. Hypotension and bradycardia

          ii. Mean arterial blood pressure (MAP) should be maintained >85 mm Hg. This may require fluids and even pressors.

   4. Disability (i.e., neurologic status)

       a. Level of consciousness and orientation

       b. Symptoms of pain, altered sensation or motor weakness

       c. Screening exam of sensory and motor function in all limbs

       d. Cranial nerve exam

       e. If all is normal, gentle cervical spine palpation

          i. Abnormal/pain: Implement cervical spine precautions

      ii. Normal/no pain: gentle active range of motion (AROM) with support

        (A) Next, AROM without support

        (B) If normal, the athlete may sit, and then stand

        (C) Full exam on sidelines/in the training room

    f. Any abnormality at any point requires cervical spine precautions

  5. Exposure

    a. Cut jersey and shoulder pads to allow access to chest for auscultation

  6. Even in patients with life-threatening cardiac or pulmonary collapse, cervical spine precautions should be maintained whenever possible.

IV. Immediate Stabilization in Neutral Position Should be Attained Without Traction

A. Primary goal is cervical spine stabilization for transport

B. Traction can cause distraction and potentially lead to further injury

C. Player may need to be log-rolled if in prone position to allow for airway management

  1. This technique requires 4–5 people

  2. This should be done directly onto a spine board if possible to avoid moving the player twice

    a. Moving the spine into neutral position should cease if any of the following occur:

      i. Movement causes increased pain

      ii. Increase or change in neurological symptoms

      iii. Airway becomes compromised

      iv. Resistance is encountered

  3. Once the body has been secured to the spine board, the helmet should then be secured to the board as well, using foam pads for support (see Figure 19.1)

    a. Sand bags are no longer recommended due to excess weight

  4. Tape is next used with a two-point system across the forehead and chin

  5. Arms should be kept free for easy intravenous access, but hands/thumbs should be taped together to prevent the arms from falling off the board during transport

D. If the athlete is supine, the lift and slide technique should be used rather than log roll, as it has been shown to cause less movement at the head and cervical spine

  a. This technique often requires at least six people (see Figure 19.2a, b, and c)

E. A vacuum mattress is another alternative. This creates a custom fit and is more comfortable for the athlete, though it still requires the stabilizing force of a long spine board underneath. It can also be used with a concomitant pelvis or femur fracture.

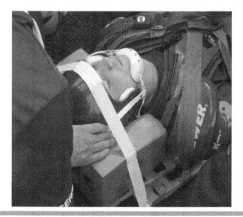

Figure 19.1   Helmet secured with tape and foam pads.

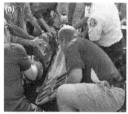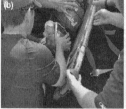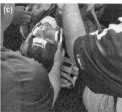

Figure 19.2 (a, b, c): Lift and slide technique (sequential pictures). Note, the rescuer who controls the head/neck is directing the rescue.

V. Sports-Specific Equipment Considerations

A. Transport should occur with helmet, chin strap, and shoulder pads in place for American football and ice hockey. The helmet and shoulder pads work together to help maintain neutral spine when they are properly fitted

1. Facemask removal should occur first for airway access (see Section V below for description of the technique)
2. Cutting of the ties of the shoulder pads can often be performed to allow for access to the chest if needed for auscultation and CPR

B. If equipment needs to be removed on the field, use the "all or nothing" principle for American football and ice hockey

1. Helmet and shoulder pads should be removed together

   a. Helmet removal with shoulder pads in place leads to hyperextension/lordosis of the cervical spine

   b. If the helmet has become dislodged, then padding should be placed under the head to maintain neutral spine until shoulder pads can be removed

C. Although the helmet and shoulder pads generally should not be removed until adequate stabilization has occurred after transport to the emergency department, there are certain situations (noted in Table 19.1) that require their removal on the field

D. In other sports, remember that the goal is maintenance of neutral spine

1. Equipment that hinders this primary goal, or that does not assist in providing stability, should be removed by a trained professional

Table 19.1　Guidelines for on-field equipment removal

Helmet and shoulder pads should generally be removed after transport to the emergency department; however, the following situations necessitate their earlier removal:
1. Helmet is not properly fitted and allows for independent movement of the head
2. The facemask cannot be removed in a reasonable period of time and is preventing airway access and control
3. Even after removal of the facemask, the helmet design is such that adequate airway control is not possible
4. Shoulder pads are preventing adequate cardiopulmonary resuscitation and require removal
5. All or none principle: helmet and shoulder pads should be removed together in American football and ice hockey

    2. Shoulder pads in lacrosse and field hockey may not be sufficient to elevate the torso to the same level as the helmeted head. In these cases both helmet and shoulder pads may need to be removed

       a. A cervical collar should then be placed before transfer to a spine board.

VI. Sports-Specific Equipment Removal

  A. This always requires at least two people; one must stabilize the spine while the other removes equipment

  B. The team physician or athletic trainer should accompany the athlete to the emergency department to ensure proper transfer of care and continued cervical spine stability during equipment removal

  C. Facemask

    1. This is removed during the initial assessment to allow for airway access

    2. Chin strap and helmet cheek pads should be left in place

    3. A combined tool approach should be utilized for facemask removal

       a. A cordless power screwdriver is often the most efficient tool and causes the least amount of movement (see Figure 19.3)

       b. Cutting tools such as a trainer's angle should always be present as backup in case of screwdriver failure (see Figure 19.4)

          i. These have been shown to cause greater head and neck movement than utilization of the cordless screwdriver

       c. Proper maintenance and donning of equipment is key to allow its prompt removal

          i. Rusted or stripped screws or improperly positioned chin straps will make removal more difficult

  D. Helmet

    1. Should be removed with the shoulder pads in American football and ice hockey. The only exception is with accidental dislodgement of the helmet at the time of the injury (see section IV above)

    2. Requires stabilization of the cervical spine from the front

    3. Ear pads inside the helmet should be removed one side at a time (see Figure 19.5)

    4. Helmets with an air inflation system will need to be deflated prior to removal. This can be accomplished with an 18-gauge needle placed in the external ports

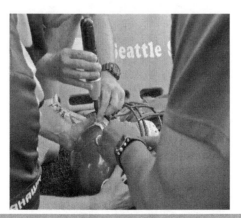

Figure 19.3 **Facemask removal with a power screwdriver.**

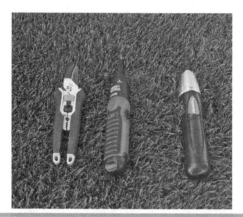

Figure 19.4   Tool options for facemask removal: a standard cutting tool and two different cordless power screwdrivers.

5. The helmet will need to be rolled forward to clear the occiput during removal (see Figure 19.6)
6. The shoulder pads should then be quickly pulled off; it is imperative that they have already been untied or cut, both anteriorly and under both arms
7. Cervical collar is put in place after helmet removal
8. Equipment may be removed before or after initial imaging of the patient in the emergency department
   a. Helmet and particularly shoulder pads make adequate visualization difficult on plain films. Computed tomography (CT) does not have this restriction
   b. MRI should not be the initial study of choice due to time constraints and artifact from metal within the helmet.

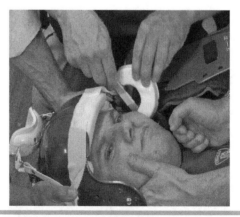

Figure 19.5   Ear pad removal with a tongue depressor in Emergency Department. Note attention to continued cervical spine stabilization.

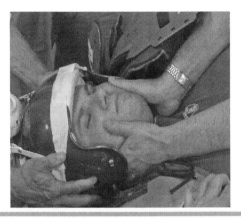

Figure 19.6   Helmet removal in Emergency Department.

VII. Airway Management

A. Management should be left to the person with the most skill and experience. As there is no clear literature on which maneuvers cause the least amount of cervical spine movement, practitioners should use the technique with which they are most comfortable

B. Jaw thrust and chin lift maneuver may be used even before facemask removal. Head tilt should be avoided to prevent further cervical spine injury

C. Mouthpiece and facemask should be removed

D. Pocket mask can sometimes be used even with the facemask in place
   1. A bag-valve device with face mask is generally adequate for on the field ventilatory support

E. Advanced airway management techniques produce less cervical spine movement but require the presence of trained personnel
   1. Indications for definitive airway management with ventilation include apnea, inability to maintain oxygenation, high-risk of aspiration, and severe closed head injuries
      a. Laryngeal mask airway may be safely inserted in the helmeted athlete
      b. Endotracheal tube (ET) is difficult to place and is often unsuccessful in the helmeted athlete
      c. Esophageal tracheal combitube (ETC) has been shown to be more easily and efficiently inserted in the helmeted athlete than ET.

VIII. Further Management Options After Transport

A. High-dose methylprednisolone has been used for the initial management of spinal cord injuries, though some authors still debate its use. There is controversy over the data analysis and conclusions of the initial studies. This can be considered a treatment option rather than a treatment requirement
   1. One survey demonstrated that 91% of neurosurgeons prescribe methylprednisolone after acute, nonpenetrating, traumatic spinal cord injury
   2. National Acute Spinal Cord Injury Study II (NASCIS II) utilized 30 mg/kg IV bolus over 15 min, followed by a 45 min rest, followed by 5.4 mg/kg/h for 23 h
      a. This showed improvements in neurological testing scores at 6 weeks and 6 months if given within the first 8 h from injury

        b. If given after 8 h from initial injury, neurological scores were not significantly different than those who received placebo

        c. Functional scores were not assessed

    3. NASCIS III suggested that the NASCIS II protocol be followed if administration is started within 3 h. In patients who received methylprednisolone within 3–8 h of injury, they suggested continuation for a total of 48 h

        a. The 48-h regimen correlated with a greater risk of pneumonia and sepsis, but not greater all-cause mortality

B. Hypothermia has also been used, though evidence remains sparse and is currently insufficient to justify its use. This is still considered an experimental treatment.

    1. Hypothermia has been shown to reduce morbidity when used in the treatment of brain injury and myocardial infarction

    2. Mechanism remains unclear, but may work by slowing metabolism, decreasing oxygen requirements and preventing the inflammatory cascade

    3. Sepsis, bleeding, and arrhythmias are all possible complications

    4. Rewarming can also be complicated by hypotension.

Recommended Reading

1. Banerjee R, Palumbo MA, Fadale PD. Catastrophic cervical spine injuries in the collision sport athlete, part 2: Principles of emergency care. *Am J Sports Med.* 2004;32(7):1760–1764.
2. Bell K. On-field issues of the C-spine-injured helmeted athlete. *Curr Sport Med Rep.* 2007;6(1):32.
3. Swartz EE, Boden BP, Courson RW, Decoster LC, Horodyski M, Norkus SA, Rehberg RS, Waninger KN. National Athletic Trainers' Association position statement: Acute management of the cervical spine-injured athlete. *J Athl Train.* 2009;44(3):306–331.
4. Waninger KN, Swartz EE. Cervical spine injury management in the helmeted athlete. *Curr Sports Med Rep.* 2011;10(1):45–49.

Lumbar Spine Injuries and Conditions

Matthew D. Maxwell and Gary P. Chimes

ANATOMY

I. General considerations

A. Diagnostic approach to lumbar anatomy is best approached by dividing the spinal canal into three columns: anterior, middle, and posterior

B. Isolated trauma to the anterior or posterior columns typically results in stable injury, while additional involvement of the middle column results in unstable injury.

II. Anterior, middle, and posterior columns (see Figure 20.1)

A. Anterior column—typically injured by spinal flexion

    1. Vertebral body (Anterior 2/3)—large to support weight of superior structures that form the anterior wall of the spinal canal

    2. Intervertebral disk (IV disk)— (Anterior 2/3)

        a. Annulus fibrosus (AF)

            i. Composed of oblique fibrocartilaginous lamellae that provide firm, circumferential support for the softer, inner portion of the IV disk

            ii. May tear allowing contained nucleus to herniate outward, particularly on posterolateral margin where the AF is thin and has no adjacent support

            iii. Tears of the AF are also pain generators without frank herniation, often correlating with the presence of a "high-intensity zone" (HIZ) seen in on T2 images of MRI. Provocation discography may have greater diagnostic accuracy than MRI for detecting an annular tear; however, discography may also hasten

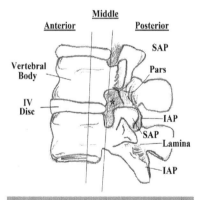

Figure 20.1 Anatomical columns of the lumbar spine. Bony anatomy of the lumbar spine divided into anterior, middle, and posterior columns. * Denotes the intervertebral foramen.

the degenerative cascade and should be reserved for cases where the diagnosis is unclear and surgical intervention is being considered

   iv. Injuries to the AF often result from repetitive forces of combined flexion, rotation, and compression (e.g., removing sports equipment from the trunk of a car)

  b. Nucleus pulposus (NP)—(Anterior 2/3)

    i. The inner core of the IV disk formed of gelatinous matrix that provides flexibility to spinal motion in normal young adults; matrix is composed primarily of water and proteoglycans, which act as a binding agent

    ii. May herniate outward through annulus, causing nerve root irritation. The NP itself, however, has no nociceptive innervation

  3. Anterior longitudinal ligament—thick, fibrous band along anterolateral vertebral bodies and IV disks, serving as the only ligament that prevents spinal hyperextension; major site of trauma after "whiplash" injury

B. Middle column—rarely injured in isolation, but will cause an unstable injury if accompanied by injury to the anterior or posterior columns

  1. Posterior third of vertebral body and IV disk (injuries to the IV disk are not considered to be unstable unless accompanied by neurological deficits)

  2. Posterior longitudinal ligament—thinner, fibrous band along posterior vertebral bodies and IV disks, serving principally as support for the posterior IV disk and adjacent soft tissues, has nociceptive nerve endings and thus can generate pain

  3. Spinal canal

C. Posterior elements—injuries are typically exacerbated by spinal extension (see Figure 20.2)

  1. Vertebral arch

    a. Pedicle—connects the vertebral body to the rest of the vertebra. The pedicles of adjacent levels form the roof and floor of the neuroforamen, through which the spinal nerves pass (e.g., the L4 nerve root passes through the L4–L5 neuroforamen, which is bordered on top by the L4 pedicle, and below by the L5 pedicle)

    b. Pars interarticularis—meaning the "part between the articular processes"—separates the superior and inferior articular processes. A defect in the pars is called a spondylolysis, and is often seen in athletes engaged in repetitive extension movements (see Section IX for details)

    c. Lamina—forms the posterior wall of the spinal canal

  2. Articular processes and zygapophyseal joints (Z-joints or "facet" joints)

    a. Extend from junction of pedicle and lamina on each side

    b. The superior articular process (SAP) of one level forms a joint with the inferior articular process (IAP) from the level above, called the zygapophyseal joint

  3. Ligamentum flavum (LF)—fibroelastic band connecting laminae of adjacent vertebrae to form the posterior wall of the spinal canal

    a. To access the vertebral canal posteriorly (e.g., for a lumbar puncture or an interlaminar epidural steroid injection), one must pierce through the LF. As one passes through the elastic LF, there is distinct feel of "loss of

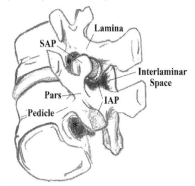

Figure 20.2 Elements of the posterior column. Posterolateral view of the posterior column bony anatomy. * Denotes the intervertebral foramen.

III. Sacrum, coccyx, and spinal column variants

A. Sacrum—Wedge-shaped bone formed by the fusion of five sacral vertebrae in most individuals, which disperses weight of spine to pelvis through the sacroiliac joints

B. Coccyx—Terminus of spine; pain generator after direct trauma—"coccydynia"

C. Spinal column variants
1. Sacralization of L5 vertebra—L5 is partially or completely fused with the sacrum; this may predispose to development of L4–L5 degenerative disease and when symptomatic is termed Bertolotti's syndrome
2. Lumbarization of S1 vertebra—S1 is NOT completely fused with the sacrum, which may result in six apparent lumbar vertebrae
3. Spina bifida occulta—incomplete closure of the vertebral arch posteriorly without clinical significance by itself, but may be associated with increased incidence of spondylolysis.

IV. Lumbar spine musculature

A. Psoas major (PM)—extends from body and transverse process of all lumbar vertebrae and all IV disks to produce spinal and hip flexion
1. In patients with tight PM, lumbar lordosis is often exaggerated to compensate for anterior pelvic tilt; this increases the load on all the posterior elements of the spine, including the Z-joints, pars interarticularis, and SI joints
2. In older athletes, this exacerbates lumbar spinal stenosis, since anything that causes the athlete to hyperextend the lumbar spine will narrow the spinal canal and potentially compress descending nerve roots. Therefore, it is important for these athletes to stretch their PM and other hip flexors

B. Erector Spinae—produce spinal extension and lateral flexion

C. Deep paraspinal muscles (specifically, the multifidi)—primarily provide dynamic segmental stabilization and serve as proprioceptors, although they also contribute to lumbar spinal rotation

D. Quadratus lumborum—extends to posterior iliac crest to produce lateral flexion

E. Abdominal musculature
1. Transversus abdominis—transversely oriented to compress abdominal contents and to provide larger radius of axial stability for lumbar spine
2. Internal/external obliques—obliquely oriented to support abdominal contents and produce spinal rotation and flexion
3. Rectus abdominis (RA)—vertically oriented to produce trunk flexion, provide counterforce to lumbar lordosis, and support pubis, modulating degree of pelvic tilt; many common causes of low back pain in athletes are made worse with flexion, for example, discogenic low back pain from an annular tear. Therefore, core strengthening programs for discogenic low back pain should initially avoid lumbar spine flexion and strengthen/reeducate the other stabilizing abdominal muscles.

EPIDEMIOLOGY, DIAGNOSIS, TREATMENT

I. General considerations

A. Epidemiology of back pain
1. Back pain affects 60–90% of people at least once during their lifetime
2. Annual incidence of 5–10% in the United States
3. Most cases are self-limited and respond well to minimally invasive treatment, although there is high recurrence rate
4. Common causes in athletes
   a. Annular tears
   b. IV disk herniation

B. Evaluation overview
  1. Demographic considerations
    a. Age
      i. Pediatric—slipped capital femoral epiphysis and other hip disorders may present as low back pain
      ii. Adolescent—greater incidence of spondylolysis
      iii. College—disk injury resulting in radiculopathy or annular tear and spondylolysis; nonspecific "muscular" pain is very common in college athletes, but most muscular pain should be self-limited. With persistent pain, one must evaluate for treatable underlying diagnoses that may cause muscle guarding and myofascial symptoms
      iv. Adult—nonspecific lumbar pain, disk injury, with increasing prevalence of facet syndrome, lumbar stenosis, and degenerative disease
      v. Senior—greater propensity for compression fractures, degenerative disease with stenosis (causing radicular pain) and facet arthropathy (causing axial back pain)
    b. Gender
      i. Women—greater propensity for SI dysfunction and compression fractures
      ii. Men—greater prevalence of pars defects in anatomic studies
  2. History
    a. Red flags that indicate emergent medical issue
      i. Bowel and bladder dysfunction and/or saddle anesthesia—cauda equina syndrome
      ii. Cancer history and/or weight loss—occult malignancy
      iii. Fever—infection, for example, epidural abscess, diskitis
    b. Yellow flags that indicate a potential poor response to basic treatment
      i. Maladaptive beliefs
      ii. Expectations and pain behavior
      iii. Reinforcement of pain
      iv. Heightened emotional activity
      v. Job dissatisfaction
      vi. Poor social support
      vii. Compensation and/or litigation issues
  3. Physical examination
    a. Neuromuscular assessment may reveal level of pathology (Table 20.1)
    b. Observe for postural preference during interview
      i. Anterior/middle column pathology is typically exacerbated by trunk flexion; patient may prefer standing or leaning backward when at rest
      ii. Posterior column pathology is typically exacerbated by trunk extension; patient may prefer sitting or leaning forward when at rest

Table 20.1 Spinal nerve assessment

Root	Muscle Action[a]	Area of Sensory Loss[a]	Associated Reflex
L2	Hip flexion	Mid-anterior thigh	
L3	Knee extension	Medial knee	Patellar
L4	Ankle dorsiflexion	Medial malleolus	Patellar
L5	Great toe extension[b]	Dorsal aspect of 3rd MTP	Medial hamstring
S1	Ankle plantarflexion[b]	Lateral aspect of calcaneus	Achilles

[a]Muscle Action and Area of Sensory Loss taken from ASIA Standard.

[b]Additional functional tests for myotomes including side-lying hip abduction (L5) and toe raises (S1).

      c. Kinetic chain assessment: examine pelvis/legs for proper ROM, strength, leg length discrepancy

C. Treatment overview

  1. Therapy programs

      a. Mechanical diagnosis and therapy (MDT) with focus on centralization of radicular pain

      b. Mobilization (e.g., of vertebral segmental dysfunction, sacroiliac dysfunction)

      c. Lumbar stabilization—typically with neutral, flexion, or extension bias

      d. Pelvic floor therapy to strengthen pelvic girdle musculature

      e. Cognitive-behavioral therapy, particularly useful when yellow flags (see Section I.B.2.b) are evident

  2. Pharmacologic treatment

      a. Most pharmacologic treatments are used empirically for symptomatic relief when the source of pain may not be clearly defined; the efficacy of oral medications in treatment of low back pain is not clearly established

      b. Anti-inflammatories—inhibit the production of cytokines that augment nociception and increase tissue swelling

         i. Oral corticosteroids

         ii. Nonsteroidal anti-inflammatory agents (NSAIDs)

      c. Opioid analgesics—act centrally at the level of the spinal cord to block nociceptive pathway

      d. Neuromodulating agents—act centrally to modulate cortical interpretation of pain

         i. Anticonvulsants—gabapentin

         ii. Antidepressants

            (A) Tricyclics—amitryptiline, nortryptiline

            (B) SNRI—venlafaxine, duloxetine

      e. Antispasmodics—no conclusive evidence of direct beneficial effect on lumbar muscle injury; however, these centrally acting medicines promote generalized muscle relaxation and sleep, providing short-term symptomatic relief

         i. Cyclobenzaprine—acts centrally by blocking serotonergic pathway, ultimately inhibiting α-motor neurons

         ii. Tizanidine—alpha 2-adrenergic agonist that increases presynaptic inhibition of motor neurons, reducing muscle spasm

  3. Interventional treatment

      a. Epidural steroid injection

         i. Injection of corticosteroid into the epidural space to reduce inflammation around the disk and spinal nerve

         ii. Transforaminal, interlaminar, and caudal approaches

         iii. Indications include radiculopathy and spinal stenosis, but sometimes used for discogenic pain (annular tears); efficacy is best proven when leg pain > axial back pain

      b. Articular steroid injection

         i. Injection of steroid into facet joints of the lumbar spine and SI joints to reduce synovitis and inflammation of joint capsules

         ii. Indications include facet syndrome and sacroiliac dysfunction

      c. Anesthetic nerve block

         i. Injection of anesthetic to block nociceptive message of medial branch afferent nerve innervating articular column

         ii. Principally used in assessment of facet syndrome and sacroiliac dysfunction when considering further treatment with radiofrequency ablation

    d. Radiofrequency (RF) ablation

      i. Electrothermal injury to block nociceptive afferent nerve innervating articular column

      ii. Provides much longer duration than anesthetic nerve block: 8–12 months

      iii. Principally used in treatment of recalcitrant facet and SI joint pain.

II. Radiculopathy

A. General considerations

  1. Herniation of the nucleus pulposus (HNP) through the annulus is the most common cause, inflaming adjacent tissues, including nerve roots and ligaments

    a. HNPs are classically divided anatomically

      i. Central/paracentral—can contribute to central spinal stenosis and can be a source of axial low back pain

      ii. Posterolateral—the affected nerve root is typically the root descending in the lateral recess (i.e., the root below the disk level)

      iii. Lateral—the affected nerve root exits at that level; this may be within the foramen (foraminal) or lateral to it (extraforaminal)

    b. >90% occur at L4–L5 or L5–S1

    c. More common in younger patients, as the nucleus desiccates with age and becomes less prone to herniate

    d. Not always symptomatic and are common on imaging of otherwise pain-free individuals

  2. Other causes of radicular/radiating leg symptoms

    a. Radiculitis without overt HNP

    b. Lumbar stenosis—degenerative disease causes mechanical compression of nerve roots, often without specific segmental findings

    c. Piriformis or "hip rotator" syndrome—mechanical stress causes irritation of the sciatic nerve as it travels adjacent to or through the piriformis; this is far less common than true radioculopathy

B. Diagnosis

  1. Pain/paresthesias radiating into the buttock or lower limb

  2. Nerve root impingement may cause neurological deficits (Table 20.1)

  3. Neural traction tests may provide clinical evidence of radiculitis (Figure 20.3)

  4. Imaging

    a. Radiographs are most often normal, but help to evaluate other causes. May show signs of segmental instability on flexion/extension views, pars defects, or narrowing of disk space

    b. MRI may show HNP or other source of compression

  5. Electrodiagnostic evaluation may support the diagnosis of radiculopathy; however, findings are often absent until 3 weeks after injury and generally absent in cases with sole sensory (without motor) involvement

C. Treatment

  1. Conservative

    a. Activity modification—relative rest and avoidance of activities that result in prolonged spinal flexion, as this often exacerbates symptoms. Absolute rest is contraindicated

    b. Rehabilitation

      i. Extension-based exercises to centralize radicular symptoms

      ii. Lumbar stabilization/strengthening to decrease mechanical stress on IV disk and vertebrae

    c. Oral medications—refer to Section I.C.2 above

2. Spinal injections
   a. Epidural injection of corticosteroids provide anti-inflammatory effect on adjacent tissues, including the inflamed spinal nerve
   b. General guidelines suggest up to three in a 6-month period, and no more than four in a year
3. Surgical
   a. Diskectomy (sometimes with fusion) or microdiskectomy of herniated disk material to decompress nerve root
   b. Decompression of neural structures by laminectomy and/or foraminotomy in cases where bony structures contribute to compression.

III. Fractures

A. Burst
1. Caused by axial loading of spine resulting in fracture of vertebral body (most commonly the superior endplate) sometimes involving the posterior elements
   a. Stable—preserved posterior elements
   b. Unstable—injury to posterior elements, typically resulting from fracture or dislocation
   c. Reports of neurologic sequelae in ~50% of patients
2. Imaging—radiographs show loss of vertebral height, possible compromise of posterior elements/alignment; cross-sectional imaging can evaluate fracture or dislocation of posterior elements and integrity of formina and contained structures

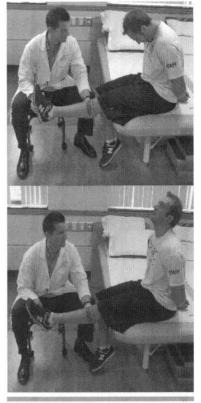

Figure 20.3   **Slump test. Full spinal flexion in the seated position accompanied by extension of each leg places tension on the lumbar nerve roots; test is interpreted as positive if it creates radicular symptoms that are alleviated by neck extension.**

3. Treatment
   a. Stable—typically treated with rest, pain control, thoraco-lumbar-sacral orthosis (TLSO) at least 3 months with close observation
   b. Unstable—surgery warranted to restore structural integrity with possible decompression of forminal or central canals
B. Compression
1. Typically caused by combined axial flexion and compression resulting in wedge fracture of the vertebral body with variable injury to more posterior elements, most often at thoracolumbar junction; compression fractures are among the most common back injuries in snowsports, followed by transverse/spinous process fractures from direct trauma
2. Compromise of middle and posterior elements increases likelihood of instability and

      3. Risk factors include osteoporosis, corticosteroid use, malignancy—most often multiple myeloma or metastatic disease

      4. Pain typically worse with flexion, valsalva, incidental postural changes

      5. Imaging—radiographs reveal wedge-shaped compression of upper lumbar/lower thoracic vertebra; CT, bone scan, SPECT may increase sensitivity when radiographs are negative with high clinical suspicion

      6. Treatment

         a. Stable—bracing with TLSO/binder with therapy focusing on spinal stability with extension bias; close observation to follow for progressive kyphosis, loss of body height, or changes in neurological status, which may necessitate surgical intervention

         b. Unstable—surgery to restore structural integrity, decompress neural structures; surgery may be needed when >40% loss of anterior body height or with >25° kyphotic deformity, both of which suggest posterior element injury

   C. Spinous and transverse process (SP and TP) fractures

      1. Typically result from direct trauma to posterior spine

      2. Forced flexion with rotation may cause a spinous process fracture

      3. Violent contraction of psoas major may cause a transverse process fracture

      4. Rarely accompanied by neurological deficits, but may have concurrent abdominal injury, such as retroperitoneal bleeding or lacerations to the spleen, liver, or kidney

      5. New onset severe back pain typically after direct trauma or forced hip extension; examine for palpable deformities, point tenderness, spasm of paraspinal muscles, and signs of contusion or ecchymosis

      6. Imaging—AP/lateral radiographs likely will reveal fracture; obtain flexion–extension films to evaluate stability; CT scan is indicated to evaluate concurrent fractures, soft tissue injury, or abdominal bleeding

      7. Treatment

         a. Symptomatic management with analgesics, antispasmodics

         b. Therapy to maintain/restore core control and proper lumbar alignment

         c. No bracing or surgery is needed for isolated SP/TP fractures

   D. Pars interarticularis fracture—see Section IX.

IV. Lumbar strain

   A. General considerations

      1. Injury to the lumbar intrinsic musculature

      2. May result from overuse, acceleration–deceleration, trauma, repetitive eccentric loading

   B. Diagnosis

      1. History typically significant for tenderness and spasm in area of pain; pain should not last longer than 7–10 days

      2. Patient may report delayed-onset muscle soreness in cases of repetitive eccentric loading

      3. No associated neurological defects or findings on imaging

   C. Treatment

      1. Symptomatic treatment with analgesics/antispasmodics/activity modification

      2. Therapy to improve lumbar stabilization strength, hip/hamstring flexibility, and possible manipulation for improved tissue mobility.

V. Facet syndrome

   A. General considerations

      1. Facet (zygapophyseal) joints are synovial joints innervated by medial branches of dorsal rami from the two spinal nerves rostral to that level (e.g., L3–L4 Z-joint is innervated by the L2 and L3 medial branches)

    2. Facet joints bear increasing weight with more caudal segments

    3. Degeneration may cause inflammation and joint hypertrophy, resulting in both irritation and compression of adjacent tissues, including spinal nerves

B. Diagnosis

    1. Pain is typically reproduced by extension and rotation, including activities such as sleeping prone or reaching overhead; no examination maneuvers are proven to be diagnostic of facet syndrome; however, lumbar extension and rotation is thought to mechanically stress the Z-joints

    2. Pain is usually just off the midline, but may be referred in nondermatomal distributions to flank, buttock, groin, or thigh

    3. Imaging

        a. Radiographs often show degenerative changes, including endplate changes, vertebral osteophytes, and facet joint sclerosis

        b. MRI may show capsule hypertrophy, foraminal stenosis, endplate changes, disk desiccation, and other degenerative changes

        c. Bone scan/SPECT are helpful to identify active inflammation and may predict better clinical response to therapeutic injection

    4. Diagnostic injection. Symptomatic relief after injection supports diagnosis:

        a. Intra-articular injection of anesthetic and/or steroid

        b. Anesthetic block of afferent nerve—medial branch of dorsal ramus

C. Treatment

    1. Physical therapy

        a. Focus on lumbar stabilization, avoiding marked lumbar extension

        b. Improve flexibility of hip flexors to reduce lumbar lordosis and adjacent musculature to reduce stress on lumbar segments

    2. Oral medications as detailed above

    3. Interventional therapeutic procedures—see Section I.C.3.

VI. Sacroiliac (SI) joint dysfunction

A. General considerations

    1. Sacrum articulates with the ilia, distributing body weight to the pelvis

    2. Innervated by the dorsal rami of L5 and sacral spinal nerves

    3. Normal SI joint function allows for mobility in pelvis

    4. Pain caused by changes in mobility, repetitive trauma, and capsular injury

B. Diagnosis

    1. Patient typically presents with low back, buttock, or groin pain. The patient will often point at the SI joint as their source of maximum pain

        a. PE typically reveals SI joint tenderness, hyper/hypomobility of SI joint on single leg stance (Gillet's maneuver), pain with iliac compression, and positive FABER maneuver

        b. Imaging

            i. While imaging may demonstrate changes in the SI joint, it is generally not diagnostically useful other than to exclude other diagnoses

            ii. Image-guided intra-articular injection of anesthetic and steroid is often used both diagnostically and therapeutically

C. Treatment

    1. Physical therapy—regimen focusing on lumbopelvic stabilization, including gluteal and pelvic floor strengthening

    2. SI joint manipulation may provide relief in cases of impaired mobility

    3. NSAID/analgesics

4. Intra-articular injection of anesthetic/steroid may resolve symptoms

5. Anesthetic block and/or RF ablation of innervating dorsal rami may also be considered in patients with persistent pain after more conservative management.

VII. Scoliosis

A. General considerations
1. Characterized by abnormal lateral curvature and/or rotation of the spine
   a. Curvature—characterized by "Cobb angle" between perpendicular lines drawn from endplates of the maximally tilted vertebrae at proximal and distal ends of the curvature (Figure 20.4)
   b. Rotation—graded by pedicle position in AP radiograph and angular orientation to midline on CT, with multiple advocated methods
2. Adolescent idiopathic scoliosis (AIS) is the most common subtype; however, scoliosis may result from underlying neuromuscular disease, bone malformation, neural tube defects, and other underlying diseases; AIS has a high chance of progression

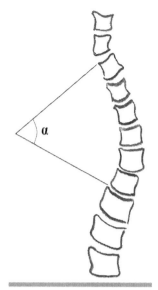

Figure 20.4 Cobb angle. Angle α formed by perpendicular lines drawn from endplates of the maximally tilted vertebrae.

B. Diagnosis
1. Pain at the site of apex is typically presenting symptom and is proportional to severity of the curve
2. Most commonly right convex curve with apex in mid-thoracic region; may present with double curve, lumbar curve, or thoracolumbar curve
3. Less common curvatures should prompt cross-sectional imaging to evaluate secondary causes
4. Imaging
   a. Radiograph and/or CT to evaluate degree of curvature/rotation
   b. Serial imaging with 4–6 month intervals until skeletally mature

C. Treatment
1. Conservative care indicated for curvature <40° (or <35° in cases where secondary to neuromuscular disease)
   a. Therapy and observation indicated when curvature <20–25°
   b. Bracing indicated for curvature 20–40°
      i. Milwaukee brace for high thoracic curves (T8 or higher)
      ii. Low-profile TLSO for lower curves
      iii. 23 h/day until bone maturation
      iv. Once spine is mature and completely grown, bracing can be gradually discontinued with careful observation and serial imaging
2. Generally, surgery (most often fusion) is indicated under the following circumstances, although other factors must be considered:
   a. Curve >40° in skeletally immature, >50° in skeletally mature
   b. Curve >35° in neuromuscular disease
   c. Progressive loss of pulmonary function.

VIII. Spinal stenosis

A. General considerations

1. Typically degenerative etiology, in which bony and soft tissue hypertrophy cause compression of canals containing neural structures, in older individuals; may also result from congenital, metabolic, and neoplastic disease

    a. Central stenosis—compression of spinal cord, conus medullaris, and/or cauda equina

    b. Foraminal stenosis—compression of nerve root, DRG, and/or spinal nerve exiting spinal canal

B. Diagnosis

1. Back, leg, or buttock pain occurs with lumbar extension, particularly while walking, and is relieved by sitting, leaning forward (pseudoclaudication)

2. Can be distinguished from vascular claudication by several findings

    a. Typically improved on bicycle (seated position), walking uphill, or upstairs

    b. Physical exam typically reveals normal pulses, normal skin/hair, muscular weakness, and atrophy in cases of long-standing pathology

3. Imaging

    a. Radiographs often show degenerative changes

    b. Further imaging with MRI/CT/myelogram will reveal extend of neural compression, soft tissue changes such as ligamentum flavum hypertrophy

C. Treatment

1. Conservative: therapy focusing on lumbar stabilization with flexion/neutral preference and oral medications

2. Interventional: epidural steroid injections may relieve radicular symptoms

3. Surgical decompression is indicated in cases of persistent pain, neurological deficit, or marked nerve root compression.

IX. Spondylolysis

A. General considerations

1. Developmental defect of pars interarticularis, most common at L5 level (85–95%) and L4 level (5–15%), resulting from incomplete ossification of cartilaginous matrix

2. Most common source of LBP in adolescent athletes, particularly those performing repeated lumbar extension, for example, wrestling, gymnastics, track and field, tennis

3. Risk of progression to spondylolisthesis (detailed in Section X)

B. Diagnosis

1. Pain worsened by lumbar extension, including athletic activity, lying prone, reaching overhead

2. Pain relieved by lumbar flexion and rest

3. Imaging

    a. Radiographs, including oblique view, may show osseous defect

       i. Standing AP and lateral films to evaluate bony abnormalities and flexion–extension views to evaluate concurrent spondylolisthesis with instability

       ii. Oblique view may show "scotty dog" with collar representing defect; may not reveal fracture in early symptomatic stress reaction (although oblique views are generally not necessary and do increase radiation exposure substantially)

    b. SPECT—bone scan

       i. May show changes ~1 week after new symptomatic stress reaction

       ii. Increased sensitivity and better correlation with symptomatic pars defect, false-positive rate around 15%

    c. CT scan provides better visualization of bony defects while evaluating adjacent structures that may also serve as pain generator; however, this has higher false-negative findings particularly when evaluating early symptomatic stress reaction. CT may distinguish acute and chronic lesions, providing information for prognosis and treatment plan

C. Treatment

1. Relative rest—allows resolution of bony matrix stress reaction; patients should avoid athletic activity and other strenuous activity not essential to daily activities. Ideal duration of relative rest is not clear; however, many argue that minimum 3 months is required for early-stage defects and longer periods to achieve full symptomatic relief when chronic features are noted

2. Physical therapy—regimen focusing on core stabilization, integrated kinetic chain principles, and hamstring/lumbar flexibility often provide the most successful return to sports; patient must demonstrate full, painless sport-specific ROM

3. Bracing—the use of rigid braces or soft corsets is advocated by some; however, evidence on the use of bracing varies widely; some evidence indicates that the primary benefit of bracing to is to promote compliance with activity restriction. For this reason, bracing may be more appropriate if patient has persistent symptoms after 2 weeks of relative rest

4. Analgesics generally not necessarily for long

5. Surgery may be needed for instability; see Section X.

X. Spondylolysthesis

A. General considerations

1. Translation of vertebral body relative to next caudal segment, defined as anterolisthesis (anterior translation) or retrolisthesis (posterior translation)

2. Increased risk in cases of bilateral spondylolysis

B. Diagnosis

1. Pain with movement, particularly extension, may result from several factors

   a. Sheer forces on IV disk may cause discogenic pain

   b. Bony translation may compress spinal nerve, causing radiculopathy

   c. Bony translation may cause increased mechanical load on Z-joints, with resulting facet syndrome

2. Concurrent hamstring tightness and paraspinal spasm are common

3. Palpable step-off noted in cases of marked translation

4. Imaging

   a. Plain films to evaluate translation; see Table 20.2 for grading

      i. Flexion–extension views to evaluate segmental stability

      ii. Radiographic instability is defined as:

Table 20.2 Grading and treatment of spondyloslisthesis

Grade	Translation	Management
1	<25%	Conservative with rest followed by therapy focusing on core stabilization
2	26–50%	Abdominal strengthening, hamstring flexibility and less likely TLSO immobilization for up to 3–6 months
3	51–75%	Asymptomatic—conservative as above Symptomatic—surgical management as below
4	76–100%	Surgical management, most often with postero-lateral fusion with decompression when indicated
Spondyloptosis	>100%	

        (A) Translation >5 mm between flex-ext films
        (B) Rotation >15° between flex-ext films
    b. CT/MRI to evaluate adjacent structures may be indicated if suspicious for other comorbid pathology or to clarify neural involvement

C. Treatment
    1. Analgesics
    2. See Table 20.2 for grade-specific treatment options.

Recommended Reading

1. Baker RJ, Patel D. Lower back pain in the athlete: Common conditions and treatment. *Prim Care.* 2005;32(1):201–229.
2. Cole AJ, Herring SA. *The Low Back Pain Handbook: A Guide for the Practicing Clinician.* 2nd ed. Philadelphia, PA: Hanley & Belfus, Inc.; 2003.
3. Curtis C, d'Hemecourt P. Diagnosis and management of back pain in adolescents. *Adolesc Med State Art Rev.* 2007;18(1):140–164.
4. Graw BP, Wiesel SW. Low back pain in the aging athlete. *Sports Med Arthrosc.* 2008;16(1):39–46.
5. Standaert CJ. Low back pain in the adolescent athlete. *Phys Med Rehabil Clin N Am.* 2008;19(2):287–304.
6. Standaert CJ, Herring SA. Expert opinion and controversies in sports and musculoskeletal medicine: The diagnosis and treatment of spondylolysis in adolescent athletes. *Arch Phys Med Rehabil.* 2007;88(4):537–540.

21

Shoulder Injuries and Conditions

Mederic M. Hall and Jay Smith

I. Anatomy

A. Bony (Figure 21.1) and muscular (Figures 21.2 and 21.3) anatomy.

II. Fractures

A. Clavicle

1. Most injuries prior to age 23–25 are actually physeal injuries.
2. Most fractures occur with direct blow, although can occur with fall on outstretched arm
3. 5–15% of all fractures, up to 50% of all shoulder fractures
4. Most mid-clavicular (80%), 15% distal, 5% medial
5. Described in terms of displaced versus nondisplaced, comminuted versus noncomminuted, and for lateral/distal fractures whether involve coracoclavicular ligaments or not.
6. Radiography
   a. AP and AP cephalic tilt (Zanca view) as well as axillary can best define triplanar orientation. CT will provide better detail as needed
   b. Shortening cannot be measured radiographically because it is a multiplanar phenomenon. Best measured clinically or with 3D CT
7. Treatment:
   a. Nonoperative: typically sling with up to 45° elevation for 4–6 weeks or until bony and clinical (nontender) healing. Then gradual return to play (RTP)
      i. Nondisplaced/minimally displaced, defined as <100% displacement and <15–20 mm shortening
      ii. Closed reduction is not recommended because the reduction never stays. Sling as good as figure-of-eight brace
      iii. Repeat radiographs as needed to ensure increased displacement has not occurred.
      iv. Nonoperative treatment results in nonunion 15–25% of the time. Of those that do heal, up to 50% may have some long-term symptom and/or activity limitation
   b. Surgical: avoid >90 elevation for 4–6 weeks, document clinical and radiographic healing, then progress. Have to consider hardware removal
      i. Operative indications for mid-clavicular fractures include:
         (A) Clinical—neurovascular compromise, open fracture, skin compromise due to deformity, multitrauma, floating shoulder, inability to tolerate/comply with sling, cosmesis
         (B) Radiographic—displacement >100%, shortening >15–20 mm, flipped butterfly fragment
      ii. Operations include use of plate and screws or intramedullary rod. All else fail or are risky. Plate and screws more commonly used but less cosmetic, risk of

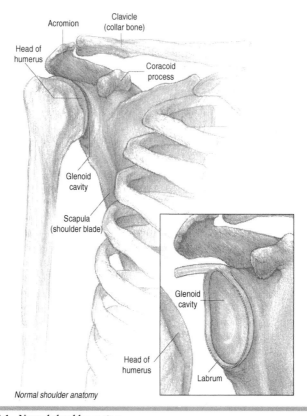

Normal shoulder anatomy

Figure 21.1   **Normal shoulder anatomy**

devascularization high, and requires second major operation to remove. Rod is harder to do, less rotational control, easier to take out. Both have similar outcomes

iii. Distal clavicular fractures (less common, older patients)

(A) Unlike mid-clavicle fractures, tend to be unstable due to loss of coracoclavicular ligament support (torn or attached to distal clavicular fragment, allowing displacement of medial clavicular fragment)

(B) Usually need the 45° cephalic tilt to accurately assess; CT as needed

(C) Treatment is controversial. If nondisplaced, some would recommend trial of sling and close observation. If displaces, then surgery. Others feel that such high rate of instability and nonunion warrant early surgery. If displaced from beginning, many would operate due to difficulty obtaining and maintaining reduction

(D) Most common surgical stabilization is coracoclavicular screw, which must be removed at a later date

B. Glenoid (see below under Traumatic Instability)

C. Humerus (see below under Traumatic Instability).

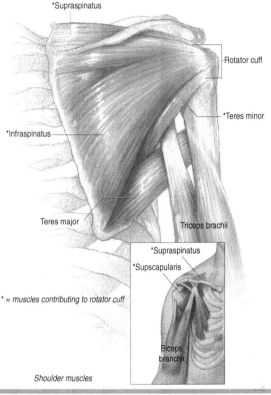

*Supraspinatus

Rotator cuff

*Teres minor

*Infraspinatus

Teres major

Triceps brachii

*Supraspinatus

*Supscapularis

* = muscles contributing to rotator cuff

Biceps branchii

Shoulder muscles

Figure 21.2   **Shoulder muscles**

III. Dislocation/Subluxation

A. Acromioclavicular joint (ACJ)

   1. Anatomy and biomechanics

      a. ACJ capsule and AC ligaments (ACL) (especially posterior) stabilize antero-posterior while coracoclavicular ligaments (CCL) stabilize supero-inferior

      b. 5–10° rotation occurs via ACJ during elevation—less than sternoclavicular joint (SCJ).

      c. Second most commonly dislocated joint (second to glenohumeral)

   2. ACJ pain syndromes

      a. Include acute traumatic separation, distal clavicular osteolysis, and degenerative joint disease (DJD)

      b. Exam: Pain over ACJ, positive scarf sign (pain with horizontal adduction at 90° elevation), positive O'Brien test with pain localizing to ACJ. May include deformity.

      c. Distal clavicular osteolysis—thought to be posttraumatic, although may be microtraumatic. Irregularity of distal clavicle with DJD. Most common in weight lifters

   3. Types of ACJ separations

      a. Type I—sprain AC ligaments, joint wide, but no increasein coracoclavicular distance (CCD)

      b. Type II—tear ACL, sprain CCL. AC joint wide, slight increase in CCD (<25%)

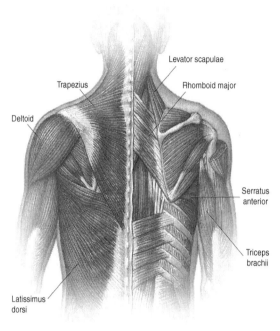

Levator scapulae

Trapezius

Rhomboid major

Deltoid

Serratus anterior

Triceps brachii

Latissimus dorsi

Scapular stabilizer muscles

Figure 21.3   **Scapular stabilizer muscles**

    c. Type III—tear ACL and CCL, but deltotrapezial fascia intact. ACJ wide, 25–100% displacement of CCD

    d. Type IV—clavicle posteriorly displaced; usually most painful

    e. Type V—100–300% increase in CCD, deltotrapezial fascia also torn

    f. Type VI—subcoracoid dislocation

4. Radiographs—AP and axillary and possibly Zanca view; stress views not useful and hurt patient; cross-body adduction view may show more dramatic instability, but often not ordered. MRI only in complicated cases

5. Treatment

    a. Type I–II—nonoperative; sling for comfort; meds; rehab

    b. Type III—controversial

        i. Initial trial of nonoperative almost never incorrect

        ii. May consider early operative intervention for Type III

    c. Type IV–VI—surgery to reduce and stabilize with wire (weaker, but does not need to be removed) or screw (stronger, but needs to be removed)

    d. Consider delayed surgery in contact sports because of the high risk of reinjury. May be better to wait until career over to reconstruct

    e. RTP dictated by symptoms in nonoperative treatment. After operative stabilization, usually sling × 4–6 weeks, followed by 6 weeks increasing activity; remove fixation at 8–12 weeks, then additional 6 weeks rehab before RTP

6. Special case for children
   a. Looks like an ACJ separation, but usually a periosteal sleeve avulsion. Ligaments usually intact with CCL attached to the periosteum and the clavicle punching through the superficial portion of the sleeve
   b. In majority of cases, treated with observation, pain control, and rehab. Nature of sleeve injury allows significant remodeling

B. Glenohumeral joint—See below under traumatic instability.

IV. Shoulder Instability

A. Symptomatic laxity of the shoulder. Laxity does not equal instability

B. May present with pain, feelings of instability, feelings of weakness, loss of speed/control/endurance with sports or work, rotator cuff syndrome (secondary impingement)

C. Classified primarily by etiology and direction of instability
   1. Traumatic unidirectional instability
   2. Atraumatic instability (often multidirectional, although may be symptomatic primarily in one direction)
   3. May also be categorized by degree (subluxation vs. dislocation), chronology (acute, chronic, recurrent), and whether voluntary sublucation/dislocation exists

D. Shoulder stabilized by balanced interaction of static and dynamic restraints
   1. Static stabilizers work primarily at end ranges of motion
      a. Bony congruency of humeral head and glenoid
      b. Capsuloligamentous structures
         i. Anterior translation resisted by the anterior band of the inferior glenohumeral ligament (IGHL) when arm is abducted and externally rotated (injured during typical anterior dislocation). The middle glenohumeral ligament (MGHL) is the restraint when the arm is in neutral
         ii. Superior glenohumeral ligament (SGHL) and coracohumeral ligament (CHL) major restraints to inferior translation when the shoulder is in neutral. Pathologic in rare cases of inferior instability (symptoms when carrying objects)
      c. Dynamic stabilizers work primarily in the mid-ranges. These include the rotator cuff, biceps tendon, and scapular stabilizer muscles. All must be evaluated and rehabilitated as part of the diagnosis and treatment

E. Traumatic instability
   1. Antero-inferior (aka anterior)—most common
      a. Fall with arm abducted and externally rotated. Arm slightly abducted and externally rotated, deltoid contour blunted, acromium prominent
      b. >90% have Bankart lesion and most include deformation of the anterior band of the IGHL. Typically need to treat both (Bankart repair and capsular plication) if surgically treated
      c. Most common nerve injury is axillary nerve (up to 7%); risk increased with dislocation duration and increasing age
      d. Relocating a dislocated shoulder
         i. No "best technique"
         ii. Always do neurovascular check before/after
         iii. Rockwood—counteraction with sheet draped around torso and traction applied to arm; may utilize slight external rotation (ER)/internal rotation (IR) to free up humeral head
         iv. Stimson—patient prone with weights (5–10 lbs) hanging from distal forearm/wrist; may combine with scapular manipulation, rotating scapula to relocate
         v. Sitting with knee flexed, fingers/hands locked around knee, lean backward to self-apply traction (recommend, patient can do himself/herself, gentle)

   e. X-ray views for instability (regardless of etiology). Must have at least two orthogonal views, preferably three

    i. At least AP and axillary lateral (West Point axillary better at identifying bony Bankart). Axillary/West Point axillary will define humeral head position relative to glenoid. AP internal rotation will identify Hill Sachs lesions, but Stryker Notch view is the best view to define Hill Sachs lesion

    ii. Supraspinatus outlet/scapular lateral/scapular Y view—lateral view also shows humeral head position relative to glenoid, and helps identify scapular body for fractures

    iii. MRI demonstrates soft tissue and osseous abnormalities, but usually not required in acute dislocations

   f. Complications (worse with increasing age and duration of dislocation)

    i. Axillary nerve injury (see above)—usuallyresolves in 3–6 months. Assess deltoid and sensation on lateral shoulder

    ii. Rotator cuff tear (RCT)—15% with acute dislocation if <40 years, over if >50 years

    iii. Proximal humerus fracture—up to 40% in patients over 50. Beware of nondisplaced greater tuberosity fractures

   g. Nonoperative treatment

    i. Bracing in external rotation may reduce recurrence risk by apposing the anterior capsule to the glenoid, but should be implemented within 24–48 h. Otherwise, immobilization has no effect on outcome

    ii. Rotator cuff and scapular stabilizer rehab program

    iii. Risk of recurrent instability following non-op treatment

        (A) Age is #1 predictor

            (1) If <20; 65–95%

            (2) If 20–40; 60%

            (3) If >40; 10%

   h. Surgical treatment

    i. Primary indication is symptomatic instability, unresponsive to appropriate nonoperative management, with documented structural pathology

    ii. Early surgery advocated for high-intensity athletes, and reduces recurrence rates. Remains controversial

    iii. Arthroscopic equal to open techniques in skilled hands, with lower morbidity Typically involves suturing detached labrum to glenoid, capsular plication, and rotator interval closure. Recurrence rates 5–15% in contact athletes

    iv. Common reason for surgical failure is failure to appropriately plicate the capsule.

    v. If there is significant bony pathology, bony stabilizing procedures may need to be performed in addition to above:

        (A) If >20–25% of gleonid is fractured (large bony Bankart), needs to be fixed or supplemented with Latarjet/Bristow procedure (coracoid bone transfer to glenoid) or Iliac Crest bone graft

        (B) A large Hill Sachs lesion (>30% humeral head) may engage the glenoid during external rotation and may need bone graft or osteotomy

2. Posterior—less common

   a. Acute dislocation—after forward fall on outstretched arm, or after grand mal seizure or electric shock (e.g., lightning strike at mass event). Arm held in significant external rotation, loss of anterior deltoid contour with dimple just lateral to coracoid (due to prominent coracoid)

   b. Chronic recurrent subluxation/dislocation—pain/symptoms with pushing objects (e.g., football linesman)

   c. PE: posterior glide with or without sulcus sign (deficient rotator interval), scapular dyskinesis, or posterior apprehension

    d. Evaluation and treatment parallels anterior instability, with the following exceptions:

        i. X-rays may demonstrate reverse bony Bankart lesion (posterior gleonid fracture) or reverse Hill Sachs lesion (in anterior humeral head)

        ii. MRI, if obtained, often demonstrate reverse Bankart lesion (posterior glenoid).

    e. Treatment:

        i. Typically nonoperative. Responds better than anterior dislocations. No definitive data on need or duration of immobilization

        ii. If surgery needed, typically perform reverse Bankart repair, capsular shift, and rotator interval closure; may be performed open or, more commonly, arthroscopically; recurrence rate 8–10%

F. Atraumatic instability

    1. Usually multidirectional, although may have symptoms primarily in one direction. May be idiopathic or acquired from repetitive use, such as in overhead athletes

    2. Pain, weakness, and/or variety of symptoms with activity

    3. PE: laxity in multiple directions (anterior and posterior glides, sulcus sign), possibly with apprehension (anterior and/or posterior)

    4. X-rays and MRI usually normal, but MRI may demonstrate large capsule (if gadolinium employed) or nonspecific findings (e.g., tendinopathy, labral fraying). This is primarily a clinical diagnosis

    5. Treatment: Rehabilitation. 80–90% of patients return to sport and activity without major symptoms. If surgery required, inferior capsular shift procedure usually successful (8–10% failure rate), although with wide variability between patients in outcome

G. Bracing for stability

    1. Used to limit "at risk" positions. Mainly for anterior instability. May not be tolerated by athletes because of restricted motion

    2. There is no hard and fast rule that players need to/should return to sport with a brace, although these are commonly prescribed. Must weigh benefits/risks as well as performance and compliance.

V. Muscle/Tendon Injuries

A. Biceps tendon, proximal

    1. May be involved with rotator cuff disease. Rarely affected in isolation.

    2. Stabilizing structures: rotator interval and subscapularis

        a. Rotator interval: contains long head of biceps tendon, coracohumeral ligament, and superior glenohumeral ligament

        b. Suspect rotator interval or subscapularis tear if biceps unstable

    3. May be affected by full spectrum of tendinopathy

    4. Symptoms/PE: Anterior shoulder pain, pain with shoulder flexion, tender over bicipital groove, positive Speed's maneuver (pain with resisted forward elevation at 90° forward elevation), positive Yergason's maneuver (pain with resisted supination with arm at side and elbow flexed to 90°)

    5. Rupture can be acute or chronic. If acute, patient may perceive a pop, and develop bruising. Patients >45 often have associated RC disease. Short head of biceps remains intact. Patient will have "Popeye" sign (i.e., bulging biceps muscle). Rupture results in loss of 20% supination and 8% flexion strength, but little functional compromise in most patients. Some continue to report cramping (particularly with rotation/supination)

        a. Radiographs usually normal. Ultrasound (US) or MRI can evaluate, depending on clinical question. US cannot evaluate intra-articular biceps or labrum reliably

        b. Treatment: Most ruptures in patients over 40 treated nonoperatively. Younger patients may elect for tenodesis, but even high-level athletes have been successful without long head biceps (e.g., John Elway)

      i. Non-op similar to RC treatment

      ii. Operative intervention may include tenotomy or tenodesis if >50% tendon affected. Tenotomy used for older, less active. If <50%, debride

      iii. Treat associated pathologies (rotator cuff, superior labral antero-posterior [SLAP])

B. Pectoralis major

  1. Multilayered attachment at lateral aspect of intertubercular groove. Clavicular portion superficial and inferior, whereas sternal portion deep (partially covered by clavicular portion) and superior

  2. Recognition of rupture is the key. Usually acute. Pain, ecchymosis, weakness in adduction and internal rotation, deformity of contour of anterior axilla due to loss of pec major

  3. MRI is probably test of choice, although US has been used

  4. Virtually all complete tears treated surgically. Usually within 2–3 months to avoid need for graft due to atrophy/retraction. Tendon tears directly repaired. Muscular or musculo-tendinous injuries may require grafting and have poorer prognosis

    a. If not repaired, adduction strength may be reduced by 50%

    b. Post-op recovery may take 4–6 months

C. Rotator cuff

  1. Rotator cuff muscles—supraspinatus, infraspinatus, subscapularis, teres minor.

    a. Long head of biceps tendon often considered the "fifth" rotator cuff muscle because of its stabilizing role

  2. Rotator cuff disease

    a. Tendinosis/tendinopathy

    b. Partial thickness tearing

      i. Articular—most common

      ii. Intrasubstance

      iii. Bursal—often more painful

    c. Full thickness (often occur after falls in patients >40 years old)

  3. Subtypes of rotator cuff pathology

    a. Primary impingement syndrome—due to structural narrowing under the anterior acromion or coracoacromial arch. Originally proposed by Neer. Thought to be uncommon in general, and rare in young people

      i. Loose association exists between the presence of a hooked (as seen on a Neer outlet view) or laterally sloped acromion and rotator cuff tear

      ii. Neer's three phases of impingement

        (A) Stage I (acute)—edema and hemorrhage

        (B) Stage II (chronic)—scarring and fibrosis

        (C) Stage III (chronic)—osteophytes, tearing

    b. Secondary impingement—pain with overhead activity and rotator cuff syndrome, but with no structural compromise. Occurs due to inability to control humeral head in glenoid. Superior humeral head migration causes dynamic narrowing of coracoacromial space and rotator cuff irritation. May be due to underlying glenohumeral instability, scapulothoracic instability (leading to glenohumeral instability), or rotator cuff dysfunction (e.g., tendinosis, tear, neurologic injury). Most common scenario for rotator cuff disease in young people, particularly athletes

    c. Posterior-superior impingement/internal impingement—pathological contact between the undersurface of the supraspinatus–infraspinatus junction and the postero-superior labrum. There is normal contact physiologically, but this can become pathological and produce symptoms. May cause partial articular side rotator cuff tear and postero-superior labral tears. Often seen in throwers during late cocking and acceleration phases of throwing

      i. Present with postero-superior shoulder pain, especially during throwing

      ii. Pain reproduced with anterior apprehension testing, reduced by scapular retraction or relocation testing

4. Calcific rotator cuff tendinitis—uncommon in athletes, most commonly affects middle-aged persons. Most often supraspinatus, but may also occur in infraspinatus and subscapularis. May be found in 6–8% of asymptomatic individuals

5. History:

    a. Insidious or traumatic. Overuse etiology common

    b. Deep achy pain over deltoid, acromion, deltoid insertion. Rule out ACJ disorders as this area is a common referral pattern for the ACJ. In internal impingement, pain may be more posterior. Acute calcific tendinitis may have a hyperacute presentation with severe pain, including pain at rest, and occasionally fever

    c. Pain increased with activity, particularly overhead (impingement syndrome). May include night pain

6. PE:

    a. Rotator cuff atrophy or fasciculations—suggests full thickness, chronic tear, or suprascapular neuropathy

    b. Tender subacromial space

    c. Mid-range painful arc of motion

    d. Pain with or without weakness

      i. Full can test—emphasizes (not isolates) supraspinatus; elevation to 90° in scapular plane with arm externally rotated (preferred over empty can)

      ii. Resisted external rotation—emphasizes infraspinatus and teres minor; arm at side and resist external rotation

      iii. Lift off test—place patient's hand on their lumbar spine, palm facing out. Lift their hand off their back and see if patient can hold position; if unable to do so, positive test and suggests subscapularis tear

    e. Impingement signs

      i. Hawkins—arm flexed 90° in sagittal plane, elbow flexed to 90°, examiner internally rotates patient's arm. Positive test = pain reproduction

      ii. Neers—arm flexed maximally in sagittal plane, internally rotated at end range. Pain reproduction = positive test

    f. Neer impingement test

      i. Reexamination for impingement after injecting lidocaine into the subacromial space. Resolution of pain confirms external impingement

7. Diagnostic evaluation

    a. X-rays—Obtain at least two orthogonal views, typically AP (ER and IR) and axillary. Outlet view may be useful to identify acromial shape and ACJ osteophytes. Evaluate for GHJ and ACJ DJD. Os acromial—unfused anterior acromial apophysis, seen best on axillary view, may cause impingement. Irregularities of greater tuberosity suggest rotator cuff disease, including tears. Narrowed acromiohumeral interval <7 mm on AP view suggestive of full thickness rotator cuff tear

    b. MRI and US excellent for evaluating rotator cuff

8. Nonoperative treatment

    a. Rest, ice, activity modification

    b. Tylenol, NSAIDs.

    c. Rotator cuff and scapular stabilizer program. Prefer to work on scapular stabilizers initially, then infraspinatus/teres minor and subscapularis, and then only later directed elevation exercises stressing the supraspinatus and deltoid

    d. Injections. Not usually first line of treatment. Recurrence rate high when used in isolation. Has been documented to improve pain and motion in short and intermediate term

9. Surgery
   a. Indicated with documented, surgically treatable structural pathology or failure of non-operative treatment. Typically repair of rotator cuff tear, bursectomy, with or without subacromial decompression
      i. Acute rotator cuff tears may be appropriate for early surgical intervention
      ii. Chronic or age-determinate cuff tears may or may not be candidates for early surgical intervention depending on tear size, number of tendons affected, and multiple patient factors. In many cases, trial of nonoperative treatment with close follow-up is reasonable
      iii. Arthroscopic rotator cuff repair produces equivalent results to open repair in experienced hands, and results in less morbidity, less pain, small incisions, and no risk of deltoid detachment (known complication of open surgery). Ultimate healing time similar to open technique
      iv. Recovery usually takes 4–6 months to return to activity, regardless of technique.

VI. Labral Tears

A. Acronyms and definitions
   1. HAGL—humeral avulsion of glenohumeral ligament
   2. Bankart—antero-inferior labral tear s/p dislocation
   3. Bony Bankart—antero-inferior glenoid fracture s/p dislocation
   4. Reverse Bankart—postero-inferior labral tear s/p posterior dislocation
   5. GIRD—glenohumeral internal rotation deficit due to posterior capsule/cuff tightness, thought to contribute to SLAP lesions in overhead athletes, as well as other pathologies
   6. Buford Complex—cord-like middle glenohumeral ligament that directly attaches to superior labrum, with absence of superior glenohumeral ligament
   7. Sublabral foramen or fovea—normal variant small foramen in antero-superior quadrant of glenoid, not to be confused with a labral tear
   8. SLAP—superior labral antero-posterior tear. Tear of superior labrum, where the long head of the biceps originates. Several varieties, but most commonly Type II (see below).
      a. Pathoetiology
         i. Peel-back phenomenon—during abduction–external rotation, the biceps anchor pulls posteriorly, placing repetitive traction forces on the labrum, eventually leading to failure
         ii. Repetitive traction forces due to the follow-through of a baseball pitch has also been implicated
      b. May be due to trauma or overuse (i.e., overhead throwers)
      c. Often occur with concomitant pathologies
      d. Types
         i. Type 1 = degenerative fraying (probably asymptomatic)
         ii. Type 2 = labral detachment, intact biceps attached to detached labral fragment
         iii. Type 3 = bucket handle tear
         iv. Type 4 = Type 2 with extension into biceps
      e. MRI arthrogram is diagnostic imaging test of choice, although often diagnosis made at arthroscopy
      f. Most can be treated successfully nonoperatively with rotator cuff and scapular stabilizer program, as well as stretching posterior capsule with sleeper stretches to correct GIRD
      g. Surgery typically involves placement of one or more suture anchors and must address all contributing pathologies. May take 3–6 months to RTP.

VII. Adhesive Capsulitis

A. Painful, restricted shoulder ROM, with early loss of ER, and normal radiographs; typically occurs in middle-aged females > males

B. Usually idiopathic, but may be associated with diabetes mellitus, inflammatory arthritis, trauma, prolonged immobilization, thyroid disease, stroke, myocardial infarction, or auto-immune disease. May also occur secondary to rotator cuff or other disease

C. Stage 1 for the first 1–3 months, pain but little motion loss initially. Stage 2 months 3–9 with reduced pain but increased motion loss, particularly ER. Stage 3 months 9–15 with gradual improvement in ROM

D. X-rays normal, but arthrogram shows significant reduction in capsule volume. Pathology thought to be due to inflammation in rotator interval > global capsule, causing capsule tightening

E. During stages 1 and 2, may use modalities, analgesics/NSAIDs, and glenohumeral joint injections to reduce inflammation and pain; facilitate rehabilitation and shorten the duration of the condition. Avoid aggressive exercise because this will exacerbate the condition

F. Generally normal/near normal function over a 12–14 month period. Patients not improved after 4–6 months may benefit from manipulation under anesthesia or arthroscopic lysis of adhesions.

VIII. Throwing Shoulder

A. Understand the phases of throwing. Motion takes about 2 s with 75% due to wind-up and cocking
   1. Wind-up
   2. Early cocking
   3. Late cocking—arm abducted (AB) and ER, scapula retracted, maximal anterior shear force due to AB–ER position, and highest shoulder torque
   4. Acceleration—transition from eccentric to concentric, only 1/3 kinetic energy stays with ball, remainder dissipated via kinetic chain; late cocking and acceleration pathetiologic in peel-back phenomenon associated with SLAP lesions
   5. Deceleration (most violent phase)—largest joint loads, including compression equal to body weight, posterior shear 400 N, inferior shear >300 N, compression >1,000 N; traction forces during deceleration implicated as one cause of SLAP lesions
   6. Follow-through

B. Rotator cuff (see prior discussion)
   1. External impingement rare
   2. Many throwers exhibit increased joint laxity and increased ROM. Laxity + overuse leads to rotator cuff dysfunction (secondary impingement)
   3. Traction forces during follow-through can acutely or chronically damage RC muscles. These same traction forces may promote cumulative tensile stress to the posterior-inferior shoulder capsule, producing a Bennet lesion (see below)
   4. Treat as previously described, surgery a consideration if failure to progress in 3–6 months.
   5. Postero-superior/internal impingement—see prior discussion; note that condition thought to be accentuated by increased shoulder ER, anterior instability, poor scapular retraction during late cocking/acceleration, and posterior capsular tightness (GIRD)

C. SLAP lesions
   1. Typically Type II
   2. Implicated during late cocking/acceleration via peel-back phenomenon and during deceleration due to traction

3. No best test to diagnose—O'Brien, Crank, Dynamic labral shear, etc
4. Many respond to rehabilitation
5. GIRD—Note relationship of posterior shoulder tightness (loss of IR and/or horizontal adduction) to accentuation of the peel-back phenomenon and etiology of SLAP lesions; treat non-op with "sleeper stretch" and if needed capsular release

D. Bennett's lesion—calcification of the posterior band of the inferior glenohumeral ligament, seen best on axillary x-rays, often an asymptomatic finding, but may be symptomatic; size does not correlate with symptoms; treat symptomatically, including injections, but may require surgical removal.

IX. Miscellaneous Conditions

A. Sternoclavicular joint
1. Only osseous connection of entire upper limb with rest of body. Supported by strong ligaments. Rarely injured acutely, but when injured usually high forces involved. Costoclavicular ligaments major stabilizers during elevation and rotation
2. Osteoarthritis—may be posttraumatic, but can occur idiopathically, postmenopausal females, dominant arm
   a. Symptomatic treatment (e.g., activity modification, NSAIDs, injections) at least 6–12 months prior to considering surgery
   b. Operation is resectional arthroplasty
3. Sepsis—IV drug users, immunocompromised; likely spread hematogenously; surgical emergency; may spread into mediastinum
4. Atraumatic instability—young, hyperlax, less common
5. Medial clavicular hyperostosis—often as part of syndromes such as SAPHO syndrome (synovitis, acne, pustulosis, hyperostosis, osteitis)
6. Traumatic instability: Most common mechanism indirect injury, fall onto lateral shoulder. Direction of force and arm position (flexed vs. extended) determine whether anterior or posterior dislocation. Direct injuries less common, but typically involve antero-to-posterior force and results in posterior subluxation/dislocation
   a. Anterior—more common (2/3), significant pain, swelling, limited ROM
   b. Posterior—less common (1/3), may suspect clinically (do not misinterpret left posterior SCJ dislocation as a right anterior SCJ dislocation); may compromise airway or adjacent vascular structures (look for venous dilatation in arm of affected side)
   c. Evaluation
      i. Radiographs should include AP and lateral of chest, but most useful is serendipity view (45° cephalic tilt centered on SCJ), will show position of clavicle relative to manubrium
      ii. CT is actually imaging modality of choice, and can be combined with CT-angiography to evaluate proximity/status of great vessels
      iii. MRI usually unnecessary and suboptimal for bone
   d. Treatment
      i. If seen within 7 days, closed reduction (CR) may be attempted
      ii. Anterior reductions usually do not remain reduced. Figure-of-eight brace preferred over standard sling
      iii. Posterior reductions should only be performed in a controlled environment, with pre- and postvascular evaluation, with emergency medical and vascular surgery on site. Immobilize for 6–10 weeks
      iv. If CR fails, need open reduction and stabilization. Putting wires, pins, other instruments into the area of the SCJ for stabilization is almost never the correct answer for any SCJ problem
      v. If chronic, anterior usually treated symptomatically for 6–12 months because many will improve. If not, resectional arthroplasty. Posterior usually open

reduction and resectional arthroplasty. May be erosion into great vessels that is controlled by displaced clavicle

   vi. In skeletally immature, more likely represents a physeal injury. Physis does not close until age 24. 80% clavicle growth arises from medial clavicle, so large amount of remodeling possible. Merely observe

B. Suprascapular neuropathy

  1. Pain (postero-superior), weakness, atrophy
  2. Noncompressive
     a. No mass lesion. Etiology?, but may be traction from repetitive overhead and adduction activities. Common in volleyball players, but seen in all overhead athletes. May be minimally symptomatic
     b. Usually affects only the infraspinatus
     c. Prognosis excellent with rest and rehab. Many asymptomatic despite marked atrophy. Uncommon need spinoglenoid notch decompression
  3. Compressive
     a. Usually paralabral ganglion cyst associated with labral tear
     b. May involve both supraspinatus and infraspinatus (compression at suprascapular notch) or just the infraspinatus (compression at spinoglenoid notch—more common)
  4. Signs/symptoms: Posterior symptoms, atrophy, weakness > pain, and preferential affecting infraspinatus; may have labral findings
  5. Evaluation: Diagnose cyst by US or MRI; MRI arthrogram better for labrum
  6. Many require surgical intervention. May percutaneously drain, but recurrence risk high.

Recommended Reading

1. Braun S, Kokmeyer D, Millett PJ. Shoulder injuries in the throwing athlete. *J Bone Joint Surg.* 2009;91:966–978.
2. Cox CL, Kuhn JE. Operative versus nonoperative treatment of acute shoulder dislocation in the athlete. *Curr Sports Med Rep.* 2008;7(5):263–268.
3. Greiwe RM, Ahmad CS. Management of the throwing shoulder: Cuff, labrum and internal impingement. *Orthop Clin North Am.* 2010;41:309–323.
4. Pujalte GG, Housner JA. Management of clavicle fractures. *Curr Sports Med Rep.* 2008;7(5):275–280.
5. Rios CG, Mazzocca AD. Acromioclavicular joint problems in athletes and new methods of management. *Clin Sports Med.* 2008;27(4):763–788.
6. Wilk KE, Obma P, Simpson CD, Cain EL, Dugas JR, Andrews JR. Shoulder injuries in the overhead athlete. *J Orthop Sports Phys Ther.* 2009;39(2):38–54.

22

Elbow and Forearm Injuries and Conditions

Steve J. Wisniewski

I. Anatomy

A. Bones of the elbow
  1. Humerus, radius, ulna
    a. Elbow is the hinge joint between the distal humerus and proximal radius and ulna.
      i. Normal range of motion is 0–140° flexion
      ii. Common for baseball pitchers to have mild flexion contracture on the dominant side
    b. Radiocapitellar and radioulnar joints allow for pronation/supination
      i. Normal range of motion is 75° of pronation and 85° of supination
      ii. The annular ligament supports the radioulnar joint

B. Ligaments of the elbow
  1. Lateral or radial collateral ligament complex
    a. Includes the radial collateral ligament, annular ligament, accessory collateral ligament, and the posterolateral (lateral ulnar) collateral ligament
    b. Provides varus support; rarely injured in the athlete
  2. Medial or ulnar collateral ligament complex
    a. Three bundles: anterior, posterior, and transverse oblique
      i. Anterior bundle is the primary restraint to valgus stress of the elbow when the elbow is flexed between 30° and 120°

C. Muscles of the elbow
  1. Elbow flexion
    a. Brachialis, brachioradialis, and biceps brachii
  2. Elbow extension
    a. Triceps and anconeus
  3. Medial flexor/pronator muscles
    a. Wrist/finger flexors
      i. Flexor carpi radialis, palmaris longus, flexor carpi ulnaris, flexor digitorum superficialis
    b. Forearm pronation
      i. Pronator teres
  4. Lateral extensor/supinator muscles
    a. Wrist/finger extensors
      i. Extensor carpi radialis longus, extensor carpi radialis brevis, extensor digitorum, extensor digiti minimi, extensor carpi ulnaris
    b. Forearm supination
      i. Supinator (biceps brachii also contributes to forearm supination)

D. Nerves

1. Median nerve
   a. Passes over the elbow anteriorly, covered by the bicipital aponeurosis. It then passes between the two heads of the pronator teres muscle and travels in the forearm deep to the flexor digitorum superficialis muscle
2. Ulnar nerve
   a. Travels posterior to the medial epicondyle and enters the cubital tunnel, which is formed by the two heads of the flexor carpi ulnaris muscle
3. Radial nerve
   a. Travels anterior to the elbow between the brachialis and brachioradialis muscles. Divides into the posterior interosseous nerve (PIN) and the superficial radial nerve. The PIN passes between the two heads of the supinator muscle into the forearm, while the superficial radial nerve runs beneath the brachioradialis muscle.

II. Epidemiology, Diagnosis, Treatment

A. Fractures

1. Radial head
   a. Mechanism of injury: fall onto an outstretch hand with forearm pronated
   b. Rule out associated collateral ligament injury
   c. Physical examination reveals tenderness over the radial head and pain with rotation of the forearm
   d. Fracture classification
      i. Type I: nondisplaced fracture
      ii. Type II: fracture with displacement, depression, or angulation
      iii. Type III: comminuted fracture
      iv. Type IV: radial head fracture with elbow dislocation
   e. Treatment
      i. Type I: Hinged elbow splinting/bracing with early range-of motion exercises
      ii. Type II: Surgical treatment—ORIF vs. excision of fragments
      iii. Type III: Excision of the radial head
      iv. Type IV: Reduction of the dislocation, treatment of fracture based on above
2. Supracondylar
   a. Mechanism of injury: usually direct trauma or fall on outstretched hand
   b. Common fracture in children
   c. Neurovascular status needs close monitoring. Observe for possible compartment syndrome.
   d. Fracture classification
      i. Type I: nondisplaced
      ii. Type II: gapping anteriorly, limited rotational malalignment
      iii. Type III: no cortical continuity, unstable
   e. Treatment
      i. Type I: Long-arm cast or splinting with frequent follow-up to ensure alignment
      ii. Type II and III: reduction and fixation
3. Olecranon
   a. Mechanism of injury: Direct blow to the posterior elbow or fall on an outstretched hand with the elbow in flexion, leading to contraction of the triceps and avulsion injury
   b. Classification: multiple classification systems have been described; the one used below is based on the amount of displacement, the amount of comminution and stability of the elbow
      i. Type I: Less than 2 mm displaced, minimal communution, elbow stable
      ii. Type II: Greater than 2 mm displaced, elbow stable
      iii. Type III: fracture associated with unstable elbow

      c. Treatment
        i. Type I: Long arm casting/splinting vs. ORIF
        ii. Type II: Surgical treatment
        iii. Type III: Open reduction and stabilization of the olecranon
    4. Radius/ulna midshaft
      a. Can occur with direct trauma or following a fall onto an outstretched hand; common fracture in children
      b. Close neurovascular evaluation and observation for compartment syndrome is important
      c. Treatment
        i. Cast immobilization if no displacement in children/adolescents; close follow-up required to observe for displacement
        ii. Adult athletes or children with displacement: open reduction internal fixation

B. Elbow dislocation
    1. Occurs most often in football, wrestling, and gymnastics. Often occurs due to a fall on an outstretched hand.
    2. Orthopedic emergency that needs reduction as soon as possible
    3. Classification
      a. Direction of dislocation: posterior (most common), posterolateral, posteromedial, medial, lateral, or divergent
      b. Termed "simple" if no fracture, and "complex" if associated fracture
    4. Pre and postreduction radiographs should be obtained to identify associated fractures
    5. Neurovascular status should be closely monitored
    6. Management depends upon degrees of instability, as injury occurs to the ulnar and radial collateral ligaments
    7. Treatment of elbow dislocations:
      a. Short-term splinting (<1 week) with the elbow in flexion
      b. Early protected range of motion with hinged brace (to prevent contracture formation)
      c. May return to activity within 4–6 weeks if no fracture or neurovascular injury; valgus instability common after dislocation
      d. Complex dislocation or recurrent dislocation: surgical referral

C. Instability/ligament injury
    1. Ulnar collateral ligament (UCL) injury
      a. Anterior bundle is primary restraint to valgus stress, especially during acceleration phase of throwing. This predisposes to acute (sudden "pop" with throwing) or chronic ligamentous injury from throwing.
      b. Symptoms: medial sided elbow pain that is worse with throwing.
      c. Physical examination: tenderness to palpation, especially at the ulnar insertion where most tears occur. Valgus stress to the elbow at 20–30° of flexion (to unlock the olecranon) may cause pain and increased laxity compared to the nonthrowing arm (although the throwing elbow in overhead athletes often has increased valgus laxity without injury).
      d. Plain radiographs may show calcifications within the UCL. Magnetic resonance imaging and/or diagnostic ultrasound may be helpful to confirm UCL tears.
      e. Chronic instability/injuries to the UCL often leads to coexisting ulnar neuropathy.
      f. Nonoperative treatment of UCL injuries
        i. May be successful in nonthrowing athletes or in athletes with mild injuries
        ii. Relative rest (i.e., no throwing), ice
        iii. A hinged elbow brace can be used to protect the elbow from valgus stress
        iv. Stretching and strengthening exercises of the elbow (especially strengthening of the wrist flexors and forearm pronators), rotator cuff, scapula stabilizer muscles, and core muscles
        v. Identify kinetic chain deficiencies, review throwing mechanics

        vi. Gradual return to throwing program when pain free, full range of motion is restored, strength has returned, and underlying deficits are properly rehabilitated

    g. Operative treatment of UCL injuries

        i. Indicated for athletes with complete UCL tears or when partial tears remain symptomatic after proper rehabilitation program

        ii. UCL reconstruction

  2. Posterolateral rotatory instability (lateral ulnar collateral ligament [LUCL] injury)

    a. Transient rotatory subluxation of the radius and ulna from the humerus secondary to injury to the lateral collateral ligament complex

    b. Symptoms: painful elbow locking and popping; possible history of previous elbow trauma or dislocation

    c. Physical examination: positive lateral pivot shift test

    d. MRI scanning can be helpful to confirm injury to the LUCL

    e. Conservative treatment: elbow bracing, rehabilitation, and avoiding provocative maneuvers. If this fails, surgical treatment focuses on reconstruction of the LCL.

D. Valgus extension overload

  1. The combination of high valgus stress and elbow extension during overhead throwing produces impingement between the posteromedial tip of the olecranon and the olecranon fossa causing synovitis, osteophyte formation, and possibly loose bodies.

  2. Symptoms: posterolateral elbow pain during follow-through phase of throwing

  3. Physical examination: pain with full elbow extension during valgus loading

  4. Nonoperative treatment

    a. Rest from throwing

    b. Rehabilitation of the elbow (including improving eccentric strength of elbow flexors), shoulder, and kinetic chain to correct strength and flexibility deficits

    c. Gradual return to throwing when symptoms resolve and following rehabilitation of the above deficits

  5. Operative treatment

    a. Indicated if failed nonoperative treatment

    b. Excision of osteophyte and exploration for loose bodies

    c. Post-op rehabilitation of elbow, shoulder, kinetic chain to correct strength and flexibility deficits

E. Muscle/tendon injury

  1. Distal biceps rupture

    a. Rupture often occurs with eccentric load to the flexed elbow

    b. Symptoms: sudden onset of anterior elbow pain and swelling, often with a "pop," followed by ecchymosis

    c. Important to distinguish between partial and complete tear as complete tears treated best with early surgical intervention

    d. Physical examination: tender to palpation over distal biceps tendon, edema, echymosis, abnormal hook test (inability to "hook" finger around distal biceps tendon when elbow is flexed and forearm supinated), supination weakness > elbow flexion weakness

    e. MRI can differentiate between partial and complete tears

    f. Nonoperative treatment for partial tears: PRICE, reestablish normal ROM, add strengthening exercises as able

    g. Surgical treatment recommended for complete ruptures

  2. Lateral epicondylitis

    a. Usually an overuse/degenerative injury (i.e., tendinosis) of the common extensor tendon. Most often involves the extensor carpi radialis brevis

    b. Symptoms: lateral elbow pain that may radiate down the forearm

    c. Physical examination: tenderness at and just distal to the lateral epicondyle. Pain exacerbated by resisted wrist extension or passive wrist flexion

       d. Treatment: rest, ice, forearm counterforce brace, physical therapy to correct underlying flexibility and strength deficits in the elbow, shoulder, and kinetic chain. Eccentric strengthening of the wrist extensors is recommended. Correction of suboptimal sporting technique/equipment is important. Occasionally, corticosteroid injections can be helpful for short-term pain relief.

       e. If no improvement with the above treatment, surgery may be indicated.

   3. Medial epicondylitis

       a. Usually an overuse/degenerative injury (i.e., tendinosis) of the common flexor tendon.

       b. Symptoms: medial elbow pain that may radiate into the proximal forearm.

       c. Physical examination: tenderness over the anterior aspect of the medial epicondyle. Pain is exacerbated by resisted wrist flexion/pronation or passive wrist extension.

       d. Treatment: rest, ice, NSAIDs, forearm counterforce brace, and physical therapy to correct underlying flexibility and strength deficits in the elbow, shoulder, and kinetic chain. Correct suboptimal sporting technique/equipment. Occasionally, corticosteroid injections can be helpful for short-term pain relief.

       e. If no improvement with the above treatment, surgery may be indicated.

   4. Triceps tendinitis

       a. Repetitive overuse injury

       b. Physical examination: tender to palpation over the distal triceps tendon as it inserts on the olecranon. Pain exacerbated by resisted elbow extension or passive elbow flexion.

       c. Treatment: ice, NSAIDs, and physical therapy to correct underlying strength and flexibility deficits. Review of sporting technique/equipment is important to prevent reoccurrence.

F. Olecranon bursitis

   1. Mechanism of injury

       a. Acute hemorrhagic bursitis due to direct trauma to the posterior elbow

       b. Chronic bursitis associated with repetitive motions or frequent irritation of the bursa (pressure)

   2. Clinical presentation

       a. Acute bursitis: rapid swelling, bursa filled with blood

       b. Chronic bursitis: bursa swelling, often have minimal pain

   3. Physical examination: extraarticular swelling/fluid collection over the olecranon

   4. Aspiration/laboratory evaluation required if concern for infection exists

   5. Treatment: compression, NSAIDs, ice, and splinting. Elbow pads. Aspiration may be performed in acute bursitis. Corticosteroid injections can be used to treat subacute/chronic cases, but may increase risk of infection.

   6. Surgical excision of the bursa rarely required

G. Acute compartment syndrome

   1. Elevation of interstitial pressure resulting in microvascular compromise

       a. Can lead to tissue necrosis and neurovascular injury if not promptly treated (Volkmann's ischemic contracture)

   2. May occur following humerus fracture or fractures of the forearm; higher incidence when combined humerus and forearm fractures

   3. Patients complain of increasing pain, tightness, and paresthesias in the forearm and hand

   4. Physical examination

       a. Reduced sensation in the hand

       b. Firm, woody feeling on palpation of the forearm

       c. Pain on passive digit extension

       d. Pallor and loss of pulses are late findings

       e. Neurologic symptoms (weakness, paresthesias)

   5. Compartment pressure measurement can confirm diagnosis

   6. Treatment consists of forearm fasciotomy.

Recommended Reading

1. Ahmad CS, El Attrache NS. Valgus extension overload syndrome and stress injury of the olecranon. *Clin Sports Med.* 2004;23(4):665–676.
2. Cain EL, Dugas JR, Wolf RS, Andrews JR. Elbow injuries in throwing athletes: A current concepts review. *Am J Sports Med.* 2003;31(4):621–635.
3. Gomez JE. Upper extremity injuries in youth sports. *Pediatr Clin North Am.* 2002;49:593–626.
4. Griggs SM, Weiss APC. Bony injuries of the wrist, forearm, and elbow. *Clin Sports Med.* 1996;15(2):373–400.
5. McFarland EG, Gill HS, Laporte DM, Streiff M. Miscellaneous conditions about the elbow in athletes. *Clin Sports Med.* 2004;23(4):743–763.
6. Rettig AC. Elbow, forearm and wrist injuries in the athlete. *Sports Med.* 1998;25(2):115–130.
7. Safran MR. Elbow injuries in athletes. *Clin Orthop Relat Res.* 1995;310:257–277.
8. Sellards R, Kuebrich C. The elbow: diagnosis and treatment of common injuries. *Primary Care: Clin Office Pract.* 2005;32:1–16.

Hand and Wrist Injuries and Conditions

Joseph Michael Ihm

I. Clinical Anatomy

A. The distal radial ulnar joint (DRUJ) allows for forearm and hand pronation and supination, with stability provided by the triangular fibrocartilage complex (TFCC), extensor carpi ulnaris, interosseous ligament, pronator quadratus, and associated forearm muscles

B. The radial portion of the DRUJ articulates with the proximal row of carpal bones, but the distal ulna does not directly articulate with the carpal bones and instead serves as an attachment for multiple stabilizing ligaments that comprise the ulnar wrist

C. The radial wrist biomechanically handles 75–80% of the axial load across the wrist.

D. Triangular fibrocartilage complex (TFCC) (Figure 23.1)

   1. The TFCC is divided into a central articular disc portion, which is relatively avascular, and the dorsal and palmar radioulnar ligaments, which are more vascular and provide stability to the DRUJ

   2. The volar ulnar carpal ligaments extend from the periphery of the TFCC and ulnar styloid to the lunate and triquetrum

   3. The TFCC is completed by the ulnar extensor muscle subsheath and the ulnar collateral ligament

   4. The triangular fibrocartilage is thinner in ulnar positive wrists, which increases the risk of injury in these individuals

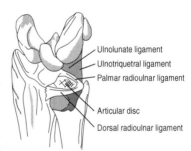

Ulnolunate ligament
Ulnotriquetral ligament
Palmar radioulnar ligament
Articular disc
Dorsal radioulnar ligament

Figure 23.1 The triangular fibrocartilage complex

E. Ulnar variance is related to the relationship between the length of the ulna and radius

   1. Neutral: the ulna and radius are the same length

   2. Positive variance: the ulna is longer than the radius

   3. Negative variance: the ulna is shorter than the radius

F. The wrist is made up of eight carpal bones (Figure 23.2)

G. Carpal tunnel (Figure 23.3)

   1. Borders of carpal tunnel

     a. Anterior border is the transverse carpal ligament, which is deep to the palmaris longus and runs from the hamate and pisiform medially to the scaphoid and trapezium laterally

     b. Posterior border is comprised of the carpal bones

   2. Contents of the carpal tunnel

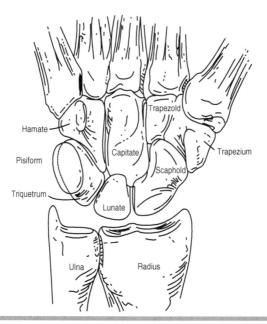

Figure 23.2   Wrist osseous anatomy

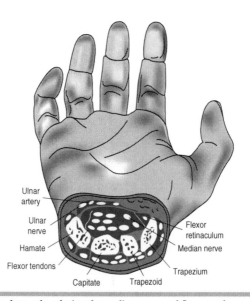

Figure 23.3   Carpal tunnel enclosing the median nerve and flexor tendons

    a. Median nerve, which provides motor innervation to the 1st and 2nd lumbricals and the thenar muscles (except the deep portion of the flexor pollicis brevis) and sensory innervation to the thenar eminence, the palmar aspect of the 1st–3rd digits and the lateral half of the 4th digit

    b. Tendons of the flexor digitorum superficialis, flexor digitorum profundus, and flexor pollicis longus

H. Ulnar nerve and artery pass through Guyon's canal

    1. Ulnar nerve provides motor innervation to the 3rd and 4th lumbricals, the palmar and dorsal interossei, the hypothenar muscles, the deep portion of the flexor pollicis brevis, and the adductor pollicis

    2. The ulnar nerve provides sensory innervation to the 5th digit and medial half of the 4th digit

    3. The radial and ulnar arteries provide the vascular supply to the hand

I. The radial nerve has no motor innervation to the hand but provides sensory innervation to the dorsum of the 1st–3rd and the lateral half of the 4th digit.

II. Epidemiology, Diagnosis, and Treatment of Specific Injuries and Conditions

A. Fractures

    1. Distal radius

        a. Often occurs as a result of a fall on an outstretched hand with hyperextension of the wrist impacting the distal radius

        b. Positive ballottement sign at the DRUJ suggests instability

        c. Plain radiographs: anteroposterior (AP), lateral and oblique views

        d. Treatment

            i. Nonsurgical: nondisplaced extraarticular fractures are treated with a long arm cast in neutral or supination for 4–6 weeks

            ii. Surgical

                (A) Displaced and comminuted

                (B) Intraarticular

                (C) Loss of radial inclination, a dorsal tilt $>20°$, or an articular step-off >2 mm

    2. Distal ulna—uncommon area for fracture, but case reports of stress reactions have been reported and are treated with immobilization

    3. Scaphoid

        a. Most commonly injured carpal bone; occurs due to a fall on an outstretched hand that causes hyperextension of the wrist

        b. Constitutes about 75% of carpal fractures in athletes, and are second only to distal radius fractures as the most common wrist fracture

        c. Most prevalent in those 15–30 years old

        d. Loss of motion, swelling, and pain over the dorsal–radial and radial–volar aspects of the wrist, with tenderness to palpation at the volar scaphoid tubercle at the scaphotrapezial joint and the anatomic snuffbox

        e. Radiographic evaluation includes an anteroposterior (AP), oblique, lateral, and an AP view with ulnar deviation

        f. If initial radiographs are negative but suspicion for fracture is high, treat presumptively by immobilizing in a thumb spica splint and reimage in 2 weeks; MRI or bone scan may be done early in the elite or professional athlete if confirmation of diagnosis is needed, but may need 1–3 days before definitively positive

        g. The definition of stability of a scaphoid fracture is an important (though controversial) concept, as treatment is dependent on stability

        h. Unstable fractures include those with more than 1 mm of displacement, malangulation, or associated carpal instability

            i. Treatment with surgical fixation is warranted to minimize risk of nonunion or malunion

      ii. Duration of postoperative splinting is dependent on degree of stability obtained intraoperatively

      i. Acute stable fractures may be treated with a short arm cast with a thumb spica extension in slight radial deviation and palmar flexion, with healing rates of 90–100% within 8–12 weeks

      j. Some stable fractures are treated surgically in order to allow the athlete to return to sport earlier with use of a cast

      k. Unprotected return to sport should be allowed only when range of motion (ROM) is normal and full healing has been confirmed

      l. Due to the vascular anatomy, proximal pole fractures have a worse prognosis for healing than more distal injuries

         i. The scaphoid receives majority of blood supply (including that to the entire proximal pole) via dorsal vessels, 70–80% of which is provided by branches from the radial artery in a retrograde fashion from the waist of the scaphoid

         ii. Due to the retrograde flow to the proximal pole of the scaphoid, a fracture in this part of the bone can adversely affect blood flow and increase the chance of avascular necrosis

4. Hamate hook fractures

    a. 2–4% of all carpal fractures; common in golf, baseball, and hockey

    b. Presents with vague complaints of pain at the volar ulnar aspect of hand, with pain provoked when attempting a tight grip

    c. Duration of symptoms may be prolonged, and some will have already seen several physicians without a diagnosis

    d. ROM is full with tenderness over the hamate hook at the hypothenar eminence

    e. Plain radiographs (including a carpal tunnel view) may not visualize fracture; thus, CT scan is considered if fracture is suspected

    f. While nonoperative management and surgical fixation may both be considered, excision of the hamate hook is considered the treatment of choice

5. Metacarpal

    a. Assessment

       i. Assess for shortening by examining metacarpal heads with metacarpophalangeal joint flexion (i.e., make a fist)

       ii. Radial or ulnar malangulation are evaluated with the fingers in extension; dorsal angulation is indicated by the presence of a "dropped knuckle"

       iii. Overlap of digits or rotation of the nail plate while assessing the volar aspect of the hand with the fingers in slight flexion indicates malrotation

       iv. Plain radiographs: posteroanterior (PA), lateral, and oblique

    b. Shaft fracture: Transverse

       i. Most common

       ii. Typical mechanism: fall onto a clenched fist while holding a ball or from a direct blow to a helmet

       iii. Unstable metacarpal shaft and neck fractures will tend to angulate with the apex directed dorsally due to the volar pull of the interosseous muscles

       iv. Treatment

          (A) Reduction required if:

            (1) Any angulation of 2nd and 3rd digits

            (2) >20° of angulation at the 4th digit

            (3) >30° of angulation at the 5th digit

          (B) Stable nondisplaced fractures are treated with buddy taping, casting, or splinting to prevent malrotation, but are followed weekly to assess for any displacement

         (C) Unstable, displaced fractures require open reduction and internal fixation (ORIF) vs. percutaneous pinning

      c. Shaft fracture: oblique and spiral

         i. High-risk fracture as these commonly rotate and shorten

         ii. Typical mechanism: fall onto open hand or direct twisting motion in wrestling

         iii. Treatment

            (A) Nonsurgical: nondisplaced fractures

            (B) Surgical: fracture with any rotation, >5 mm shortening, or comminution

      d. Neck fracture

         i. Boxer's fracture: 5th digit

         ii. Often present with dorsal angulation

            (A) Can treat with buddy taping 4th and 5th digits

            (B) >20° in the 2nd or 3rd digits commonly requires surgery

         iii. Angulation and malrotation at the index and long fingers can be corrected with buddy taping or surgical fixation

      e. First metacarpal fractures

         i. Bennett fracture

            (A) Intraarticular noncomminuted fracture at the base of the 1st metacarpal

            (B) >1/4 of all metacarpal fractures

            (C) Generally treated with ORIF

         ii. Rolando fracture

            (A) Intraarticular comminuted fracture at the base of the 1st metacarpal

            (B) Worse prognosis compared to the Bennett fracture

            (C) Generally treated with internal or external fixation

         iii. Extraarticular fracture: generally treated with closed reduction followed by spica splinting for 4–6 weeks

      f. Professional or elite athletes may be able to return to sport within 2 weeks with a cast or splint in place, but risks of returning to sport this early, such as loss of fixation or reoperation, need to be discussed

   6. Phalangeal (Figure 23.4)

      a. May be associated with tendon injuries, such as a mallet finger (Section D.4) or boutonniere deformity (section D.6)

      b. Due to the effect of the extensor mechanism and dorsal translation of the lateral bands, a fractured proximal phalanx will tend to angulate with the apex directed volarly

      c. Due to the influence of the flexor digitorum superficialis insertion into the middle phalanx, a proximal fracture of a middle phalanx will involve angulation with the apex dorsal, and a distal fracture will involve angulation with the apex volar

      d. Fractures of the distal phalanx that lie between the points of extensor insertion and flexor insertion, as well as physeal fractures, will frequently be unstable due to the opposing forces of the two tendons

      e. Distal phalangeal fractures may be treated with a splint unless unstable, which then require reduction and fixation

   7. Volar plate—after a dorsal metacarpophalangeal (MCP) joint dislocation, the distal aspect of the plate remains attached to the proximal phalanx and the remaining component flaps dorsal to the metacarpal head, which may ultimately block a closed reduction and if present would need to be treated surgically

B. Dislocations

   1. Distal radioulnar joint

      a. Often occurs secondary to a fall onto an outstretched, pronated forearm, resulting in a dorsal dislocation

      b. Falling onto a supinated forearm results in volar instability

      c. Plain radiographs are obtained to assess for associated fractures

      d. If not complicated by a fracture, treatment is closed reduction with immobilization for 6 weeks

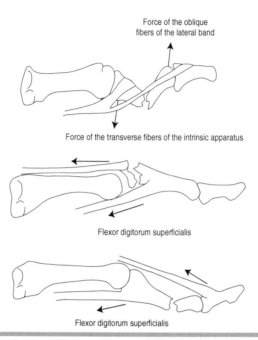

Figure 23.4 **How location of fracture affects angulation in phalangeal fractures.**

    e. Inability to reduce the joint should prompt a search for interposed soft tissue such as the extensor carpi ulnaris tendon

  2. Lunate and perilunate

    a. Perilunate or volar lunate dislocation at the wrists results from excessive radiocarpal hyperextension and ulnar deviation plus intercarpal supination; compression of the median nerve is frequently a complication

    b. Diagnosis is readily made on a true lateral plain radiograph

      i. With perilunate dislocations, the capitate is dorsally displaced on the lunate

      ii. With volar lunate dislocations, the lunate is displaced volarly into the carpal tunnel

    c. Surgical treatment with closed or open reduction is recommended

  3. Metacarpophalageal joint

    a. Dorsal dislocation of the MCP joint is uncommon and usually occurs at the index finger or thumb

      i. Sometimes called the "irreducible dislocation" since the metacarpal head is pushed through the volar plate of the MCP joint and is caught between the lumbrical and long flexor tendons with a button-holing effect; the single most important element in preventing a closed reduction is the interposition of the volar plate between the base of the proximal phalanx and the metacarpal head

      ii. Suspect this injury when examination reveals hyperextension of the involved MCP joint with ulnar deviation of the finger overlapping the adjacent finger

      iii. Plain radiographs are needed to assess for associated fracture

      iv. While closed reduction may be successful, open reduction may be required

      v. After reduction, athlete should wear a splint for 5–6 weeks, allowing full flexion but preventing the last 30° of MCP joint extension

      vi. Recurrent dislocations are rare and near complete ROM is usually achieved

     b. Coronal plane dislocations and volar dislocations are very rare; the former may be reduced by closed means, but the latter generally needs reduction with open treatment

  4. Proximal interphalangeal (PIP) joint (e.g., coach's finger or jammed finger)

     a. Common in contact sports that involve catching or hitting a ball; athlete will generally report jamming or catching a finger while blocking a fall or catching or tapping a ball, sustaining a hyperextension and angular injury to the PIP joint

     b. Dorsal dislocation is much more common than volar dislocations

        i. Generally, one of the collateral ligaments is injured in conjunction with the volar plate

        ii. Plain radiographs (with some preferring fluoroscopy) should be obtained to identify associated fractures and to assess stability, with a small avulsion fragment often seen at the volar lip of the middle phalanx, which is attached to the volar plate

        iii. Treatment is dictated by stability, with stable injuries treated symptomatically and managed by buddy taping the injured digit to noninjured digit adjacent to the compromised ligament

        iv. Unstable injuries are usually associated with an intraarticular fracture of the base of the middle phalanx affecting 40% or more of the joint surface and may be treated with a dorsal extension-block splint, with incremental extension of the splint and digit performed on a weekly basis for 4 weeks or until full extension is achieved

           (A) ROM should be performed actively and passively within the constraint of the splint to minimize scar adhesion

           (B) Unstable injuries are treated with surgery if reduction cannot be achieved or sustained by closed means

     c. Volar dislocations of the PIP are uncommon and surgical reduction is usually required; these dislocations are frequently associated with an injury to the central slip of the extensor mechanism and should be treated like a boutonniere deformity (see section D.6)

  5. Distal interphalangeal (DIP) joint

     a. Often seen in ball-handling and contact sports

     b. Usually occur dorsally and are commonly associated with a volar skin laceration; most often caused by a ball hitting the finger into hyperextension; mallet finger (see section D.4) can occur with a volar dislocation of the DIP joint

     c. Collateral ligament injuries at the DIP joint are rare; flexor tendon function must be assessed as avulsion can occur with this injury

     d. Plain radiographs should be obtained to assess for fracture

     e. Immediate and stable reduction is often achieved with traction and flexion, with the joint splinted for 3 weeks in 10° of flexion, though some consider buddy taping sufficient

C. Instability (ligament injury without dislocation)

  1. Scapholunate/dorsal intercalated segmental instability

     a. Most common wrist ligament injury

     b. Occurs with excessive wrist extension and ulnar deviation with intercarpal supination, such as falling on a pronated hand; thus, scaphoid palmar flexes, lunate dorsiflexes, and capitate moves proximally

     c. Wrist ROM and load-bearing capacity may be compromised after such an injury, with pain occurring secondary to shearing of the articular cartilage and synovitis

     d. Pain with the scaphoid shift test (Watson's sign—Figure 23.5): apply a dorsal load to the distal pole of the scaphoid as the wrist is moved from ulnar to radial deviation; reproduction of pain ± hearing a pop constitutes a positive test and suggests scapholunate ligament insufficiency

     e. Plain radiographs (should be compared to the uninjured wrist)

        i. AP and pronated clenched fist views

            (A) Positive when a gap of more than 2–3 mm exists

            (B) Shortened appearance of the scaphoid with the ring sign, which may be present as a result of the cortical projection of the distal pole in a more vertical position

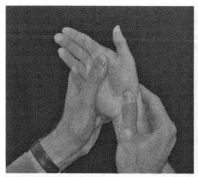 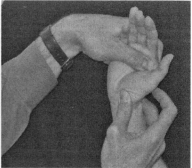

Figure 23.5 Watson's sign: begin with the patient's wrist in ulnar deviation and slight extension. While applying AP pressure to the scaphoid tuberosity move the wrist from ulnar to radial deviation. If pain is provoked then test is positive.

      ii. Lateral view
         (A) Normal scapholunate angle: 30–60°
         (B) Increased scapholunate angle (>70°)
   f. While an MR arthrogram may be helpful some consider wrist arthroscopy the standard method of diagnosing intercarpal ligament injuries
   g. Treatment
      i. Acute (3–4 weeks): open surgical treatment is recommended
      ii. Chronic (>3 months): surgical repair may be performed when anatomic reduction is possible; if anatomic reduction is not possible or osteoarthritis is present then a partial wrist arthrodesis may be performed
2. Lunotriquetral/volar intercalated segmental instability
   a. Much less common than scapholunate injuries and are a result of an axial load with the wrist extended and radially deviated
   b. Lunotriquetral shear test—apply a dorsally directed force over the pisiform (and triquetrum) and a palmar-directed force on the lunate, with reproduction of pain with a click indicating a positive test
   c. If imaging not diagnostic and symptoms persist after immobilization, wrist arthroscopy is pursued
   d. Treatment consists of immobilization ± corticosteroid injection initially; if no improvement, then surgical treatment is pursued
3. First MCP ulnar collateral ligament (UCL) (skier's thumb, gamekeeper's thumb)
   a. Mechanism of injury is hyperabduction and radial deviation of the 1st MCP joint
   b. Tenderness to palpation above the UCL, frequently at its insertion into the base of the proximal phalanx
   c. Need to determine presence of Stener lesion
      i. Occurs when the UCL detaches from the base of the proximal phalanx and is transposed dorsal to the adductor aponeurosis, thus facing proximally (Figure 23.6)
      ii. Visible and/or palpable mass ± gross instability is noted
      iii. Present in 50–70% of suspected cases
      iv. Best treated acutely with open anatomic repair but can be delayed for 3–4 weeks after the injury
   d. Plain radiographs
      i. Obtain AP and lateral prior to stress views to assess for fracture
      ii. Stress views if no fracture seen on initial films

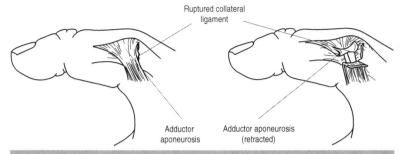

Figure 23.6   Complete rupture of the ulnar collateral ligament resulting in a Stener lesion; the distal attachment has been avulsed from the bone.

      iii. Radial deviation applied with the MCP joint in extension and at 30° of flexion
          (A) If the joint opens more than 30° (or more than 15° compared to the noninjured side) with both flexion and extension views, complete rupture has occurred
      iv. If laxity with flexion only, then closed treatment may be adequate
   e. Treatment
     i. Nonoperative for stable (clinically and radiographically)
       (A) Short arm thumb spica cast for 4 weeks
       (B) After short arm cast removed then removable spica splint for 2–4 months
     ii. Surgical
       (A) Unstable
       (B) Stener lesion
       (C) Larger displaced avulsion fractures at the base of the proximal phalanx
D. Muscle/tendon injuries
  1. DeQuervain's tenosynovitis (stenosing tenosynovitis of the first dorsal compartment)
    a. Most common tenosynovitis about the wrist in the athlete, and is a result of repetitive gliding of the abductor pollicis longus (APL) and the extensor pollicis brevis (EPB)
    b. Occur in activities requiring forceful gripping with ulnar deviation, such as golf, fly fishing, and some racquet sports
    c. High incidence of EPB tendon traveling in a separate compartment from the APL
    d. Pain is reproduced over the radial aspect of the wrist with palpation and with Finkelstein's test (Figure 23.7)—positive when there is pain reproduced at the APL and EPB at the distal radial forearm and wrist with passive ulnar deviation of the wrist with the thumb inside a closed fist

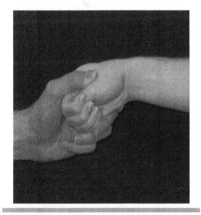

Figure 23.7 Finkelstein's test: with patient actively holding the thumb in a closed fist the examiner moves the wrist into ulnar deviation. If pain is provoked over lateral wrist and/or distal forearm then suggestive of DeQuervain's tenosynovitis.

    e. Treatment
       i. Rest and immobilization are initial treatments, with 25–72% experiencing resolution of symptoms
       ii. Corticosteroid injections are helpful for most
       iii. Surgical treatment is used rarely in recalcitrant cases
2. Intersection syndrome (extensor tenosynovitis)
    a. Located at the crossing points of the APL and EPB with the radial wrist extensors 4–6 cm proximal to the radiocarpal joint/Lister's tubercle
    b. Frequently seen in sports requiring repetitive wrist extension: oarsmen, weight training, and those playing racquet sports
    c. Symptoms generally respond to rest, splinting, and NSAIDs, with use of corticosteroid injections in recalcitrant cases
3. Jersey finger
    a. Flexor digitorum profundus (FDP) avulsion, often at the distal phalanx; often occurs in football when a player tries to grab an opponent's jersey while tackling, and the finger is forced into extension while the DIP is actively flexed
    b. Ring finger most commonly involved (75%) but any digit can be injured
    c. Inability to flex the DIP actively, which is tested while holding the PIP in extension; tenderness may be focal at the site of injury or as proximal as the palm since the flexor tendon sheath may retract
    d. Plain radiographs to assess for fractures
    e. Surgery is treatment of choice in acute cases and should be considered within 7–10 days; in chronic cases, functional impairment and pain is often minimal so observation is preferred
4. Mallet finger (Figure 23.8)
    a. Results from a disruption of the terminal extensor tendon at its insertion on the distal phalanx, which occurs most often due to impact of the fingertip on a ball or other object resulting in flexion force to the DIP joint, but can occur from an extension axial force
    b. Common in baseball, basketball and with football receivers
    c. Inability to extend the DIP actively
    d. Treatment
       i. Splint DIP in extension (PIP can be free) for 6 weeks; then for 4 additional weeks at night
       ii. Surgery is considered for fracture subluxation injuries
5. Trigger finger (flexor tenosynovitis)
    a. Often occurs in racquet and club sports
    b. Nodule forms from overuse or direct pressure at the flexor tendon sheath, which leads to mechanical catching under the A1 pulley at the MCP level
    c. A corticosteroid injection into the nodule or thickened tendon sheath can improve symptoms in up to 90% of cases; modification of the racquet handle or grip may facilitate recovery
6. Boutonniere deformity (Figure 23.9)
    a. Rupture of the central slip of the extensor mechanism at its insertion into the base of the middle phalanx
    b. Results from direct trauma to the dorsum of the PIP joint, an acute flexion force at the DIP, or more commonly following a lateral volar dislocation of the PIP joint that results in injury to the central slip and collateral ligament

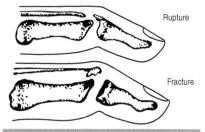

Figure 23.8 Mallet finger: mechanism of injury either rupture or avulsion fracture.

c. Inability to extend the flexed PIP joint actively, but ability to maintain the extended posture if the finger is placed there passively
d. Common finger posture: PIP is flexed and DIP is extended
e. Treatment
   i. If full passive extension (i.e., no flexion contracture) at PIP is present: splint PIP in extension (DIP free) for 6 weeks
   ii. In chronic cases serial casting or splinting for a longer period may be needed to correct flexion contracture

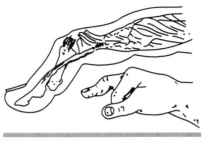

Figure 23.9   **Boutonniere deformity**

E. TFCC injury
 1. May be a result of acute trauma, such as from a fall on an outstretched hand, or from overuse or repetitive trauma (e.g., in racquet sports)
 2. Must be differentiated from other causes of ulnar wrist pain, such as lunotriquetral injuries and ulnar extensor tendon disorders
 3. Symptoms
    a. Pain with palpation over the hollow between the pisiform and ulnar styloid on the ulnar border of the wrist
    b. Pain is reproduced with lifting an object with the forearm in full supination or while pushing off the palm of the hand with the wrist extended
 4. Diagnostic imaging
    a. Plain radiographs may show positive ulnar variance
    b. MRI arthrogram of the wrist may be diagnostic
 5. Treatment
    a. Neutral wrist splinting for 4–6 weeks
    b. Surgical
       i. Central tear (most common): debridement
       ii. Peripheral tear: consider repair
       iii. More chronic injuries and those with positive ulnar variance: ulnar shortening procedure

F. Gymnast's wrist
 1. Seen in young gymnasts (12–14 years old) from repetitive dorsiflexion (>35 h/week of training) creating injury to the distal radial physis
 2. Plain films may demonstrate radial epiphyseal widening or metaphyseal irregularity; if normal, consider bone scan or MRI to assess physis further
 3. Treatment
    a. Modify activity
    b. Resist hyperextension: splint or tape
    c. Surgery is rarely necessary

G. Nail bed injuries
 1. With any of the following nail bed injuries, plain radiographs should be performed to look for fractures of the phalanx
 2. Subungual hematoma—accumulating painful hematoma that can be decompressed using cautery or an 18-gauge needle
 3. Simple and complex nail bed lacerations
    a. Simple: repaired by removing the nail plate to suture, then replacing the nail plate after repair
    b. Complex often occur with a distal phalanx fracture, so both need to be addressed

   4. Avulsion of the nail and complex injury with loss of nail bed—both treated with surgical repair
H. Ganglion cysts
   1. Synovial cyst communicating with the joint space, most commonly at the scapholunate space, often painless; occur at any age
   2. Main complaint is wrist pain and decreased ROM
   3. Swelling may be present but should not be relied upon to make the diagnosis
   4. History of wrist trauma in 15% with a dorsal ganglion
   5. Ultrasound or MRI to confirm diagnosis if necessary
   6. Treatment includes observation, aspiration with corticosteroid injection, or surgical removal for persistent symptoms.

Recommended Reading

1. DeLee JC, Drez D, eds. *DeLee and Drez's Orthopedic Sports Medicine: Principles and Practice*. 2nd ed. Philadelphia: Saunders; 2003.
2. Morgan WJ, Slowman LS. Acute hand and wrist injuries in athletes: Evaluation and management. *J Am Acad Orthop Surg* 2001;9:389–400.
3. Rettig AC. Athletic injuries of the wrist and hand: Part I: traumatic injuries of the wrist. *Am J Sports Med* 2003;31:1038.
4. Rettig AC. Athletic injuries of the wrist and hand: Part II: overuse injuries of the wrist and traumatic injuries to the hand. *Am J Sports Med*. 2004;32:262.

24

Pelvis, Hip, and Thigh Injuries and Conditions

Heidi Prather and Devyani Hunt

I. Hip Dislocation

A. Hip dislocation
1. Orthopedic emergency (requires rapid reduction to reduce chance of avascular necrosis [AVN]); often have associated fractures, dislocations usually occur posteriorly
2. History: fall on hip or posterior directed blow to flexed knee
3. Physical exam (PE): hip pain, leg internally rotated/shortened
4. Diagnosis: Anteroposterior (AP) and lateral hip radiographs. Post reduction computed tomography (CT) recommended to identify fractures or loose bodies
5. Treatment: early reduction (often requires sedation), protected weight bearing, progressive rehabilitation program as pain resolves; surgical treatment often required for associated fractures/loose bodies.

II. Pelvic and Hip Fractures

A. Femoral neck stress fractures
1. Five percent of all stress fractures, usually occur in adults, due to repetitive abductor muscle contraction
2. Classification: insufficiency-type (normal physiologic stress on abnormal bone) and fatigue-type (excessive physiologic stress on normal bone)
3. Two locations: Compression side (inferior femoral neck), tension side (superior femoral neck)
4. History: insidious onset groin or lateral hip pain, worse with weight bearing, possible recent change in activity intensity or volume, or change in equipment/environment
5. PE: Antalgic gait, pain with Patrick's/FABER test (hip flexion, abduction, and external rotation) and hip log roll (see Figure 24.1)
6. Diagnosis: AP and oblique hip radiographs, but often negative first 2–3 weeks after symptom onset, after which time may show periosteal reaction, fracture line, or sclerosis; 3-phase bone scan (bone scan) = increased uptake at fracture site, sensitive but not specific; magnetic resonance imaging (MRI) = bone edema ± fracture line, sensitive and specific.
7. Treatment: Compression-side: reduced weight bearing to allow healing and then rehabilitation. Tension side: often progress to displacement even with limited weight bearing, may require surgical intervention to prevent displacement. Displaced fractures require open reduction and internal fixation (ORIF).

B. Pelvic and sacral stress fractures
1. 1.25% of all stress fractures in runners.
2. History: insidious onset pelvic/sacral pain worse with weightbearing activity
3. PE: antalgic gait, pain with single leg stance/hopping

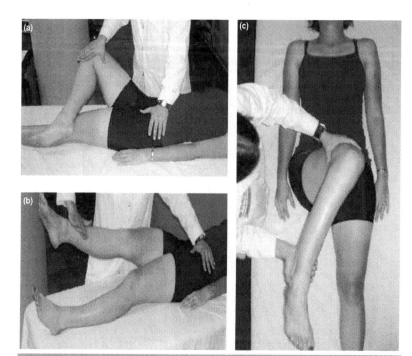

Figure 24.1 Hip physical exam. (a) FABER's, (b) resisted straight leg raise, (c) Hip impingment test.

4. Diagnosis: radiographs (AP pelvis), bone scan or MRI (see hip stress fracture section)
5. Treatment: modified weight bearing to allow healing, then progressive rehabilitation.

C. Avulsion fractures
   1. A failure of the bone at the origin or the insertion of the tendon. More common in adolescent athletes. Can occur at the anterior superior iliac spine (Sartorius), the anterior inferior iliac spine (rectus femoris), lesser trochanter (iliopsoas) and the ischial tuberosity (hamstring)
   2. History: Acute onset of pain after a forceful muscle contraction. Is associated with painful ambulation and localized swelling
   3. PE: Swelling and tenderness with muscle weakness and pain inhibition. An antalgic gait is common
   4. Diagnosis: X-rays usually demonstrate the avulsion and the degree of displacement. MRI if diagnosis is questionable
   5. Treatment: Minimally displaced fractures (<3 mm) heal well with conservative treatment—relative rest, protected weight bearing and analgesics. Return to sport after progressing through rehab. Initially starting with pain free range of motion (ROM) to static contraction, to concentric exercises and eccentric training. Displaced fractures >5 mm or symptomatic patients after appropriate rehab may require surgical treatment.

D. Apophysitis about the hip region
   1. Traction apophysitis most common at the anterior inferior iliac spine at the attachment of the rectus femoris, anterior superior iliac spine at the attachment of the Sartorius, or lesser trochanter at the attachment of the iliopsoas
   2. Treatment: reduce activity, and treat predisposing factors such as muscle tightness.

III. Pubic Symphysis Disorders

A. Pain may be due to trauma (macro or repetitive micro-trauma), instability, stress fracture/reaction, osteoarthritis (OA)

B. Osteitis pubis

1. Degenerative pubic symphyseal changes related to repetitive overload, trauma, pregnancy, rheumatologic disorders or postinfection. More common with limited hip range of motion (ROM), sports that require repetitive forceful rotation and kicking (e.g., soccer)

2. History: Insidious or acute onset of groin pain ± radiation to medial/anterior thigh or abdomen, increased with activity, relieved by rest

3. PE: Tenderness to palpation (TTP) over the pubic symphysis or pubic ramus, pain with passive hip internal rotation or passive or active hip adduction

4. Diagnosis: AP pelvis radiographs = normal, widened, or narrowed pubic symphysis with bony sclerosis/cystic changes. Single leg weightbearing radiographs may detect pelvic instability. Bone scan = increased uptake in pubic bones. MRI = bony edema in pubic bones, helps rule out other causes of pubic pain

5. Treatment: relative rest, sacroiliac joint belt, correction of strength/flexibility imbalances around the pelvis, occasionally pubic symphyseal corticosteroid injections.

IV. Intra-Articular Hip Disorders

A. Prearthritic intra-articular hip disorders

B. Intra-articular hip problems prior to the onset of degenerative changes includes abnormalities to the acetabular labrum, articular cartilage, ligamentum teres, synovium, osseous structures, and loose bodies in the joint.

C. Acetabular labral tears

1. Acetabular labrum is a fibrocartilage ring that surrounds the joint, seals the joint and aids in transferring forces away from the articular surfaces (see Figure 24.2).

2. History: Labral abnormalities are a common cause of anterior hip and groin pain in athletes. The labrum can be injured with a traumatic event but more commonly occur insidiously due to cumulative microtrauma. Sports activities with repetitive pounding, pivoting, and torsional force across the hip can damage the labrum. Symptoms include anterior hip, groin or lateral hip pain, mechanical symptoms of popping, clicking or locking, pain worsened with walking, pivoting, and impact

3. PE: Antalgic to normal gait, normal to decreased, painful hip flexion and internal rotation, and a positive hip impingement and FABER tests (see Figure 24.1)

4. Diagnosis: Radiographic assesses for fracture or deformity (see Figure 24.3)
   a. Suggested views include: standing AP pelvis, AP hip, frog-leg lateral, Dunn, cross-table lateral, and false profile view
   b. Studies report a 49–90% association of osseous structural abnormalities in patients undergoing hip arthroscopy for an acetabular labral tear

5. MR arthrograms (MRA) are more specific and sensitive than plain MRI to detect labral and chondral abnormalities. Most labral tears occur in the anterior superior labrum and 15–20% of labral tears are not seen on MRA

6. Image-guided intra-articular diagnostic hip injections are used to confirm pain is intra-articular and if reduction in pain is correlated with MRA findings

7. Treatment: Options include a trial of conservative care and progression to surgery if necessary
   a. Conservative treatment: relative rest, nonsteroidal anti-inflammatory drugs (NSAIDs), and off loading; focused physical therapy aimed at improving the femoral head motion within the joint, and improving the biomechanics around the hip
   b. Image-guided intra-articular steroid injection considered if there is chondrosis or wearing of the articular cartilage

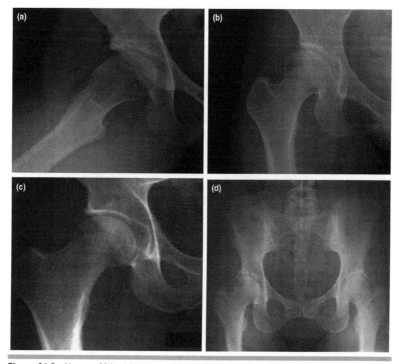

Figure 24.2   X-rays of hip. (a) normal, (b) CAM FAI, (c) Pincer FAI, and (d) DDH.

    c. Surgical intervention should be consider after failure of a conservative trial and include
       i. Hip arthroscopy to debride or repair the labrum
      ii. Underlying osseous hip deformities should be addressed and may require an open procedure
     iii. Poor prognosis is associated with a higher degree of chondrosis or articular cartilage wearing.

  D. Femoral acetabular impingement (FAI)
    1. FAI results from morphological abnormalities of the proximal femur and/or acetabulum which produce abnormal abutment of the acetabular rim and femoral head–neck junction. Symptomatic FAI typically occurs in young, active individuals
    2. There are three categories of FAI (see Figure 23.2)
      a. CAM impingement occurs when an abnormal femoral head–neck junction (i.e., decreased femoral head–neck offset distance, "pistol grip deformity") is driven into the acetabulum during flexion/internal rotation producing damage to the labrum/articular cartilage in the region of the anterosuperior rim
      b. Pincer impingement occurs when a normal femoral neck impinges against an overhanging anterosuperior acetabulum, compressing the labrum and creating circumferential microtrauma
      c. A combination of CAM and Pincer also occurs
    3. If untreated and symptomatic, FAI is thought to be a common cause of secondary OA of the hip

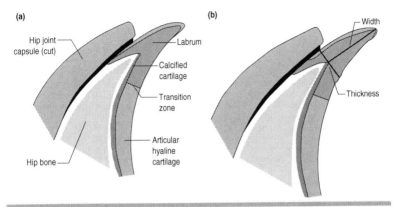

Figure 24.3 Illustration of the acetabular labrum. Cross section of acetabular labrum. (a) Labral attachment. (b) Labral width and thickness. (From Lewis CL, Sahrmann SA. Acetabular labral tears. *Phys Ther* 2006;*86*:112; with permission.)

4. The history and PE: Consistent with an intra-articular hip disorder and is associated with pain/decreased hip flexion and internal rotation
5. Diagnosis: AP, oblique, lateral, axial radiographs are essential to characterize the extent of deformity and the presence of associated OA
   a. CAM type: Pistol grip deformity, femoral head–neck offset distance of less than 7 mm of AP or oblique radiographs, alpha angle (line from femoral head/neck junction to center of femoral head, then from center of femoral head along axis of femoral neck on axial radiograph) >50°
   b. Pincer type: Protrusio acetabulae (femoral head extends medial to ilioischial line on AP of pelvis), coxa profunda (acetabular fovea extends medial to ilioischial line on AP of pelvis), lateral center edge angle (line from lateral margin of acetabulum to center of femoral head, then from center of femoral head vertically to center the cephalad portion of the femoral head on AP of pelvis) >40°
6. Treatment: Options include a trial of conservative measures depending on the severity of deformity. Joint preservation surgeries are indicated for young athletes with well-maintained joint surfaces and no articular cartilage damage.

E. Developmental dysplasia of the hip (DDH)
   1. Acetabular dysplasia is insufficient anterolateral coverage of the femoral head, superolateral inclination of the articular surface and a lateral hip joint center (see Figure 24.2).
   2. The inadequate coverage of the femoral head causes excessive loading of the acetabulum and can lead to degeneration of the cartilage overtime and secondary OA
   3. History and PE: Findings are consistent with an intra-articular hip disorder. Excessive range of motion of hip flexion, internal and external rotation is common in DDH
   4. Diagnosis: Radiographic analysis is essential to characterize the extent of deformity and the presence of OA
   5. Treatment: Options include a trial of conservative measures depending on the severity of the deformity. Joint preservation surgeries indicated for young athletes with well-maintained joint spaces without articular cartilage damage.

F. Slipped capital femoral epiphysis (SCFE)
   1. Salter–Harris type I fracture through the proximal femoral physis

2. Results in slippage of the metaphysis and femoral neck typically superiorly and anteriorly relative to the femoral head

3. It is the most common hip disorder in adolescents and more common in obese, prepubescent, African American males

4. Also associated with endocrine abnormalities such as hypogonadism, or thyroid disorders

5. 20–30% of cases occur bilaterally, often within 6 months

6. History: Usually insidious onset of anterior groin and hip pain and/or knee pain. Delayed diagnosis (and therefore poorer outcomes) is associated with athletes who present with only knee pain

7. PE: Findings consistent with an intra-articular process and include a waddling gait with an externally rotated foot, decreased and painful hip range of motion, leg length discrepancy with the involved limb shorter
   a. Positive Whitman's sign; hip flexion past 90° causes hip to externally rotate

8. Diagnosis: Radiographic evaluation with AP pelvis and frog-leg lateral
   a. AP pelvis demonstrates widening and irregularity of the growth plate and the height of the femoral head above the growth plate appears shortened as compared to the contra-lateral side
   b. Frog–leg lateral view may be contraindicated with acute slips, as this position can increase the slip
   c. The most sensitive indicator of a mild slip is the loss of lateral overhang of the femoral epiphysis
   d. Klein's line on AP view—slip is suspected if a straight line drawn up lateral surface of femoral neck does not touch the femoral head

9. Classification systems (see Table 24.1)

10. Treatment: Once a SCFE is suspected nonweight bearing and strict bed rest is advised to decrease the chance for further slippage
    a. Considered an orthopedic emergency
    b. Requires surgical pinning to prevent further slippage
    c. Head of the femur is pinned "as is." Attempts at correcting the slippage by moving the femur back in place has been associated with avascular necrosis and chondrolysis.
    d. Delayed treatment can lead to avascular necrosis, early degenerative joint disease, chronic limp, and chronic pain
    e. Resultant deformity can be a cause of CAM-type FAI in the future.

V. Advanced Intra-Articular Hip Disorders

A. Avascular necrosis (AVN)

1. AVN of the hip is the disruption of blood supply to the femoral head resulting in necrosis. The hip is the most common site of AVN.

2. Etiologies: Trauma, SCFE, Legg–Calve–Perthes disease, corticosteroids, excessive alcohol use, blood dyscrasias, extremes in barometric pressure (deep-sea divers), femoral neck stress fractures

3. History: Typically insidious onset of anterior hip, groin, or lateral hip pain with a painful limp or inability to weight bear

4. PE: Consistent with an intra-articular hip disorder

5. Diagnosis: Radiographic evaluation with standing AP pelvis, frog-leg lateral, and cross table lateral. Can take 3 months for x-rays to be positive, (+) crescent sign (radio-lucent arc below rim of femoral head), 90% of lesions are in the anterior, superior femoral head

6. Bone scans are sensitive but not specific. MRI has 95% sensitivity and specificity. CT is best for determining the extent of the lesion and bone infarction

7. Consider laboratory evaluation for etiology of AVN with lipid levels, protein C and S, antithrombin III, plasminogen activator inhibitor-1

Table 24.1   Classification chart

SCFE classifications	AVN classifications	OA classifications
Wilson classification	**ARCO (Association Research Circulation Osseous)**	**Tonnis classification**
Grade I—displacement of epiphysis less than 30% of width of femoral neck	Stage 0—X-rays, MRI, bone scan normal, bone biopsy demonstrates AVN	Grade 0—No signs of OA
Grade II—slip between 30% and 60%	Stage I—Radiographics normal, bone scan or MRI positive	Grade 1—Increased sclerosis, slight narrowing of the joint space, no or slight loss of head sphericity
Grade III—includes slips of greater than 60% the width of neck	Ia— < 15% femoral head involvement	Grade 2—Small cysts, moderate narrowing of the joint space, moderate loss of head sphericity
	Ib—15–30%	Grade 3—Large cysts, severe narrowing or obliteration of the joint space, severe deformity of the head
	Ic— > 30%	
	Stage II—Radiographics show sclerosis, cystic changes, osteopenia or mottled femoral head without subchondral collapse or acetabular involvement, bone scan/MRI positive	
	IIa— < 15% femoral head involvement	
	IIb—15–30%	
	IIc— > 30%	
	Stage III—Radiographics show a crescent sign, bone scan/MRI positive	
	IIIa— < 15% femoral head involvement or < 2 mm femoral head depression	
	IIIb—15–30% or 2–4 mm depression IIIc— > 30% or > 4 mm depression	
	Stage IV—Radiographs show flattened articular surface, joint space narrowing, acetabular changes, osteophytes	
Loder classification	**Ficat staging**	**Kellgren Lawrence classification**
Stable SCFE—If child is able to walk with or without crutches	Stage 0—Asymptomatic hip with no radiographic changes	Grade 0—No osteophytes, normal joint space
Unstable SCFE—If child is not able to walk with or without crutches	Stage I—Slight patchy osteoporosis, subtle loss of clarity	Grade 1—Minute osteophytes, doubtful significance
	Stage IIa—osteoporosis, sclerosis, cysts	Grade 2—Definite osteophyte, unimpaired joint space
	Stage III—crescent sign indicating subchondral collapse, flattening of femoral head	Grade 3—Moderate dimunition of joint space
	Stage IV—flattened femoral head, articular surface collapse, degenerative change	Grade 4—Joint space greatly impaired with sclerosis of subchondral bone

8. Classification systems (see Table 24.1)
9. Treatment: Depends on stage, presence of subchondral collapse, articular surface involvement and degree of arthritic change
    a. Conservative treatment is considered for asymptomatic lesions, lesions prior to x-ray or MRI findings and small lesions without articular collapse that are asymptomatic with restricted weight bearing. Nonoperative treatment is also indicated in young patients with significant subchondral collapse and articular involvement not amenable to core decompression or free-vascularized fibular graft (FVFG) and too young to consider total hip arthroplasty (THA). Electromagnetic bone stimulator can be a helpful adjunct to conservative care
    b. Bisphosphonates such as Alendronate 70 mg weekly for 3 months has been shown to improve nonoperative outcomes. Correct lipid and coagulation abnormalities if present
    c. Protected weight bearing is essential until symptom free and then progress weightbearing status and return to sport after rehab for reconditioning and sport-specific training
10. Surgical treatment with core decompression. The prognosis is improved in athletes treated earlier and with smaller lesion. Indicated when no degenerative change is seen in the hip
    a. Six weeks protected weightbearing post-op with return to sport after rehab for reconditioning and sport-specific training
11. Free vascularized fibular graft (FVFG) can be considered in early and later stages of AVN
    a. Healthy bone with intact vascular structures are harvested from the fibula and implanted into the femur after removal of the necrotic bone
12. Osteotomy considered only for symptomatic patients without subchondral collapse
13. Hip resurfacing or THA if athletes demonstrate significant subchondral collapse with advanced degenerative changes and other conservative measures are ineffective.

B. Osteoarthritis
1. The degeneration of articular cartilage of the hip with associated changes to the synovium, subchondral bone, and joint margins
2. Primary OA is less common and due to a genetic predisposition
3. Secondary OA has been implicated in some studies to account for 80% of cases
    a. SCFE, Legg-Calve Perthes disease, trauma, FAI, DDH, labral tears, chondral injury, inflammatory arthritis, AVN, infection
4. History: Typically insidious onset of groin pain, anterior hip, lateral hip, and less commonly buttock pain
5. PE: Consistent with an intra-articular process with painful and decreased hip range of motion, especially internal rotation and flexion
6. Diagnosis: Radiographic evaluation with standing AP pelvis, frog leg-lateral and cross table lateral views demonstrates joint space narrowing, sclerosis, subchondral cysts, and osteophytes
7. Classification systems (see Table 24.1)
8. Conservative treatment options include
    a. Relative rest with avoidance of internal rotation, end range hip flexion and pivoting
    b. NSAIDs
    c. Supplementation with glucosamine/chondroitin could be considered. Studies show mediocre to no improvement in pain and functioning.
    d. Physical therapy for pelvic strengthening with special consideration to work within a pain-free range of motion
    e. Intra-articular, image-guided hip injections of corticosteroids have been found to transiently improve the symptoms of hip OA
    f. Although not Food and Drug Administration (FDA) approved in the United States, intra-articular injection of viscosupplementation has inconsistent results and remains controversial
9. Surgical treatment is considered when conservative measures fail

VI. Extra-Articular Hip Disorders

A. There are many sources for extra-articular hip pain originating from the pelvic girdle. Some extra-articular disorders may be the primary source of pain while others are a result of adaptations or guarding mechanisms for an intra-articular hip or pelvic girdle disorder. Recognizing and differentiating the primary disorder versus secondary adaption can be difficult and analogous to the old adage of the "chicken or the egg": which came first?

B. Iliopsoas muscle–tendon complex disorders

1. The iliopsoas muscle–tendon complex consists of three muscles; the psoas major, the psoas minor, and the iliacus.

2. The proximal fibers of the psoas muscles originate on the bodies of the 12th thoracic vertebrae and the lumbar vertebrae, cross into the pelvis and join with the fibers of the iliacus to make the iliopsoas tendon and insert on the lesser trochanter

3. The iliopsoas is the primary hip flexor and provides functional stability to the hip, pelvis, and spine. (Figure 24.1b)

4. History: Anterior hip pain or groin pain that is worse with concentric or eccentric contraction of the hip flexor. Pain with sports activities that require forceful hip flexion or adduction. Painful ambulation or rising from a seated position

   a. Runner's may describe anterior groin pain when trying to lengthen their stride during speed training, or with uphill running.

5. PE: Key finding of a tender tendon with palpation and pain with eccentric or concentric activation. Range of motion is painful and positive FABERs

   a. Secondary dysfunction of the hip flexor muscle–tendon complex due to an underlying intra-articular disorder commonly occurs. It is also important to examine the hip in weight bearing during dynamic motion to further assess for abnormal motor patterns that contribute to repetitive overuse injuries

6. Diagnosis: AP and frog-leg lateral radiographs can be used to rule out underlying osseous abnormalities. An MRI or ultrasound can evaluate the tendon and underlying psoas bursa for pathology

7. Treatment: See treatment for internal snapping hip syndrome below.

C. Snapping hip syndrome

1. The key feature for snapping hip syndrome is the audible snap heard at or around the hip joint

2. The syndrome has been classified into three types: external, internal, and intra-articular.

3. External snapping hip is the most common type. It occurs when the gluteus maximus tendon or iliotibial band snaps over the greater trochanter

4. Internal snapping hip occurs when the iliopsoas tendon glides across the iliopectineal prominence, the femoral head or the lesser trochanter causing an audible snap

   a. The snap or pop occurs as the hip moves from flexion to extension and is often associated with pain

   b. The tendon is commonly normal, but not at its optimal length. Less commonly the tendon is thickened

   c. It is most likely a part of the continuum of iliopsoas chronic dysfunction

5. The intra-articular type refers to an intra-articular source for the audible or palpable snap often associated with pain

   a. Intra-articular sources include: loose bodies, synovial osteochondromatosis, labral tears, cartilage flaps, or osteochondral fractures, or transient hip subluxation

6. Diagnosis: Radiographs should be performed to assess for fracture, deformity, avascular necrosis, and OA. Ultrasound can assess muscle tendon integrity, bursitis, and dynamic snapping of the tendon across the iliopectineal prominence. MRI can assess muscle tendon integrity and provide basic assessment of intra-articular or bony abnormalities

7. A diagnostic injection under image guidance (fluoroscope or ultrasound) of anesthetic into the bursa or tendon can be useful when the diagnosis remains in question. A diagnostic

intra-articular injection should also be considered if an intra-articular abnormality needs to be excluded

8. Treatment:
   a. Internal snapping hip: Initial conservative treatment of iliopsoas muscle–tendon complex disorders is relative rest by reducing activities that activate or stretch the tendon complex
      i. A course of oral or topical anti-inflammatory medications is recommended
      ii. Physical therapy should focus on the iliopsoas tendon with the goal of optimizing the length and strength of the muscle–tendon complex
      iii. If the athlete fails a 3-month period of conservative treatment, an image-guided lidocaine and corticosteroid injection into the psoas bursa or iliopsoas tendon sheath should be considered. Caution should be used as tendon ruptures have occurred after steroid injections
      iv. Surgical treatment for painful iliopsoas muscle–tendon complex disorders is used for recalcitrant cases of internal snapping and include lengthening or release of the iliopsoas tendon. A positive response to an image-guided diagnostic injection of the tendon can predict the response to surgical release. Return to full activity is generally allowed after 3–6 months
   b. External snapping hip: stretch the iliotibial band (ITB), gluteus maximus, and tensor fascia lata. Strengthen the lumbopelvic musculature with a focus on the hip abductor and external rotators. Occasionally and injection into the greater trochanteric bursa is warranted. Surgical release of the ITB is rarely required.

D. Adductor strains
   1. Adductor strains are a significant cause of groin pain in athletes involved in sports that require a strong eccentric contraction
   2. The adductor muscle group consists of six muscles in the medial thigh and originate at various points along the pubis and insert in the medial femur
   3. In the open chain activation, the primary function of this muscle group is hip adduction. In the closed chain activation, they, with the lower abdominals, stabilize the pelvis and lower extremity. The individual muscles have secondary roles including femoral flexion and rotation
   4. The adductor longus is the most commonly strained muscle due to its poor mechanical advantage and it is hypothesized that its low tendon to muscle ratio at its origin predisposes it to injury
   5. History: Athletes with adductor strains present with groin pain and or medial thigh pain that is worse with activity and commonly insidious in onset
   6. PE: Adductors are tender to palpation and exhibit pain with passive stretch or activation. In cases of direct trauma, acute rupture or osseous avulsion should be considered. Swelling of the muscle group and weakness of hip adduction can occur
   7. Diagnosis: Hip radiographs often do not confirm the diagnosis, but can identify associated bony abnormalities of the pelvis and hip such as osteitis pubis or pelvic or hip stress fracture. Musculoskeletal ultrasound evaluation can further visualize the tendon and bony attachment sites, muscles, ligaments, and nerves. MR confirms can evaluate soft tissue and osseous structures of the hip
   8. Treatment: Relative rest, ice, and analgesia. Rehabilitation focused on balancing muscle length and strength of the adductors and other pelvic girdle muscles such as lateral hip rotators and hamstrings
   9. Surgical treatment: In cases of acute rupture, surgery is considered. An open repair with suture anchors has been described with good results.

E. Athletic pubalgia/sports hernia
   1. Etiology: Debatable. Some describe a hyperextension injury to the rectus abdominus insertion at the pubic symphysis. Others described an occult hernia of the posterior inguinal wall without signs of a visualized tear

2. Gilmore's groin is a tear in the external oblique aponeurosis and conjoint tendon
3. Sports and exercise that require repetitive rotation of the upper leg and torso such as ice hockey, soccer, and rugby are at risk for sports hernias. Repetitive trunk hyperextension and thigh hyper-abduction causes shearing at the pubic symphysis
4. Muscle imbalances between strong proximal thigh muscles and relatively weaker abdominal muscles also pose additional risks for injury
5. History: Insidious onset of groin pain with activity. Worsened with coughing or sneezing or explosive contractions. Pain associated with sprinting or kicking
6. PE: Tenderness to palpation of the superficial inguinal ring, posterior inguinal canal, pubic tubercle, or the conjoined tendon without a palpable hernia is commonly found on physical examination. Resisted sit ups, active hip adduction or Valsalva may provoke pain
7. Diagnosis: MRI is the recommended imaging study with good sensitivity and specificity.
8. Treatment: Surgical exploration is considered after failure of at least 6–8 weeks of conservative management. Both open and laparoscopic approaches are used. The surgical procedure depends upon the underlying etiology. True hernias are repaired with or without the use of mesh and the athlete is allowed to return to play in 6 weeks with a laparoscopic repair and 6 months for an open repair. Other surgical procedures include repair of the adductor/rectus abdominus aponeurotic plate and adductor longus tenotomies or releases.

F. Lateral extra-articular hip pain
1. Lateral hip pain has been commonly diagnosed as greater trochanteric bursitis. Current literature is beginning to refute that bursitis is the primary diagnosis. More likely a continuum of disorders can develop and is referred to as greater trochanteric pain syndrome (GTPS)
2. GTPS has been termed by some the "Great Mimicker" because it is often mistaken for or seen in conjunction with other sources of pain such as lumbar radiculopathy or intra-articular hip pathology
3. Studies have found GTPS to be associated with a number of other conditions which can alter the shearing and tension forces of the hip abductors due to weakness or altered gait mechanics
4. GTPS involves the tendons and bursa of the lateral hip region including the gluteus medius and minimus
5. Typically there are three main bursae in the trochanteric region: subgluteus medius, subgluteus minimus, and subgluteus maximus bursae. The subgluteus maximus bursa is often implicated as the source of pain in greater trochanteric bursitis
6. Tears of the gluteus medius and gluteus minimus are becoming more recognized as a source of lateral hip pain
7. Lateral hip pain can also be related to intra- and extra-articular hip disorders. Intra-articular sources such as labral disorders, hip deformity, and OA. Extraarticular sources include referred pain from the sacroiliac joint (SIJ), and hip girdle musculotendinous units
8. History: Pain when sleeping on the affected side, climbing stairs, getting up and down from a chair, crossing the affected leg or single leg weight bearing on the affected limb. The pain can radiate down along the outside of the hip to the knee
   a. GTPS is more common in women with approximately a 3:1 or 4:1 female-to-male predominance. It is also more common in the fourth and sixth decades of life
9. PE: Lateral hip pain with weight bearing, resisted hip abduction, palpation over the region of the greater trochanter, and passive hip internal rotation
10. Diagnosis: Imaging studies are useful to assess acute trauma and chronic repetitive overload but are not uniformly positive. Bone scan or MRI helps to rule out stress fracture. MRI and US can also be used to detect soft tissue (MRI and US) or osseous (MRI) pathology such bursitis, tendonopathy, enthesopathy, and partial and complete hip external rotator or abductor tears.

G. Thigh compartment syndrome

1. Compartment syndrome occurs when the pressure within the compartment of the thigh exceeds capillary filling pressure (12–32 mm Hg). If untreated, can lead to muscle necrosis, fibrosis, and neurologic injury

2. Acute compartment syndrome of thigh is usually a result of direct trauma and affects the anterior compartment and is a surgical emergency

3. History: Progressive pain and swelling, increasing tissue turgor and further provocation with passive range of motion

4. Diagnosis: Intra-compartmental pressures testing (>15 mm Hg at rest is abnormal)

5. Early surgical consultation is imperative to minimize long-term injury.

VII. Posterior Pelvic Pain

A. Piriformis pain is thought to be related to muscle inhibition or dysfunction while piriformis syndrome includes entrapment of the sciatic nerve. The diagnosis can be confirmed with electromyography (EMG) or image-guided intramuscular injection.

B. Hamstring strains, incomplete, and complete tears are another source of extra-articular hip and posterior pelvic pain that can be insidious in onset or a result of trauma

1. The hamstring strain, like other muscles, likely occurs on a continuum. Overuse can occur with intramuscular strain and/or inefficiencies that results in friction at the insertion site that leads to bursitis. The inflammation resolves and tendinopathy can develop. This can eventually lead to repetitive pain with use and even tears

2. A direct trauma causing a stretch of the hamstring beyond its physiological barrier during flexing of the knee or extension of the hip can result in an incomplete or complete tear. These tears occur at the myotendinous junction or insertion at the ischium

3. Water skiers report the most hamstring injuries but sprinters, middle distance runners, and contact sports athletes are also at risk. However, the injury can occur with any sport with the mechanism as described above

4. History: With acute tears, athletes often report feeling a "pop" and may visualize a bruise in the posterior thigh

5. PE: Localized tenderness and at times, a muscle defect can be felt on palpation with the athlete in the prone position. Pain may also be provoked with resisted knee flexion or hip extension

6. Treatment: Rest, ice, and crutch use for 3–5 days followed by rehabilitation to reestablish strength and flexibility of the hamstring

7. Surgical treatment: Acute traumatic tears can be surgically treated if there is no bony ischial avulsion, the tendon integrity is healthy and the repair is completed within weeks of the initial injury.

C. The sacroiliac joint (SIJ)

1. Athletes that participate in activities that require single leg stance and torsion are at risk. These include skaters, bowlers, racket sport athletes, and rowers

2. History: Some athletes may report a fall or direct blow to the pelvis as the inciting event. Commonly, patients with SIJ pain present with gluteal pain near or surrounding the posterior superior iliac spine. Pain occurs with transitional activities such as getting up from a chair or with sport-specific activities that require unilateral loading or torsion through the pelvis and lower extremity. Associated popping and/or clicking can occur

3. PE: No single test has been found to be sensitive and/or specific for SIJ pain. Rather, several positive tests can be a better indicator of SIJ pain

4. Confirmation of the diagnosis can be completed by an image-guided SIJ injection

5. Treatment: The rehabilitation needs to include pelvic and lumbar stability, improved neuromuscular control prior to advancing to sport-specific activities. SIJ belting can be useful during the rehabilitation.

Recommended Reading

1. Anderson K, Strickland SM, Warren R. Hip and groin injuries in athletes. *Am J Sports Med.* 2001;29(4):521–533.

2. Burnett RS, Della Rocca GJ, Prather H, Curry M, Maloney WJ, Clohisy JC. Clinical presentation of patients with tears of the acetabular labrum. *J Bone Joint Surg Am.* 2006;88(7):1448–1457.

3. Byrd JW. The role of hip arthroscopy in the athletic hip. *Clin Sports Med.* 2006;25(2):255–278, viii.

4. Clohisy JC, Beaule PE, O'Malley A, Safran MR, Schoenecker P. AOA symposium Hip disease in the young adult: Current concepts of etiology and surgical treatment. *J Bone Joint Surg Am* 2008;90(10):2267–2281.

5. Clohisy JC, Knaus ER, Hunt DM, Lesher JM, Harris-Hayes M, Prather H. Clinical presentation of patients with symptomatic anterior hip impingement. *Clin Orthop Relat Res.* 2009;467(3):638–644.

6. Lesher JM, Dreyfuss P, Hager N, Kaplan M, Furman M. Hip joint pain referral patterns: A descriptive study. *Pain Med.* 2008;9(1):22–25.

7. Peterson L, Renström P. Groin and thigh. In: RP Peterson L, ed. *Sports Injuries: Their Prevention and Treatment.* London, England: Taylor & Francis; 2001:247–266.

8. Prather H, Hunt D. Conservative management of low back pain, part I. Sacroiliac joint pain. *Dis Mon.* 2004;50(12):670–683.

9. Prather H, Hunt D. Hip and pelvic injuries in sports medicine. *Sacroiliac Joint Problems.* G. C. Philadelphia, PA: Lippincott, Williams & Wilkins; 2010:200–206.

Knee Injuries and Conditions

Marla S. Kaufman

I. Clinical Anatomy

A. Tibiofemoral joint ("knee joint"): Modified hinge joint
   1. ROM: generally 5–10° of hyperextension normal, 135° of flexion, 10° internal/external rotation
   2. Screw home mechanism: With extension, there is automatic external rotation of tibia with anterior glide, occurs between 0° and 20° of knee flexion, stable position of the knee. With flexion, the reverse occurs, popliteus "unlocks" joint, full extension to 20° flexion, internal rotation of tibia with posterior glide.

B. Patello-femoral joint: modified plane joint (see Figure 25.1)
   1. Patellar excursion controlled by quadriceps, especially vastus medialis. As flexion increases, greater area of patellar articular surface is in contact with the femur. With full extension: the patella lies lateral to the femoral trochlea. With flexion, the patella moves medially (J-sign) to engage the intercondylar groove. At ~130° of flexion, the patella moves laterally again. Patellar stability depends upon the depth of intercondylar groove, proper contour of patella, adequate muscular control
   2. Patellar loading with activity
      a. Walking: 0.3–0.5 × body weight
      b. Ascending stairs: 2–4 × body weight
      c. Descending stairs: 3.5 × body weight
      d. Squatting: 7–8 × body weight.

C. Ligaments
   1. Anterior cruciate ligament (ACL)
      a. Originates at the posteromedial aspect of lateral femoral condyle and courses antero-medially to insert on the anterior tibial spine
      b. Two bundles
         i. Anteromedial: tight in flexion
         ii. Posterolateral: tight in extension
      c. Function
         i. Primary—prevents anterior displacement of tibia on femur
         ii. Secondary—limits varus/valgus stress and rotation, prevents hyperextension, assists in screw home mechanism and proprioception
   2. Posterior cruciate ligament (PCL)
      a. Originates at the anterolateral aspect of the medial femoral condyle, courses postero-lateral to insert on the posterior surface of the tibial spine
      b. Two bundles
         i. Anterolateral: ~65% of substance of PCL, tight in flexion
         ii. Posteromedial: ~35% of substance of PCL, tight in extension

  c. Function
     i. Primary—prevents pos-
        terior displacement of
        tibia on femur
    ii. Secondary—limits varus/
        valgus stress, assists in
        proprioception and screw
        home mechanism
  3. Meniscofibular ligament: inserts
     on the body of the PCL
  4. Medial collateral ligament
     (MCL)
     a. Originates at medial femoral
        condyle and inserts on prox-
        imal medial tibia
     b. Two components
        i. Superficial: tibial collat-
           eral ligament

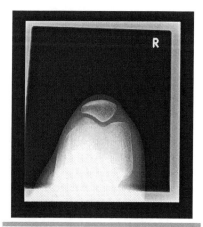

Figure 25.1   X-ray sunrise view demonstrating normal patellofemoral alignment.

       ii. Deep: medial capsular
           ligament (contiguous
           with medial meniscus;
       limits meniscus rotation and thus puts medial meniscus at increased risk of tear)
       (A) Function: provides ~80% of valgus stability, helps secure medial meniscus
           to tibia
     c. Lateral collateral ligament (LCL)
        i. Originates at lateral femoral condyle and inserts on fibular head
       ii. Function: although it is thin, provides ~70% of varus stability.
 D. Menisci
     1. Fibrocartilage: Outer 1/3 has good blood supply ("red zone") and ability to heal, avascu-
        lar inner 2/3 ("white zone"). Thick and convex peripherally, thin centrally.
     2. Lateral: circular ("O"-shaped), covers 70–80% of lateral tibial plateau, equal thickness
        throughout, excursion of ~10 mm
     3. Medial: semi-circular ("C"-shaped), covers 50–60% of medial tibial plateau, thicker pos-
        teriorly, excursion of ~2 mm, attaches to ACL and MCL, more susceptible to injury
        than lateral
     4. Terrible triad: injury to the medial meniscus, ACL, and MCL
     5. Function: joint lubrication/nutrition, load transmission, shock absorption, knee stability
        (increase concavity of tibia)
     6. Discoid meniscus variant:
        i. More common laterally, incidence: 3.5–5%
       ii. Discoid menisci without associated tears are often asymptomatic; though with or
           without associated tears, discoid menisci can cause popping and/or reduced
           knee flexion
      iii. Surgery is recommended for those that are symptomatic, regardless of whether or not
           a tear is present.
 E. Capsule: Composed of ligaments and tendons surrounding the knee joint. Lined with syno-
    vium and secretes synovial fluid
     1. Synovial plicae: during fetal development, plicae are membranes that separate the knee
        into compartments. They typically diminish in size during 2nd trimester of development,
        but may resorb incompletely. Four locations for these redundant synovial folds: mediopa-
        tellar (most common), suprapatellar, lateral, infrapatellar.

II. Knee injuries and conditions

A. Fractures

1. Patellar fracture
   a. Direct trauma (e.g., fall onto patella or hit with hockey puck): usually causes commi-nution, but typically not displaced, damage to articular cartilage
   b. Indirect trauma (e.g., forceful quadriceps contraction from jumping or rapid flexion): less likely than direct trauma to be comminuted, but more likely displaced fragments, less damage to articular cartilage
   c. Most patellar fractures are a combination of direct and indirect trauma
   d. Plain radiographs
      i. Anterior–posterior view (AP): difficult to visualize patella well and peripheral fractures may be mistaken for bipartite patella (check bilateral films as bipartite patella is common bilaterally)
      ii. Lateral view: reveals comminution or displacement
      iii. Merchant view: reveals vertical fractures better
   e. Treatment
      i. Nonoperative: minimal or nondisplaced fractures with minimal disruption of articular surface, preserved extensor mechanism
         (A) Splint in extension
         (B) Gradually increase flexion range as healing progresses
      ii. Operative: avulsion of extensor mechanism, displaced transverse fracture
   f. Complications: infection (communicates with knee joint), avascular necrosis, chondro-malacia patellae and/or posttraumatic arthritis of patellofemoral compartment, quad-riceps weakness, extensor lag

2. Tibial plateau fracture
   a. Valgus force with axial loading: low energy—osteoporotic bone, typically depressed fracture; high energy—secondary to MVA, typically bicondylar fracture
   b. Majority involve lateral plateau, about 1/4 bicondylar
   c. May also be accompanied by partial or complete ligamentous injury (15–45%) and/or meniscal injury (5–35%)
   d. Treatment
      i. Nonoperative: minimal displacement or depression, nonweight bearing/brace × 6 weeks
      ii. Operative
         (A) Absolute indications—open plateau fractures, associated compartment syn-drome, associated vascular injury
         (B) Relative indications—displaced bicondylar fractures, displaced medial condy-lar fractures, lateral fractures with joint instability

3. Segond fracture
   a. Small capsular avulsion fracture of lateral tibial plateau
   b. Results from abnormal varus stress to the knee combined with internal rotation of the tibia
   c. Likely to be associated with ACL tear (75–100%), and/or meniscal injury (66–75%)
   d. Can also be associated with avulsion of fibular head or Gerdy's tubercle
   e. Treatment—typically requires surgical intervention given concomitant injuries

4. Stress fractures
   a. Patella: rare
   b. Medial tibial plateau: commonly misdiagnosed as pes anserine bursitis.

B. Dislocation

1. Patellar dislocation
   a. Patella displaced laterally out of the femoral groove
      i. Traumatic, usually with hemarthrosis, often associated with twisting or jumping

    ii. Atraumatic, occurs mainly in young females with generalized ligamentous laxity, less swelling

    iii. Osteochrondral fracture occurs in one-third of cases

    iv. Usually reduces spontaneously with knee extension

    v. Risk factors include: shallow femoral groove, generalized ligamentous laxity, patella alta, femoral anteversion, loose medial or tight lateral retinaculum

   b. Imaging

    i. X-rays should be obtained postreduction to evaluate for osteochrondral fracture or avulsion (AP, lateral, and patellar views)

    ii. If osteochondral lesion noted on x-ray or suspicion is high given persistence of symptoms, obtain MRI to evaluate integrity of articular surfaces

   c. Treatment

    i. Nonsurgical treatment is routine

     (A) Consider knee brace/immobilizer to maintain extension for 3–6 weeks, then progress rehabilitation program, specifically to include quadriceps strengthening

    ii. Recurrent patellar dislocations require surgical repair (of medial stabilizers)

    iii. Surgical consultation should also be considered for those with associated displaced osteochrondral lesions

 2. Knee dislocation

   a. High force injury often associated with ligament injury (ACL, PCL), nerve injury (fibular nerve), vascular injury (popliteal artery—medical emergency), fracture

    i. Described by position of tibia relative to femur

     (A) Anterior: occurs with hyperextension

     (B) Posterior: dash-board type injuries

     (C) Also medial, lateral, rotatory

   b. Thorough neurovascular examination to evaluate the integrity of the popliteal artery and fibular nerve and to evaluate for compartment syndrome

   c. Early arteriography is considered to evaluate for popliteal artery injury and thus defines knee dislocation as a medical emergency

   d. Treatment

    i. Emergent surgical intervention: open dislocation, popliteal artery injury, irreducible dislocations, compartment syndrome

    ii. Delayed: ligamentous reconstruction.

C. Muscle/tendon injuries

 1. Iliotibial band (ITB) friction syndrome

   a. Often seen in runners, but can also occur in other sports, including cycling and tennis

   b. Caused by abnormal biomechanics (such as genu varum) causing excess friction between ITB and lateral epicondyle of femur

   c. Friction maximal at 30° of knee flexion

   d. Pain over lateral knee, usually absent at rest

   e. Physical examination

    i. Tenderness over IT band, commonly at insertion and 3 cm proximal to the lateral joint line (friction at the lateral epicondyle of the femur)

    ii. Positive Ober's test (see Figure 25.2): demonstrating ITB tightness

    iii. Positive Noble's test (see Figure 25.3): knee extended from 90° of flexion to 30° of flexion precipitating lateral knee pain

   f. Treatment

    i. Rehabilitation focusing on correction of abnormal biomechanics, especially ITB, hamstring, and hip external rotator stretching, hip abductor and quadriceps strengthening

    ii. Cross-friction massage and self-massage with foam roller

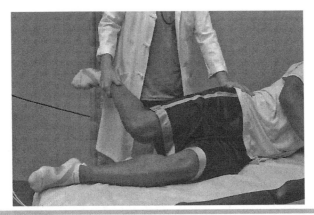

Figure 25.2   Ober's test. The patient lies on his/her side with the bottom leg flexed in order to minimize lumbar lordosis. With the upper leg flexed ~90° at the knee, the examiner grasps the ankle lightly with one hand and stablizes the hip with the other. The upper leg is then abducted widely and extended so the thigh is in line with the body. A positive test is when the leg remains passively abducted.

   iii. Foot orthotics
   iv. Surgical intervention: recalcitrant cases, excision of posterior portion of IT band that overlies lateral epicondyle of femur
  2. Patellar tendinopathy (jumper's knee)
   a. Mechanism
    i. Usually insidious onset
    ii. Repetitive knee flexion/extension, such as with jumping (e.g., volleyball, basketball)
    iii. Younger athletes

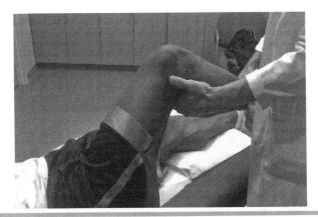

Figure 25.3   Noble's test. The knee is flexed and extended between 90° and 30° of flexion, with the examiner's thumb over the lateral epicondyle of the femur. Reproduction of lateral knee pain is considered positive.

    b. Treatment

      i. Relative rest

      ii. NSAIDs

      iii. Cross friction massage

      iv. Functional rehabilitation

      v. Patellar tendon strap

      vi. Rarely surgical intervention (debridement) for recalcitrant cases

3. Popliteus tendinopathy

    a. Originates at lateral femoral condyle and inserts at proximal tibia

    b. Posterolateral knee pain

    c. Typically chronic/overuse injury, excessive downhill walking or running

    d. Physical examination: tenderness to palpation over popliteus tendon

      i. Place leg in figure four/cross-legged position and palpate just posterior to the LCL while resisting tibial internal rotation

    e. Treatment: relative rest, NSAIDs, functional rehabilitation

4. Extensor mechanism rupture

    a. Biomechanics

      i. At >45° of knee flexion, patellar tendon is at a mechanical advantage and thus less susceptible to injury

      ii. At <45° of knee flexion, quadriceps tendon is at a mechanical advantage and thus less susceptible to injury

      iii. Rupture more likely to occur at insertion than intra-substance and typically with a rapid eccentric contraction

      iv. Patellar tendon rupture

        (A) Usually acute injury, <40 years old, often associated with sports such as soccer or basketball, may report a "pop" heard with acute injury, unable to actively extend knee

        (B) Patella alta on physical exam and imaging

      v. Quadriceps tendon rupture

        (A) Often degenerative, typically older athletes (>40 years old), may have pain prior to rupture, more common than patellar tendon ruptures

        (B) Patella baja on physical exam and imaging

    b. Treatment for both patellar and quadriceps tendon ruptures

      i. Partial tears: can be treated with cast/brace in full extension × 4–6 weeks, then rehabilitation

      ii. Complete tear: surgically repaired immediately.

D. Instability/ligament injuries

1. Anterior cruciate ligament (ACL)

    a. Most common knee ligament injured in sports, females experience ACL tears 9 × more often than males

    b. > 50% of ACL injuries occur with a meniscal tear

      i. Even more common with a chronic ACL tear

    c. "Terrible triad:" concomitant tears of ACL, MCL, and medial meniscus

    d. Studies have suggested that ACL injuries are an important risk factor for the development of osteoarthritis

    e. Mechanism

      i. Typically occurs with external rotation of the femur and a valgus load on fixed tibia/foot planted

      ii. Cutting, deceleration, hyperextension

      iii. Contact vs noncontact injuries (see Chapter 50 regarding female predisposition to noncontact ACL injuries)

f. Initial presentation
  i. Often report a "pop"
  ii. Instability/give-way: especially with twisting movements
  iii. Hemarthrosis typically forms within several hours of injury
g. Diagnosis
  i. Physical examination
    (A) May be difficult to perform complete examination due to pain and swelling
    (B) Effusion (hemarthosis)
    (C) Positive Lachman test (Sensitivity: 95–99%)
      (1) Grade 1+: 0–5 mm displacement
      (2) Grade 2+: 5–10 mm
      (3) Grade 3+: >10 mm
    (D) Positive anterior drawer (sensitivity 22–95%, specificity 53–97%) and pivot shift tests (sensitivity 35–98%, specificity 98–100%)
  ii. Imaging
    (A) Plain radiographs: evaluate for bony injuries such as tibial spine avulsion, tibial plateau, or Segond fracture (see section IIAiii)
    (B) MRI
      (1) Sensitivity 86–100%, specificity 95–100%
      (2) Often demonstrate bony contusions (anterior lateral femoral condyle and posterior lateral tibial plateau)
      (3) Also evaluate for concomitant injuries
  iii. Arthroscopy
h. Treatment
  i. Acute/initial
    (A) Rest, ice, compression, elevation (RICE)
    (B) Knee immobilizer or hinged knee brace, crutches
    (C) Early gentle knee ROM exercises
    (D) Exercises to prevent quadriceps inhibition/atrophy
  ii. Subacute/long-term
    (A) Depends on activity requirements
      (1) Consider surgical reconstruction for athletes who participate in cutting sports (i.e., soccer, basketball) and/or those with associated repairable meniscal injuries or severe tears of other ligaments, instability with daily activities
        (a) Surgery too soon after ACL injury increases the risk of arthrofibrosis; thus, early rehabilitation to regain range of motion and decrease swelling is helpful in the preoperative period
        (b) Surgery may help to decrease chance of developing posttraumatic osteoarthritis (OA). A recent study, however, demonstrated a notable rate of OA in those who had undergone prior ACL reconstruction. Thus, the initial trauma may be responsible for the development of OA and ACL reconstruction may not prevent the degenerative process.
        (c) Increase knee stability
        (d) Typically reconstruction using autograft over allograft
        (e) Postsurgical rehabilitation program × 6–9 months
      (2) Aggressive rehabilitation for sedentary patients or athletes participating in noncutting sports (i.e., cycling) who wish to avoid surgery or those without significant instability (key component: hamstring strengthening to compensate for loss of ACL)
      (3) Bracing for ACL-deficient athletes, though commonly used, is controversial. Recent review found no evidence that pain, range of motion, graft stability, or protection from subsequent injury were affected by brace use

2. Posterior cruciate ligament (PCL)

    a. Less common than ACL injuries: PCL is ~2× as strong and thick as ACL

    b. Majority associated with injury to other structures, need to evaluate posterolateral corner (see Section 5) when PCL injury is suspected

    c. Mechanism: impact to anterior tibia in knee flexion (e.g., dashboard injury), less common hyperextension

    d. Presentation: less significant functional limitations than ACL injury

    e. Diagnosis

        i. Physical examination

            (A) Positive posterior drawer test

                (1) Grade 1+: 0–5 mm displacement

                (2) Grade 2+: 5–10 mm

                (3) Grade 3+: >10 mm

            (B) Positive quadriceps active test (sensitivity 54–98%, specificity 97–100%): Patient is supine with knee flexed to 90°, foot is stabilized by the examiner, and subject is asked to slide foot gently down the table. In PCL-deficient knee, quadriceps contraction results in anterior shift of tibia of ≥2 mm

            (C) Positive reverse Lachman's test

            (D) Posterior sag sign (quadriceps spasm may cause false negative)

        ii. Imaging

            (A) Plain radiographs

                (1) Usually negative in isolated PCL injuries

                (2) Can evaluate for concomitant avulsion injury from tibial insertion

            (B) MRI

                (1) Useful to diagnose PCL injury and evaluate for associated injuries

        iii. Arthroscopy

    f. Treatment

        i. Acute/initial

            (A) RICE

            (B) Early ROM exercises

            (C) Consider knee brace (in full extension)/crutches × 1–2 weeks if significant disability

        ii. Subacute/long-term

            (A) Functional rehabilitation, especially quadriceps strengthening. Typically have good recovery

            (B) Surgical reconstruction of PCL rarely required for ongoing instability and/or functional limitations; but useful if there is persistent instability or other surgically repairable injuries

3. Medial collateral ligament

    a. Mechanism: impact to lateral knee, causing valgus stress, especially with foot planted in knee flexion

    b. Diagnosis

        i. Physical examination

            (A) Tenderness along course of MCL

            (B) Positive valgus stress test

                (1) Grade 1: pain but no laxity

                (2) Grade 2: some laxity but clear endpoint

                (3) Grade 3 (complete disruption of ligament): laxity with gapping of medial joint line without clear endpoint

            (C) No effusion in isolated injury (MCL is extra-articular)

ii. Imaging
   (A) X-ray usually normal: antero-posterior and lateral views can rule-out associated bony injury (epiphyseal fracture).
      (1) Pellegrini–Stieda sign (see Figure 25.4): posttraumatic ossification in or near the MCL margin of the medial femoral condyle, can be seen in those with a history of MCL injury. This is typically asymptomatic
   (B) MRI: usually obtained if there are other suspected injuries

c. Treatment
   i. RICE
   ii. Consider hinged knee brace × 1–2 weeks
   iii. Early gentle knee ROM exercises (within 1–2 weeks)
   iv. Gradual advance to higher level activities as tolerated (next 1–4 weeks)
   v. Isolated MCL injuries rarely require surgery. In cases with tibial-sided avulsion, acute repair is indicated

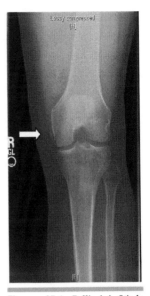

Figure   25.4   Pelligrini–Stieda sign

4. Lateral collateral ligament (LCL)
   a. Mechanism: direct varus stress
   b. Rarely injured in isolation
   c. Physical examination
      i. Positive varus stress test
      ii. Evaluate for associated fibular nerve injury
   d. Treatment
      i. RICE
      ii. Early knee ROM exercises
      iii. Functional rehabilitation
      iv. Surgical intervention typically depends upon concomitant injuries

5. Posterolateral corner (PLC)
   a. Many structures in this region: posterolateral joint capsule, biceps femoris tendon, LCL, popliteus tendon, fibular nerve, gastrocnemius (lateral head), posterior meniscofemoral ligament, lateral meniscus
      i. Injury to part/all of these structures may be associated with severe injury to other structures (especially PCL or ACL)
   b. Diagnosis
      i. Physical examination: may not be able to clearly differentiate focal etiology. Need to evaluate fibular nerve function
         (A) Dial test—assess external rotation (ER) of tibia compared to the contralateral knee at 30° and 90° of knee flexion
            (1) Increased ER at 30°, but not 90°, indicates isolated PLC injury
            (2) Increased ER at both angles suggests injury to both the PLC structures and the PCL
      ii. MRI to determine specific structures involved
   c. Treatment: If injury is associated with cruciate ligament tear, typically recommend surgical intervention, although there is some debate regarding the timing of surgical intervention. Typically, surgery within several weeks of injury is recommended. Reasons for

this include: less scar tissue proliferation, higher tissue quality, less proximal retraction of musculotendinous structures. Complications of early surgery include a higher risk of arthrofibrosis, so ROM exercises and modalities to decrease joint effusion should be initiated preoperatively and continued postoperatively.

E. Plica syndrome
   1. Most synovial plicae are not symptomatic. May become painful, inflamed, and eventually hypertrophy (mediopatellar most commonly involved)
   2. Physical examination: taut articular band that reproduces concordant pain with palpation
   3. Imaging: plain radiographs or MRI to rule-out more common sources of pain.
   4. Treatment
      a. RICE, NSAIDs, consider steroid injection
      b. Functional rehabilitation
      c. Arthroscopic removal reserved for recalcitrant cases and may have high rate of failure.

F. Fat pad impingement ("Hoffa's syndrome")
   1. Located deep to patellar tendon, can become inflamed/swollen due to direct trauma, hyperextension, or chronic irritation
   2. When inflamed, it may impinge between the inferior pole of patella and femoral condyle.
   3. Presentation: pain in anterior/inferior knee, exacerbated by knee extension, more commonly irritated by transitioning from sit to stand in contrast to patellofemoral pain (see G below) which is more symptomatic with prolonged sitting (knee flexion)
   4. Physical examination
      a. May have genu recurvatum
      b. Positive Hoffa's test (see Figure 25.5): patient lies supine with knee bent, and the examiner presses both thumbs along the sides of the patellar tendon, just distal to the patella. The patient is then asked to actively extend the knee. Pain and/or apprehension are considered positive
   5. Treatment
      a. RICE
      b. Patellar taping
      c. Surgical removal of fat pad in recalcitrant cases.

G. Patellofemoral syndrome
   1. Anterior knee pain in region of patella
      a. Typically insidious onset, worse with prolonged sitting (positive theater sign) or activities that load patellofemoral joint (such as walking down stairs)
   2. Likely combination of poor patellar tracking/malalignment within femoral groove and also peripatellar synovial irritation/inflammation
   3. Chrondromalacia patellae: degeneration of patellar cartilage, may cause patellofemoral syndrome, but not all subjects with patellofemoral syndrome have chrondromalacia
   4. Risk factors: weak vastus medialis, tight lateral structures, femoral anteversion, excessive pronation, poor femoral control (i.e., excessive femoral adduction and internal rotation), overtraining
   5. Patellar subluxation and/or patellar hypermobility noted on examination, may be related to shallow intercondylar groove
   6. Diagnosis
      a. Physical examination
         i. Evaluate patellar position in static positions and dynamically
            (A) J-sign: the inverted J pathway the patella takes—laterally at terminal extension and medially with early flexion
         ii. Evaluate kinetic chain (including hip and ankle/foot) to assist with biomechanical treatment and direct functional rehabilitation

   iii. Positive patellofemoral grind/compression
        test
   b. Imaging—rarely necessary
7. Treatment
   a. RICE, activity modification
   b. Rehabilitation program, especially focusing on
      vastus medialis strengthening, stretching of
      lateral structures (IT band, lateral retinaculum),
      pelvic control (hip rotators and abductors), cor-
      rection of underlying biomechanical deficits/
      malalignment issues
   c. Taping: based upon position of patella in
      relation to femur—need to evaluate tilt, glide,
      and rotation
   d. Bracing: to maintain medial glide of patella
      in flexion
   e. Massage therapy: to assist with stretching of
      lateral structures
   f. Orthotics: consider correction of overpronation
   g. Surgical intervention (lateral release) rarely
      indicated.

H. Meniscal tears
   1. Medial more common than lateral meniscal tears
      a. Medial meniscus injury: cutting activity,
         tibial rotation with knee flexion during weight
         bearing (i.e., soccer, football). Commonly
         associated with ACL injury
      b. Lateral meniscus injury: squatting, full flexion
         with rotation (i.e., wrestling)
   2. Degenerative: >40 years old, minimal trauma
   3. Physical examination
      a. Effusion ± restricted ROM
      b. Pain with squatting
      c. Joint line tenderness
      d. Provocative maneuvers

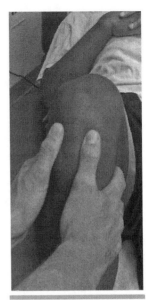

**Figure 25.5 Hoffa's test.
Patient lies supine with knees
bent. Examiner presses both
thumbs along the sides of the
patellar tendon, just distal to
the patella. The patient then
actively extends the knee. Pain
and/or apprehension are
considered positive.**

         i. McMurray test—audible and palpable click; though more commonly pain is
            solely elicited
         ii. Apley grind—pain with flexion, rotation, and axial compression
         iii. Bounce home test—pain with terminal extension
         iv. Duck walking
   4. Imaging:
      a. Plain radiographs: to evaluate for degenerative changes, loose body
      b. MRI: evaluate for meniscal pathology and surrounding structures. See Figure 25.6
         i. True tear: abnormal signal extends to the articular surface
         ii. False positive: abnormal signal may be seen in up to one-third of asymptomatic
             patients without history of knee injury
   5. Treatment
      a. Nonoperative for those with minor tears without significant functional disability
      b. Surgical intervention—if symptoms interfere with daily activities, work, sports and/or
         have not responded to nonsurgical treatment, or in cases of large tears causing mech-
         anical symptoms (catching, locking)

i. Attempt to maximize preservation of meniscus. Inner two-third of meniscus not well vascularized, may need surgical removal of damaged tissue. Outer one-third can often be repaired

ii. More favorable outcomes
   (A) Surgery within 4 months of injury
   (B) Smaller tears confined to the outer third
   (C) Age <30
   (D) No articular cartilage damage
   (E) Simultaneous ACL reconstruction
   (F) Tear of the lateral meniscus

iii. Postsurgical rehabilitation important.

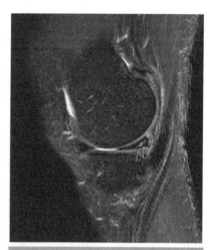

Figure 25.6 Complex tear posterior horn medial meniscus.

I. Degenerative joint disease
   1. Medial (most common), lateral, patellofemoral, or combination of compartments all possible
   2. History of joint trauma/previous acute ligamentous injury is common
   3. Plain radiographs: weight bearing to evaluate for joint space narrowing
      a. Hallmarks: joint space narrowing, subchondral cysts, sclerosis, and osteophytes
   4. Treatment
      a. Activity modification, weight loss, rehabilitation (quadriceps strengthening), unloader bracing, assistive devices (cane in contralateral hand), heel wedge (lateral wedge for medial compartment offloading), oral medications (acetaminophen/NSAIDs)
      b. Intra-articular injections: corticosteroids vs. hyaluronic acid compounds (see Procedures in Sports Medicine, Chapter 7)
      c. Indications for knee arthroplasty
         i. Failure of nonsurgical management in the setting of significant functional limitations with notable radiographic degenerative changes.

J. Bursitis
   1. General principles
      a. Bursae typically provide an interface between bony surfaces and ligaments or tendons in areas of friction
      b. Acute traumatic injury, infection, or systemic disease, abnormal biomechanics or chronic overuse can cause bursitis/ irritation of bursa
      c. Examination typically demonstrates focal tenderness and swelling
         i. Warmth or erythema may indicate infection
      d. Treatment typically consists of RICE, NSAIDs, and sometimes aspiration with corticosteroid injection
   2. Prepatellar bursitis—"housemaid's knee"
      a. Due to trauma or chronic irritation from extensive kneeling (wrestling)
      b. May have urate crystals due to gout

3. Pes anserine bursitis
   a. Difficult to differentiate between bursal pathology and tendon (sartorius, gracilis, semitendinosis) insertional pathology
4. MCL bursitis—"Voshell's bursitis"
   a. MCL bursa located between superficial and deep portions of MCL.

Recommended Reading

1. Earl J, Hoch AZ. A proximal strengthening program improves pain, function, and biomechanics in women with patellofemoral pain syndrome. *Am J Sport Med.* 2011;39(1):154–63.

2. Howells NR, Brunton LR, Robinson J, Porteus AJ, Elridge JD, Murray JR. Acute knee dislocation: An evidence based approach to the management of the multiligament injured knee. *Injury.* December 12, 2010 (epub ahead of print).

3. Kennedy J, Jackson MP, O'Kelly P, Moran R. Timing of reconstruction of the anterior cruciate ligament in athletes and the incidence of secondary pathology within the knee. *JBJS Br.* 2010;92-B(3): 362–366.

4. Lohmander LS, Englund PM, Dahl LL, Roos EM. The long-term consequence of anterior cruciate ligament and meniscus injuries: Osteoarthritis. *Am J Sports Med.* 2007;35(10):1756–69.

5. Maffuli N, Longo UG, Gougoulias N, Loppini M, Denaro V. Long-term health outcomes of youth sports injuries. *Br J Sports Med.* 2010;44(1):21–5.

6. Marchant MH Jr, Tibor LM, Sekiya JK, Hardaker WT Jr, Garret WE Jr, Taylor DC. Management of medial-sided knee injuries: Part 1: Medial collateral ligament. *Am J Sports Med.* December 8, 2010 (epub ahead of print).

7. O'Keeffe SA, Hogan BA, Eustace SJ, Kavanagh EC. Overuse injuries of the knee. *Magn Reson Imaging Clin N A.* 2009;17(4):725–739.

8. Tibor LM, Marchant MH Jr, Taylor DC, Hardaker WT Jr, Garrett WE Jr, Sekiya JK. Management of medial-sided knee injuries: Part 2: Posteromedial corner. *Am J Sports Med.* December 20, 2010 (epub ahead of print).

9. Woo SL, Debski RE, Withrow JD, Janaushek MA. Biomechanics of knee ligaments. *Am J Sports Med.* 1999;27:533–43.

Lower Leg Injuries and Conditions

John P. Metzler

I. Anatomy

A. Four fascial compartments (Figure 26.1)

   1. Anterior compartment

      a. Muscles: Extensor hallucis longus, extensor digitorum longus, peroneus tertius, anterior tibialis

      b. Deep peroneal nerve

   2. Lateral compartment

      a. Muscles: Peroneus longus and brevis

      b. Superficial peroneal nerve

   3. Deep posterior compartment

      a. Muscles: Flexor hallucis longus, flexor digitorum longus, posterior tibialis

      b. Posterior tibial nerve

   4. Superficial posterior compartment

      a. Muscles: Gastrocnemius, soleus

      b. Sural nerve

B. Proximal tibiofibular joint

   1. Diarthrodial joint

   2. Communicates with the knee in 10% of adults

   3. Stabilized by the tibiofibular ligaments, biceps femoris tendon, and lateral collateral ligament

   4. Functions to diminish torsional stresses at the ankle joint.

II. Fractures: Tibia

A. Epidemiology

   1. Uncommon injury in athletes.

   2. High incidence of major complications: associated soft-tissue injuries, compartment syndrome, delayed union, malunion, or nonunion

   3. Mechanism: contact during a tackle or a collision

B. Diagnosis

   1. Tender at fracture site

   2. Evaluate for neurovascular, knee, or ankle injuries

   3. Radiographs—anteroposterior, lateral, oblique

C. Treatment

   1. Nondisplaced: immobilization (splint, then cast)

   2. Displaced: closed reduction and casting versus open reduction and internal fixation or intramedullary nail.

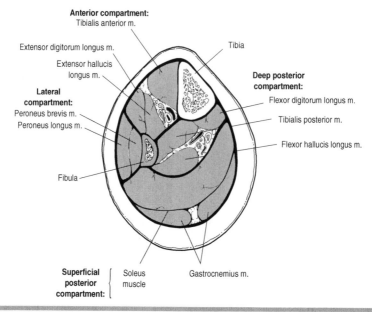

Figure 26.1   Four fascial compartments. (This figure was published in *Sports Medicine: A Comprehensive Approach*, Chapter 24, Edward Brown III and Michael Kelly, MD, p. 389, Elsevier/Mosby; 2005.)

III. Fracture: Fibula

A. Mechanism: direct blow to the lateral leg

B. Maisonneuve fracture (Figure 26.2)
   1. Fracture of proximal fibula
   2. Mechanism: ankle eversion/external rotation causing medial malleolar fracture or deltoid ligament injury, anterior–inferior tibiofibular ligament sprain, and syndesmotic membrane injury

C. Diagnosis
   1. Tender proximal fibula.
   2. Radiographs—anteroposterior, lateral, oblique of fibula

D. Treatment
   1. Nondisplaced with insignificant associated injury: short leg walking cast or walking boot for 6–8 weeks
   2. Displaced or with significant associated injury: Nonweight bearing cast immobilization or surgical treatment.

IV. Stress Fractures: Tibia

A. Epidemiology
   1. Medial tibia (compression side): most common stress fracture site in athletes. Highest incidence seen in runners.
   2. Anterior tibia (tension side): Usually seen in repetitive jumping athletes

B. Diagnosis
   1. Insidious onset of pain, worse with activity, better with rest

2. Recent history of change in training volume or surface
3. Localized pain with palpation over a confined area
4. Radiographs (Figure 26.3): anteroposterior, lateral, oblique. Often normal in first 2–3 weeks, later show periosteal reaction or fracture line
5. Bone scan: High sensitivity, poor specificity
6. MRI: Highly sensitive and specific. See fracture line surrounded by edema
7. Treatment
   a. Medial tibial stress fracture: relative rest (i.e., avoid painful activities), avoid NSAIDs, core/lower extremity strengthening, gradual return to activity as pain resolves
   b. Anterior tibial stress fracture: High risk of delayed or nonunion, athlete should be nonweightbearing and placed in a cast. Bone grafting or intramedullary tibial nailing is indicated when closed treatments are unsuccessful or to facilitate quicker return to sport

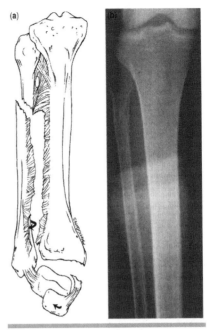

Figure 26.2 Maisonneuve fracture. (This figure was published in *Fracture Management for Primary Care*, Chapter 13, M. Patrice Eiff, Robert Hatch, Walter Calmbach, p. 201, W.B. Saunders Company; 1998.)

C. Fibula
   1. Usually seen in distance runners in distal one-third of the fibula
   2. Diagnosis and treatment similar to medial tibial stress fracture.

V. Instability/Dislocation: Fibular Head

A. Injury to the proximal tibiofibular joint is uncommon and can occur in isolation or with associated trauma

B. Diagnosis
   1. Usually a traumatic onset with a "popping sensation"
   2. Tender over the fibular head, more mobile than contralateral fibula, may lack of full knee extension
   3. Classification (Figure 26.4)
      a. Subluxation
         i. Seen with underlying connective tissue disorder and generalized hypermobility
      b. Anterolateral dislocation
         i. Most common type
         ii. Seen with sliding as the athlete falls on an inverted and plantar flexed foot with the knee flexed and the leg adducted
      c. Posterior medial dislocation
         i. Caused by direct trauma or twisting motion
         ii. Concomitant injuries may include the peroneal nerve or lateral collateral ligament

        d. Superior dislocation
          i. Extremely rare
          ii. Usually associated with severe trauma to the lower extremity
    4. Radiographs: leg in internal rotation will maximize the distance between the lateral tibia and fibula. Compare with contralateral extremity
    5. Treatment
        a. Acute injuries—closed reduction and 3 weeks of immobilization
        b. Chronic instability—often requires ligamentous reconstruction.

VI. Muscle/Tendon Injury: Gastrocnemius Tear

A. Medial head tears ("Tennis Leg") more common than lateral due to larger size and more oblique fiber orientation of the medial head

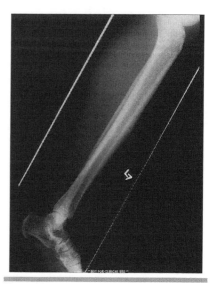

Figure 26.3 Stress fracture of the anterior tibia in a 16-year-old female.

B. Diagnosis
    1. Middle-aged recreational athlete who experiences a sharp, acute pain in the posterior calf during activity
    2. Pain and tenderness at the musculotendinous junction with swelling and ecchymosis that may track distally to the ankle
    3. MRI or ultrasound can be used to confirm diagnosis.

C. Treatment
    1. Rest, ice, compression, elevation
    2. Ultrasound-guided aspiration can be considered if there is significant fluid collection
    3. Stretching and strengthening with sports specific activities as symptoms allow.

VII. Medial Tibial Stress Syndrome

A. Repetitive traction of the muscular attachments to the periosteum creates a periostitis

B. Most commonly seen in runners. Presents bilaterally in 50% of cases

C. Diagnosis
    1. History: Aching pain over tibial shaft, worse with exertion but athlete may be able to "run through the pain," better with rest, recent change in training volume/intensity, early in athletic season
    2. Physical exam: Diffuse medial tibial tenderness, often elicited with resisted plantar flexion
        a. Evaluate for biomechanical abnormalities and muscle imbalances
    3. Imaging
        a. Radiographs: usually normal, but may show periosteal or cortical thickening.
        b. MRI or bone scan: can differentiate from stress fracture
          i. Bone scan—linear uptake on delayed images (versus a localized uptake seen on all three phases with a stress fracture)

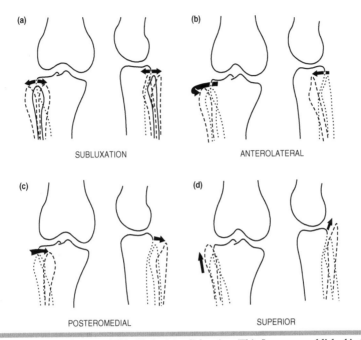

Figure 26.4   Classification of tibio-fibular joint dislocation. (This figure was published in the *Journal of Bone and Joint Surgery Amercian*, 1974, 56, Subluxation and dislocation of the proximal tibiofibular joint, Ogden, pp. 145–154, Figure 26.1.)

D. Treatment

    1. Relative rest with appropriate cross training, correction of biomechanical deficits, arch supports in athletes with overpronation, correction of training errors.

VIII. Acute Compartment Syndrome

A. Increased pressure in a fascial compartment causing impaired tissue perfusion, ischemic pain, and tissue necrosis if not urgently treated

B. Diagnosis

    1. Suspect with persistent or progressive severe pain after fracture or soft-tissue injury.

    2. Paresthesia, weakness of affected compartments

    3. Late findings can include pulselessness and palor

    4. Compartmental pressure testing

        a. Not necessary if clinical picture is unequivocal

        b. Intra-compartmental pressure >30 mm Hg

C. Treatment—Emergency surgical decompression via fasciotomy.

IX. Chronic Exertional Compartment Syndrome

A. Recurrent episodes of reversible ischemia due to transient elevations in intracompartmental pressure due to activity, which subsides with rest or cessation of activity

B. Runners most commonly affected

   C. Diagnosis

     1. History: Tight, cramping leg pain in a specific leg compartment (see anatomy section) that occurs with exercise at a predictable intensity and duration and is relieved with rest. Paresthesias and weakness may occur due to nerve compression

     2. Physical exam and radiologic studies are normal.

     3. Diagnosis confirmed when pre- and postexercise compartment pressure testing demonstrates one of the following:

       a. Preexercise $\geq$ 15 mm Hg

       b. 1 min postexercise $\geq$ 30 mm Hg

       c. 5 min postexercise $\geq$ 20 mm Hg

   D. Treatment

     1. Cessation or alteration of symptom-inducing activity

     2. Cross training with nonaggravating activity

     3. If the athlete is unwilling to change or alter the level of activity then surgical referral for fasciotomy is appropriate.

X. Popliteal Artery Entrapment

   A. Congenital deviation of the popliteal artery leading to entrapment by the medial or lateral gastrocnemius or the popliteus

   B. Condition is rare

   C. Diagnosis

     1. Most common in athletic males under the age of 40

     2. History: claudication symptoms in the calf and foot (unilateral or bilateral)

     3. Physical exam may demonstrate decreased posterior tibial or dorsalis pedis artery pulses with provocative maneuvers (i.e., passive ankle dorsiflexion or active ankle plantar flexion). Popliteal bruit may be present

       a. Arteriography with provocative maneuvers provides definitive diagnosis. Most common finding is medial displacement of the popliteal artery beneath the origin of the medial gastrocnemius

   D. Treatment—surgical release and if necessary vascular reconstruction.

Recommended Reading

Eiff MP, Hatch R, Calmbach WL. *Fracture Management for Primary Care*. Philadelphia: Saunders; 1998; *x*, 283pp.

Garrett WE Jr, Kirkendall DT, Squire DL, eds. *Principles and Practice of Orthopaedic Sports Medicine*. Philadelphia: Lippincott Williams & Wilkins; 2000: *xix*, 1062pp.

Gill CS, Halstead ME, Matava MJ. Chronic exertional compartment syndrome of the leg in athletes: Evaluation and management. *Phys Sportsmed. 38*(2):126–32.

Harrast MA, Colonno D. Stress fractures in runners. *Clin Sports Med*. 2010 Jul;*29*(3):399–416.

O'Connor FG, et al. *Textbook of Running Medicine*. New York: McGraw-Hill, Medical Publishing Division; 2001:*xxiv*, 696p.

Pedowitz RA, Hargens AR, Mubarak SJ, Gershuni DH. Modified criteria for the objective diagnosis of chronic compartment syndrome of the leg. *Am J Sports Med*. 1990 Jan–Feb;*18*(1):35–40.

Scuderi GR, McCann PD. *Sports Medicine: A Comprehensive Approach*. 2nd ed. Philadelphia: Mosby-Elsevier; 2005:*xvii*, 782pp.

Touliopolous S, Hershman EB. Lower leg pain. Diagnosis and treatment of compartment syndromes and other pain syndromes of the leg. *Sports Med.*, 1999;*27*(3):193–204.

Tucker AK. Chronic exertional compartment syndrome of the leg. *Curr Rev Musculoskelet Med*. 2010 Sep 2; *3*(1–4):32–7.

27

Ankle and Foot Injuries and Conditions

Gerard Malanga, Ricardo Vasquez-Duarte,
and Michael Esrick

I. Relevant Anatomy

A. Bones: Tibia, fibula, tarsals (e.g., calcaneus, talus), metatarsals, phalanges

B. Ligaments: Anterior inferior tibiofibular (AITFL), deltoid, anterior talofibular (ATFL), calcaneofibular (CFL), posterior talofibular (PTFL), calcaneonavicular (spring ligament)

C. Joints: Ankle, subtalar, mid-tarsal, tarsal–metatarsal (Lisfranc), metatarsophalangeal (MTP), proximal interphalangeal (PIP), distal interphalangeal (DIP)

D. Tendons: Anterior: tibialis anterior, extensor hallucis longus (EHL), extensor digitorum longus (EDL); posteromedial: tibialis posterior, flexor digitorum longus (FDL), flexor hallucis longus (FHL); posterior: Achilles; foot intrinsic muscles

E. Nerves: Tibial nerve, medial and lateral plantar nerves, deep and superficial peroneal nerves, sural nerve, saphenous nerve

F. Blood vessels: tibial artery, dorsalis pedis artery.

II. Fractures

A. Ankle
1. Classification system
   a. Danis–Weber: Based solely on fibula and location of fracture in relationship to ankle mortise
      i. Type A—fibular fracture below ankle mortise
      ii. Type B—fibular fracture at the level of ankle mortise
      iii. Type C—fibular fracture above the ankle mortise
2. Diagnosis
   a. Radiographs: Anteroposterior (AP), lateral, mortise view
3. Treatment
   a. Type A: if avulsion fracture (fx) of fibula is undisplaced or minimally displaced, and if there is no medial lesion (by exam and x-ray), then apply a walking cast until fibula has healed (usually 6–8 weeks);
   b. Patients with possible unstable injury (Danis–Weber classification types B or C) or those with bimalleolar fractures should be referred to an orthopedist.

B. Talus
1. 1% of foot fractures
2. Fracture sites: neck (most common), talar dome, posterior process, lateral process (snowboard fracture)

   3. Diagnosis:
     a. Radiographs: AP, lateral, mortise views of ankle
     b. Computed tomography (CT) if fracture suspected but x-rays normal
   4. Treatment:
     a. Nondisplaced: cast immobilization × 6–8 weeks
     b. Displaced: open reduction, internal fixation (ORIF)

C. Calcaneus
   1. Mechanism: Axial load with/without plantar or dorsiflexion
   2. Diagnosis:
     a. Radiographs: AP, lateral, mortise, 45° oblique
     b. CT if high index of suspicion but negative radiograph
   3. Treatment
     a. Nondisplaced: cast immobilization/nonweightbearing × 6–8 weeks
     b. Displaced: ORIF

D. Metatarsals
   1. Common fracture sites: diaphysis (traumatic or stress fracture), base of 5th (Jones fracture or avulsion fracture)
   2. Diagnosis:
     a. Radiographs: AP, lateral, oblique
     b. Magnetic resonance imaging (MRI) if stress fracture suspected and x-ray normal
   3. Treatment
     a. Nondisplaced: walking boot or postoperative shoe × 6–8 weeks, Jones fracture requires cast and nonweightbearing (NWB) × 8–12 weeks versus surgical treatment (possible faster recovery)
     b. Displaced: ORIF

E. Phalanges
   1. Common: 8–9% of fractures involve the toes
   2. Diagnosis: AP, lateral, oblique radiographs
   3. Treatment: Nondisplaced: walking boot/postoperative shoe × 3–4 weeks, then buddy tape for 4–6 additional weeks

F. Os trigonum
   1. Accessory ossicle formed by lack of fusion of the posterior talar process
   2. Present in 10% of population
   3. Causes posterior ankle pain with ankle plantar flexion
   4. Diagnosis: AP, lateral radiographs
   5. Treatment: relative rest, occasionally a steroid injection, surgical excision if nonoperative treatments ineffective

G. Stress fractures
   1. 0.7–20% of all sports injuries, most common in running athletes and female athletes.
   2. History: progressive pain with activity, training errors, female athlete triad, history of stress fractures
   3. Physical examination (PE): localized tenderness and swelling, (+) hop test, (+) pain with tuning fork
   4. Diagnosis:
     a. Radiographs: usually negative within 2–3 weeks of symptom onset, usually positive (fracture or periosteal reaction) 6 weeks after symptom onset
     b. Bone scan: sensitive, not specific. (+) 2–8 days after symptom onset
     c. MRI—Sensitive and specific. Graded as follows:
       i. Grade 1—abnormal STIR
       ii. Grade 2—abnormal T2

        iii. Grade 3—abnormal T1

        iv. Grade 4—fracture line on T1

  5. Treatment

    a. Relative rest, avoid nonsteroidal anti-inflammatory drugs (NSAIDS), correct biomechanics, change shoes every 300–500 miles, strengthen legs/core, possibly use orthotics

  6. Critical vs. noncritical stress fractures

    a. Critical: anterior tibial cortex, navicular (may require CT to define fracture), proximal 5th metatarsal, proximal 2nd metatarsal, sesamoids

    b. Noncritical: fibular, medial tibia, calcaneus, distal metatarsal diaphysis.

III. Dislocations

  A. Ankle dislocations (tib/fib and talus)

    1. Frequently have associated fractures

    2. Direction: posterior (most common), anterior, lateral, superior

    3. Treatment: surgical repair of capsular/ligamentous tears and fractures.

  B. Interphalangeal dislocation

    1. Mechanism: hyperflexion or hyperextension

    2. Dorsal PIP joint dislocation most common

    3. Diagnosis: AP, lateral, oblique radiographs

    4. Treatment: reduction, splint immobilization × 3 weeks, then buddy tape × 3–6 additional weeks.

IV. Tendinopathy: Usually Degenerative (-Osis) Rather than Inflammatory (-itis)

  A. Achilles tendinopathy

    1. Athletes (24% lifetime incidence) >nonathletes, incidence 7:100,000 general population, men >women, most common site 2–6 cm above insertion (watershed zone/poor vascular supply)

    2. History: insidious onset, pain with activity, relieved with rest, occasional edema/crepitus

    3. PE: tender to palpation at tendinopathy site, ±edema

    4. Diagnosis: usually clinical, but can be confirmed with ultrasound (US) or MRI

    5. Treatment: activity modification, correct training errors/biomechanical deficits, heel lift, glyceryl trinitrate patch, eccentric strengthening program. Surgery if nonoperative treatment fails.

  B. Tibialis posterior tendinopathy

    1. Inverts the subtalar joint, stabilizes the hind foot and arch

    2. More common in middle-aged/older individuals, can cause pes planus.

    3. History: Insidious or acute onset medial ankle pain, acute or gradual development of flat foot deformity, sometimes associated with underlying inflammatory condition

    4. PE: Tender posterior/inferior to medial malleolus, ±edema, pes planus, calcaneal valgus, too many toes sign (see >2 toes from behind), unable to perform single leg heel raise

    5. Diagnosis: AP, lateral, mortise view radiographs to identify arthrosis, MRI or US to evaluate posterior tibialis tendon

    6. Treatment: Rule out inflammatory condition, protection/rest/ice/compression/elevation (PRICE) principles, rigid orthosis to control pronation, medial heel flare, firm heel counter, eccentric exercises. Walking boot for severe cases. Surgery if nonoperative treatment fails.

  C. Peroneal tendinopathy and subluxation

    1. Usually insidious, but can be traumatic

2. History: Posterolateral ankle pain (insidious or acute/posttraumatic), snap/pop (tendon subluxation), ±edema, ankle instability, pain increased with forceful ankle plantar flexion or walking on uneven surface

3. PE: Posterolateral ankle edema, ±ecchymosis (posttraumatic), tenderness posterior/inferior to lateral malleolus, click/pain with active ankle ROM (tendon subluxation), pain with resisted ankle plantar flexion/eversion, tendon subluxation with ankle-eversion-plantar flexion to ankle-eversion-dorsiflexion against resistance

4. Diagnosis: AP, lateral, mortise view radiographs to evaluate for osseous abnormality; MRI to evaluate for tendinopathy; US to evaluate for tendinopathy or subluxation (dynamic imaging)

5. Treatment
   a. Tendinopathy: PRICE, heel lift, eccentric exercises. US-guided injection in refractory cases. Surgery if nonoperative treatment fails.
   b. Tendon subluxation: Immobilization in walking boot/cast with heel lift. Nonweight-bearing (NWB) × 2 weeks, weightbearing as tolerated (WBAT) × 4 weeks, then reestablish range of motion (ROM), strength, proprioception. Nonoperative treatment frequently fails. Surgical treatment can be performed before nonoperative treatment or after nonoperative treatment fails

D. Plantar fasciopathy
   1. Men = women, bilateral in up to 1/3 of cases, chronic >acute
   2. Clinical presentation
   3. History: insidious onset of sharp, medial, or inferior heel pain; most severe with first step out of bed in the morning or after a period of inactivity, lessens with gradually increased activity, worsens toward end of day with increased duration of weightbearing activity, often associated with a recent increase in intensity of walking or running regimen, change in footwear, exercised on different surface
   4. PE: Localized area of maximal tenderness over the anteromedial aspect of the plantar heel surface, gastroc-soleus tightness
   5. Diagnosis: radiographs to rule out other causes of heel pain (e.g., stress fracture, osseous lesion), bone scan to rule out stress fracture, MRI or US to evaluate plantar fascia (>5 mm thickness on US is abnormal)
   6. Treatment: 80% will resolve within 1 year regardless of treatment, conservative treatment within 6 weeks hastens recovery, PRICE, stretch gastroc-soleus complex and plantar fascia, strengthen foot intrinsics and ankle support muscles, NSAIDs for pain control, night splint, orthotics, or arch taping, proper foot wear (runners should replace shoes every 300–500 miles), corticosteroid or platelet-rich plasma (PRP) injection (palpation or US guided), extra-corporeal shock wave therapy (ECSWT). Surgery if refractory to nonoperative treatment × 6 months

E. Tibialis anterior tendinopathy
   1. Primary dorsiflexor of the foot; also adducts and supinates the foot
   2. Due to overuse of ankle dorsiflexors (e.g., downhill running, over striding), excessive pronation, restricted ankle ROM, athletes who wear a fixed boot (e.g., skiers, skaters), excessive tightness of strapping or shoelaces over area of tendon (e.g., runners, "weekend" athletes who do not maintain a consistent level of training), sports requiring abrupt change in direction
   3. History: Anteromedial ankle pain, edema, stiffness, increased with activity, especially running or walking down hills
   4. PE: Localized tenderness, swelling, occasional crepitus along tendon, pain with resisted dorsiflexion
   5. Diagnosis: MRI or US can be used to confirm diagnosis and exclude tendon rupture

6. Treatment: Eccentric strengthening, soft-tissue therapy, ankle mobilization, correction of biomechanical errors, orthotics, correct shoe wear (soft heel), mobilization of ankle joint, US-guided injections for refractory cases

F. Flexor hallucis longus tendinopathy

1. Assists with plantar-flexion of ankle
2. Due to overuse, large or medially positioned os trigonum, posterior ankle impingement (Ballet Dancer's tendinosis due to en pointe position) or trauma; wearing large shoes.
3. History: posteromedial ankle pain with radiation along medial arch, worse on toe-off or forefoot weightbearing, may report snap/pop or triggering
4. PE: Tender to palpation (TTP) over posteromedial ankle or under sustentaculum tali at medial longitudinal foot arch, aggravated with resisted first toe flexion or passive first toe and ankle dorsiflexion
5. Diagnosis: AP lateral, mortise view ankle radiographs, and lateral view with foot in full equinus (fully plantar-flexed and inverted) to rule out bony abnormalities; MRI or US to diagnosis tendon abnormalities
6. Treatment: PRICE, occasional walking boot progressing to rigid shoe insert, avoid en pointe temporarily, tape 1st metatarsophalangeal (MTP) joint to restrict dorsiflexion, US-guided corticosteroid injection in refractory cases. Surgery if nonoperative treatment fails—may need to excise os trigonum.

V. Tendon Tears

A. Achilles

1. Peak age 30–40 years old, male >female, usually 2–6 cm above insertion (decreased blood supply/watershed zone), left >right, usually have underlying tendinopathy (sometimes asymptomatic), 80% occur during recreational "stop-go" sports (e.g., basketball), type O blood, fluoroquinolone exposure, anabolic–androgenic steroid use, corticosteroid exposure (oral or injected), obesity
2. History: sudden sharp pain with/without "pop" during "stop-go" sport, reported as "someone hit me with a bat in the back of my leg," unable to weight bear
3. PE: ecchymosis, edema, palpable defect, (+) Thompson test (no plantar flexion of ankle when calf squeezed)
4. Diagnosis: MRI or ultrasound
5. Treatment:
   a. Surgical for active/young athlete
   b. Some literature suggests nonoperative treatment with dynamic splinting may be as good as surgery in active individuals.

VI. Ligament Injury/Instability

A. Lateral ankle sprain

1. Most common sports injury, accounting for 14–21% of all sports injuries, most common injury presenting to ER or primary care office: 25,000 occur daily; estimated 1.5 million ER visits annually in the United States, 85% of ankle injuries are ankle sprains. Eighty-five percent of ankle sprains are lateral ankle sprains, most commonly occurs in basketball, volleyball, soccer, football (i.e., sports that require rapid direction changes)
2. Mechanism of injury: inversion of plantarflexed foot
3. Most commonly injured ligaments: Anterior talofibular ligament (ATFL) > Calcaneofibular Ligament (CFL) > Posterior Talofibular Ligament (PTFL)
4. History: inversion ankle injury, "giving way," lateral ankle pain, possible "pop" at time of injury, ecchymosis, edema; usually able to bear weight immediately after injury with subsequent increase in pain and swelling later

5. PE: lateral ankle ecchymosis, edema, restricted ROM, TTP over injured ligament (usually ATFL), no bony tenderness, poor proprioception (if able to weight bear), (+) ankle anterior drawer test (assesses ATFL—more laxity when pulling ankle anteriorly relative to tibia), (+) talar tilt (assesses CFL—increased inversion with inversion ankle stress)

6. Diagnosis: **radiographs** of ankle or foot if (+) Ottawa ankle or foot rules, respectively (**Ottawa ankle rules**: TTP over posterior aspect of distal 6 cm of tibia or fibula or distal tip of medial or lateral malleolus, or inability to walk four steps immediately after injury and in the emergency department; **Ottawa foot rules**: TTP over base of fifth metatarsal, navicular bone, or inability to walk four steps immediately after the injury and in the emergency department). **CT scan** for occult fractures. **MRI** for occult fractures, osteochondritis dessicans (OCD), chondral injury, or soft-tissue injury

7. Treatment: PRICE (including crutches until can walk without a limp), over the counter (OTC) analgesics, AROM, isometric progressing to isotonic strengthening, proprioceptive exercises when able to weight bear, ankle bracing or taping during normal ambulation until ankle feels stable then just with sports for 6–12 months, functional exercises prior to return to sport

B. Medial ankle sprain
1. Due to eversion injury, injures deltoid ligament, isolated medial ankle sprain very uncommon due to deltoid ligament strength, often have associated with medial malleolus fracture
2. History: anteromedial ankle pain, ecchymosis, and edema following eversion ankle injury
3. PE: TTP over injured ligament
4. Diagnosis: Radiographs indicated if (+) Ottawa ankle rules; other diagnostic studies as above.
5. Treatment: Same as lateral ankle sprain, but may take longer to return to play.

C. Syndesmotic sprain (anterior inferior tibiofibular ligament [AITFL] sprain, also known as a "High Ankle Sprain")
1. Usually due to ankle dorsiflexion and external rotation. 10% of all ankle sprains. Most common in collision sports. May also involve posterior inferior tibiofibular ligament or syndesmotic membrane. Can lead to Maisonneuve fracture (fracture of proximal fibula).
2. History: Anterior ankle pain after above mechanism
3. PE: TTP over AITFL (be sure to palpate proximal fibula to evaluate for Maisonneuve fracture), (+) squeeze test (syndesmotic pain with tibiofibular compression in the mid-leg), (+) external rotation stress test (syndesmotic pain with external rotation of the ankle in a neutral dorsiflexion/plantar flexion position)
4. Diagnosis: Radiographs of entire tibia and fibular, and AP, lateral and mortise views of the ankle. Ideally should be weightbearing. A (+) mortise view for a syndesmotic injury would be indicated by any of the following: tibiofibular clear space of >5 mm (same measurement for AP view), tibiofibular overlap of <1 mm (<5 mm on AP view) or medial tibiotalar clear space of >4 mm. CT can identify small osseous abnormalities. MRI is 100% sensitive and 93% specific for AITFL ruptures
5. Treatment:
   a. Grade I (pain, negative radiographs): Rest, ice, immobilization for comfort ×2–4 weeks. Progress to functional ankle brace that limits eversion and external rotation, and begin progressive strengthening program (isometrics to isotonics to proprioceptive and plyometrics)
   b. Grades II–III (pain, positive radiographs): Warrant surgical evaluation. If can be reduced and maintained in reduction, can use posterior molded splint with sugar tong addition, nonweightbearing (NWB), elevation, and ice until edema subsides. If reduction maintained, switch to short leg cast for 6–8 weeks. Progress to walking cast and then a soft ankle brace. Rehabilitation should reestablish ROM, strength and proprioception. Serial radiographs should be performed q 2 weeks to ensure

maintenance of reduction. If cannot be reduced or reduction cannot be maintained, surgical treatment is warranted

D. Chronic ankle instability
   1. Due to functional and/or mechanical instability
      a. Mechanical instability—caused by structural damage to the connective tissue that supports that joint
      b. Functional instability—due to neuromuscular deficits
   2. Due to poorly healed/rehabilitated ankle sprains—ligaments heal in a lengthened position, persistent ankle support muscle weakness, poor proprioception. Hereditary hypermobility/connective tissue disorder may contribute
   3. History: Prior ankle injuries, recurrent ankle "give way" episodes, edema, pain, potentially mechanical symptoms (e.g., clicking and popping)
   4. PE: ±TTP over injured area, hypermobility of ankle (i.e., positive talar tilt test, anterior drawer test, etc.), poor proprioception (e.g., difficulty with single leg balance), poor strength
   5. Diagnosis: AP, lateral, mortise ankle radiographs while weightbearing. Consider stress views: Anterior drawer (positive if >3 mm anterior excursion), Talar tilt (positive if >15° side-to-side difference). MRI can identify osseous and soft-tissue lesions contributing to ankle instability
   6. Treatment: Ankle muscle strengthening, proprioceptive exercises, taping, bracing, orthotics, heel wedge (lateral for lateral ankle instability, medial for medial ankle instability). Surgical intervention considered if nonoperative treatment fails

E. Lisfranc joint injury
   1. Sprain of the tarsal–metatarsal joint at the base of the 1st and 2nd metatarsals.
   2. Two mechanisms
      a. Direct: Crush injury
      b. Indirect: Longitudinal force sustained while foot plantar-flexed and slightly rotated (e.g., opponent roles onto plantar aspect of plantar flexed foot of football linemen causing hyperplantar flexion)
   3. History: Mechanism above, mid-foot pain aggravated by weightbearing (particularly when weightbearing through forefoot), severity of injury often underestimated at time of injury. Suspect if pain persists >5 days
   4. PE: TTP over dorsal mid-foot, ±edema, pain with combined eversion and abduction of forefoot, pain with passive pronation/supination of tarso-metatarsal joint
   5. Diagnosis: AP, 30° oblique, and lateral weightbearing radiographs of foot. Positive x-rays = displacement >2 mm between 1st and 2nd metatarsal bases. "Fleck Sign" = avulsion fracture near base of the 2nd metatarsal or medial cuneiform in AP view. Medial cortex of 2nd metatarsal base should line up with medial border of intermediate cuneiform on AP x-ray. Medial cortex of 4th metatarsal base should line up with medial border of cuboid on 30° oblique x-ray. Dorsal cortex of 1st metatarsal and medial cuneiform should line up on lateral weightbearing x-ray. MRI: more sensitive than x-ray for ligament injury. CT scan may demonstrate small avulsion fracture
   6. Nunley and Vertullo Grading System
      a. Stage 1
         i. Able to bear weight but could not return to play
         ii. Local point tenderness over medial aspect of 1st TMT joint
         iii. No radiographic diastasis between 1st and 2nd metatarsals on AP weightbearing x-ray and no medial longitudinal arch on weightbearing lateral x-ray
      b. Stage 2
         i. Similar physical findings to Stage 1
         ii. Diastasis 2–5 mm (normal = 1–2 mm) between 1st and 2nd metatarsals on A-P weightbearing x-ray but no collapse of arch on weightbearing lateral x-ray

    c. Stage 3

      i. Diastasis 2–5 mm between 1st and 2nd metatarsals on A-P weightbearing x-ray and collapse of medial longitudinal arch on weightbearing lateral x-ray evidenced by displacement of dorsal cortical line between 1st metatarsal and medial cuneiform

  7. Treatment

    a. Stage 1: Nonweightbearing cast or cast boot immobilization×2 weeks. Repeat x-ray at 2 weeks to rule out diastasis. If follow-up x-ray shows stability and patient is nontender, then can begin weightbearing and progressive functional rehabilitation program of foot and ankle with orthotic to provide arch support. If nondisplaced but still tender at 2 weeks, transition to walking boot/cast×4 weeks, then begin progressive functional rehabilitation program with orthotic to provide arch support

    b. Stage 2 or 3: Surgical treatment with ORIF

F. First metatarsophalangeal joint sprain ("Turf Toe")

  1. Hyperextension injury to 1st metatarsophalangeal (MTP) joint causing damage to plantar plate, joint capsule, and 1st MTP joint ligaments. Risks include playing on artificial turf, pes planus, poor ankle dorsiflexion ROM, poor 1st MTP joint extension ROM, flexible shoes

  2. History: Hyperextension injury to 1st MTP causing pain with weightbearing and great toe movement. Ecchymosis and edema are often present

  3. PE: Plantar (and occasionally dorsal) 1st MTP joint tenderness, 1st MTP joint effusion, pain with passive and active 1st MTP ROM, decreased 1st MTP joint ROM

  4. Diagnosis: Radiographs usually unremarkable, but may show small plantar avulsion fracture of MTP capsule. MRI may demonstrate soft tissue injuries to capsule, ligaments, or plantar plate

  5. Treatment: WBAT in post-op shoe, rest, ice, compression, elevation, taping. As pain resolves, gradually work on re-establishing 1st MTP joint ROM. Transition from post-op shoe to running shoe with carbon fiber insert and Morton's extension to decrease 1st MTP joint dorsiflexion. Often takes 3–6 weeks to recover. Can be complicated by the development of hallux rigidus.

VII. Bursitis

A. Retro-Achilles (subcutaneous calcaneal)

  1. Located posterior to Achilles tendon

  2. Caused by excessive friction posterior to insertion of Achilles tendon on calcaneus. Seen in athletes who wear heel tabs, shoes that are too tight or too large, stiff boots (i.e., ice skates, cricket), Haglund deformity (bony prominence at the posterosuperior aspect of the calcaneus)

  3. History: Posterior heel pain aggravated by direct pressure, weightbearing activity and at the beginning of activity (i.e., warm-up phenomenon). May cause limp. ±edema ("pump bump")

  4. PE: TTP retro-Achilles region, ±edema

  5. Diagnosis: Radiographs may demonstrate a Haglund deformity or stress fracture. MRI and US can demonstrate bursitis.

  6. Treatment: Ice, reduce pressure (i.e., widen/press out heel of shoe), doughnut pad around area, heel cup to raise area over heel counter, NSAIDs, iontophoresis. Occasionally corticosteroid injections are warranted, but be aware of tendon rupture risk. Surgical treatment for Haglund deformity can be considered if nonoperative treatment fails

B. Retro-calcaneal (subtendinous)

  1. Located between the Achilles tendon and calcaneus

2. Predisposing factors: training errors, tight Achilles tendon, Haglund's deformity, Achilles enthesopathy, underlying seronegative spondyloarthropathy
3. History: Posterior ankle pain, ±edema, aggravated by weightbearing activity (particularly when weightbearing on forefoot), may report limp
4. PE: ±limp, TTP between calcaneus and Achilles tendon, possible "pump bump"
5. Diagnosis: Radiographs usually normal but may reveal evidence of enthesopathy (e.g., enthesophytes) or Haglund's deformity. MRI or US can demonstrate the bursopathy, but rarely required
6. Treatment: Ice, reduce pressure on area (e.g., stretch calf, wear shoes that do not press on area), modify training/activities, heel lift, NSAIDs, and iontophoresis. Occasionally a walking boot is beneficial. May consider corticosteroid injection if unresponsive to other treatments, but beware of increased tendon rupture risk. Surgical treatment of Haglund's deformity of nonoperative treatment fails.

Recommended Reading

1. Alfredson H, Cook J. A treatment algorithm for managing Achilles tendinopathy: New treatment options. *Br J Sports Med*. 2007;41:211–216.
2. Bennell KL, Malcom SA, Thomas SA, Reid SJ, Brukner PD, Ebeling PR, Wark JD. Risk factors for stress fractures in track and field athletes. A twelve-month prospective study. *Am J Sports Med*. 1996;24(6):810–818.
3. Bozelle J, Kirshner S. Orthopedic surgery: Foot and ankle: recurrent ankle sprains. *Emedicine*. www.emedicine.com. April 9, 2010.
4. Bruckner P, Khan K. *Clinical Sports Medicine*. Revised 3rd ed. New York, NY: McGraw-Hill Companies; 2010.
5. Buchbinder R. Plantar fasciosis. *N Engl J Med*. 204;350:2159–2166.
6. Dyck D, Boyajian-O'Neill L. Plantar fasciosis. *Clin J Sport Med*. 2004;14:305–309.
7. Foye P, Stitick T, Nadler S. Physical medicine and rehabilitation: Retrocalcaneal bursosis." *Emedicine*. www.emedicine.com. August 31, 2010.
8. Fredericson M, Jennings F, Beaulieu C, Metheson GO. Stress fractures in athletes. *Top Magn Reson Imaging*. 2006;17(5):309–325.
9. Fu FH, Stone DA. *Sports Injuries: Mechanisms, Prevention, and Treatment*. 2nd ed. Philadelphia: Lippincott Williams & Wilkins; 2001
10. Gudemann SD, Eisele SA, Heidt RS Jr, Colosimo AJ, Stroupe AL. Treatment of plantar fasciitis by iontophoresis of 0.4% dexamethasone: A randomized, double-blind placebo controlled study. *Am J Sports Med*. 1997;25(3):312–16.
11. Hatch R. Achilles tendon rupture: A challenging diagnosis: Discussion. *J Am Board Fam Med*. 2000;13(5). Medscape Family Medicine. wwww.medscape.com.
12. Hoch AZ. Dx, Mx, Rx of sports-related injuries and conditions: Lower leg/Ankle/foot. *AAPM&R Sports Medicine Board Examination Review Course Self Study Material* pp. 315–331.
13. Jensen SL, Andresen BK, Mencke S, Nielsen PT. Epidemiology of ankle fractures. A prospective population-based study of 212 cases in Aalborg, Denmark. *Acta Orthop Scand*. 1998;69(1):48–50.
14. Kader D, Sazena A, Movin T, Maffulli N. Achilles tendinopathy: Some aspects of basic and clinical management. *Br J Sports Med*. 2002;36:239–249.
15. Kelsey JL, Bachrach LK, Procter-Gray E, Nieves J, Greendale GA, Sowers M, Brown BW Jr, Matheson KA, Crawford SL, Cobb KL. Risk factors for stress fractures among young female cross-country runners. *Med Sci Sports Exercise*. 2007;39(9):1457–1463.
16. Lake C, Trexler G, Barringer W. Posterior tibial tendon dysfunction: a review of pain and activity level of twenty-one patients. *J Prosth Ortho*. 1999;11(1):2–5.
17. Maughan K. Ankle sprain. UpToDate Online. May 2010.
18. *Netter's Orthopaedics* by Walter Greene Chapter 19, pp. 428–453.
19. Premkmar A, Perry MB, Dwyer AJ, Gerber LH, Johnson D, Venzon D, Shawker TH. Sonography and MR imaging of posterior tibial tendinopathy. *AJR Am J Roentgenol*. 2002;178:223–32.
20. Renstrom PA, Konradsen L. Ankle ligament injuires. *Br J Sports Med*. 1997;31:11–20.

21. Roth J, Tayler W, Whalen J. Peroneal tendon subluxation: The other lateral ankle injury. *Br J Sports Med.* 2010;*44*:1047–1053.

22. Sherman KP. The foot in sport. *Br J Sports Med.* 1999;*33*:6–13.

23. Sorosky B, Press J, Plastaras C, Rittenber J. The practical management of Achilles tendinopathy. *Clin J Sport Med.* 2004;*14*:40–44.

24. Young C. Sports medicine: Ankle sprain: *Emedicine.* www.edmedicine.com. April 28, 2009.

Pediatric Musculoskeletal Injuries and Conditions

Andrew John Maxwell Gregory

PEDIATRIC MUSCULOSKELETAL INJURIES AND CONDITIONS

I. Fractures

A. Plastic deformation—bending of bone without fracture propagation
1. Ulna/fibula most common

B. Buckle (torus)—compression failure of cortex/periosteum
1. Metaphyseal/diaphyseal junction

C. Greenstick—tension failure causing single cortex separation and buckling opposite

D. Complete—fracture propagates through both cortices
1. Spiral—rotational, low velocity, associated with child abuse
2. Oblique—diagonal to diaphyseal bone, unstable
3. Transverse—three-point bending

E. Epiphyseal fractures—fractures that involve the physis (growth plate) at the end of long bones
1. Distal radius is most common
2. Potential for deformity—angular, limb length discrepancy or joint incongruity
3. Salter–Harris (SH) classification (see Figure 28.1)
   a. SH I—through the physis only (x-ray normal or widened physis), growth disruption is unusual, treatment is generally cast immobilization
   b. SH II—through the metaphysis and the physis, most common, growth disruption is unusual, treatment is generally cast immobilization
   c. SH III—through the epiphysis and the physis, intraarticular, anatomic reduction required
   d. SH IV—through the metaphysis and epiphysis, intraarticular, anatomic reduction required
   e. SH V—crush injury to the physis, difficult to recognize as initial films will appear similar to SH I, high risk of growth disturbance, often diagnosed retrospectively after growth arrest is obvious

F. Slipped capital femoral epiphysis—Salter Harris I of the femoral head
1. Boys aged 13, girls aged 11, African American (AA), obese
2. Bilateral 30–40%
3. Endocrine disorders
4. Groin, thigh or knee pain and limp
5. Loss of internal rotation with flexion

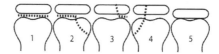

Figure 28.1   Cartoon depiction of the Salter–Harris classification schema.

    6. AP and frogleg pelvis x-rays—posteromedial displacement of the epiphysis

        a. Klein's line—line drawn along the superior femoral neck should intersect with the femoral head (see Figure 28.2)

    7. Immediate nonweight bearing

    8. Prompt referral for open reduction and internal fixation (ORIF).

II. Apophyseal/epiphyseal avulsion fractures—traction injury of the bony attachment of the tendon or ligament from its origin/insertion; general treatment is conservative, however, marked displacement may indicate surgical management

    A. Shoulder

        1. Coracoid—origin of short head of the biceps and coracobrachialis

            a. Adolescents

            b. Fall

            c. Anterior pain, pop

            d. Anterior tenderness

            e. Rest, sling, ice

    B. Elbow

        1. Medial epicondyle—humeral origin of the ulnar collateral ligament and wrist flexor tendons

            a. School-age children

            b. Fall, throwing

            c. Medial pain, pop, swelling

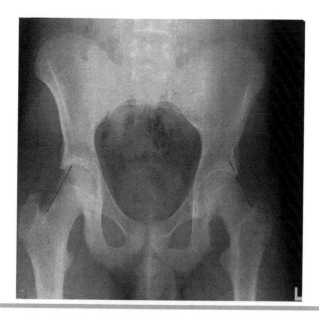

    d. Medial tenderness, pain with valgus stress

    e. X-ray—displacement of medial epicondyle

    f. Long arm splint/cast, surgery for significant displacement (>5 mm)

C. Wrist/Hand

  1. Proximal phalanx (PP) of the thumb—insertion of the ulnar collateral ligament

    a. Adolescents

    b. Fall

    c. Pain, swelling

    d. Tenderness ulnar side of the base of the PP, pain with valgus stress

    e. X-ray—SH III fracture

    f. Thumb spica splint/cast

  2. Middle and distal phalanges (MP, DP)—insertion of the flexor and extensor tendons or collateral ligaments (see Figure 28.3)

    a. Adolescents

    b. "Jammed finger"

    c. Pain, swelling

    d. Tenderness at the base of the MP, DP

    e. Pain with varus/valgus stress, flexor/extensor tendon testing

    f. X-ray—SH III fracture

    g. Flexion splint for volar plate avulsion, extension splint for extensor tendon avulsion, ice, acetaminophenm tape for collateral injuries

D. Spine

  1. Superior/inferior endplate—attachment of the annulus fibrosus of the intervertebral disc (Limbus Vertebrae)

    a. Adolescents

    b. Olympic weight lifting (squats)

    c. Pain with sitting, bending

    d. Decreased forward flexion with pain, positive straight leg raise

    e. CT X-ray, CT MRI—displacement of endplates

    f. Rest, avoid flexion, extension exercises

E. Pelvis and hip

  1. Iliac crest—origin of the iliotibial (IT) band/tensor fascia lata (TFL) (palpable)

  2. ASIS—origin of the sartorius (palpable)

  3. AIIS—origin of the rectus femoris just superior to the acetabulum (not palpable)

  4. Ischial tuberosity—pelvic origin of the adductors and hamstrings (palpable)

  5. Greater trochanter—femoral insertion of the gluteus medius (palpable)

  6. Lesser trochanter—femoral insertion of the iliopsoas (not palpable)

  7. General

    a. Adolescents

    b. Painful pop with sprinting, kicking or doing the splits

    c. Tenderness over the apophysis

    d. X-ray—widening of the apophysis

    e. Rest, crutches, stretching, ice, acetaminophen

F. Knee

  1. Superior pole patella—patellar insertion of the quadriceps tendon

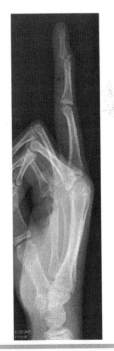

Figure 28.3 Distal phalanx epiphyseal avulsion fracture

    2. Inferior pole patella—patellar origin of the patellar tendon
    3. Tibial tubercle—tibial insertion of the patellar tendon
    4. General
      a. Adolescents
      b. Painful pop with jumping or landing
      c. Tenderness over the patella or tibial tubercle
      d. X-ray—widening of the apophysis, ossicle
      e. Knee immobilizer, rest, crutches, ice, acetaminophen
G. Foot
    1. Base of the fifth metatarsal—insertion of the peroneal brevis tendon
      a. Adolescents
      b. Inversion injury with pop
      c. Swelling, pain on the lateral foot
      d. Tenderness at the base of the 5th metatarsal
      e. X-ray—widening of the apophysis
      f. Walking boot, ankle brace, ice, acetaminophen.

III. Apophysitis/epiphysitis—overuse traction injury to the apophysis or epiphysis

A. Little league shoulder
    1. Humeral head epiphysis—insertion of rotator cuff musculature
      a. Age 8–15 years
      b. Pitchers, catchers
      c. Shoulder pain with throwing
      d. Tenderness of the proximal humerus
      e. X-rays—normal or widening of epiphysis, sclerosis, cystic changes
      f. Rest from throwing until pain free, ice, acetaminophen, rehabilitation to correct biomechanical faults that may predispose to injury
      g. Adhere to age-based pitch counts when returning to pitching (see Chapter 4, Table 4.1)
B. Little league elbow
    1. Medial epicondyle apophysis—humeral origin of the ulnar collateral ligament
      a. Age 8–15 years
      b. Pitchers, catchers
      c. Medial elbow pain with throwing
      d. Tenderness of the medial epicondyle
      e. X-rays—normal or widening of apophysis, ossicle
      f. Rest from throwing until pain free, ice, acetaminophen, rehabilitation to correct biomechanical faults that may predispose to injury
      g. Adhere to age-based pitch counts when returning to pitching (see Chapter 4, Table 4.1)
C. Gymnast's wrist
    1. Distal radial epiphysis—compression from weight bearing on the arms
      a. Age 8–15 years
      b. Gymnasts, cheerleaders
      c. Wrist pain with tumbling
      d. Tenderness of the distal radius
      e. X-rays—normal or closing of epiphysis, shortening of the radius (positive ulnar variance)
      f. Rest from tumbling until pain free, ice, acetaminophen, rehabilitation, wrist braces
D. Pelvis
    1. Iliac crest—origin of the IT Band/TFL
    2. ASIS—origin of the sartorius
    3. AIIS—origin of the rectus femoris just superior to the acetabulum
    4. Ischial tuberosity—pelvic origin of the adductors and hamstrings

a. General
   i. Adolescents
   ii. Hip/groin pain with activity
   iii. Tenderness over the apophysis
   iv. X-rays—normal or widening of apophysis
   v. Rest from activity until pain free, ice, acetaminophen, stretching

E. Sinding–Larsen–Johannson disease
  1. Superior pole patella—patellar insertion of the quadriceps tendon
  2. Inferior pole patella—patellar origin of the patellar tendon
    a. Adolescents, typically during periods of rapid growth
    b. Anterior knee pain with activity
    c. Tenderness of the apophysis
    d. X-rays—normal or widening of the apophysis
    e. Rest from activity until pain free, ice, acetaminophen, stretching, Cho-Pat strap, reassurance

F. Osgood–Schlatter disease (see Figure 28.4)
  1. Tibial tuberosity—tibial insertion of the patellar tendon
    a. Adolescents, typically during periods of rapid growth
    b. Anterior knee pain with activity
    c. Tenderness of the apophysis
    d. X-rays—normal or widening of apophysis
    e. Rest from activity until pain free, ice, acetaminophen, stretching, Cho-Pat strap, reassurance

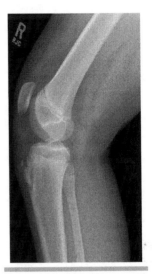

Figure 28.4 O-S Disease with ossicle-A

G. Sever's disease
  1. Posterior calcaneus—insertion of the Achilles tendon
    a. School-age children
    b. Soccer, baseball
    c. Heel pain with activity
    d. Tenderness of the posterior calcaneus
    e. X-rays—normal apophysis, often multipartite
    f. Rest from activity until pain free, ice, acetaminophen, calf stretching, heel cups, walking boot for severe cases

H. Iselin's disease
  1. Base the fifth metatarsal—insertion of the peroneus brevis tendon
  2. Adolescents
  3. Lateral foot pain with activity
  4. Tenderness at the base of the 5th metatarsal, supination
  5. X-rays—normal or widening of apophysis
  6. Rest from activity until pain free, ice, acetaminophen, stretching, lateral heel wedge, walking boot for severe cases.

IV. Osteochondritis dessicans (OCD)—subchondral bone and cartilage fragment that loses its blood supply due to trauma or vascular insult, most commonly seen in elbow, knee, and ankle, 2nd decade

A. General

1. Tend to heal well in the skeletally immature
2. Surgery for unstable lesions or skeletally mature.
3. MRI classification (Berndt and Harty)—stable (attached fragment) vs. unstable (detached fragment)
   a. Stage I—subchondral compression, cartilage still attached, edema and signal changes seen on MRI (stable)
   b. Stage II—partially detached with breach in articular cartilage, fluid leaking under articular cartilage (low signal rim underneath fragment indicating fibrous attachment) (stable)
   c. Stage III—completely detached fragment but still in crater with a breach in articular cartilage but with high signal on MRI underneath fragment and subchondral bone (unstable)
   d. Stage IV—completely detached fragment loose in joint (loose body) (unstable)

B. Elbow
   1. Capitellum—compression from valgus stress from throwing or tumbling
      a. Adolescents
      b. Pain, swelling with activity
      c. Effusion, lateral tenderness, loss of motion
      d. X-rays—sclerosis, fragmentation, collapse
      e. Rest from activity, physical therapy for stable lesions
      f. Surgery—removal of loose bodies

C. Knee (see Figure 28.5)
   1. Femoral condyles (medial 80%; lateral 15%), patella (5%), trochlea
      a. Male adolescents
      b. Pain, swelling with activity
      c. Effusion, joint line tenderness
      d. Tunnel view x-ray—semilunar lucency, fragmentation
      e. Rest, physical therapy, unloader brace for stable lesions
      f. Surgery for unstable lesions

D. Ankle
   1. Talar dome
      a. Pain, swelling with activity, associated with ankle sprain
      b. Effusion, joint line tenderness
      c. AP x-ray—semilunar lucency, fragmentation, typically in the supermedial corner of talar dome
      d. Rest, physical therapy
      e. Surgery for unstable lesions.

V. Osteonecrosis—avascular necrosis of the apophyseal center

A. Elbow
   1. Panner's disease—capitellum
      a. Children under age 10; throwing, gymnastics
      b. Good prognosis
      c. Lateral elbow pain
      d. X-rays—sclerosis, fragmentation, collapse
      e. Self-limited process, thus conservative management is warranted: rest, range of motion

B. Wrist/Hand
   1. Kienbock's disease—carpal lunate
      a. Men aged 20–40
      b. X-rays—increased density, fragmentation, collapse
      c. Tenderness to palpation of the lunate
      d. Osteoarthritis develops

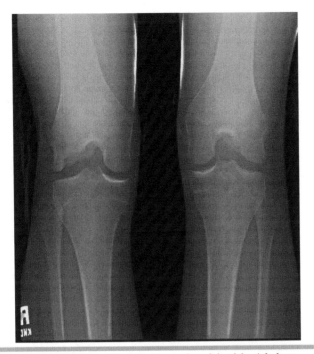

Figure 28.5 Large OCD lesion of the lateral femoral condyle of the right knee

    e. Treatment with a cast or splint initially, surgery for bone grafting, osteotomy, excision or fusion if chronic/recalcitrant

C. Spine
  1. Scheuermann's disease—vertebral superior or inferior endplates:
    a. Male adolescents
    b. Poor posture, pain
    c. Rigid kyphosis
    d. Diagnosis via x-ray—three adjacent vertebrae with 5° of anterior wedging, kyphosis of 45°, Schmorl's nodes, irregular endplates
    e. Treatment—physical therapy, extension exercises, brace, surgery for severe deformity

D. Hip
  1. Legg–Calve–Perthe's disease—femoral head
    a. Boys aged 4–8
    b. 90% unilateral
    c. Limp with groin, thigh, or knee pain
    d. Limited hip abduction
    e. AP and frog leg pelvis x-rays—sclerosis, fragmentation, crescent sign
    f. Osteoarthritis can develop, especially if >10 years old
    g. Better prognosis for those < 10 years old
    h. Physical therapy for range of motion maintenance, crutches or walker with decreased weight bearing to limit femoral head deformity
    i. Abduction brace

E. Knee
  1. Blount's disease (tibia varum)—medial tibial epiphysis

    a. Adolescent—obese, AA
    b. Infantile—unilateral,   distinguish   from physiologic varus
    c. Genu varus (bow leg)
    d. Lateral thrust with gait
    e. X-rays—beaking of the proximal medial tibia, metaphyseal–diaphyseal angle
    f. Weight loss, bracing (effective in infantile form)
    g. Surgery—osteotomy

F. Foot/Ankle

  1. Freiberg's infraction—second or third metatarsal (see Figure 28.6)
    a. Adolescent females
    b. Tenderness at the metatarsal head
    c. X-rays—flattening of the metatarsal head
    d. If diagnosis is early, conservative management often successful: orthotic (metatarsal pad, graphite shank), relative rest
    e. Surgery—debridement, loose body removal

  2. Kohler's disease—tarsal navicular
    a. Children aged 4–8
    b. Arch pain and limp
    c. Tenderness over the medial navicular
    d. X-rays—sclerosis, collapse, fragmentation
    e. Walking boot, short leg cast.

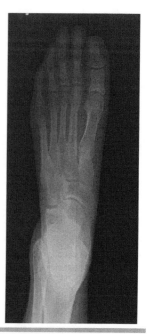

Figure 28.6 Freiberg's infraction of the second metatarsal head

Recommended Reading

1. Bracker MD, eds. *The 5-Minute Sports Medicine Consult*. 2nd ed. Philadelphia, PA: Wolters Kluwer; 2011:596–597.
2. Green MD, Swiontkowski MD, eds. *Skeletal Trauma in Children*. 3rd ed. Philadelphia, PA: Saunders; 2003.
3. Harris SS, Anderson SJ, eds. *Care of the Young Athlete, Harris*. 2nd ed. Elk Grove Village, IL: American Academy of Pediatrics; 2010:315–321.
4. Kibler B, eds. *Orthopaedic Knowledge Update, Sports Medicine*. Rosemont, IL: American Academy of Orthopaedic Surgeons; 2009:389–431.
5. Metzl MD, eds. *Sports Medicine in the Pediatric Office*. Elk Grove Village, IL: American Academy of Pediatrics; 2008.
6. Micheli MD, eds. *The Sports Medicine Bible for Young Athletes*. Naperville, IL: Sourcebooks, Inc.; 2001.
7. Snider RK, eds. *Essentials of Musculoskeletal Care*. Rosemont, IL: American Academy of Orthopaedic Surgeons; 1999.

29

Environmental Illness

Cara C. Prideaux and Jonathan T. Finnoff

I. Heat Illness

A. Thermoregulation = balance between heat production and dissipation
1. Metabolism: contributes to heat production, greater with exercise than rest
2. Radiation = exchange of heat via electromagnetic waves
   a. Heat gain in partially clothed athlete > fully clothed athlete
   b. Heat absorption in pigmented skin > nonpigmented skin
3. Convection = heat transfer between the body and circulating medium (air, water)
   a. Greater rate of medium movement → more rapid heat exchange
   b. High thermal conductivity → more rapid heat transfer (water > air)
4. Conduction = transfer of heat between warmer and cooler object via direct contact
5. Evaporation: Sweat vaporization → heat loss
   a. Primary heat dissipation mechanism if ambient temperature >68 °F or with vigorous exercise
   b. High humidity, lack of wind → reduced sweat vaporization
   c. Wearing hat and coat → impaired evaporative cooling

B. Body temperature regulated by preoptic area of hypothalamus
1. Exercise → blood decreased to viscera and skin, increased to exercising muscles
2. Rise in core temperature >38 °C detected by hypothalamus → activation of efferent fibers of autonomic nervous system → cutaneous vasodilation and increased rate of sweating → heat loss

C. Risk factors predisposing to heat-related injury
1. Hot, humid, no clouds, no wind; males > females; improper clothing; acute illness (fever, URI, GI); poor fitness; lack of acclimatization; dehydration; heavier weight, shorter height, higher body mass index; extremes of age; cardiovascular disease; skin injury; previous heat-related illness; sickle cell trait
2. Medications: diuretics, β-blockers, anticholinergics, alcohol, phenothiazines, butyrophenones, benztropine, ephedra, amphetamines, cocaine, ecstasy

D. Heat-related disorders
1. Miliaria rubra (heat rash—a pruritic papulovesicular rash)
   a. Due to occluded sweat glands on skin covered by clothing
   b. Treatment: good hygiene; cooling and drying the skin
2. Heat edema
   a. Dependent edema in athletes undergoing heat acclimatization
   b. Due to increased plasma volume associated with acclimatization
   c. Treatment: elevation of the extremity; resolves with acclimatization

3. Sunburn
   a. Predominantly caused by ultraviolet B (UV B) rays
   b. Risk factor for heat illness (reduced heat transfer in sunburned skin)
   c. Prevention: Cover skin with clothing or sunscreen
4. Heat tetany—carpopedal spasms
   a. Due to compensatory hyperventilation from acute heat exposure
   b. Treatment: remove athlete from heat, breathe in a paper bag
5. Heat cramps—muscle cramps in large muscle groups
   a. Due to heat exposure and electrolyte loss in sweat
   b. Treatment: rest, prolonged static stretching of muscle group, rehydration, electrolyte replacement, cooling
   c. Intravenous (IV) normal saline if severe. IV benzodiazepines administered as the last option.
6. Heat syncope—orthostasis
   a. Due to peripheral vasodilation and venous pooling
   b. Treatment: elevate legs, rehydrate, cool
7. Heat exhaustion
   a. Profuse sweating, headache, nausea, weakness, malaise, mild mental status changes, inability to continue exercise. No end-organ damage.
   b. Core (i.e., rectal) temperature $<40\ °C$ (104 °F)
   c. Assessment/Treatment:
      i. Mild symptoms: treat on site
      ii. Place athlete supine in cool, shaded area with legs elevated
      iii. Assess vitals, rectal temperature; begin oral fluid replacement
      iv. Rapid cooling: remove excess clothing; wet with water; direct fan over them; ice packs in axilla, neck, groin; "ice-cube burrito"—lay athlete on wet blanket, pour ice water over them and wrap blanket around them; submersion in tub of ice water.
8. Exertional heat stroke (EHS)
   a. Core (i.e., rectal) body temperature $\geq 40\ °C$ (104 °F)
   b. Multiple organ system failure (renal failure, hepatic necrosis, cardiac damage, rhabdomyolysis, ischemic colitis, adult respiratory distress syndrome, and endotoxic shock from gut cell breakdown, disseminated intravascular coagulation) or central nervous system dysfunction
   c. Hot, pale, and wet skin (dry skin in sick and elderly)
   d. Disorientation, dizziness, inappropriate behavior, headache, loss of balance, collapse, fatigue, vomiting, hyperventilation, delirium, seizures, coma
   e. Assessment/treatment
      i. Early recognition, rapid cooling → reduced morbidity and mortality
      ii. Activate emergency services; transport to medical facility
      iii. Airway, breathing, circulation; monitor vitals (rectal temperatures)
      iv. Same cooling techniques as described in heat exhaustion section
      v. Oral rehydration preferred. If not able, IV fluids (normal saline)
      vi. Assess for electrolyte abnormalities (e.g., hyponatremia)
E. Return to sport
   1. Sustaining heat injury predisposes to a subsequent heat-related injury
      a. Do not allow return to sport immediately following heat injury
      b. Gradually reintroduce exercise in a nonheat-stressed followed by heat-stressed environment
   2. Mild heat exhaustion
      a. No return to exercise ≥ 24–48 h after athlete is asymptomatic
      b. If symptoms arise, activity should stop and athlete reevaluated

3. Severe heat exhaustion or heat stroke
   a. No exercise until physician follow-up 7 days after hospitalization
   b. If no signs or symptoms → gradual reintroduction of exercise over 2 weeks
F. Prevention of heat-related illness
   1. Heat acclimatization: allows athlete to exercise at higher level for longer time in a hot environment while maintaining a lower core body temperature
      a. Physiologic adaptations: increased plasma volume, earlier onset of sweating and increased sweating rate, reduction in electrolyte content of sweat/urine
      b. Initially decrease exercise duration and intensity in hot environment
      c. Gradually increase to normal duration/intensity over 10–14 days
   2. Adequate hydration (maintain ability to sweat)
      a. Drink 5–7 mL/kg of fluid 4 h prior to exercise
      b. If urine output is low or dark in color—drink additional 3–5 mL/kg 2 h prior to exercise
      c. During exercise—drink enough to prevent >2% weight loss during activity
      d. Fluid: 20–30 mEq/L sodium, 2–5 mEq/L potassium, 6–8% carbohydrate
      e. IV fluids: severe dehydration >7% body weight loss, cannot rehydrate orally
   3. Preexercise cooling: cold water or air; drink cold fluids
G. Quantification of environmental heat stress: Wet bulb globe temperature (WBGT)
   1. Takes into account humidity (T_w), solar radiation (T_g), and heat (T_d) using the following equation: WBGT $= 0.7T_w + 0.2T_g + 0.1T_d$
   2. Table 29.1 shows the ACSM recommendations for exercise in a heat-stressed environment utilizing the WBGT[11].

II. Cold Illness

A. Body temperature regulated by preoptic area of hypothalamus
   1. Body temperature <36 °C detected by hypothalamus → stimulate sympathetic nervous system → epinephrine and norepinephrine release, peripheral vasoconstriction, tachycardia, increased cardiac output, increased cellular metabolic rate → heat production
   2. Stimulation of primary motor center → shivering → increased metabolic rate
      a. Produces heat for ~4–6 h, then declines
B. Risk factors for hypothermia
   1. Environment: cold temperature, wind, moisture, clouds, high altitude; intoxication, substance abuse; lack of adequate clothing; lack of fitness; fatigue; dehydration; hypoxia; infection; diabetes; hypoglycemia; hypopituitarism; hypoadrenalism; hypothyroidism; peripheral vascular disease; psychiatric illness, mental impairment; trauma, cutaneous injury (burns, open wounds); central nervous system dysfunction; females > males; amenorrheic > eumenorrheic women
C. Hypothermia
   1. Core body temperature ≤35 °C (95 °F) (rectal thermometer)
   2. Mild hypothermia: core temperature 35°–32 °C
      a. Ataxia, dysarthria, apathy are often present
      b. Athlete will shiver and skin will be pale and cool
   3. Moderately severe hypothermia: core temperature 32–28 °C
      a. Core temperature <30 °C → body loses the ability to compensate
      b. Apathy, impaired judgment, ataxia, slowed reflexes, slurred speech, weakness, fatigue, hypotension, slowed respiratory rate
      c. Possible progressive decline in level of consciousness
      d. Shivering will decrease in intensity and eventually stop
      e. Bradycardia; arrhythmias (atrial fibrillation, ventricular arrhythmias); EKG changes (prolonged PR, QRS, QT intervals; J (Osborn) waves) (Figure 29.1)

TABLE 29.1 Modifications or cancellations of athletic events based on WBGT

WBGT (°F)	WBGT (°C)	Continuous activity and competition	Training and noncontinuous activity	
			Nonacclimatized	Acclimatized
≤50	≤10	Safe	Normal activity	Normal activity
50.1–65	10.1–18.3	Generally safe	Normal activity	Normal activity
65.1–72	18.4–22.2	Risk of EHS rises; monitor high-risk individuals closely	Increase rest:work ratio	Normal activity
72.1–78	22.3–25.6	Risk for all competitors increased	Increase rest:work ratio, decrease total duration	Normal. Monitor fluids
78.1–82	25.7–27.8	Risk for unfit, nonacclimatized individuals is high	Increase rest:work ratio, decrease duration and intensity	Normal. Monitor fluids
82.1–86	27.9–30	Cancel level for EHS risk	Increase rest:work ratio, decrease duration and intensity, watch at risk individuals closely	Plan intense or prolonged exercise with discretion. Watch at risk individuals closely
86.1–90	30.1–32.2		Cancel or stop practice or competition	Limit intense exercise and heat exposure. Monitor for signs and symptoms of heat illness
≥90.1	≥32.3		Cancel exercise	Cancel exercise

4. Severe hypothermia: core temperature <28 °C
   a. Athlete unresponsive with muscular rigidity, fixed and dilated pupils
   b. Ventricular fibrillation or asystole frequently occur
D. Assessment/treatment of cold-related injury
   1. Mild hypothermia treatment
      a. Body's compensatory warming capabilities remain functional
      b. Remove from the cold, change to dry clothes, and add layers
      c. Exercise to generate heat; drink warm fluids

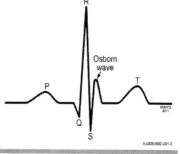

Figure 29.1 The Osborn wave is a positive deflection occurring at the S point (also known as the J point) located between the QRS complex and the ST segment.

    d. Apply external heat source (heat to torso, warmed air), but beware of:
        i. Impaired shivering, reduced peripheral vasoconstriction → heat loss
        ii. Afterdrop: when cold blood flows from the limbs back to the core → drop in core temperature
        iii. Rewarming shock: hypovolemic hypotension may result when dehydration combined with venous pooling

2. Treatment of more significant hypothermia
    a. Activate emergency personnel, early transport to medical facility
    b. Remove from cold environment, provide insulation
    c. Assess airway, breathing, circulation, rectal temperature
        i. If no carotid pulse or respirations for 1 min → CPR
    d. Beware of potential for inducing fatal cardiac arrhythmia
        i. Minimize movement, consider leaving clothing in place
        ii. If any pulse is present, CPR is not indicated
    e. Active external rewarming (avoid burns, watch for rewarming shock)
        i. Warm water immersion, hot packs, heat lamps
    f. Active internal rewarming (access to advanced life support available)
        i. Rewarming rate $\leq 2\,°C/h$
        ii. Warm fluids for IV or body cavity lavage (peritoneal, bladder)
        iii. Others: extracorporeal blood warming; hemodialysis; cardiopulmonary bypass; heated humidified oxygen

3. Treatment of ventricular fibrillation
    a. Core temperature $<30\,°C$: Defibrillatory shocks should be limited to three attempts; most antiarrhythmetic medicines (other than bretylium) not helpful
    b. Core temperature $\geq 30\,°C$: Administer defibrillations and cardiac medications as per advanced cardiac life support protocols

4. Prevention of cold illness
    a. Recognize risky environments (wet, windy, cold, exposed); stay dry
    b. Adequate nutrition and hydration status and wear appropriate clothing

E. Frostbite: freezing of tissues in temperature at or below freezing
  1. Grade 1: numb, red patch of skin with white or yellow firm plaques
  2. Grade 2: blisters with clear fluid and erythematous and edematous base
  3. Grade 3: large, deep blisters with purple fluid (penetrate dermal vascular plexus)
  4. Grade 4: freezing of underlying muscle and bone
  5. Treatment of frostbite
    a. Mild: remove from cold; rewarm with warm air or water; avoid burning; do not rub
    b. More severe: avoid rewarming until you can ensure no refreezing, then rapid rewarming (40 °C water) until thawing complete; débride clear blisters but not hemorrhagic blisters; *Aloe vera*; daily hydrotherapy debridement in 40 °C water
    c. Elevate the injured region; consider splinting
    d. Antiinflammatory medications; Narcotic medications; Tetanus

F. Chilblains (pernio or cold sores): due to cold-induced vasoconstriction
  1. Local erythema; cyanosis; nodules; plaques; occasional vesicles, bullae, ulceration
  2. Treatment: Rewarming, elevation, dry bandaging, anti-inflammatory medications

G. Trench (immersion) foot: due to prolonged vasoconstriction
  1. Due to prolonged exposure to sustained wet, nonfreezing conditions
  2. Painful paresthesias, erythema, and edema of the foot. Eventually the foot becomes numb, pale or mottled, and edematous with vesicles, ulcers, and gangrene
  3. Treatment: Anti-inflammatory medications, keep feet warm, dry, and elevated

    H. Other cold illnesses: Cold-induced urticaria, angioedema, anaphylaxis

        1. Treatment: Prevention—proper clothing; avoid exercise in the cold; prophylactic antihistamines, tricyclic antidepressants, or leukotriene modifiers.

        2. Epinephrine for anaphylaxis.

III. Altitude Illness

    A. Cold exposure (discussed in the last section)

    B. Hypoxia

        1. Lower partial pressure of oxygen (decreased barometric pressure)

        2. Carotid body detects decreased partial pressure of arterial oxygen

        3. Hypoxic ventilatory response

            a. Hyperventilation → increased PaO_2, decreased $PaCO_2$, respiratory alkalosis → compensatory renal bicarbonate excretion (within 24–48 h of altitude exposure)

        4. Other acclimatization changes: Increased alveolar ventilation, arterial oxygen extraction, hemoglobin, hematocrit, capillary density, mitochondrial numbers, myoglobin concentration, 2,3-diphosphoglycerate concentration, fatty acid mobilization, glucose utilization, glycogen sparing, and improved buffering

        5. Pulmonary vasoconstriction, pulmonary hypertension

            a. Due to hypoxemia and increased sympathetic activity

            b. Dysfunction of alveolar-capillary barrier → extravasation of intravascular volume into lung tissue → high-altitude pulmonary edema (HAPE)

        6. Cerebral blood flow changes

            a. Hypoxemia → failure of cerebral ion pumps, cerebral vasodilation

        7. Increased intravascular pressure → extravasation of fluid → high-altitude cerebral edema (HACE). Can cause cerebral herniation and death

    C. Other factors to consider at high altitudes

        1. Risk of dehydration increases at altitude → decreased ambient humidity

        2. High sunburn risk—UV radiation increases 4% per 300 m elevation gain

        3. Exercise performance (VO_{2max}) decreases by 1% per 100 m over 1500 m

        4. Higher perceived exertion due to increased ventilation rate and blood lactate

            a. Lactate paradox: peak blood lactate in acclimated athlete < nonacclimated

    D. Acute mountain sickness (AMS)—often occurs within 6–12 h

        1. Headache, insomnia, anorexia, nausea, vomiting, dizziness, fatigue

        2. Often nonaccclimatized individuals, altitude >2500 m, rapid altitude gain

        3. Due to cerebral vasodilation and mild cerebral edema

        4. Other risk factors: history of AMS; higher altitudes; higher sleeping altitudes; heavy exertion; age <50; sedative drug and/or alcohol consumption

        5. Prevention of AMS

            a. Slowly increase elevation to allow for acclimatization

            b. Acetazolamide (carbonic anhydrase inhibitor)

                i. Reduces formation of bicarbonate → reduced alkalosis

                ii. Side effects: paresthesias and diuresis

            c. Dexamethasone: effective but risk of rebound AMS if stopped at altitude

            d. NSAIDs and aspirin: prophylaxis for headaches associated with AMS

        6. Treatment of AMS

            a. Descent 500–1000 m can cause dramatic improvement

                i. Portable hyperbaric chamber if not able to descend

            b. Mild cases may resolve by stopping ascent, resting for few days

            c. Oxygen at 1–2 L/min can be helpful

            d. Acetazolamide 500 mg PO bid

            e. Dexamethasone 8 mg initially followed by 4 mg q 6 h

E. HACE
1. Signs/symptoms: Ataxia, drowsiness, decline in the level of consciousness, can progress to coma or death over hours to days
2. Treatment:
   a. Avoid Nifedipine (reduced cerebral perfusion pressure)
   b. Rapid descent (or hyperbaric chamber); oxygen (goal saturation $\geq 90\%$)
   c. Dexamethasone 8 mg PO × 1, then 4 mg PO q 6 h
F. HAPE
1. Signs/symptoms: fatigue, dyspnea, cough, chest tightness, cyanosis, tachycardia, tachypnea, and rales
2. Can rapidly progress to hypoxia-induced coma and death
   a. Most common cause of altitude-related death
3. Prevention: Acclimatization, avoidance of sedative drugs and alcohol, Salmeterol 125 µg inhaled bid can reduce the incidence of HAPE
4. Treatment
   a. Rapid descent (or hyperbaric chamber); oxygen (goal saturation $\geq 90\%$)
   b. Nifedipine 10 mg (decrease pulmonary vascular resistance)
   c. Acetazolamide 250 mg PO q 6 h or Dexamethasone 8 mg PO × 1 followed by 4 mg PO q 6 h.

IV. Diving Medicine

A. Decompression illness
1. Henry's Law of physics: Amount of gas dissolved in a liquid is directly proportional to the partial pressure of the gas
   a. Increased diving depth → increased pressure → more oxygen and nitrogen dissolved in the blood and extravascular fluids
   b. Return to surface → oxygen and nitrogen released from body fluids, can cause nitrogen bubbles in blood that may occlude blood flow to the limbs and viscera
2. Type I decompression illness: pruritus, arthralgias, urticarial rash
   a. Usually resolves within 30 min of dive completion
3. Type II decompression illness: weakness, sensory deficits, headache, postural instability, labyrinth, and vestibular dysfunction, "chokes" due to occlusion of pulmonary vasculature
   a. Usually occurs within 30 min; early recognition important
   b. Treatment: immediate oxygen; place in recompression chamber to dissolve nitrogen bubbles
4. Prevention
   a. Follow decompression table recommendations for ascent rate
   b. Lower depth dives—usually does not occur if dive <10 m
   c. No breath holding during ascent (continuously breath out)
   d. Do not ascend faster than smallest exhaled air bubbles toward the surface
B. Barotrauma
1. Boyle's Law of Physics: Gas volume inversely related to pressure
2. Ascent → reduced pressure → expansion of gas in gas-filled body spaces
3. Most common area for barotrauma is the middle ear
4. Pulmonary barotrauma → pneumothorax or air embolism
5. Treatment: hyperbaric oxygen
C. Nitrogen narcosis ("rapture of the deep")
1. Pleasant drowsy sensation from increased partial pressure of nitrogen in brain
2. Risk factors: alcohol, fatigue, increased CO_2 tension, cold water
3. Treatment: ascent to diving depth <100 feet

D. Contraindications to diving include: history of spontaneous pneumothorax, COPD, asthma (requiring medications), pulmonary blebs, pregnancy

E. Wait ≥ 12 h after a dive before flying on an airplane.

Recommended Reading

1. Armstrong L, Casa DJ, Millard-Stafford M, Moran DS, Pyne SW, Roberts WO. Exertional heat illness during training and competition. *Med Sci Sports Exerc.* 2007;*39*(3):556–572.
2. Castellani J, Young AJ, Ducharme MB, Giesbrecht GG, Sallis RE. American College of Sports Medicine positions stand: Prevention of cold injuries during exercise. *Med Sci Sports Exerc.* 2006;*38*(11):2012–2029.
3. DeFranco M, Baker CL, DaSilva JJ, Piasecki DP, Bach BR. Environmental issues for the team physician. *Am J Sports Med.* 2008;*36*(11):2226–2237.
4. Giesbrecht G. Emergency treatment of hypothermia. *Emerg Med.* 2001;*13*:9–16.
5. Levine B, Stray-Gundersen J. Exercise at high altitude. In: Mellion M, ed. *Sports Medicine Secrets.* 3rd ed. Philadelphia: Hanley & Belfus; 2003:120–125.
6. Madden C. Safe exercise in the cold and cold injuries. In: Mellions M, ed. *Sports Medicine Secrets.* 3rd ed. Philadelphia: Hanley and Belfus; 2003:108–119.
7. McArdle W, Magel JR, Spina RJ, Gergley TJ, Toner MM. Thermal adjustment to cold-water exposure in exercising men and women. *J Appl Physiol.* 1984;*56*:1572–1577.
8. Rodway G, Hoffman LA, Sanders MH. High-altitude-related disorders—Part I: Pathophysiology, differential diagnosis, and treatment. *Heart Lung.* 2003;*32*:353–359.
9. Sawka M, Burke LM, Eichner ER, Maughan RJ, Montain SJ, Stachenfeld NS. ACSM position stand: Exercise and fluid replacement. *Med Sci Sports Exerc.* 2007;*39*(2):377–390.
10. Seto C, Way D, O'Connor N. Environmental illness in athletes. *Clin Sports Med.* 2005;*24*:695–718.
11. Torres J. Scuba and diving medicine. In: Mellion MB, ed. *Sports Medicine Secrets.* 3rd ed. Philadelphia: Hanley and Belfus; 2003:126–129.
12. Trojian T. Environment. In: McKeag D, Moeller JL, eds. *ACSM's Primary Care Sports Medicine.* 2nd ed. Philadelphia: Lippincott, Williams, and Wilkins; 2007:279–291.
13. Yeo T. Heat stroke: A comprehensive review. *AACN Clin Issues.* 2004;*15*(2):280–293.

30

Exercise-Associated Collapse

Daniel V. Colonno and Mark A. Harrast

EXERCISE-ASSOCIATED COLLAPSE

I. Emergency Evaluation

    A. Athlete unable to stand or walk secondary to lightheadedness, faintness, dizziness, or syncope

        1. In running events, if the collapse occurs:

            a. BEFORE crossing the finish line—more likely an ominous source of collapse

            b. AFTER crossing the finish line—more likely a benign source of collapse

    B. Differential diagnosis of the medical causes of exercise-associated collapse (see the below table). (Special note: many of these topics are covered in more detail in separate chapters; they are reviewed here specifically as they relate to the emergency assessment and care of the collapsed athlete.)

Postural hypotension (benign exercise-associated collapse)
Cardiac insult and arrest
Heat-related illness and heatstroke
Hypothermia
Hypoglycemia
Hyponatremia
Anaphylaxis

    C. Further assessment is based on history and physical examination with particular attention to level of responsiveness and vital signs. Consider obtaining:

        1. Rectal temperature—imperative to check with other vitals signs, given heat stroke is a medical emergency

        2. Blood glucose—to rule out hypoglycemia

        3. Blood sodium—to rule out hyponatremia and choose appropriate intravenous fluids if needed

        4. Cardiac rhythm—if cardiac source is considered, particularly to determine if the potential arrhythmia is a "shockable" rhythm

        5. Orthostatics—when evaluating postural hypotension from venous pooling

II. Differential Diagnosis and Treatment

A. Benign exercise-associated collapse/postural hypotension
  1. Presentation
     a. Often in the setting of endurance activities/competition
     b. Generally occurs AFTER crossing the finish line of a running race/event
     c. Symptoms: Lightheadedness, dizziness, nausea, confusion, collapse
  2. Epidemiology
     a. Eighty-five percent of runners admitted to a medical tent after finishing a marathon were reported to have postural hypotension.
  3. Pathophysiology
     a. Postural hypotension from venous pooling
     b. While running, an athlete's contracting leg muscles act as a venous pump facilitating blood return to the central circulation. Upon cessation of exercise, this "pump" is no longer active which can lead to venous pooling, decreased venous return, decreased cerebral perfusion, and collapse.
     c. More common in warmer conditions: as ambient temperature increases, blood flow is shunted from the core to the skin (cutaneous vasodilation) and thus there is less blood volume in the central circulation increasing the chance of syncope from less cerebral perfusion
  4. Treatment
     a. Place athlete in supine position and elevate legs and pelvis relative to head
     b. Oral rehydration as tolerated
     c. Observe mental status and monitor HR and BP for 15–30 min
     d. If not clearing within this time interval, and other sources of EAC have been ruled out, may consider intravenous fluid (IVF) replacement (though this is rarely necessary)
        i. Blood sodium concentration needs to be confirmed before administering IVF in order to choose the proper fluids (see Hyponatremia, section F)
  5. Prevention
     a. Keep runners walking after crossing the finish line
B. Cardiac arrest (see Sports Cardiology Chapter 33 for more details)
  1. Patients are generally asymptomatic prior to the collapse
  2. Epidemiology and pathophysiology
     a. In the young population, structural abnormalities represent the leading cause of death
     b. Hypertrophic cardiomyopathy accounted for 26% of sudden cardiac arrests (SCA) in a cohort of 387 athletes. Commotio cordis and coronary artery anomalies accounted for 20% and 14%, respectively
     c. In athletes over the age of 35, coronary artery disease is by far the most common cause of SCA accounting for 75%
  3. Survival
     a. The probability of survival rapidly declines over time: 7–10% per minute for every minute defibrillation is delayed
        i. Factors leading to delay in defibrillation include mistaking agonal breathing or gasping for respirations, false identification of a pulse, myoclonic activity falsely identified as seizure
     b. Single greatest factor affecting outcome for out-of-hospital arrests is time interval from arrest to defibrillation
  4. Treatment
     a. Early recognition and early defibrillation (within 3–5 min) with CPR
     b. Automated external defibrillators (AED) need to be easily accessible at sporting event practices and competitions
     c. All potential first responders need to be skilled in CPR and AED use

C. Heat-Related Illness (see Environmental Illness, Chapter 29 for more details)
  1. Heat exhaustion
     a. Inability to continue to exercise in the heat
     b. Represents failure of the cardiovascular system to respond to exercising in the heat
     c. No known chronic or harmful effect
     d. Signs and symptoms
        i. Not hyperthermic (if the athlete is hyperthermic and symptomatic, the athlete has heatstroke, not "heat exhaustion")
        ii. Headache
        iii. Weakness
        iv. Dizziness
     e. Risk factors
        i. Exertion at or near maximum
        ii. Dehydration
        iii. Inadequate conditioning
        iv. Not acclimatized to heat
     f. Treatment
        i. Rest
        ii. Oral rehydration
  2. Exertional Heat Stroke (EHS)
     a. EHS occurs in the otherwise healthy population and is associated with exertion in varying environments as opposed to "classic" heat stroke which occurs in sick and compromised populations during heat waves
        i. Untreated EHS has greater morbidity and mortality than "classic" heat stroke
     b. Defined as multiorgan system failure (initially manifested by CNS dysfunction) secondary to hyperthermia from strenuous exercise and/or environmental heat exposure with a core temperature > 40 °C/104 °F
        i. Core (e.g., rectal) temperature assessment is a necessity
     c. Medical emergency
        i. Causes multiorgan system failure
        ii. Mortality rate and organ damage are proportional to the length of time between core temperature elevation and onset of cooling therapy
     d. Potential etiologies
        i. Not solely due to high ambient temperatures, as heat stroke can occur in cooler environments
        ii. Excessive endothermy (endogenous heat production)
        iii. Metabolic heat production from exercise exceeds heat loss (inadequate heat losing mechanisms)
        iv. Environmental and exercise heat stress lead to diversion of blood flow from viscera to skin and vital organs. Reduced blood flow to intestines can result in ischemia and endotoxemia which can then lead to a systemic inflammatory response syndrome (similar to sepsis) and multiorgan system failure
     e. Other contributing factors
        i. Medications (ACE inhibitors and diuretics), caffeine, ephedra, other sympathomimetics
        ii. Concomitant infection
           (A) Recent or concurrent illness increases risk of dehydration and increased thermal load. In one study, 13% of heat-related casualties had recent GI or respiratory illness
        iii. In a study of six fatal cases of exertional heat stroke, the following two factors were identified in all cases: physical effort unmatched to physical fitness and absence of proper medical triage. Other factors identified in at least 2/3 of the

cases included: low physical fitness, sleep deprivation, improper acclimatization, high solar radiation, improper work/rest cycles, training during the hottest hours.

   f. Physical exam differences between classic and exertional heat stroke

      i. Classic heat stroke: skin is hot and dry (due to impaired sweating or anhydrosis)

      ii. Exertional heat stroke: skin is moist with sweat

      iii. Both: altered sensorium (a spectrum from mildly depressed mental status to coma), tachycardia, rectal temperature is typically >40 °C

   g. Treatment

      i. Whole body cooling to decrease core temperature as quickly as possible. There are several possible methods. Chosen method should be simple and safe and should not prevent other necessary treatments (CPR, defibrillation, IV cannulation)

         (A) Ice or cold water immersion has cooling rate of 17 °F/h

         (B) Rotating ice water towels with ice packs to the neck, groin, and axilla has cooling rate of 15 °F/h

         (C) "Burritto" method: lay athlete on a wet/cool sheet, pour ice over the athlete, then wrap the athlete in the wet sheet and ice, frequently changing the sheet and adding ice

         (D) Stop active cooling at 102 °F to prevent rebound hypothermia

      ii. Monitor vital signs and frequent assessment of ABCs

D. Hypothermia (see Environmental Illness, Chapter 29 for more details)

   1. Core temperature less than 32 °C/90 °F

   2. Generally occurs in colder environments, but variable and dependent on clothing and equipment. Wet conditions are also a risk factor due to additional evaporative heat loss

   3. Presentation

      a. Mild (35–32 °C)

         i. Tachypnea, tachycardia, hyperventilation, mental status change, shivering, dysarthria, diuresis

      b. Moderate (32–28 °C)

         i. Reduced pulse, hypoventilation, central nervous system depression, shivering stops, arrhythmias, paradoxical undressing.

      c. Severe (<28 °C)

         i. Pulmonary edema, hypotension, bradycardia, coma, ventricular arrhythmias (including VF), asystole

   4. Assessment

      a. Obtain core temperature with low reading rectal thermometer

   5. Treatment

      a. Passive external rewarming with blankets and added insulation is appropriate for mild hypothermia. Active external warming may be appropriate for the athlete not responding to passive means or for those who are unstable

      b. Active external rewarming with heated blankets, forced heated air devices (Bair Huggers), heating pads and other sources of externally applied heat are appropriate for moderate-to-severe hypothermia (<32 °C). Patients with moderate hypothermia may require transfer to the Emergency Department (ED)

      c. Active internal rewarming with warmed oxygen, irrigation of body cavities with warmed fluid, or extracorporeal blood rewarming is appropriate for severe hypothermia (<28 °C). Patient with severe hypothermia will require transfer to the ED

      d. Caution: Physical agitation and rewarming of the severely hypothermic patient increases the risk of ventricular arrhythmia and thus should be performed in a setting with advanced cardiopulmonary monitoring and treatment

E. Hypoglycemia

   1. Usually diabetic (type 1 or 2 can be affected)

2. Exercise often a mainstay of treatment in diabetes, but can increase risk of hypoglycemia and serious hypoglycemic events
3. Signs and symptoms
   a. Adrenergic: caused by sympathomimetic mediators
      i. Hunger, palpitations, anxiety, sweating, tremor, tachycardia, feeling of impending doom
   b. Neuroglycopenic: inadequate glucose available to support brain activity
      i. Weakness, fatigue, slow or slurred speech, impaired performance, mental status change, vertigo, parasthesias, blurred vision, stupor. Severe hypoglycemia can lead to seizure and loss of consciousness
      ii. Nondiabetic athletes do not feel symptomatic until blood glucose drops to 50–55 mg/ dL, whereas diabetic patient typically feel symptomatic at 65–70 mg/dL
   c. In general, presentation is similar to that of postural hypotension and heat-related illness (see sections IIA and IIC)
4. Assessment/monitoring
   a. Capillary glucose monitor
      i. Athletes with diabetes should become familiar with their typical glucose levels during exercise
      ii. Should be checked in the setting of exercise-associated collapse, particularly in diabetic patients
   b. Continuous glucose monitor
      i. Limited availability, but may be highly beneficial in some diabetic athletes
5. Treatment
   a. Best strategy is prevention
   b. Mild hypoglycemia
      i. If suspected, remove athlete from play
      ii. Check capillary glucose
      iii. Administer 15–20 g of fast-acting carbohydrate (glucose tablets)
      iv. Recheck capillary glucose and repeat as necessary
   c. Severe hypoglycemia involving loss of consciousness or seizure is a medical emergency
      i. Glucagon injection if previously prescribed or otherwise available
      ii. Parenteral D50W, 1–3 ampules in field
      iii. Transfer to ED

F. Exercise-associated hyponatremia (EAH)
   1. Hypervolemic hyponatremia
   2. Epidemiology
      a. In a study of 488 runners after completion of a marathon, 13% had blood sodium concentration (Na) <135. 0.6% had Na <120
   3. Etiology
      a. Largely related to over-consumption (above the amount of fluid lost by sweating) of hypotonic fluids during prolonged exercise. More recent evidence suggests a correlation with the Syndrome of Inappropriate Antidiuretic Hormone (SIADH) which may exacerbate the hyponatremia in those who consume too much fluid
      b. Relationship to SIADH
         i. In the setting of hyponatremia or hypervolemia, ADH should be maximally suppressed
         ii. However, exercise is a known mild stimulus to ADH secretion and elevated ADH levels have been found in athletes with EAH
         iii. Thus ("inappropriately") circulating ADH will cause the kidneys to retain fluid and exacerbate the hypervolemia and subsequent hyponatremia
      c. Risk factors
         i. Weight gain during race (ingested too many fluids)

      ii. Race time greater than 4 h
      iii. Low body mass index
      iv. Possibly female gender
   4. Symptoms
     a. Early: lightheadedness, nauseated feeling
     b. Mid: headache, vomiting, confusion
     c. Late: obtundation, seizure, death
   5. Pathophysiology
     a. Fluid shifts occur due to low osmotic pressure in the blood leading to cerebral edema followed by neurogenic pulmonary edema
   6. Treatment
     a. If Na <135 and volume overloaded with minimal symptoms
       i. Allow natural diuresis
       ii. Close observation
       iii. Fluid restriction
       iv. If Na is very low and not reversing, may need hospital monitoring
     b. If Na <135, volume overloaded, and symptomatic with progressive encephalopathy
       i. 100 mL of 3% NaCl over 10 min × 2
       ii. High flow oxygen
       iii. Transfer to ED
     c. If Na <135 and dehydrated
       i. Rehydrate with IV normal saline
         (A) If encephalopathic, use 3% NaCl on site prior to transfer to ED
       ii. Check electrolytes after each liter administered
       iii. Consider transfer to ED
   7. Prevention
     a. Educate athletes about risk of over-drinking during endurance races. Prior to the race athletes should become familiar with their fluid needs for a given distance, level of exertion, and specific environmental conditions (i.e., understand individual fluid needs)
     b. Sodium or electrolyte replacement generally is not needed for most athletes during competition to prevent hyponatremia, but can be helpful to facilitate fluid absorption in the gut.
     c. On-course water stations should be placed no closer than every 1.5 miles
     d. General fluid replacement guidelines in a marathon
       i. Drinking according to thirst (ad libidum) is generally safe
       ii. 400–800 mL (14–27 ounces) per hour of racing depending on size and speed of the athlete (individualized according to the athlete and race conditions)
  G. Anaphylaxis (see Chapter 42, Sports Allergy and Immunology, for more details.)
   1. Bee stings
     a. Important to be aware of preexisting allergy
     b. Treatment is administration of epinephrine, antihistamines, and/or systemic corticosteroids. May require transfer to ED
   2. Exercise-induced anaphylaxis (EIA)
     a. Broad range of triggering activities including mild exertion
     b. EIA is not necessarily repeatable
       i. The same exercise does not always trigger anaphylaxis
       ii. Prophylaxis includes avoiding exercise in hot, cold, and humid weather, aspirin and NSAIDs during exercise, as well as exercising during pollen season
   3. Food-dependent, exercise-induced anaphylaxis (FDEIA)
     a. The combined ingestion of sensitizing food and exercise is necessary to induce symptoms.
     b. Prophylaxis includes the measure listed above as well as avoiding eating before and after exercise

    c. Treatment of EIA and FDEIA is immediate termination of activity, administration of epinephrine, antihistamines, and/or systemic corticosteroids. May require transfer to ED

H. Sickle cell trait (see Chapter 38, Sports Hematology, for more details)

    1. Sickling is induced by heat and hypoxia, thus sickling risk factors include:

        a. High environmental temperatures

        b. Exertional heat stroke

        c. Exercise at altitude

    2. Sickling causes vaso-occlusion and ischemia in working muscles which can lead to rhabdomyolysis, cardiogenic collapse, and ultimately sudden cardiac death

    3. Presents with muscle cramping, shortness of breath, mental status changes, collapse

    4. Early recognition and avoiding overexertion are key preventive strategies.

Recommended Reading

1. Armstrong LE, Casa DJ, Millard-Stafford M, Moran DS, Pyne SW, Roberts WO. American College of Sports Medicine position stand. Exertional heat illness during training and competition. *Med Sci Sports Exerc.* 2007;39(3):556–572.

2. Barg W, Medrala W, Wolanczyk-Medrala A. Exercise induced anaphylaxis: An update on diagnosis and treatment. *Curr Allergy Asthma Rep.* 2011;11:45–51.

3. Hew-Butler T, Ayus JC, Kipps C, Maughan RJ, Mettler S, Meeuwisse WH, Page AJ, Reid SA, Rehrer NJ, Roberts WO, Rogers IR, Rosner MH, Siegel AJ, Speedy DB, Stuempfle KJ, Verbalis JG, Weschler LB, Wharam P. Statement of the Second International Exercise-Associated Hyponatremia Consensus Development Conference, New Zealand, 2007. *Clin J Sports Med.* 2008;18:111–121.

4. Kirk SE. Hypoglycemia in athletes with diabetes. *Clin Sports Med.* 2009;28(3):455–468.

5. Moritz MM, Ayus JC. Exercise-associated hyponatremia: Why are athletes still dying? *Clin J Sports Med.* 2008;18(5):379–381.

6. Noakes TD. Reduced peripheral resistance and other factors in marathon collapse. *Sports Med.* 2007;37(4–5):382–385.

7. Noakes TD. A modern classification of exercise-related heat illnesses. *J Sci Med Sport.* 2008;11(1):33–39.

8. Roberts WO. Exercise-associated collapse care matrix in the marathon. *Sports Med.* 2007;37(4–5):431–433.

31

Head, Ears, Eyes, Nose, and Throat Injuries and Conditions

Michael P. Schaefer

I. Anatomy

A. Eye structures (Figure 31.1)
  1. Cornea/sclera
  2. Aqueous humor (anterior chamber)
  3. Iris
  4. Lens (and attached ciliary process, ligaments)
  5. Vitreous humor (posterior chamber)
  6. Retina
  7. Choroid
  8. Optic nerve (at optic disc)

B. Neck structures
  1. Thyroid/parathyroid
  2. Larynx
  3. Hyoid
  4. Thyroid and cricoid cartilage
  5. Trachea
  6. Larynx
  7. Esophagus
  8. Lymphatics
  9. Muscles: Sternoclycomastoid (SCM), scalenes, platysmus, cervical paraspinals
  10. Great vessels (note close proximity to clavicle)
  11. Brachial plexus
  12. Cervical spine and roots
  13. Recurrently laryngeal nerve

C. Facial structures
  1. Parotid gland
  2. Stensen's duct—leads from medial border of parotid to oral cavity

D. Facial nerve—Exits skull via stylomastoid foramen and travels between the superficial and deep lobes of the parotid gland. Provides motor innervation to muscles of facial expression
  1. Five major branches:
    a. Temporal
    b. Zygomatic
    c. Mandibular

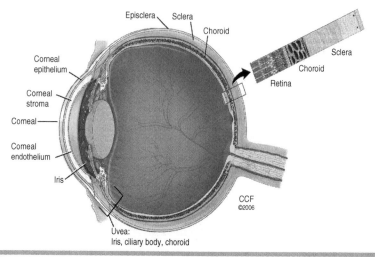

Figure 31.1 Eye anatomy. Sagittal section of the globe showing anterior and posterior chamber structures. Cut-out section depicts layers of the globe.

    d. Cervical

    e. Buccal

  2. Lacerations lateral to the lateral canthus should be explored with intention of finding and repairing any major facial nerve or branch injuries

  3. Lacerations of the medial (distal) ends of the nerve branches are expected to reinnervate spontaneously

E. Trigeminal nerve—Supplies majority of sensory innervation of the face. Divides into three major branches

  1. V1—Supratrochlear and supraorbital

  2. V2—Infraorbital

  3. V3—Buccal and mental

F. Vascular anatomy of face

  1. Supplied by both internal and external carotid systems.

  2. Multiple branches and presence of many collaterals make ischemia rare.

  3. Vessels follow nerves and ducts.

II. Epidemiology, Diagnosis, Treatment

A. Epidemiology

  1. Facial trauma represents 2–3% of all sports injuries.

  2. Sports injuries account for 12% of all maxillofacial traumas.

  3. Incidence has declined over past 20–30 years due to improved equipment; rules and technique but continue to be serious injuries

B. General principles

  1. Beware of associated major trauma—Head (brain), neck, and chest

  2. Airway must be protected, and may easily become compromised—have appropriate devices available—laryngoscope, ET tube, mask

  3. Infection should be prevented—use copious dilution, explore wound, consider antibiotics, administer tetanus toxoid if needed

C. Soft-tissue injury—most common injury type
   1. Contusions—usually minor, treated with ice
   2. Abrasions—often have impregnated particles that need to be debrided or risk tattooing. Treat with antibiotic ointment and daily cleansing
   3. Simple lacerations
      a. Shallow without injury to deep structures
      b. Skin margin should be debrided to smooth edge and beveled
      c. Sutures placed subdermally (absorbable)
   4. Complex lacerations
      a. Involve deeper structures with crush injury and structural deformity
      b. Need thorough irrigation
      c. Layered repair with careful approximation, may need realignment periodically
      d. Plastic surgery referral needed for very complex injuries, those involving major facial landmarks, or those with tissue loss

D. Skeletal injury
   1. Skull fractures
      a. Indicate severe trauma, especially if open.
      b. May lacerate meningeal arteries (especially middle) and cause epidural hematoma.
      c. Often (but not necessarily) involve loss of consciousness, penetrating injury, and post-traumatic neurological symptoms
      d. Basal skull fracture may present with ecchymosis behind the ear (Battle's sign) or under the orbits (Raccoon eyes), hemotympanum, or cerebrospinal fluid (CSF) leak.
      e. Classification
         i. Linear-hairline—most common, loss of skull curve
         ii. Comminuted—usually due to focal impact with bone fragmentation
         iii. Depressed—indents, may displace or entrap meninges
      f. Treatment
         i. Requires neurosurgical consultation
   2. Zygomatic fractures
      a. May include temporal bone (zygomatic arch), maxillary buttress, and infraorbital rim.
      b. Underlying temporalis muscle may be involved
      c. Treatment is elevation without instrumentation
   3. "Tripod" fracture (Zygomaticomaxillary complex)
      a. Always includes posterior orbital wall and maxillary sinus
      b. Treatment is nonoperative for nondisplaced fractures, but often requires internal fixation due to displacement
   4. Frontal sinus fracture
      a. Most only involve the frontal wall
      b. If posterior wall involved, may have CSF rhinorrhea and pneumocephaly due to direct association of posterior wall with dura mater
      c. Anterior wall fracture indicated by frontal depression
      d. Supraorbital nerve involvement causes numbness
      e. Sinus drains into nasal cavity causing increased rhonorrhea
      f. Treatment requires exploration and repair of dura mater if CSF leak, and often requires internal fixation
   5. Nasal fractures
      a. Bony or cartilaginous
      b. Signs of fracture include crepitance, airway obstruction, deformity
      c. Septal injury—causes deformity and airway obstruction
      d. Early evaluation may show deformity, which is obscured by edema
      e. Nondisplaced fracture treated conservatively

    f. Displaced fracture should be relocated immediately (within hours) or after swelling resolves (within 4 days for children and 12 days for adults)

    g. Protective splinting is usually difficult to keep in place due to perspiration. However, participation in a collision or contact sport requires facial protection. Therefore, a full-face shield may be fabricated at a substantial cost. For simple nondisplaced fractures, it is acceptable to treat with a simple splint or without a splint in limited-contact sports.

  6. Orbital blow-out fracture

    a. May include frontal, zygomatic, nasal, and maxillary bones

    b. Medial and lateral canthal ligaments suspend the globe

    c. Ocular muscles and their pulleys attach to the orbit

    d. Usually involve fracture of inferior orbital floor

    e. May entrap ocular muscles, infraorbital nerve

    f. Medial fractures may involve nasolacrimal duct with excess tearing

    g. Findings include diplopia gaze palsy, subconjunctival hemorrhage, enopthalmos

    h. Operative treatment is required for structure entrapment, but this may be easily confused with mass effect from swelling

  7. Le Fort-type facial fractures

    a. Common patterns of facial fractures, usually with high-velocity injuries.

    b. Almost all are treated with internal fixation

      i. Le Fort I—transverse through maxilla

      ii. Le Fort II—midface, through nose, orbital floor/inferior rim

      iii. Le Fort III—craniofacial disjunction, through suture line between zygoma and frontal bones, inferior orbits, and nasofrontal junction

  8. Mandible fractures and dislocations

    a. Subcondylar, body or angle fractures

      i. Presents with dental mal-occlusion

      ii. Trigeminal (V3) numbness may result

      iii. Mucosal laceration may be present—requires antibiotics

      iv. Treatment is conservative unless mal-aligned

    b. Dislocation (without fracture)

      i. Should be promptly reduced with downward and backward force

      ii. Pre- and postreduction x-rays are recommended

      iii. After reduction, relative jaw rest with soft diet and avoidance of extreme jaw opening is recommended for 1–2 weeks

      iv. Surgical referral is necessary for recurrent dislocations

  9. Return to play after fractures of skull and face

    a. Highly individualized

    b. Neurological clearance must accompany bony healing

    c. Typically takes 3–6 months after ORIF

    d. Consider permanent use of facial shield and helmets (even in practices)

E. Ear injury

  1. Auricular hematoma

    a. Usually from contusive injury.

    b. Blood accumulates in the subperichondrial layer

    c. Will from organized fibrosis ("cauliflower ear") if not treated appropriately

    d. Immediate drainage with 18-guage needle or late incision and drainage, reaspiration may be needed

    e. Compressive dressing immediately applied

    f. Collodion pack, silicone mold—sutured in place

    g. Monitor frequently for infection

  2. Tympanic membrane rupture

    a. Blow to ear or violent fall followed by "pop"

    b. May include severe pain or dizziness due to vestibular stimulation

    c. Usually managed conservatively

    d. Ossicle dislocation may require surgical intervention

    e. Prophylactic antibiotics are controversial

    f. Athlete should be withheld from sports that may cause barotrauma until healed, but may play other sports when vestibular symptoms resolve

    g. Water sports may be played with custom plugs

F. Nose injury

  1. Epistaxis

    a. Most from Kisselbach's plexus on anterior septum

    b. More serious if from ethmoidal artery (away from septum) and can be an emergency

    c. Athlete should lean forward to clear one nostril at a time with gentle blowing, and apply a light pinch

    d. Beware occult posterior blood flow into pharynx

    e. May require packing with nasal tampon, which may be soaked with neosynephrine

    f. Commercial products available for medical kits, but feminine hygiene products may be used in emergencies

    g. May return to play when bleeding stops

    h. If no resolution, referral for A-P packing or electrocautery is required.

    i. Secondary prevention may include petroleum jelly application, discontinuation of decongestants and avoidance of dry air (and cocaine)

  2. Septal hematoma (Figure 31.2)

    a. Blue-colored bulge on one or both sides of nasal septum

    b. Should be drained and packed to avoid ischemic cartilage loss

  3. Nasal fracture (see section II, D, 5 above)

    a. Check for deformity before swelling develops

    b. Closed reduction should occur either immediately or after initial swelling subsides (within 4 days for children and 12 days for adults)

    c. X-rays are usually negative but may show other facial fractures, although CT is gaining favor

    d. Deformity may cause septal deviation and Eustachian tube malfunction

    e. Return to play after 1–2 weeks, but usually hard to keep nasal splint in place with sweating. Require custom or off the shelf polycarbonate face shield to protect the fracture if returning to high-risk sports (e.g., basketball)

G. Eye injury

  1. Foreign body

    a. May be hard to visualize without special equipment such as a slit lamp

    b. Remove from play/out of wind

    c. Use anesthetic solution and moistened sterile swab to remove any foreign body

    d. Invert lid if necessary

    e. Evaluate for corneal abrasion when clinically indicated

  2. Conjunctivitis

    a. Allergic—Try to identify allergen such as new pet exposure, topical agents, soaps, and so on. Treatment includes

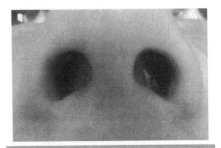

Figure 31.2 Septal hematoma. Traumatic septal hematoma in a young child, requires prompt evacuation.

isolation from triggering causes and corticosteroid drops if severe

b. Posttraumatic/abrasive— Have history of trauma. Treatment is comfort measures only, including patch and antibiotic ointment if severe (see #3 below)

c. Viral or bacterial—may become purulent or crusted in later stages, Treatment includes patch and antibiotic ointment, and frequent reevaluation. Avoid steroid solutions when chance of infection exists. Wash hands frequently. Avoid contact with others to avoid spreading infection

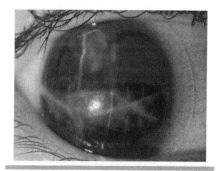

Figure 31.3 Corneal abrasion. Large lesion best seen under fluorescein stain

3. Corneal abrasion (Figure 31.3)
   a. Very common
   b. May produce foreign body sensation, photophobia, and lacrimation
   c. Anesthetic solution (proparacaine) allows exam
   d. Remove foreign bodies, invert lid, and examine conjunctiva
   e. Fluorescein stain on cornea will reveal abrasion/laceration
   f. Treat with antibiotic and mydriatic drops
   g. Eye patch is for comfort only
   h. Monitor in 24–48 h for improvement and refer to ophthalmologist if not improving quickly

4. Orbital blunt trauma
   a. May produce pain, swelling, surrounding edema, and ecchymosis
   b. Usually treated conservatively but rule out other conditions (see below).

5. Subconjunctival hemorrhage (Figure 31.4)
   a. Usually from blunt trauma, sometimes spontaneous.
   b. Rule out other lesion
   c. Check coagulation status
   d. Treat with observation, resolves in 2–3 weeks

6. Peri-orbital hematoma
   a. Blood collection around or behind the globe
   b. Usually self-limited
   c. If large enough may displace globe, increase intraocular pressure, expose cornea, and therefore may require referral

7. Hyphema (Figure 31.5)
   a. Hemorrhage into the anterior chamber of the eye, appears as a red layer of blood in the anterior chamber, of varying size

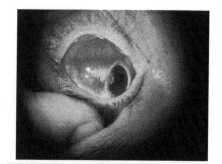

Figure 31.4 Subjunctival hemorrhage. Uncomplicated injury typically resolves with observation only.

b. Pain, swelling, pupillary constriction or dilatation
c. Usually results from blunt trauma to the eye with microvascular injury to the ciliary mechanism
d. May be associated with severe eye trauma
e. Requires prompt evaluation by ophthalmologist
f. Initial treatment is rigid, nonocclusive shield, bed rest, and discontinuation of aspirin (ASA), nonsteroidal antiinflammatory drugs (NSAIDs), or other anticoagulants

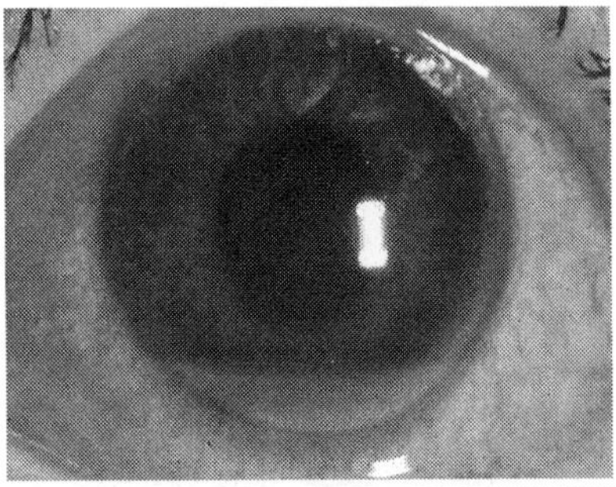

Figure 31.5 Hyphema. Hemorrhage into the anterior chamber. Requires prompt evaluation by an ophthalmologist.

g. Complications include glaucoma and particulate accumulation in the anterior chamber
h. May re-bleed. Requires close follow-up
8. Vitreous hemorrhage
   a. Due to trauma, aneurysm rupture, retinal tear, retinal detachment, neovascularization, or underlying disease (e.g., sickle cell anemia, diabetes, carotid artery disease)
   b. Usually presents with "floaters" and cloudy vision, but may present with severe vision loss
   c. May be sign of major orbital trauma
   d. Cold compresses help with pain
   e. Stop anticoagulants
   f. Withhold from play and refer to ophthalmologist
9. Retinal detachment
   a. Presents with visual aberrations: floating objects, flashing lights, or (most commonly) a "curtain" effect moving through the field of view
   b. May occur slowly after trauma with retinal tearing
   c. Genetic predisposition (i.e., check family history)
   d. Large lesions require prompt re-attachment or may result in blindness.
10. Scleral laceration
    a. May be due to blunt or penetrating trauma
    b. Need to rule out foreign body or ruptured globe
    c. Requires referral to ophthalmologist
11. Ruptured globe
    a. Seen after high-impact trauma, and often associated with extensive swelling, leaking of vitreous fluid, pupillary deformity, and circumferential subconjunctival hemorrhage
    b. Ophthalmologic emergency
    c. Use eye shield (instead of patch) to avoid placing excess pressure on the globe
12. Lid lacerations
    a. Consider repair if they are superficial (partial thickness) do not extend to the lid margin, and do not involve the inner (medial) one-third of the lid
    b. Otherwise should be referred to ophthalmologist
H. Dental injury
   1. Tooth fractures
      a. Often associated with lip laceration

    b. Deciduous tooth fractures or dislodgements may be ignored but should still be examined for root injury or socket widening

    c. Nondeciduous tooth fractures should be referred to a dentist or oral surgeon within 24 h (see #2 for dislodged tooth)

    d. If exposed pulp is bleeding usually required temporary filling/capping with $CaOH_2$ and dental referral

    e. Impacted teeth should be left in place and referred to a dentist or oral surgeon within 24 h

2. Dislodged teeth

    a. Have 35–40% save rate

    b. Should be promptly placed in warm saline or "tooth saver" compound

    c. Handle only by crown to protect the root

    d. May be packed back in socket but risk contamination, aspiration, or swallowing

    e. X-rays should be done to rule out mandibular or alveolar fracture

3. Lip lacerations

    a. Should be referred for repair if they are full thickness, irregular, or if they involve the vermilion border or corner of the mouth

    b. May require antibiotics if deep (full thickness) and/or associated with contamination (soil, foreign bodies, other player's saliva).

Acknowledgments

Dr. Tomas Steinemann, MetroHealth Medical Center Division of Ophthalmology, Associate Professor of Ophthalmology, Case Western Reserve University, and Dr. Joe Hollyfield, Cole Eye Institute, Cleveland Clinic Foundation are acknowledged for providing original images.

Recommended Reading

1. Bord SP. Trauma to the globe and orbit. *Emerg Med Clin North Am.* 2008;26(1):97–123.

2. Grindel SH. Ch 24—Head and neck. In: McKeag DB, Moeller JL, eds. *ACSM's Primary Care Sports Medicine.* 2nd ed. Philadelphia: Wolters Kluwer/Lippincott Williams & Wilkins; 2007.

3. Hatef DA. Contemporary management of pediatric facial trauma. *Curr Opin Otolaryngol Head Neck Surg.* 2009;17(4):308–314.

4. Hollier LH Jr. Facial trauma: General principles of management. *J Craniofac Surg.* 2010;21(4):1051–1053.

5. Kaufman BR, Heckler FR. Sports-related facial injuries. *Clin Sports Med.* 1997;16(3):543–562.

6. MacEwen CJ. Eye injuries in sport. *Scott Med J.* 2010;55(2):22–24.

7. Rozsasi A. Persistent inner ear injury after diving. *Otol Neurotol.* 2003;24(2):195–200.

8. Ziccardi VB. Management of nasal fractures. *Oral Maxillofac Surg Clin North Am.* 2009;21(2):203–208.

32

Chest Trauma: Thoracic Injuries and Conditions

Constance Marie Lebrun

ANATOMY

I. General considerations

A. Skin and soft tissues
1. Breast tissue—modified sudoriferous (sweat) glands
   a. Nipple surrounded by areola (containing sebaceous glands)
   b. Larger mammary glands (milk-producing); drained to the nipples by lactiferous ducts
   c. Remainder of breast tissue: connective tissue (collagen and elastic), adipose tissue (fat), and Cooper's ligaments (suspensory)
   d. Underlying pectoralis major muscle—from 2nd to 6th rib
   e. Arterial blood supply: internal thoracic artery, lateral thoracic artery, thoraco-acronial artery, and posterior intercostal arteries; venous drainage—mainly to axillary vein; lymphatic system

B. Chest wall—musculoskeletal structures
1. Twelve ribs—seven (true) ribs articulate anteriorly with sternum via the costochondral cartilage; eighth to tenth (false) ribs articulate with adjacent ribs via the costochondral cartilage; eleventh and twelfth (floating) ribs—no articulations anteriorly
2. Posteriorly—ribs 2–10 articulate with vertebral bodies and transverse processes of two adjacent vertebrae via costovertebral and costotransverse joints; remaining ribs articulate with only one vertebra
3. Anteriorly—sternum, manubrium, and xiphisternum—attached to body of sternum by fibrocartilage; sternum articulates proximally with clavicles via synovial joints (sterno-clavicular joints)
4. Each clavicle articulates distally with acromion process of scapula (acromioclavicular joint)
5. Thoracic musculature: internal and external intercostal muscles, overlying serratus anterior, latissimus dorsi, trapezius muscles
6. Neurovascular bundle lies inferior to each rib—intercostal arteries and veins, intercostal nerves supply thoracic wall
7. Referred pain to the chest can come from cervical or visceral structures; posterior vertebrae can refer pain to anterior chest wall

C. Thoracic spine:
1. Vertebrae, discs, ligaments
2. Zygoapophyseal or "Z" joints (facet joints), costovertebral junctions

D. Lung structures:
1. Pleura—parietal (attached to chest wall) and visceral (covering lungs), pleural cavity in between; chest wall surrounding, diaphragm below
2. Trachea, bronchi, bronchioles, alveoli; bronchovascular system
3. Lung parenchyma—alveolar tissue

E. Mediastinum:
1. Bordered by sternum anteriorly, vertebral column posteriorly, thoracic inlet superiorly, and diaphragm inferiorly
2. Cardiovascular structures:
   a. Myocardium
   b. Heart chambers and valves
   c. Ascending aorta, aortic arch, descending thoracic aorta
   d. Right innominate (brachiocephalic) artery and veins, left common carotid and left subclavian arteries (come directly off aortic arch) and veins; pulmonary arteries and veins
   e. Vena cava (superior and inferior), azygos vein
3. Gastrointestinal structures:
   a. Esophagus
   b. Gastroesophageal junction
   c. Stomach and duodenum
4. Other structures:
   a. Pancreas
   b. Liver and gall bladder
   c. Kidneys (retro-peritoneal).

EPIDEMIOLOGY, DIAGNOSIS, TREATMENT

I. General considerations

A. Epidemiology of chest/thoracic pain
1. Can occur due to:
   a. Trauma (usually acute onset)
   b. Overuse (more chronic insidious onset)
   c. Can be "acute on chronic" injury—that is, underlying stress fracture with sudden excess load or trauma causing fracture
2. "Atypical" chest pain can be due to:
   a. Musculoskeletal causes: bone/cartilage, joints, myofascial
   b. Gastrointestinal disorders: gastrointestinal esophageal reflux disease (GERD), esophagitis or rupture, Boerhaave's syndrome (esophageal rupture from vomiting), esophageal motility disorders, hiatal hernia, peptic ulcer, biliary colic/cholecystitis, pancreatitis
   c. Respiratory conditions: lower respiratory tract infection, asthma, exercise-induced bronchospasm (EIB), spontaneous or traumatic pneumothorax, hemothorax, pneumohemothorax, pulmonary embolus (single or multiple), pulmonary contusion
   d. Cardiac conditions: myocardial infarction, myocardial contusion, myocarditis, pericarditis, pericardial effusion, cardiac tamponade, pneumopericardium, aortic aneurysm/dissection
   e. Miscellaneous: malignancy, herpes zoster, spontaneous pneumomediastinum, Mondor's disease (idiopathic thrombosis of subcutaneous veins of anterior chest wall)
3. History
   a. Penetrating trauma
   b. Blunt trauma
   c. Barotrauma (i.e., scuba diving) or "blast" trauma
   d. Insidious onset—overuse mechanism

4. Physical examination
   a. Neuromuscular assessment may reveal level of pathology
   b. "Observe"—ecchymosis, active bleeding, "splinting," signs of respiratory distress (use of accessory muscles), cyanosis (lips and nail beds), bulging neck veins, plethoric facies
   c. "Palpate"—areas of tenderness, rib "springing," paradoxical motion of "flail chest" segment, carotid and peripheral pulses, tracheal deviation, subcutaneous emphysema
   d. "Listen"—hoarseness, dysphonia, quality of breath sounds (or lack of), wheezing/ stridor, cardiac sounds/rhythm, blood pressure.

II. Fractures

A. General considerations
   1. Usually due to blunt trauma, history of injury mechanism is important
B. Rib fractures
   1. Rib cage is a circle—trauma to one area may cause rib fracture in another, check for pain with "rib-springing"—compression of the rib cage between the examiner's two hands in an antero-posterior or side-to-side direction will cause discomfort at the site of the rib fracture
   2. Solitary or multiple—multiple rib fractures in two places can give "flail" chest—unstable segment—"paradoxical" motion with breathing
   3. Fractures to the first rib require a great amount of force—high risk of injuries to nearby structures—brachial plexus, Horner's syndrome, subclavian artery or vein; later—thoracic outlet syndrome due to callus
   4. Can also fracture through synchondrosis of first rib—due to compressive force applied to posterolateral aspect of upper thorax or shoulder girdle, same mechanism as posterior sternoclavicular dislocation
   5. Rib fractures can have many associated injuries—pulmonary contusion, pulmonary laceration, hemothorax, pneumothorax, hemopneumothorax, pneumomediastinum, subcutaneous emphysema
   6. Diagnosis—usually plain radiographs will suffice—chest x-ray—AP and lateral (possibly in inspiration and expiration if pneumothorax is suspected); dedicated rib views, CT scan for suspected 1st rib fracture
   7. Management
      a. Usually conservative, including analgesics
         i. Intercostal nerve blocks for severe pain
      b. Avoid "rib strapping"—may cause atelectasis of underlying lung due to inadequate inspiratory efforts
      c. Exception is "flail chest"—need to stabilize unstable segment; hospitalization
      d. Normally heal within 6–8 weeks, follow with serial radiographs; return to activity as tolerated
C. Sternum
   1. Blunt trauma, large amount of force needed
   2. Danger of trauma to underlying cardiac structures and lungs
   3. Manubrium, body of sternum, xiphi-sternum, or xyphoid process
   4. Can fracture through bony sections or through fibrocartilageous areas
   5. Treatment is conservative, pain management
D. Thoracic vertebrae
   1. Vertebral body fractures
      a. Burst-type fracture
         i. Stable (posterior elements intact) or unstable—with retropulsion of fragments of posterior elements into spinal canal, damaging or compressing spinal cord—can cause neurological sequelae in ~50% of patients

      b. Compression fracture

         i. Combined axial flexion and compression resulting in anterior wedge fracture of the vertebral body

         ii. Most often at thoracolumbar junction, followed by transverse/spinous process fractures from direct trauma

         iii. Among the most common back injuries in snow sports

         iv. Also more common in athletes with long-term corticosteroid use; postmenopausal women or athletes with osteopenia or osteoporosis (Female Athlete Triad)

      c. Imaging—plain radiographs, may need SPECT bone scan if negative x-ray and clinical suspicion, or CT scan for anatomy

      d. Fractures of T11 and T12 can easily be missed on x-ray, because of overlying shadow of the diaphragm

  2. Treatment

      a. Stable—rest, pain control, thoraco-lumbar-sacral orthosis (TLSO) at least 3 months with close observation

      b. Unstable—surgery warranted to restore structural integrity with possible decompression of foraminal or central canals; surgery may be needed with >40% loss of anterior body height or >25 degrees kyphotic deformity, suggestive of posterior element injury

  3. Spinous process fracture

      a. Direct trauma to posterior spine, forced flexion with rotation

  4. Transverse processes and floating ribs (11 and 12)

      a. Can also occur from violent contraction of psoas major

      b. Need to rule out concurrent retro-peritoneal bleed or injury to intra-abdominal and retro-peritoneal contents: liver, spleen, pancreas, stomach, duodenum, kidney (renal contusion, hematuria)

  5. Diagnosis

      a. Severe back pain after direct trauma or forced hip extension

      b. Palpable deformities, point tenderness, spasm of paraspinal muscles, and signs of contusion or ecchymosis

  6. Imaging

      a. AP/lateral radiographs; flexion–extension films for stability

      b. CT scan for concurrent fractures, soft tissue injury, retro-peritoneal or intra-abdominal bleeding

  7. Treatment

      a. Symptomatic management with analgesics, antispasmodics

      b. Maintain/restore core control and proper alignment

  8. Costovertebral subluxation—seen in rowers, swimmers

      a. Localized tenderness, pain increased with side flexion of thoracic spine, rotation away from or into painful side

      b. Treatment is by manipulation, prevention by therapeutic exercises and ballistic rotational stretches away from painful side

  9. "Slipping rib" syndrome—abdominal and/or thoracic pain—due to hypermobility of anterior ends of false rib costal cartilages—leads to slipping of affected rib under superior adjacent rib (usually ribs 8–10)

      a. Diagnose with "hooking manuever"—clinician slips fingers under lower costal margin and pulls anteriorly; pain and clicking

      b. Treatment primarily conservative (avoidance of postures that cause symptoms); may require nerve block, surgical resection.

III. Stress fractures

  A. General considerations

    1. Overload mechanism—need to understand specific stresses of sport; usually occur with increases in training, change in equipment or technique

B. Sternum—uncommon
   1. One case reported in manubrium due to repetitive strenuous abdominal exercises—combination of forward flexion of thoracic spine, and muscle pull from sternal heads of sternocleidomastoid and pectoralis muscles
C. Ribs
   1. First rib
      a. Common in golfers, overhead athletes (i.e., volleyball)
      b. Also reported in male ballet dancers—combination of weight-training (deadlifting, military press), partner lifting, rapid pirouettes, and turning of head while "spotting"
      c. Most commonly found at subclavian sulcus—anatomically the thinnest portion, between insertions of scalenus anterior and medius and serratus anterior muscles—"fatigue failure"
      d. Diagnose with "trapezius squeeze" test—focal tenderness
      e. Can develop painful hypertrophic pseudoarthrosis
   2. Other rib stress fractures
      a. Can be seen in golfers (posterolateral ribs 4–6)
         i. Due to repeatedly striking ground (novice players)
      b. Most common in rowers (6–12%), other paddlers (kayak, canoe, Dragon boat, outrigger canoe):
         i. 5th–9th ribs posterolaterally—most common location; but also seen in anterior axillary line
         ii. Site of rib cage compression (bending) with isometric cocontraction of serratus anterior muscles and trapezius during the "drive" phase, and/or opposite pull of external abdominal oblique muscle—various theories
      c. Training on ergometers (winter, bad weather) ~1/3 of time
      d. Increased incidence since introduction of larger blades in 1992
      e. Long (>10 K) slow (stroke rate ~16–18/min) steady-state rows early in season (more load on ribs with lower stroke rates)
      f. Sudden change in training or competition—increased training load, bad weather (wind and waves), "Big Blades"
      g. No specific side or location, seen in both sweep rowers and scullers, low bone mineral density may be additional risk factor
   3. Diagnosis
      a. High index of suspicion in appropriate sport setting
      b. Insidious onset, localized tenderness, pain with "rib springing," deep inspiration, cough, even rolling over in bed
      c. X-rays negative early on, show callus with healing (see Figure 32.1)
      d. Technicium[99] bone scan is diagnostic (see Figure 32.2)
   4. Treatment
      a. Rest from aggravating activities—may take 4–6 weeks

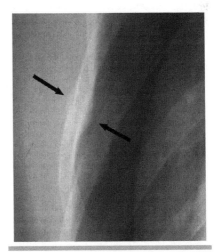

Figure 32.1 Healing rib fracture with callus formation

b. Pain management—analgesics, NSAIDs

c. Physiotherapy—correction of underlying biomechanics

d. Appropriate strength training; preventive exercises—scapular stabilizing and protraction strengthening for serratus anterior

e. Alternate cardiovascular activities to maintain fitness

f. May require correction of technique, equipment (blade size, weight, rigging of boat), training load (role of coach)

g. Prevention: for long "pieces" on ergometer, at low stroke rate—damper should not be set higher than 3; for long steady-state rows (especially against a current or into a headwind)—use "clams" on blades to "lighten" the load (by decreasing "outboard" of blade). Entire ergometer can be placed on "slides"—allows movement of ergometer relative to the rower—thereby decreasing the load.

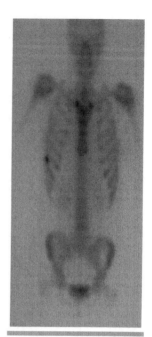

Figure 32.2 Bone scan showing a stress fracture of the 7th right lateral rib in a rower.

IV. Fractures/dislocations

A. Sternoclavicular joint

1. General considerations

a. Synovial joint, epiphysis does not fuse until age 22–25

b. Posterior dislocations are rare (less than 1% of all joint dislocations and 3% of all shoulder girdle injuries) but are a *medical emergency* due to the presence of the great vessels and the airway immediately posterior to the joint

c. Anterior/superior dislocations can also occur and are treated conservatively

d. Sternoclavicular subluxation common in overhead sports and swimming—may be unilateral or bilateral

2. Diagnosis

a. History consistent with injury

b. Physical examination—localized swelling/tenderness over sternoclavicular joint; may have deformity, arm paresthesias, respiratory distress

c. X-rays—oblique views may be helpful, Rockwood's "serendipity" view, chest x-ray to rule out other conditions; gold standard is spiral CT; angiography if suspect vascular injury to underlying subclavian artery/vein

3. Treatment

a. Posterior dislocations—reduction—immediate if possible—supine position, sandbag between shoulder blades, traction on arm; otherwise in OR (closed or open), may require operative fixation

b. Anterior/superior dislocations—reduction is less urgent

c. Sternoclavicular subluxation—can be chronic—can alter technique or stroke or side, surgical repair not commonly done.

V. Penetrating trauma

A. General considerations

1. Indoor sports—that is, fencing foil or fixed stationary object

2. Outdoor sports—field events (javelin); archery (arrow)

B. Diagnosis

1. Can be obvious (protruding object); less obvious—puncture wound
2. Associated injuries may be presenting feature—laceration to blood vessels, lung, cardiac structures; pneumothorax, hemothorax
3. X-ray will show metal objects, including ones that have broken off

C. Management

1. Leave object in place until in hospital ER for more definitive care
2. May require surgical exploration, treatment of associated injuries.

VI. Pneumothorax and pneumomediastinum (spontaneous and traumatic)

A. General considerations

1. Can be due to congenital blebs; phenotype is tall, thin person
2. Traumatic—usually due to penetrating or direct blunt trauma, blast injuries—perforation of pharynx or esophagus or lung parenchyma
3. Underlying asthma is a risk factor; also Marfan's syndrome
4. Occurs after episodes of increased intrathoracic pressure—coughing, straining, vomiting, Valsalva manuever (weight lifting), breath-holding
5. Spontaneous pneumomediastinum or mediastinal emphysema (free air in mediastinal structures)—can occur by same mechanisms)
   a. Cases have been reported after intense physical activity (sprints), high-altitude or underwater activity (scuba-diving, synchronized swimming), contact sports (football, rugby)
   b. Recreational inhalational drug use (cocaine, methamphetamine, ecstasy, marijuana) also a risk factor
   c. Concurrent pneumothorax in 6–32% of cases

B. Diagnosis

1. Symptoms: dyspnea or shortness of breath (SOB), sore throat, dysphagia, nonspecific pleuritic chest pain, cough, hemoptysis
2. Physical examination: pneumothorax—increased respiratory rate, tachycardia, hypotension; diminished breath sounds, amphoric breathing
3. Tension pneumothorax—rapidly expanding pneumothorax with laryngeal shift, tracheal deviation, and acute respiratory distress
4. Pneumomediastinum—subcutaneous emphysema (crepitus on palpation of soft tissues over chest wall and in neck region); reduced or muffled heart sounds, and systolic crepitation (Hamman's auscultatory sign)—best heard in left lateral decubitus position
5. X-ray diagnosis—may need inspiration/expiration views for small pneumothorax; pneumomediastinum—para-aortic air stripe and subcutaneous emphysema show up as lucent black areas
6. CT scan helpful; barium study to rule out esophageal rupture
7. Sonographic diagnosis is possible—supine and/or sitting position
8. Treatment—>15% pneumothorax—needs decompression with chest tube or valve (Heimlich valve); smaller pneumothoraces can be left to resorb on their own; follow with serial x-rays
9. Tension pneumothorax is a *medical emergency*—treatment involves immediate decompression with a large bore (16G) needle into second intercostal space in mid-clavicular line
10. Recurrent spontaneous pneumothorax may require some sort of pleurodesis—either with talc or chemicals (tetracycline, poviodine); video-assisted thorascopic surgery (VATS)
11. Spontaneous pneumomediastinum usually treated conservatively, should resolve within several weeks, often in 2–4 days

12. Restriction from athletic and strenuous activity, analgesics, (occasionally antibiotics if suspicion of rupture of esophagus)
13. Rest in comfortable position (usually sitting or semireclined)
14. Full return to activity is dependent on radiographic resolution; resumption of vigorous cardiovascular activity may take 6–8 weeks
15. Needs resolution and clearance by physician prior to air travel.

VII. Hemothorax

A. General considerations
1. Can occur with blunt or penetrating chest trauma, or in association with pneumothorax or injuries to great vessels, cardiac structures
B. Diagnosis and treatment
1. Physical examination: dullness to percussion, diminished breath sounds at lung bases
2. X-ray—upright and lateral decubitus, blunting of costo-phrenic angle
3. Requires drainage with chest tube if compromising respiratory function; need to find and stop source of bleeding.

VIII. Pulmonary embolus

A. General considerations
1. Fat embolus—from trauma/surgery to long bone elsewhere
2. From deep venous thrombosis (DVT)—usually from leg veins, rarely reported after shoulder arthroscopy
B. Diagnosis
1. High level of suspicion, predisposing clinical setting
2. Symptoms—chest pain, dyspnea, tachypnea, cough (may be nonproductive), hemoptysis, diaphoresis
3. Physical examination—tachycardia, increased respiratory rate, coarse breath sounds (rhonchi, wheezing, rales), pleural rub, cyanosis
4. Chest x-ray (Hampton's hump—shallow wedge-shaped opacity in periphery of lung with base against pleural surface)—usually not helpful
5. ECG—may show T wave inversions in leads V1 and V2 characteristic of right ventricular outflow obstruction or volume or pressure overload
6. D-dimer blood test (normal is less than 451 ng/mL)
7. Ventilation–perfusion (V/Q) scan; gold standard—CT pulmonary angiography
C. Treatment
1. Supportive—supplemental oxygen, analgesia
2. Anticoagulation
   a. Immediate—subcutaneous low-molecular-weight heparin
   b. Long-term (3–6 months) with warfarin
   c. Monitor with INR (international normalized ratio)
   d. Caution with contact sports—increased risk of bleeding from injuries while anticoagulated; wait 2 weeks after stopping
3. Discontinue oral contraceptives—especially preoperatively
4. Hypercoagulability evaluation includes homocysteine, antithrombin III, anticardiolipin antibody, prothrombin 20210A, factor V Leiden, and lupus anticoagulant levels (antithrombin mutations, prothrombin mutations).

IX. Heart and great vessels

A. General considerations
1. Commotio cordis—possible with direct trauma to anterior chest/heart
2. Pericardium and pericardial space—pericarditis, pericardial effusion, cardiac tamponade

3. Heart muscle—laceration, ventricular rupture, myocardial contusion
4. Great vessels—Ascending and descending aorta, vena cava, jugular, and subclavian veins; aortic dissection/intimal tear from blunt trauma—can also have damage from penetrating trauma; usually occurs at transition from mobile to fixed aorta—aortic isthmus (ligamentum arteriosum)
5. Coronary artery dissection—left anterior descending under sternum

B. Pericardial effusion and cardiac tamponade
1. Cardiac sounds may be muffled in simple pericardial effusion; with cardiac tamponade—neck veins engorged—increased jugular venous pressure (JVP), hypotension, arterial pulsus paradoxus, face plethoric, athlete may have dysphonia and dysphagia
2. Right-sided tension pneumothorax can mimic symptoms of cardiac tamponade
3. ECG—electrical alternans or cyclical variation in QRS voltage specific for cardiac tamponade
4. Troponin I and T elevation may reveal evidence of cardiac injury
5. Chest x-ray—enlarged cardiac silhouette, "flask-like" configuration
6. Echocardiogram is useful for definitive diagnosis
7. Treatment
   a. Percutaneous pericardiocentesis, ultrasound guided—decompress heart, increase stroke volume, filling pressure, restore adequate circulation
   b. Surgical exploration to repair any laceration/rupture that resulted in bleeding and tamponade

C. Aortic dissection
1. Aortic dissection/intimal tear may present with vague chest discomfort and/or back pain (interscapular); hypotension is a *late* sign
2. Pulse deficits or absences—in 50% of patients with proximal aortic dissection; also variation in blood pressure between right and left arms
3. Chest x-ray may be diagnostic—widening of mediastinum, obscured aortic knob, loss of paraspinous stripe, and/or aortopulmonary window, left bronchial depression; need spiral CT and/or angiography (gold standard) if mechanism suspicious for injury
4. Traumatic injury to the ascending aorta is typically fatal; more stable patients may have an incomplete laceration near the ligamentun arteriosum.

X. Injuries to the breasts

A. Breast contusion: direct trauma

B. Breast protection
1. For contact sports—chest protectors—may be modified for women

C. Breast support
1. Some women refrain from physical activity due to pain and/or embarrassment associated with excessive breast motion, especially during exercises involving running and jumping; deep-water running is better
2. Halter-style bras without cups (e.g., Jogbra®) compress rather than support the breasts; not recommended for athletes with large breasts
3. Large-breasted women—special encapsulating sports bras are best
4. Breast reduction procedures may be necessary to decrease discomfort

D. Considerations for lactating women
1. Breasts will be more engorged and tender; breast-feed or pump regularly to minimize discomfort
2. No significant risks for breast-feeding infant

E. Breast cancer survivors—may have specific issues
1. Tissue scarring, and "pulling" with activity—treat with physiotherapy

2. Lymphedema—may need to modify activity—that is, "side" in rowing, Dragon boat—keep affected arm elevated to improve lymphatic drainage
3. Overall positive effects on health, physical fitness, muscular strength, flexibility, and self-esteem, and the benefits of teamwork and social engagement far outweigh any risk of musculoskeletal injury.

XI. Costochondritis

A. Diagnosis
   1. Costochondral junction—localized pain, rarely swelling
   2. Inflammation, pain—overuse (increase in muscle pull from adjoining ribs) or idiopathic (Tietze's syndrome with painful, localized swelling)
   3. X-ray not helpful—need bone scan for diagnosis, if necessary
B. Management
   1. Rest from aggravating activities, analgesics, reassurance
   2. Physiotherapy—manual therapy, mobilization of costochondral and costovertebral joints; modalities; rehabilitative exercises (scapula).

Recommended Reading

1. Al-Mufarrej F, Badari J, Gharagozloo F, Tempesta B, Strother E, Margolism. Spontaneous pneumomediastinum: Diagnostic and therapeutic interventions. *J Cardiothorac Surg* 2008;3:59–62.
2. Best R, Niess A, Schlemmer H, Striegel H. Exercise dependent pleurisy in a soccer athlete. *Int J Sports Med.* 2009;30:834–838.
3. Choi JD, McFadden DP, Nanavatie VN, O'Connor FG. Acute dyspnea in a 10-year-old boy after a fall. *Curr Sports Med Rep.* 2008;7(2):66–69.
4. Gregory PL, Biswas AC, Batt ME. Musculoskeletal problems of the chest wall in athletes. *Sports Med.* 2002;32(4):235–250.
5. Karmy-Jones R, Jackson N, Long W, Simeone A. Current management of traumatic rupture of the descending thoracic aorta. *Curr Cardiol Rev* 2009;5:187–195.
6. Russi EW. Diving and the risk of barotrauma. *Thorax* 1998;53(Suppl 2):S20–S24.
7. Sadarangi S, Patel DR, Pejka S. Spontaneous pneumomediastinum and epidural pneumatosis in an adolescent precipitated by weight lifting: A case report and review. *Phys Sports Med.* 2009;37(4):147–153.
8. Sakellaridis T, Stamatelopoulos A, Andrianopoulos E, Kormas P. Isolated first rib fracture in athletes. *Br J Sports Med.* 2004;38(3):e5.
9. Sik C, Batt ME, Heslop LM. Atypical chest pain in athletes. *Curr Sports Med Rep.* 2009;8(2):52–58.
10. Vinther A, Kanstrup I-L, Christiansen E, Alkjaer T, Larsson B, Magnusson SP, Ekdahl C, Aagaard P. Exercise-induced rib stress fractures: Potential risk factors related to thoracic muscle co-contraction and movement patterns. *Scand J Med Sci Sports.* 2006;16:188–196.

Sports Cardiology

Irfan M. Asif and Jonathon A. Drezner

I. Sudden Cardiac Death (SCD)

A. Epidemiology
1. Leading cause of sudden death during sport and exercise in young athletes
   a. Usually a result of undiagnosed structural or electrical cardiovascular disease (Figure 33.1)
2. SCD incidence
   a. Initial reports estimated SCD to occur in 1:200,000 athletes per year; likely an underestimate due to the lack of a mandatory reporting system and incomplete identification of all cases
   b. More recent estimates have found an incidence of 1:43,000 NCAA athletes per year
3. Gender
   a. Initial reports found a male to female ratio as 9:1
   b. A more recent report in NCAA athletes found that SCD was only 2.3 times higher in male than female athletes
4. Sports
   a. Occurs most often in basketball and football
5. Race
   a. More common in African American athletes
6. Presentation
   a. In up to 80% of cases, the athlete is asymptomatic and SCA is the first presentation of their underlying cardiac disorder
   b. Symptoms (if present) of cardiac disease may include:
      i. Palpitations
      ii. Exertional chest pain
      iii. Syncope or pre-syncope
      iv. Dyspnea
      v. Reduced exertional tolerance
      vi. Disproportionate fatigue compared to peers or level of exertion
7. Prevention
   a. Preparticipation screening
      i. Personal and family history, as well as, thorough physical exam
      ii. No studies have demonstrated that the traditional preparticipation exam (PPE) based on history and physical exam alone reduces SCD
   b. ECG screening greatly increases the sensitivity of the preparticipation evaluation to identify cardiac disorders that predispose to SCD.

Disease of the Myocardium	• Hypertrophic cardiomyopathy • Arrhythmogenic right ventricular cardiomyopathy • Dilated cardiomyopathy • Left ventricular non-compaction
Coronary Artery Disease/ Anomalies	• Anomalous origin of coronary arteries • Artherosclerotic coronary artery disease
Cardiac Conduction Tissue Abnormalities	• Wolff-Parkinson White syndrome
Valvular Heart Disease and Disorders of the Aorta	• Aortic Stenosis • Marfan's Syndrome • Aortic dissection • Mitral Valve Prolapse
Ion-channelopathies	• Long QT syndrome • Short QT syndrome • Catecholeaminergic polymorphic ventricular tachycardia • Brugada syndrome
Acquired heart disease	• Myocarditis • Trauma (Commotio cordis)

Figure 33.1   Causes of sudden cardiac death in athletes

II. Congenital/Structural Cardiac Disease

A. Hypertrophic cardiomyopathy (HCM)
  1. Epidemiology
    a. Most common cause of SCD in young competitive US athletes (approximately one-third of cases)
    b. Inheritance pattern is autosomal dominant
    c. Most common genetic mutations occur in β-myosin heavy chain and myosin binding protein C
    d. Prevalence in adult general population is approximately 1:500; prevalence in younger athletes may be lower
    e. Involves asymmetric left ventricular hypertrophy
      i. Wall thickness ≥16 mm
      ii. Septum to free wall ratio of >1.3
      iii. Nondilated LV <45 mm with impaired diastolic function
    f. Histology shows disorganized cellular architecture and myocardial disarray
  2. Symptoms
    a. Eighty percent of athletes are asymptomatic until sudden death
    b. May have exertional chest pain, lightheadedness, syncope, dyspnea, poor exertional tolerance, or palpitations
  3. Physical exam
    a. Only 25% have systolic ejection murmur from left ventricular outflow tract obstruction
      i. Murmur increases in intensity with maneuvers that decrease venous return such as Valsalva or going from squatting to standing position
      ii. Murmur decreases in intensity with maneuvers that increase venous return such as lying down or going from standing to squatting

4. Diagnostic tests
   a. ECG pattern may include:
      i. Prominent Q waves
      ii. Deep negative T waves
      iii. ST depression
      iv. Left axis deviation
      v. Marked increase in QRS voltage
   b. Echocardiogram is currently the standard to diagnose HCM
   c. Cardiac MRI helpful in borderline cases to distinguish pathologic hypertrophy from athlete's heart, and to delineate apical or anterolateral hypertrophy not well visualized on echocardiography
5. Return to play
   a. No participation in competitive athletics, except possibly low static sports

B. Arrhythmogenic right ventricular cardiomyopathy
   1. Epidemiology:
      a. Leading cause of SCD in the Venetto region of Italy
      b. Accounts for <5% of SCD in U.S. athletes
      c. Caused by genetic mutations encoding myocyte desmosomal (adhesive) proteins
      d. Results in myocyte replacement by fibro-fatty tissue in the right ventricle (RV), which predisposes the athlete to arrhythmias
   2. Symptoms
      a. Syncope, chest, pain, palpitations, or sudden death
   3. Physical exam does not yield any specific findings
   4. Diagnosis
      a. ECG pattern may include
         i. Epsilon wave
            (A) Small terminal notch just after QRS complex in leads V1 or V2
         ii. T wave inversion beyond V1 (i.e., V2–V4)
         iii. Prolonged QRS >110 ms
         iv. Preventricular contractions with left bundle branch block pattern
      b. Echocardiography does not detail RV very well but may show:
         i. RV dilatation, wall thinning, aneurysms, or regional wall motion abnormalities
      c. Cardiac MRI
         i. Best modality to visualize RV and fibro-fatty infiltration
   5. Return to sports
      a. Athletes are disqualified from competition and require long-term follow-up with a cardiologist

C. Dilated cardiomyopathy (DCM)
   1. Epidemiology
      a. Prevalence is 1:2,500
      b. Accounts for 4% of SCD in athletes
      c. Characterized by progressive LV dilatation and systolic dysfunction
   2. Symptoms
      a. Progressive exercise intolerance
      b. Dyspnea
      c. Orthopnea
      d. Edema
   3. Physical exam
      a. Possible S3
   4. Diagnostic tests
      a. Echocardiogram is diagnostic with dilated LV and reduced ejection fraction

5. Treatment

    a. ACE inhibitors and β-blockers should be considered in all athletes with DCM

6. Return to play

    a. Athletes should abstain from vigorous activity

    b. Activity such as brisk walking or gentle cycling can have prognostic benefit

D. LV Noncompaction

  1. Epidemiology

    a. Newly recognized disorder with currently unknown incidence

    b. Characterized by prominent trabeculations with deep intratrabecular recesses leading to LV dilatation or hypertrophy, which may be seen on echocardiogram

  2. Return to play

    a. Currently little information is available, but *36th Bethesda Conference* recommends restriction from athletic competition

E. Anomalous origin coronary artery

  1. Epidemiology

    a. Second leading cause of SCD in young competitive athletes in the United States.

    b. Most common anomaly leading to SCD is an anomalous left coronary artery origin arising from the right sinus of Valsalva.

  2. Symptoms

    a. Exertional syncope, chest pain, or palpitations

  3. Physical exam

    a. No findings to suggest disease

  4. Diagnosis

    a. ECG: may show pathologic Q waves from prior infarction

    b. Echocardiogram: sensitivity to detect coronary ostia is approximately 80–90% and dependent on sonographer experience, patient body habitus, and transducer quality

    c. Cardiac MRI or CT angiography: very accurate

      i. Radiation exposure in children and women is of concern for use of CT angiography

    d. Coronary angiography: makes a definitive diagnosis

  5. Return to play

    a. If a congenital coronary artery anomaly is found, then the athlete should be removed from sport

    b. If the athlete undergoes correction of the defect and is asymptomatic, participation can be considered 6 months after correction

F. Marfan's syndrome

  1. Background

    a. Eighty-five percent of cases are inherited in an autosomal dominant pattern

    b. Genetic disorder involving fibrillin, a connective tissue protein

      i. Leads to cystic medial necrosis of the aortic root and degeneration of mitral or aortic valves

      ii. Most worrisome complications is aortic dissection/rupture leading to sudden death

      iii. Valvular dysfunction may also occur

  2. Symptoms

    a. Typically asymptomatic

    b. Chest and back pain can occur from aortic dissection

    c. Valvular dysfunction can lead to decreased exertional tolerance or heart failure

  3. Physical exam—see Figure 33.2

  4. Diagnostic tests

    a. ECG: no specific findings

    b. Echocardiogram

      i. Aortic root dilation, aortic or mitral valve insufficiency

Major and Minor Criteria for Diagnosis of Marfan's Syndrome				
Skeletal findings	Cardiovascular findings	Ocular findings	Family/genetic history	Other findings
Major manifestations	**Major manifestations**	**Major manifestations**	**Major manifestations**	**Major manifestations**
Need 4 of the following:	Need 1 of the following:	Need 1 of the following:	Need 1 of the following:	Need 1 of the following:
Reduced upper to lower segment ratio (<0.85)	Dilatation of the ascending aorta	Ectopia lentis	A parent, child or sibling who meets criteria independently	Dural ectasia affecting the lumbosacral spinal canal
Arm span exceeding height	Dissection of the ascending aorta		Presence of a mutation in FBN1 known to cause Marfan syndrome	
Arachnodactyly of fingers and toes				
Scoliosis >20° or spondylolisthesis				
Pectus carinatum				
Pectus excavatum needing surgery				
Reduced extension of elbows (<170°)				
Pes planus				
Protrusio acetabulae (deep socket protruding into pelvis)				
Minor manifestations	**Minor manifestations**	**Minor manifestations**	**Minor manifestations**	**Minor manifestations**
Pectus excavatum (moderate severity)	Mitral valve prolapse	Flat cornea		Spontaneous pneumothorax
Joint hypermobility	Mitral regurgitation	Increased axial globe length (measured by ultrasound)		Apical blebs
High arched palate	Dilatation of the pulmonary artery	Hypoplastic iris		Cutaneous striae distensae
Dolichocephaly	Calcification of mitral annulus	Myopia		Recurrent hernias
Malar hypoplasia		Retinal detachment		
Enophthalmos				
Retrognathia				
Down-slanting palpebral fissures				

Figure 33.2   Diagnosis of Marfan's syndrome

        c. Slit lamp: to detect ectopia lentis (lens dislocation)

        d. Lumbosacral MRI or CT: to evaluate for dural ectasia

    5. Return to play

        a. If aortic root diameter is >4.0 cm, then only low static sports are recommended

        b. No contact or collision sports

G. Valvular

    1. Aortic stenosis

        a. Epidemiology

            i. Congenital narrowing of aortic valve, often associated with bicuspid aortic valve

            ii. Causes pressure gradient: <20 mmHg—mild, 21–29 mmHg—moderate, >50 mmHg—severe

            iii. Leads to LV hypertrophy

                (A) Ischemia secondary to increased LV mass

                (B) Decreased diastolic compliance, exacerbated by decreased filling time with exertion

        b. Usually asymptomatic

        c. Physical exam reveals systolic ejection murmur at the right upper sternal border with apical ejection click

            i. Murmur decreases with decreased venous return (i.e., Valsalva)

        d. Diagnostic tests

            i. ECG can show LV hypertrophy with LV strain pattern (high QRS voltage with ST and T wave changes)

            ii. Echocardiogram will show narrowing of aortic valve and elevated pressure gradient

        e. Return to play

            i. Mild AS patients may participate in sports but need serial evaluations

            ii. Symptomatic AS with moderate disease or severe AS patients should not participate in competitive athletics

    2. Mitral valve prolapse

        a. Role in SCD in athletes is controversial

        b. Symptoms: no specific findings

        c. Physical exam

            i. Mid-systolic click

            ii. Systolic ejection murmur if mitral regurgitation is present

        d. Diagnostic tests

            i. ECG: no specific findings

            ii. Echocardiogram will show prolapsed mitral valve

        e. Return to play

            i. Can participate in sports, unless one of the following is present

                (A) History of syncope with documented arrhythmia

                (B) Family history of sudden death

                (C) Supraventricular tachycardia

                (D) Moderate-to-severe mitral valve regurgitation

                (E) Prior embolic events.

III. Primary Electrical Disease

    A. Long QT syndrome (LQTS)

        1. Background

            a. Most common ion channel disorder

            b. Prolongation of ventricular repolarization and QT interval corrected for heart rate (QTc)

    c. Family history may include unexplained sudden death (drowning, motor vehicle accident, or sudden infant death syndrome)

  2. Symptoms: syncope (often multiple episodes) associated with physical or emotional stress

    a. Subtypes of LQTS associated with triggers for ventricular arrhythmias

      i. LQTS 1: emotion, exercise, swimming

      ii. LQTS 2: emotion, exercise, auditory stimuli

      iii. LQTS 3: sleep

  3. Diagnostic tests

    a. ECG

      i. QTc > 0.47 s (99% males)

      ii. QTc > 0.48 s (99% females)

      iii. QTc > 0.50 s (unequivocal long QT)

  4. Return to play

    a. No competitive athletics is recommended

    b. Placement of an internal cardioverter defibrillator is recommended in symptomatic patients

    c. β-Blockers can reduce mortality for certain types of LQTS

    d. Asymptomatic athletes that are genotype positive for LQTS but phenotype negative are typically not restricted from athletics due to lack of data; however, swimming is not recommended for asymptomatic genotype positive LQTS 1 athletes due to the high association of SCD with swimming

B. Short QT syndrome

  1. Epidemiology

    a. Characterized by hyperfunctioning potassium channel

  2. Symptoms

    a. Palpitations

    b. Syncope

    c. Sudden death

  3. Diagnostic tests

    a. ECG shows QTc ≤ 340 ms

  4. Return to play

    a. Restriction from competitive athletics

    b. Consider antiarrhythmic or AICD

C. Brugada syndrome

  1. Epidemiology

    a. Autosomal dominant sodium channelopathy

    b. Incidence of 1:2,000–5,000

    c. Higher prevalence in south Asians

  2. Symptoms

    a. Syncope

    b. Sudden death

  3. Diagnostic tests

    a. ECG

      i. High take off and down-sloping ST segment elevation in V1–V3

  4. Treatment

    a. AICD placement

  5. Return to play

    a. Restricted from prolonged exercise

D. Catecholaminergic Polymorphic Ventricular Tachycardia (CPVT)

  1. Epidemiology

    a. Hereditary ion channel disorder that leads to adrenergically mediated polymorphic ventricular tachycardia

      b. SCD triggered by emotional stress or exercise

   2. Diagnostic tests

      a. ECG and Echo may be normal

      b. Exercise stress testing may show multifocal premature ventricular contractions

         i. Ventricular tachycardia with a beat to beat 180° alternating QRS axis (bi-directional ventricular tachycardia) is considered highly characteristic of CPVT, but is extremely rare

   3. Treatment

      a. β-Blockers

   4. Return to play

      a. Avoidance of moderate-to-high intensity exercise

 E. Wolff–Parkinson–White (WPW) Syndrome

   1. Ventricular preexcitation

      a. Background:

         i. Tachyarrhythmias possible due to accessory conduction pathway in the Bundle of Kent (between the atrium and ventricle)

         ii. Aberrant reentrance cardiac conduction pathways (such as in WPW) are more commonly found in those with high resting vagal tone

         iii. This conduction pathway is more concerning in the athlete with atrial fibrillation due to the possibility of very rapid conduction through the accessory pathway which can lead to ventricular fibrillation

      b. Symptoms may include palpitations or syncope/near syncope

      c. Diagnostic tests:

         i. ECG

            (A) Short PR interval (<120 ms)

            (B) Delta wave (slurred upstroke of QRS complex)

            (C) Prolonged QRS complex (>120 ms)

      d. Return to play

         i. In young athletes and those with symptoms, electrophysiologic study and catheter ablation of the accessory pathway should be considered

            (A) In older athletes (>25 years old) with no symptoms, return to play without intervention can be considered.

IV. Acquired Heart Disease

 A. Myocarditis

   1. Epidemiology

      a. Inflammation of the myocardium, often accompanied by a flu-like illness

      b. Etiologies

         i. Infectious: Most common pathogens include parvovirus B19, human herpes virus 6 and coxsackie virus, echovirus, adenovirus, influenza, *Chlamydia pneumonia, Mycoplasma, and Borrelia burgdoferi* (lyme disease)

            (A) Myocardium becomes infiltrated by lymphocytes leading to necrosis or degeneration with subsequent ventricular dysfunction and electrical instability

         ii. Eosinophilic myocarditis: may occur with hypersensitivity, parasitic infection, or malignancy

         iii. Autoimmune: lupus, sarcoid

   2. Symptoms

      a. Symptoms can vary greatly from asymptomatic changes on an ECG to fulminate heart failure

      b. Prodromal viral illness: fever, cough, myalgias, muscle tenderness

         i. Eighty-nine percent of patients in the United States. Myocarditis Treatment Trial reported symptoms consistent with a viral prodrome

     c. Eosinophilic myocarditis may present with rash, fever, and peripheral eosinophilia

     d. Progressive exercise intolerance

     e. More advanced cases present with clinical manifestations of heart failure (i.e., dyspnea, cough, orthopnea) due to dilated cardiomyopathy

  3. Physical exam

     a. S3 gallop

     b. Heart failure signs: edema, crackles at lung bases

  4. Diagnosis

     a. ECG

        i. Electrical changes may be nonspecific including Q waves, ST-T wave changes, AV or bundle branch blocks, and tachy or brady arrhythmias

     b. Echocardiogram may show regional or diffuse wall motion abnormalities, LV dysfunction, and reduced ejection fraction

     c. Endomyocardial biopsy may be needed in some cases

  5. Treatment

     a. Majority of cases are self-limiting with no short- or long-term sequelae.

     b. Those with more severe ECG changes (i.e., Q waves, high degree AV block, or bundle branch block) often have worse long-term clinical outcomes.

     c. Specific therapy should aim at the potential cause

        i. Azithromycin in cases of suspected *C. pneumoniae*

        ii. New experimental therapies consist of ribavarin, interferon, or immunosuppressive treatments

        iii. Animal models have shown that NSAIDs are not effective and may actually enhance the inflammatory process

     d. Nonspecific therapies for heart failure symptoms

        i. Low salt diet, cautious diuresis, and ACE inhibitors

     e. Exercise limitation

        i. Electrical instability during acute myocardial inflammation or late myocardial scar places athletes at risk for sudden death

        ii. Return to exercise or sport should be guided by a cardiologist

           (A) Athletes require normal echocardiography, stress testing, and ambulatory monitoring

  6. Complications

     a. Limitations in cardiac reserve or conduction disturbances may persist for months to years due to scar tissue formation

        i. May need ICD implantation or a pacemaker for life-threatening arrhythmias

     b. Thromboembolic complications may occur with severe heart failure

B. Commotio cordis

  1. Epidemiology

     a. Caused by blunt trauma to chest during vulnerable phase of ventricular repolarization (prior to peak of T wave) leading to ventricular fibrillation

        i. Can be caused by a direct blow or projectile

        ii. More common in baseball, hockey, lacrosse, ice-hockey, karate, and judo

     b. Higher incidence in young males (mean age 13)

     c. Collapse is instantaneous or after short delay (seconds)

  2. Treatment

     a. Prompt recognition, CPR, and defibrillation (AED) is necessary for survival

C. Arteriosclerotic coronary artery disease

  1. Epidemiology

     a. Most common cause of sudden cardiac death (SCD) in older athletes over age 30

     b. Risk of exercise-related SCD is one in 15,000–18,000 adult runners per year

    c. Usually caused by atherosclerotic plaque disruption
      i. Plaque formation is progressive
      ii. Approximately half of patients with an acute coronary syndrome have no prior symptoms
      iii. Related to coronary risk factors
        (A) Hypertension
        (B) Tobacco use
        (C) Dyslipidemia
        (D) Diabetes
        (E) Family history of early heart disease (women age <55, men age <45)
  2. Symptoms
    a. Exertional chest pain
    b. Angina
    c. Lightheadedness
    d. Palpitations
    e. Acute coronary syndrome (myocardial infarction)
    f. Sudden death
  3. Physical exam
    a. Evaluate for CAD risk factors (HTN, tobacco use, dyslipidemia, diabetes, family history)
    b. In advanced CAD, possible signs of ischemic heart failure
      i. S3 or S4
      ii. Increased jugular venous pressure
      iii. Crackles in lower lung fields
  4. Diagnosis
    a. Indications for screening older athletes
      i. One or more known risk factors for CAD and engaged in competitive athletics or starting a new exercise program
        (A) Exercise treadmill test
        (B) Stress echocardiogram
        (C) Nuclear stress test
    b. Acute coronary syndrome
      i. Increased cardiac enzymes
        (A) Troponins
        (B) CK-MB
    c. Electrocardiogram (ECG)
      i. ST segment changes
        (A) ST elevation: infarction
        (B) ST depression: myocardial ischemia
      ii. T wave inversion
      iii. New left bundle branch block (LBBB)
    d. Coronary angiography
      i. Determine extent of vessel narrowing and need for surgical revascularization
      ii. Potential for percutaneous revascularization
  5. Treatment
    a. Acute coronary syndrome
      i. Oxygen, aspirin, establish IV access
      ii. β-Blockers, nitroglycerin, heparin, morphine
      iii. Thrombolytic therapy
    b. Revascularization
      i. Coronary artery bypass grafting (CABG)

    ii. Percutaneous coronary intervention (PCI)

      (A) Angioplasty

      (B) Stent placement.

V. Athletic Heart Syndrome

A. Describes normal, physiologic cardiac adaptations due to regular exercise training

B. Extent of changes dependent upon the frequency, duration, and intensity of exercise

  1. Physiologic changes

    a. Decrease in resting HR due to increased vagal tone and larger stroke volume (cardiac output = heart rate × stroke volume)

  2. ECG changes seen in the athlete's heart

    a. Due to increased parasympathetic tone

      i. Sinus bradycardia

      ii. Sinus arrhythmia

      iii. First-degree AV block

      iv. Early repolarization/ST segment elevation

    b. Changes consistent with increased cardiac mass

      i. Isolated voltage criteria for LVH

      ii. Incomplete right bundle branch block

  3. Morphologic changes

    a. Left ventricle (LV) may enlarge, thicken, or increase in mass

    b. LV changes occur according to Laplace's law: wall stress = (pressure × radius)/(wall thickness × 2)

      i. Isotonic exercise, such as running and cycling, present a volume load to the heart leading to eccentric thickening

      ii. Isometric exercise, such as weightlifting, place a pressure load on the heart that leads to concentric hypertrophy

      iii. Most sports are a combination of both isotonic and isometric exercises

    c. LV wall thickness

      i. Normal ≤12 mm

      ii. Pathologic ≥16 mm

      iii. Borderline "Gray Zone" 13–15 mm

    d. LV cavity dimensions and LV function may help distinguish pathologic hypertrophy from athlete's heart

      i. Small, noncompliant LV <45 mm with impaired diastolic function suggests HCM

    e. Consider a period of deconditioning (4–6 weeks) with repeat echocardiography as athletic heart changes may resolve while pathologic hypertrophy would remain unchanged

    f. Cardiac MRI is also helpful in distinguishing athlete's heart versus HCM

      i. Cardiac MRI provides a more accurate assessment of LV wall thickness, especially in the apex of the heart where echocardiogram measurements are limited

      ii. Delayed gadolinium enhancement suggests myocardial scar/fibrosis consistent with HCM.

VI. Hypertension

A. Background

  1. Most common cardiovascular disease in athletes

  2. Elevated blood pressure found in approximately 5% of athletes during preparticipation screening

B. Classification
1. Adults (Guidelines of JNC-7: The Seventh Report of the Joint National Committee on Prevention, Detection, Evaluation, and Treatment of High Blood Pressure (2003))
   a. Normal: systolic <120 mmHg, diastolic <80 mmHg
   b. Prehypertension: systolic 120–139 mmHg, diastolic 80–89 mmHg
   c. Stage 1 hypertension: systolic 140–159 mmHg, diastolic 90–99 mmHg
   d. Stage 2 hypertension: systolic >160 mmHg, diastolic 100 mmHg
2. Adolescents (Fourth Report)—adjusted for age, sex, and height
   a. Normal: <90th percentile
   b. Prehypertension: 90th–95th percentile or >120/80
   c. Stage 1 hypertension: 95th–99th percentile + 5 mmHg
   d. Stage 2 hypertension: >99th percentile + 5 mmHg

C. Pathophysiology
1. Primary versus secondary hypertension
   a. Primary hypertension
      i. Accounts for 95% of cases
      ii. Age of onset typically 25–55 years old
   b. Secondary hypertension
      i. Usually in patients <20 years old or >50 years old
      ii. Consider in cases where hypertension is sudden in onset, severe, or less responsive to traditional therapies
      iii. Causes
         (A) Renal
            (1) Renal vascular disease
               (a) Examples: atherosclerosis, fibromuscular dysplasia
            (2) Renal parenchymal disease
         (B) Endocrine
            (1) Adrenal: pheochromocytoma, Cushing's syndrome, primary hyperaldosteronism
            (2) Thyroid disorders
         (C) Other
            (1) Oral contraceptives
            (2) NSAIDs
            (3) Coarctation of the aorta
            (4) Obstructive sleep apnea
2. End-organ effects
   a. Cardiac
      i. Left ventricular hypertrophy
      ii. Coronary artery disease and congestive heart failure
   b. Vascular: aortic aneurysm or dissection, peripheral vascular disease
   c. Renal: proteinuria or renal insufficiency
   d. Neurologic: stroke or aneurysm
   e. Ocular: retinopathy

D. Risk factors
1. Family history
2. Gender: more common in males
3. Race: more common in African Americans
4. Stress
5. High sodium diet
6. Excessive alcohol intake
7. Drug abuse

    8. Steroids

    9. Dietary supplements: mua huang, caffeine, guarana, ephedra

E. Symptoms

    1. Often asymptomatic

    2. May have headache, fatigue, dyspnea, or chest pain

F. Physical exam

    1. Identify potential secondary causes

        a. Renal: bruits or masses

        b. Thyroid

    2. Look for possible end-organ damage

        a. Cardiovascular: murmurs, bruits, pulses

        b. Abdominal: auscultate and palpate for masses

        c. Eye exam for hemorrhages, exudates, or papilledema

G. Diagnosis

    1. At least two blood pressure readings, in a seated position, with arm at heart level

    2. Correct cuff size bladder encircles at least 80% arm circumference

H. Lab evaluation

    1. Serum: Hematocrit, electrolytes, glucose, lipids, and TSH

    2. Urinalysis

    3. ECG to evaluate for LVH

    4. Echocardiography in young athletes with stage 1 or 2 HTN

    5. Further workup to evaluate for secondary causes as needed

I. Treatment

    1. Nonpharmacologic

        a. Optimize diet

            i. Reduction in dietary sodium ($\sim$2–2.5 g/day)

            ii. Emphasize fruits, vegetables, and low fat diet

        b. Limit alcohol consumption to 1–2 drinks per day

        c. Weight reduction

        d. Regular exercise

    2. Pharmacologic

        a. Angiotensin-converting enzyme inhibitors (ACE inhibitors) and angiotensin receptor blockers (ARBs)

            i. Mechanism of action

                (A) Blocks conversion of angiotensin I into angiotensin II

                    (1) Decreases vasoconstriction

                    (2) Lowers sodium retention

            ii. Benefits

                (A) Often used as first-line therapy in athletes, due to lack of major impairments on cardiac function

                (B) Renal protective agent that decreases microalbuminuria and preserves renal function

                (C) Induces remodeling in heart failure and can potentially reverse ventricular hypertrophy

            iii. Adverse effects

                (A) Dry cough (ACE inhibitors; usually not ARBs)

                (B) Hyperkalemia

                    (1) Check potassium baseline and 2 weeks after drug initiation and periodically thereafter

                    (2) Caution in patients taking NSAIDs, which can worsen hyperkalemia

                (C) Contraindicated in pregnancy due to adverse effects to the fetus

    b. Calcium channel blockers

      i. Mechanism of action

        (A) Reduces calcium in vascular smooth muscle, which allows for peripheral vasodilation

      ii. Two classes

        (A) Dihydropyridines (e.g., amlodipine)

          (1) Does not affect heart rate so preferred in athletes over nonhydropyridines

        (B) Nonhydropyridines (e.g., verapamil, diltiazem)

          (1) Not as effective on vascular smooth muscle as dihydropyridines

          (2) More effective on cardiac AV node suppression, leading to decreased heart rate

          (3) May be banned substance in certain sports

      iii. Adverse effects

        (A) Lower extremity edema

        (B) Reflex tachycardia

        (C) Lightheadedness

    c. β-Blockers

      i. Mechanism of action

        (A) Noncardioselective decrease heart rate and contractility while causing peripheral vasodilatation

        (B) Cardioselective decreases heart rate, but have less effect on peripheral vasodilatation

      ii. Benefits

        (A) Cardio-protective in patients with history of coronary artery disease

        (B) May play a role in patients with performance anxiety

      iii. Adverse effects

        (A) Can decrease VO_2 max and reduce endurance

        (B) Banned substance in precision sports

    d. Thiazide diuretics

      i. Mechanism of action: inhibit sodium reabsorption in renal tubules causing increased urine excretion

      ii. Benefits

        (A) Inexpensive

        (B) Cardio-protective

      iii. Adverse effects

        (A) Can cause electrolyte imbalances leading to cramps, arrhythmias, or rhabdomyolysis, especially when dehydrated

        (B) Banned by athletic associations because of urinary dilution, which can hide steroids or drugs in urine specimens

J. Participation in sports

  1. Prehypertension

    a. No restriction in activity

    b. Encourage lifestyle modification

  2. Stage 1 hypertension

    a. No end-organ damage

      i. No restriction from sports participation

      ii. Encourage lifestyle modification

      iii. Recheck blood pressure in 2–4 months

      iv. If BP not improving consider pharmacologic therapy

    b. End-organ damage

      i. Limit participation in sports until blood pressure is controlled and end-organ changes resolved by either lifestyle modification or pharmacologic therapy

3. Stage 2 hypertension
   a. Limit participation in sports, even if no end-organ damage, especially in high static sports
   b. Pharmacologic therapy likely
   c. Can resume sports participation when blood pressure is controlled and end-organ changes resolved (if present)
K. Long-term follow-up recommended.

VII. Supraventricular Arrhythmias

A. Atrial fibrillation

1. Background
   a. Overall prevalence in general population is approximately 1%
   b. More common with increasing age and in men
   c. Some studies suggest distance runners are at higher risk due in part to increased vagal tone
   d. Leads to decreased cardiac output and susceptibility to atrial thrombi
   e. May be paroxysmal, persistent, or permanent
   f. Risk factors
      i. Hypertension
      ii. Alcohol consumption
      iii. Hyperthyroidism
      iv. Cardiac valvular disease
2. Symptoms
   a. Palpitations
   b. Fatigue
   c. Decreased exercise tolerance
   d. Dyspnea
   e. Chest pain
   f. Syncope
3. Physical exam
   a. Irregularly irregular rhythm
4. Diagnostic tests
   a. ECG
   b. Chest X-ray
   c. Echocardiogram
   d. TSH
   e. 24 h Holter monitor (paroxysmal atrial fibrillation)
   f. Stress testing to evaluate rate control with exercise or exercise-induced atrial fibrillation
5. Treatment
   a. Cardioversion: DC or pharmacologic
      i. Presence of atrial fibrillation >48 h requires anticoagulation for 6 weeks prior to cardioversion, or evaluation by trans-esophageal echocardiogram to rule out atrial thrombi
      ii. Cardioversion should be followed with anticoagulation for at least 4 weeks
      iii. Only 20–30% maintain sinus rhythm for over 1 year
   b. Rate control
      i. β-Blockers or calcium channel blockers
   c. Rhythm control with pharmacologic agents or electrophysiologic ablation should be considered for patients who are cardiovascularly unstable in atrial fibrillation, patients with inadequate exercise capacity for desired activities, or when adequate rate control cannot be achieved

    d. Anticoagulation

        i. CHADS 2 score

          (A) 1 point for each: history of heart failure, hypertension, age ≥ 75, diabetes

          (B) 2 points for history of thromboembolic event

          (C) Low-risk patients with score of 0 or 1 can be treated with aspirin

          (D) High-risk patients with score ≥ 2 should be treated with warfarin (goal INR 2–3)

  6. Athletic participation

    a. Athletes whose heart rate increases and slows appropriately without therapy can safely participate in competitive sports

    b. β-Blockers, used for rate control, are prohibited in certain competitive sports

    c. Athletes using warfarin should refrain from contact and collision sports

    d. If an electrophysiologic ablation is performed, return to participation may be considered in 4–6 weeks after an exercise stress test confirms noninducibility.

VIII. Screening and Electrocardiogram (ECG) Interpretation

  A. Background

    1. No proven efficacy that history and physical exam alone adequately identifies athletes at risk or decreases the rate of SCD

    2. The Italian screening model utilizing history, physical exam, and ECG and has shown a 90% reduction in SCD over a 25-year period

    3. The European Society of Cardiology and International Olympic Committee endorse ECG screening in athletes

  B. Current controversy

    1. ECG changes resulting from regular intense physical training must be distinguished from those associated with cardiac pathology

    a. False-positive rate is dependent on ECG criteria used to distinguish normal from abnormal findings

    b. False-positive results may lead to unnecessary diagnostic workups and temporary disqualification

    2. History and physical exam have up to an 8% false-positive rate in competitive young athletes

    3. Modern studies using contemporary criteria for ECG interpretation suggest ECG screening is more cost-effective than history and physical exam alone

    4. Normal and training-related ECG changes

    a. Athletic conditioning leads to a physiologic increase in cardiac vagal tone

        i. Sinus bradycardia

        ii. Sinus arrhythmia

        iii. First-degree AV block

    b. Athletic conditioning leads to morphologic adaptations in cardiac size

        i. Isolated increases in left ventricular voltage

    5. Abnormal and training unrelated ECG changes

    a. ST-T repolarization abnormalities (ST depression, T-wave inversion, "strain" pattern)

    b. Pathologic Q waves

    c. Ventricular preexcitation

    d. Left axis deviation ($< -30°$)

    e. Complete left or right bundle branch block (QRS >120 ms)

    f. Intraventricular conduction defects (QRS >120 ms)

    g. Prolonged QTc interval.

IX. Management of Sudden Cardiac Arrest (SCA)

A. Initial response
   1. SCA should be suspected in any collapsed and nonresponsive athlete
      a. Commotio cordis should be suspected if the athlete has been struck in the chest prior to collapse
   2. Prompt recognition of SCA is critical to avoid delays in resuscitation
      a. SCA can be mistaken for a seizure as nearly 50% of young athletes with SCA have seizure-like activity shortly after collapse
      b. Agonal breathing or gasping, and inaccurate rescuer assessment of a pulse can also mislead responders
   3. Apply an AED (automated external defibrillator) as soon as possible for rhythm analysis and defibrillation if indicated
   4. New 2010 CPR guidelines
      a. Changes made to simplify CPR and to minimize interruptions in chest compressions
      b. Shift in the basic life support sequence of steps from "A-B-C" (Airway, Breathing, Chest compressions) to C-A-B (Chest compressions, Airway, Breathing)
         i. Ventilation is only minimally delayed until completion of the first cycle of chest compressions
      c. Chest compressions should be provided at a rate of 100/min (push hard, push fast)
      d. Hands-only (compression only) CPR is recommended for the lay rescuer
         i. For a witnessed arrest, blood in the victim still has modest oxygenation for several minutes; thus the emphasis on chest compressions to promote circulation
         ii. Hands-only (compression only) CPR appears to achieve similar outcomes to those of conventional CPR (compressions with rescue breathing)
         iii. New changes may encourage more bystanders to help
         iv. New changes do not apply to infants, children, or a nonwitnessed collapse, in which case, 30 chest compressions, alternated with two rescue breaths and repeated are still indicated
      e. Chest compressions should be provided until an AED is available, then the AED applied as soon as possible
      f. Restart chest compressions immediately after any shock delivery
      g. CPR with repeat rhythm analysis every 2 min should be provided until the victim is responsive or advanced cardiac life support is available
   5. Emergency response plan
      a. Each school or institution that sponsors an athletic program needs a written emergency response plan for SCA, including:
         i. Establishing an effective and efficient communication system to call 9-1-1 and activate the local response team
         ii. Identifying and training likely responders in CPR and AED use (i.e., coaches)
         iii. Ensuring access to early defibrillation through on-site AEDs (goal <3–5 min from collapse to first shock)
         iv. Integrating and registering AEDs with the local EMS system
         v. Practicing and reviewing the response plan with potential first responders at least annually.

Recommended Reading

1. Campbell RM, Berger S, Drezner J. Sudden cardiac arrest in children and young athletes: The importance of a detailed personal and family history in the pre-participation evaluation. *Br J Sports Med*. 2009;43(5):336–341.
2. Corrado D, Basso C, Schiavon M, Thiene G. Screening for hypertrophic cardiomyopathy in young athletes. *N Engl J Med*. 1998;339(6):364–369.

3. Corrado D, Basso C, Pavei A, Michieli P, Schiavon M, Thiene G. Trends in sudden cardiovascular death in young competitive athletes after implementation of a preparticipation screening program. *JAMA.* 2006;*296*(13):1593–1601.

4. Corrado D, Pelliccia A, Heidbuchel H, Sharma S, Link M, Basso C, Biffi A, Buja G, Delise P, Gussac I, Anastasakis A, Borjesson M, Bjornstad HH, Carre F, Deligiannis A, Dugmore D, Fagard R, Hoogsteen J, Mellwig KP, Panhuyzen-Goedkoop N, Solberg E, Vanhees L, Drezner J, Estes NA 3rd,, Iliceto S, Maron BJ, Peidro R, Schwartz PJ, Stein R, Thiene G, Zeppilli PP, McKenna WJ. Recommendations for interpretation of 12-lead electrocardiogram in the athlete. *Eur Heart J.* 2010;*31*:243–259.

5. Drezner J, Corrado D. Is there evidence for recommending ECG as part of the pre-participation examination. *Clin J Sport Med.* 2011;*21*(1):18–24.

6. Drezner JA. Contemporary approaches to the identification of athletes at risk for sudden cardiac death. *Curr Opin Cardiol.* 2008;*23*(5):494–501.

7. Drezner JA. Preparing for sudden cardiac arrest—The essential role of automated external defibrillators in athletic medicine: A critical review. *Br J Sports Med.* 2009;*43*(9):702–707.

8. Drezner JA, Rao AL, Heistand J, Bloomingdale MK, Harmon KG. Effectiveness of emergency response planning for sudden cardiac arrest in United States high schools with automated external defibrillators. *Circulation.* 2009;*120*(6):518–525. Epub 2009 Jul 27.

9. Harmon K, Asif I, Klossner D, Drezner J. Incidence of sudden cardiac death in NCAA athletes. *Circulation.* 2011;*123*:1594–1600.

Sports Pulmonology

Darlene R. Nelson, Brian P. Williams,
and Paul D. Scanlon

I. Asthma

  A. Common chronic inflammatory disorder of the airways
  1. Occurs in 5–15% of the population
  2. Characterized by airway hyperresponsiveness that leads to recurrent episodes of wheezing, breathlessness, chest tightness and coughing, particularly at night or in the early morning

  B. Pathogenesis
  1. Variable airflow obstruction within the lungs that is often reversible either spontaneously or with treatment
  2. Factors contributing to airway narrowing
   a. Airway inflammation
    i. Eosinophilia common but not universal
   b. Airway smooth muscle contraction
    i. Due to multiple bronchoconstrictor mediators and neurotransmitters
    ii. Predominant mechanism of airway narrowing and is largely reversed by bronchodilators
   c. Airway edema
    i. Due to increased microvascular leakage in response to inflammatory mediators, particularly important during acute exacerbation
   d. Airway wall thickening
    i. Due to structural changes often termed "remodeling," more important in more severe disease and not fully reversible by current therapies
   e. Mucous hypersecretion
    i. May lead to luminal occlusion "mucous plugging" and is a product of increased mucous secretion and inflammatory exudate

  C. Diagnosis
  1. Acute symptoms include episodic breathlessness, chest tightness, coughing, wheezing and sputum production
   a. Patterns of symptoms that strongly suggest a diagnosis of asthma are:
    i. Variability (seasonal, after allergen exposure)
    ii. Precipitation by nonspecific irritants (smoke, fumes, strong smells, or exercise)
    iii. Worsening at night
    iv. Response to appropriate asthma therapy
  2. Measurements of lung function (spirometry or peak expiratory flow) provide an assessment of the severity of airflow limitation, its reversibility by bronchodilators, its variability and provide confirmation of the diagnosis

D. Acute exacerbations
   1. Transient worsening of asthma that may occur as a result of exposure to risk factors for asthma symptoms or "triggers" such as exercise, air pollutants, and even certain weather conditions, for example, thunderstorms
E. Treatment
   1. Medications are divided into two major categories: controllers and relievers
      a. Controllers: taken daily on a long-term basis to keep asthma under clinical control through their anti-inflammatory effects
         i. Inhaled glucocorticoids—most effective controller medications currently available
         ii. Long-acting inhaled β-2 agonists—should not be used as monotherapy in asthma, most effective when combined with inhaled glucocorticoids
         iii. Leukotriene modifiers—may be used as an alternative treatment in adults with mild persistent asthma or as an add on in those with moderate-to-severe asthma
      b. Relievers: used on an as-needed basis that act quickly to reverse bronchoconstriction and relieve symptoms
         i. Rapid-acting inhaled β-2 agonists are the medication of choice for relief of bronchoconstriction
F. Exercise-induced asthma
   1. Physical activity is the most common trigger of bronchospasm in those who are known to be asthmatic
   2. 50–90% of individuals with asthma are hyperreactive to exercise.

II. Exercise-Induced Bronchoconstriction (EIB)

A. Acute transient airway narrowing that may occur during or after exercise, characteristic of asthma, but may occur in athletes without a diagnosis of chronic asthma
   1. Symptoms
      a. Coughing, wheezing, chest tightness, dyspnea, fatigue, poor performance for level of conditioning, avoidance of activity
      b. Range from postexercise cough or chest tightness, mild performance impairment to severe bronchoconstriction and respiratory failure (less commonly)
   2. Exercise duration of at least 5–8 min at a workload representing at least 80% of the maximal oxygen consumption is required to generate bronchospasm in most athletes
   3. Symptoms usually peak 5–10 min after exercise ceases (or intensity is reduced) and remain significant for 30 min if no bronchodilator therapy is provided
   4. Some patients with asthma present only with exercise-induced symptoms
B. Epidemiology
   1. Prevalence ranges from 8% to 80% of athletes
      a. Varies depending on sport with largest proportion in cold weather sports
   2. Athletes who compete in high ventilation or endurance sports with exposure to cold or dry air (e.g., cross-country running, soccer, ice-hockey, swimming, and cross-country skiing) are most likely to experience symptoms
   3. EIB occurs very frequently in subjects who are not known to be asthmatic and it is likely under diagnosed clinically
   4. Despite EIB, athletes have been shown to compete and perform at elite levels
      a. 1984 USA Olympic team members with asthma outperformed those without asthma (determined by number of medals won)
   5. Risk of death with EIB in athletes
      a. Overall risk of death is low
      b. One study identified 61 deaths over a 7-year period met criteria of asthma death occurring in close association with a sporting event or physical activity (Becker et al., *J Allergy Clin Immunol* 2004;113:264–267)

C. Pathogenesis
1. Likely multifactorial and is not completely understood
2. Two competing hypotheses:
   a. Loss of water leading to a change in airway osmolarity that initiates epithelial cell and mast cell activation, leading to a release of vasoactive and inflammatory mediators (e.g., histamine from mast cell degranulation, leukotrienes) in the airways that cause bronchoconstriction
   b. Loss of heat from airway epithelium leads to vascular engorgement as the airways re-warm after exercise initiating bronchoconstriction
3. Role of inflammation in EIB is not clear
   a. Significant correlation between the severity of EIB and the degree of peripheral blood eosinophilia and eosinophilic inflammation in induced sputum
   b. Inflammatory cells documented in the airways of nonasthmatic individuals, may play a role in development of bronchial hyperresponsiveness
      i. Unknown whether this contributes to pathogenesis of asthma
4. Environmental factors may increase bronchial hyperresponsiveness
   a. Increased incidence in winter sport athletes
      i. High minute ventilation of cold or dry air for extended periods
      ii. Twenty-five percent of 1998 USA Winter Olympic Athletes, and 50–60% of cross country skiers (up to 80% in some surveys)
   b. Environmental pollutants may also act as triggers
      i. Chlorine compounds in swimming pools, chemicals (NO_2) related to Zamboni, environmental ozone, and NO_2
D. Diagnosis
1. Symptoms are nonspecific and may be subtle
   a. Cough (often postexercise), dyspnea, chest tightness, sputum production
   b. Poor performance levels given level of conditioning
   c. Reduced participation
   d. Avoidance of a specific physical activity
2. Careful history and physical in each athlete with respiratory complaints, requires diagnostic testing to confirm clinical impression
3. Differential diagnosis: deconditioning, overtraining, vocal cord dysfunction, cardiac arrhythmias, pulmonary or cardiac shunts
E. Testing
1. Spirometry shows a decline of 10% or greater in FEV1 (forced expiratory volume in 1 s) after appropriate exercise challenge
2. Field exercise challenge—preferably in the environment-specific and sport-specific conditions—have been reported to be more accurate than laboratory exercise challenges
3. The World Anti-Doping Agency (WADA) and the International Olympic Committee-Medical Commission (IOC-MC) consider eucapnic voluntary hyperpnea (EVH) the best method to confirm EIB
   a. Indirect challenge
      i. EVH—hyperventilation of a gas mixture of 5% CO_2 and 21% O_2 at 85% of maximum voluntary ventilation for 6 min and the assessment of FEV_1 at specified intervals after the test
      ii. This test is technically difficult and not widely available
4. Direct challenge
   a. Methacholine challenge is also widely accepted and used as a test for asthma
   b. Indirect challenge (EVH or challenge with hypertonic aerosols) correlate better with exercise challenge than do direct challenge

   5. Exercise challenge and spirometry are required for diagnosis of EIB in elite athletes because of the poor relationship between symptoms and diagnosis
      a. Identifies athletes who need β-2 agonists
   6. Other forms of pulmonary function testing (e.g., carbon monoxide diffusing capacity [DLCO]) have more limited role in evaluation of symptomatic athletes
F. Treatment
   1. Prophylaxis
      a. Premedication
         i. Short-acting β-2 agonists 10–15 min prior to exercise
         ii. Long-acting bronchodilators (LABAs) are also beneficial but take longer to be effective
            (A) Formoterol effective in approximately 10 min
            (B) Salmeterol effective in approximately 30 min
            (C) LABAs generally not used in absence of inhaled corticosteroids for preventing EIB
      b. Warm-up period
         i. Should include 10–15 min of calisthenics with stretching exercises with an objective of reaching 50–60% of maximum heart rate
         ii. Precompetition warm-up reduces the occurrence of EIB during or after competitive activity
         iii. "Refractory period" — after occurrence of EIB, athletes can be refractory to a second episode of EIB for several hours
         iv. Thought to be due to a depletion of pre-formed mediators of bronchospasm such as histamine
   2. Inhaled corticosteroids (ICS)
      a. Recommended as first-line therapy as controller medications for athletes who have persistent asthma and experience EIB
   3. Leukotriene modifiers
      a. Second-line controller therapy
      b. Not as effective in most patients, but selected patients seem to derive great benefit (e.g., those with aspirin sensitivity).

III. Cystic Fibrosis

A. Epidemiology
   1. Most common fatal autosomal recessive disorder among Caucasians
B. Frequency
   1. Caucasians: 1:3,000
   2. Hispanics: 1:9,200
   3. Native Americans: 1:10,900
   4. African Americans: 1:15,000
   5. Asian Americans: 1:30,000
C. Definition
   1. Two of the following must be met (any of the criteria from i and one from ii, iii, or iv):
      a. Clinical symptoms of organ dysfunction
         i. Pulmonary disease (chronic cough, recurrent infections, obstruction on PFTs, etc.)
         ii. Sinus disease (chronic sinus infection, complete opacification of sinuses on CT)
         iii. Pancreatic insufficiency
         iv. Meconium ileus
         v. Biliary disease (focal biliary cirrhosis, portal hypertension)
         vi. Male infertility
         vii. Decreased bone mineralization
         viii. Recurrent venous thrombosis

    b. Elevated sweat chloride

    c. Presence of two disease-causing mutations

    d. Abnormal nasal potential difference

2. Pathophysiology

    a. Genetic mutations of cystic fibrosis transmembrane conductance regulator protein (CFTR) on chromosome 7

        i. Recessive trait (clinical disease requires both copies of the gene to be abnormal)

    b. CFTR is a regulated chloride channel

    c. Defective c-AMP-dependent chloride secretion results in highly viscous secretion in the airway

    d. Chronic obstruction of airways leads to inflammation and bacterial overgrowth

        i. Leads to recurrent respiratory infections and bacterial antibiotic resistance

3. Treatment

    a. Survival is substantially improved by regular care in a certified CF specialty center

    b. Antibiotics

        i. Chronic suppressive antibiotics not recommended

        ii. Antibiotics for acute pulmonary infections selected based on susceptibilities of colonizing bacteria

        iii. Periodic hospitalizations for "tune up" IV antibiotics have not been shown to improve overall outcomes

    c. Agents used to promote airway secretion clearance

        i. Hypertonic saline—administered via a nebulizer

        ii. DNAse 1—inhaled enzyme protein that cleaves DNA strands and thereby reduces viscosity of respiratory secretions

    d. Chest physiotherapy

        i. Chest vibration vest to improve mobilization of thickened secretions

        ii. Exercise:

            (A) Shown to play an important role in secretion mobilization

    e. Bronchodilators:

        i. Major respiratory complication is airway obstruction from chronic inflammation, mucus plugging, and airway destruction

        ii. Short-acting β-2 agonists should be used on a regular basis prior to exercise

    f. Inhaled corticosteroids (ICS)

        i. Recommended therapy as controller medications for athletes who have CF and asthma symptoms

4. Special considerations for athletes with cystic fibrosis

    a. Majority of acute respiratory complications are due to airway obstruction and hyperresponsiveness of the airways

    b. Many CF patients have asthma-like symptoms

    c. Symptoms associated with exercise can be abated with inhaled bronchodilator prior to or during exercise

    d. Acute respiratory issues should be treated the same as with asthmatic patients.

IV. Acute Airway Compromise

  A. Rare in most sporting events

  B. Etiology

    1. Anaphylaxis (vocal cord edema)

    2. Laryngotracheal fracture (contact and extreme sports)

    3. Upper airway hemorrhage

    4. Foreign body aspiration

    5. Loss of consciousness and inability to protect the airway

C. Evaluation
1. Basic life support (BLS) techniques are essential for all sports-related physicians
2. Use ABCs
   a. Airway—Is the airway patent? Are there signs of tracheal trauma, hemorrhage, or foreign body? If the athlete can talk then the airway is open
   b. Breathing—Are there spontaneous respirations? Bilateral chest wall movement? Respiratory distress?
   c. Circulation—Evaluate heart rate, peripheral pulses, and skin perfusion
D. Treatment
1. Establishing an open airway
2. Head tilt and jaw lift can be adequate enough to open up a narrowed or compromised air way (use jaw thrust for suspected C-spine injury patients)
3. If aspirated foreign body is suspected then the Heimlich maneuver should be performed
4. If signs of anaphylaxis are present then intramuscular (IM) epinephrine (EpiPen) should be administered if available
5. In an unconscious patient without a gag reflex an oropharyngeal airway may be placed
6. Nasopharyngeal airways may be placed as an alternative (not to be used in facial trauma or suspected skull base fractures)
7. Advanced airway devices such as a CombiTube and laryngeal mask airway (LMA) can be placed blindly to protect the airway as well as to provide ventilation (should not be considered a secured airway)
8. Endotracheal intubation via direct laryngoscopy can be performed in the field for airway protection and ventilation (requires a trained operator and advanced cardiac life support [ACLS] level equipment)
9. In cases where endotracheal intubation is not possible such as extrinsic compression of the trachea from hemorrhage or anaphylaxis, acute surgical airway may be needed
   a. Should be performed by trained personnel only
   b. Commercial kits are available for needle cricothyrotomy
10. After initial intervention, athletes with airway compromise should be transferred to the nearest trauma center for further evaluation and management.

V. Vocal Cord Dysfunction
A. Definition
1. Paradoxical vocal cord motion—inappropriate adduction of the vocal cords resulting in air way obstruction (inspiratory or expiratory stridor)
   a. Can mimic asthmatic wheezing and is often misdiagnosed as asthma, though typically stridor is inspiratory, whereas wheezing is usually expiratory
B. Diagnosis
1. Clinical presentation
   a. Commonly presents at ages 20–40, occasionally in adolescence
   b. More common in women than men
   c. Usually respiratory distress associated with wheezing or stridor and is frequently misdiagnosed as asthma and acute asthma exacerbation
   d. May be associated with throat tightness, choking sensation, dysphonia, or cough
   e. Physical exam
      i. Stridor that is loudest over the neck or upper chest with less transmission through the lung fields
      ii. Bronchodilators have no effect on symptoms
      iii. Dysphonia may be present
   f. Etiology
      i. Exercise induced—most common in young female athletes with high-achieving personality traits

      ii. Psychosocial disorders and stress may contribute

      iii. Gastroesophageal reflux disease (GERD)

      iv. Inhaled irritants

      v. Postsurgical or postintubation vocal cord damage

  2. Diagnostic studies

    a. Radiographic images are unremarkable—may be of benefit to rule out other causes of upper airway obstruction or pulmonary parenchymal diseases

    b. Pulmonary function testing with inspiratory and expiratory flow volume loops

      i. Inspiratory flow volume loop may show dynamic vocal cord closure or flattening consistent with variable extrathoracic airway obstruction

    c. Direct or video laryngoscopy—may be able to visualize abnormal vocal cord motion

    d. Exercise testing with simultaneous laryngoscopy

      i. Performed in specialized centers when vocal cord dysfunction is suspected and resting laryngoscopy is unremarkable and pulmonary function testing has been nondiagnostic

      ii. Graduated cardiopulmonary exercise testing (cycle-ergometer is preferred over treadmill) with direct vocal cord visualization to examine vocal cord motion during exercise

C. Treatment

  1. Acute management:

    a. Reassurance during exercise-induced episode

    b. Breathing techniques can be of help (in through nose and out through the mouth)

    c. Deep diaphragmatic breathing

    d. Panting may abort an episode by activation of the posterior cricoarytenoid muscles resulting in abduction of the true vocal cords

  2. Long-term management

    a. Reassurance about the diagnosis and absence of underlying asthma

    b. Speech therapy may be beneficial

    c. Psychological counseling may be needed in high stress or highly competitive individuals for biophysical feedback and management of performance-related anxiety and stress

    d. Treat underlying GERD if evidence of vocal cord inflammation is seen on laryngoscopy even if there are no symptoms of GERD

      i. Esophageal or hypopharyngeal pH monitors may help identify some cases.

VI. Chronic Obstructive Pulmonary Disease (COPD)

A. Sports-related issues

  1. COPD in young athletes is rare—disease usually occurs after the age of 35, but may develop earlier such as in alpha-1-antitripson deficiency

  2. May be encountered by the physician as part of general physical examination prior to starting an exercise program

  3. The physician will have a role in pulmonary rehabilitation and initiation of an exercise program

  4. Aging athletes are more common than in the past, so COPD may become more commonly seen in the athletic population

B. Definition

  1. Airflow obstruction seen on pulmonary spirometry, that is not fully reversible with bronchodilator, usually related to cigarette smoking

  2. Most common preventable smoking-related disease (more deaths and morbidity than smoking-related heart disease)

3. Three main categories
   a. Chronic bronchitis—daily productive cough for at least 3 months in two successive years
   b. Emphysema—abnormal and permanent enlargement of the airspaces distal to the terminal bronchiole
   c. Chronic asthma—chronic inflammation of the airways and hyperresponsiveness to inflammation and environmental exposures

C. Epidemiology
  1. Third leading cause of death in the United States in the year 2010. In 2000, accounted for 119,000 deaths with increasing mortality particularly among women
  2. Mortality data are likely under reported
  3. Death rate has increased more in the female population when compared to male
  4. Almost exclusively a tobacco smoking-related disease in developed countries
    a. Rarer causes include alpha-1-antitrypsan deficiency, heavy cannabis (marijuana) smoking, in home exposure to biomass fuels for heating and cooking (especially in undeveloped countries)

D. Diagnosis
  1. Clinical features
    a. Generally insidious in the onset with symptoms gradually developing over many years
    b. Often present with dyspnea, cough with or without production or wheezing
    c. May first present as a COPD exacerbation
      i. Increased sputum production
      ii. Increased wheezing
      iii. Fevers and chills
      iv. Increased shortness of breath
    d. Some patients have extremely sedentary lifestyle so present late in the course of disease
  2. Physical examination
    a. Early in the disease, physical exam may be unremarkable
    b. Pulmonary exam:
      i. Hyperinflation
      ii. Decreased breath sounds
      iii. Wheezing
      iv. Course or medium crackles in the lung bases
      v. Prolonged phase of expiration
      vi. Increase in the anteroposterior diameter of the chest
      vii. Use of accessory muscles during quiet breathing
  3. Diagnostic studies
    a. Pulmonary function studies required for the diagnosis
    b. Spirometry
      i. Will show obstruction defined as a reduced FEV1 to FVC ratio less than lower limit of normal (~0.7, but lower in the elderly)
      ii. Degree of reduction of the FEV1 defines the severity and stage of disease
        (A) Mild obstruction—reduced FEV1:FVC ratio with postbronchodilator FEV1 $\geq$80% of predicted value
        (B) Moderate obstruction—reduced FEV1:FVC ratio with FEV1 <80% and $\geq$50% of predicted value
        (C) Severe obstruction—reduced FEV1:FVC ratio with FEV1 <50% and $\geq$30% of predicted value
        (D) Very severe obstruction—reduced FEV1:FVC ratio with FEV1 <30% of predicted value
    c. Other

        i. Reduced DLCO correlates with presence of emphysema
       ii. Lung volumes show air trapping and hyperinflation
   d. Radiographic studies
        i. Plain film chest X-ray poor diagnostic study for identifying COPD, may show hyperinflation
       ii. Chest CT more sensitive for the diagnosis of emphysema and bronchial wall thickening

E. Treatment
   1. Avoidance of irritants and smoking
   2. Keep immunizations up to date (i.e., Pneumovax and yearly influenza)
   3. Pulmonary rehabilitation and exercise
      a. Exercise is an essential part of maintaining good quality of life for patients with COPD at any stage
      b. Patients may be enrolled in a formal and structured pulmonary rehabilitation program which consists of upper and lower extremity muscle training as well as aerobic/cardio-vascular exercise training in a gradually increasing fashion
   4. Medications
      a. Pharmacotherapy indicated to reduce symptoms and exacerbations, and improve exercise tolerance
      b. Bronchodilators—consist of inhaled β-agonists and anticholinergics
        i. Definition
           (A) β-agonist—activates β-2 receptors on smooth muscles within the airway
             (1) Available in both short- and long-acting
           (B) Anticholinergic—blocks the cholinergic activation of smooth muscle contraction within the airway
             (1) Available in both short- and long-acting
       ii. Main therapy
           (A) Short acting used for intermittent symptoms and mild disease as well as for immediate relief of symptoms
           (B) Long acting used for persistent symptom relief in moderate-to-very severe disease (FEV1 $\leq 65\%$)
             (1) Improves exercise tolerance, quality of life, pulmonary function, and survival
             (2) Decreases frequency of acute exacerbations
      c. Inhaled corticosteroids—decrease airway inflammation
        i. Used to prevent exacerbation of symptoms
       ii. Recommended for patients who have frequent or recurrent COPD exacerbations (more than one event per year)
       iii. Little value as a single agent in COPD
       iv. Should be used in combination with long-acting bronchodilators (β-agonist or anticholinergic)
   5. Exercise-related issues
      a. Patients with COPD tend to be very sedentary, but need to exercise as part of pulmonary rehabilitation and for preservation of functional status
      b. Short-acting bronchodilators should be used prior to exercise and as needed during exercise to control symptoms of wheezing and worsening dyspnea
      c. Oxygen supplementation may be used during exercise for patients who are shown to have exercise-induced hypoxia (SaO$_2$ $\leq 88\%$)
        i. Improves exercise performance and decreases symptoms but has not been shown to improve survival.

Recommended Reading

1. Bateman ED, Boulet LP, Cruz AA, et al. *Global Strategy for Asthma Management and Prevention 2009 (update).*
2. Celli BR, MacNee W. Standards for the diagnosis and treatment of patients with COPD: A summary of the ATS/ERS position paper. *Eur Respir J.* 2004;23:932–946.
3. Global Initiative for Chronic Obstructive Lung Disease strategy for the diagnosis, management and prevention of chronic obstructive pulmonary disease: An Asia-Pacific perspective. *Respirology.* 2005;10:9–17.
4. Parsons JP, Mastronarde JG. Exercise-induced bronchoconstriction in athletes. *Chest.* 2005;128:3966–3974.
5. Ratjen F, Doring G. Cystic fibrosis. *Lancet.* 2003;361:681–689.
6. Ries AL, Bauldoff GS, Carlin BW., et al. Pulmonary rehabilitation: Joint ACCP/AACVPR evidence-based clinical practice guidelines. *Chest.* 2007;131:4S–42S.
7. Weiler JM, Bonini S, Coifman R, et al. American Academy of Allergy, Asthma & Immunology Work Group report: Exercise-induced asthma. *J Allergy Clin Immunol.* 2007;119:1349–1358.

35

Sports Gastroenterology and Abdominal Injuries and Conditions

Ashwin Rao

I. Anatomy and Function

A. Abdominal musculature

  1. Anatomy:

    a. The muscular layer of the abdomen is made up of four flat muscles: the external obliques, the internal obliques, the transversus abdominis, and the rectus abdominis

    b. Rectus sheath

      i. The rectus sheath consists of the rectus abdominis muscle, an enveloping fascial sheath, and their blood supply via the epigastric arteries and veins

      ii. The rectus abdominis includes two parallel muscle groups, arising from the pubic symphysis medially and pubic crest laterally. They insert onto the ventral aspects of the fifth, sixth, and seventh costal cartilages and the xyphoid process, and are separated in the middle by the linea alba, with lateral borders consisting of the linea semilunaris

      iii. Innervation of the rectus abdominis comes from the lower six thoracic nerves.

  2. Function

    a. Abdominal wall musculature can be defined in terms of stabilizing and mobilizing function

    b. Stabilizers, including the internal oblique and transversus abdominis muscles, maintain posture and function against gravity

      i. The internal oblique assists in providing additional support to the abdomen and pelvis during spine rotation and flexion

      ii. The transversus abdominis is a key pelvic stabilizer, trunk stabilizer, and assists in stabilizing running and throwing activities

        (A) Contracts prior to lower limb musculature during foot strike

        (B) Contracts prior to arm and shoulder cocking during throwing activity

    c. Mobilizers, specifically the rectus abdominis and external oblique, function to accomplish ballistic movements

      i. The rectus abdominis principally flexes the spine and acts to compress the abdominal and pelvic cavities. Secondarily, it aids in respiration by depressing the lower rib cage and pulling the chest downward

      ii. The external oblique muscles are responsible in assisting spine flexion and rotation

B. Liver

  1. Anatomy

    a. Largest solid organ in the body—four-lobed structure

        b. Enclosed anteriorly and laterally by the rib cage in the right upper quadrant of the abdomen

        c. It's relatively fixed position, friable parenchyma, and thin capsule leave it prone to injury

        d. Two blood supplies

          i. Portal vein (70%)—carries blood from the GI tract

          ii. Hepatic arteries (30%)—carries oxygenated blood to the liver

    2. Function

        a. Assists in a wide variety of functions, including

          i. Glycogen storage

          ii. Plasma protein synthesis

          iii. Decomposition of red blood cells

          iv. Bile production

          v. Detoxification

        b. Function is both catabolic (breaking down of metabolites, insulin, hormones, toxic substances) and anabolic (gluconeogenesis, glycogenolysis, lipogenesis, coagulation cascade)

C. Spleen

    1. Anatomy

        a. Functionally complex organ situated in the left upper quadrant of the abdomen, surrounded anteriorly, posteriorly, and laterally by the 9th–11th ribs

        b. The position of the spleen is secured by the gastrosplenic, splenorenal, splenocolic, and splenophrenic ligaments

        c. Splenic artery

          i. Divides into >5 smaller branches that do not anastamose

          ii. Damage to one branch will result in segmental splenic infarction

    2. Function

        a. Mechanically filters red blood cells and is active in the immune system.

        b. The most vascular organ in the body, with an average pass through of 350 L of blood per day

        c. The spleen contains approximately 1 unit of blood at any given time

D. Gall bladder

    1. Small organ which stores bile produced by the liver and aids in the digestion of ingested fats

    2. Sits immediately below the liver, measuring approximately 8 cm in length and 4 cm in diameter when distended

    3. Rarely the cause of exercise-related symptoms, though gallstones can become symptomatic in the context of exercise

E. Small intestine

    1. The component of the gastrointestinal tract connecting stomach and colon, where the majority of digestion takes pace

    2. Measures 3–7 m in length

    3. Three segments: the duodenum, jejenum, and ileum

    4. Food contents move from the stomach into the duodenum through the pyloric sphincter

    5. Food contents are processed and passed through the small intestine via peristalsis

    6. Nutrient absorption occurs through microscopic fingerlike projections along the mucosal lining of the small intestine known as villi

F. Large intestine

    1. Principal organ in the GI tract responsible for water reabsorption and final processing of indigestible food matter

    2. Consists of the cecum and colon

    3. Typically 1.5 m long

G. Pancreas
1. Organ of the digestive tract serving both endocrine (insulin, glucagon, and somatostatin) and exocrine (production of digestive enzymes which aid in processing food) function
2. Exercise-associated pancreatitis is rarely reported in individuals with hypertriglyceridemia, prior pancreatic anatomic abnormality or variant, or with history of prior surgery of the sphincter of Oddi.

II. Epidemiology, Diagnosis, and Treatment

A. Overview
1. Exercise can have a significant influence on GI physiology, which in turn can cause a myriad of GI complaints in the athlete
2. Potential sources of exercise associated GI symptoms
    a. Decreased splanchnic blood flow
        i. Produces changes in intestinal permeability
            (A) Intra-luminal substrates (bile, pancreatic juices, or bacteria) may enter through the intestinal wall into the circulation
    b. Carbohydrate solutions ingested by athletes will increase osmotically driven intraluminal fluid resulting in bloating or diarrhea
    c. Mechanical compression of the gut by the psoas muscle
    d. A potential alteration in GI-related hormones (somatostatin, glucagon, secretin, vasoactive intestinal peptide) during exercise
B. Exercise-related transient abdominal pain (ETAP)
1. Background
    a. Nearly every person engaged in recreational or competitive exercise has experienced side stitches, side cramps, or side aches, which are encompassed in the phenomenon of ETAP
    b. Incidence is highest in runners, with nearly 20% annual reported incidence, with a 10–20% recurrence rate
2. History
    a. Patient typically reports a well localized pain in any area of the abdomen, typically sharp, stabbing, or cramping
    b. Pain usually localizes laterally, more commonly on the right side in adults and more commonly left-sided in children aged 7–16 years old
    c. Seen in activities other than running, which involve repetitive torso movement (vertical translation or rotation)
    d. Etiology is unclear, with postulates including transient diaphragmatic ischemia or spasm, peritoneal ligament stress, exertional peritonitis, or pleural irritation
3. Physical exam
    a. Patients usually present when asymptomatic, as symptoms are closely linked to exercise and resolve immediately following cessation of offending activity
4. Diagnosis and treatment
    a. Diagnosis is typically clinical and must be differentiated from other causes of abdominal pain such as abdominal wall strain, renal or gall stones, ischemic colitis, pancreatitis, or splenic dysfunction
    b. Prevention and treatment strategies are less apparent, due to a lack of clear understanding of physiology of the process
    c. Avoid offending foods high in sugar, fatty foods, or fruit/fruit juices, dairy products immediately prior to exercise
    d. Avoid larger meals or fluid consumption prior to exercise
    e. Reduce exercise pace and intensity.
    f. Stretch right arm over head and exhale through pursed lips

C. Liver laceration and contusion
1. Background
   a. Majority of injury to the liver is blunt abdominal trauma (i.e., helmet to the abdomen)
      i. The liver accounts for 15–20% of blunt abdominal trauma
      ii. Liver trauma accounts, however, for 50% of deaths from blunt abdominal trauma
   b. One of the two most common organs to be injured by blunt trauma, along with the spleen
   c. Due to its proximity to the rib cage, the right side of the liver is more prone to laceration than the left
   d. More than 85% of liver injury occurs to segments 6, 7, and 8 of the liver
   e. The liver's ligamentous attachment to the diaphragm and posterior abdominal wall may act as sites of shearing injury during rapid deceleration
      i. This can be seen in field sports requiring rapid changes in position (i.e., football, soccer, hockey, lacrosse)
   f. Liver injury is more common in children, given increased flexibility of the ribs and resultant increased force transmittal to the liver parenchyma, coupled with less developed framework of liver parenchyma in the pediatric population
2. History
   a. More common in athletes participating in contact sports
   b. Direct abdominal trauma is the usual mechanism
   c. Typically right upper quadrant (RUQ) pain with referred shoulder pain
3. Physical exam
   a. Tenderness in the RUQ, which may become more generalized and diffuse
   b. Patient may present with an acute abdomen, with substantial guarding and rebound tenderness
   c. Patient may be unable to stand straight due to increased abdominal pressure in this position
   d. Nausea and vomiting may be presenting symptoms
   e. Pulse may be elevated due to pain and/or blood loss
   f. Blood pressure may begin to drop if significant bleeding occurs (hypovolemic shock)
4. Diagnosis and treatment
   a. Inpatient treatment is generally required for monitoring and potential intervention
   b. Diagnosis is confirmed by computed tomography imaging (CT scan) and/or diagnostic peritoneal lavage
   c. Monitoring for intraabdominal blood loss may be performed through serial hematocrit checks
   d. Unstable cases may require surgical exploration and to identify laceration and achieve hemostasis
   e. The majority of cases (80% adults, 97% children) resolve with observation (i.e., without surgical intervention)
   f. Complications—Liver trauma may result in any of the following resultant complications
      i. Subscapular or intrahepatic hematoma
      ii. Contusion and hematoma
      iii. Hepatic vascular disruption
      iv. Bile duct injury
D. Spleen laceration and contusion
1. Background
   a. Laceration of the spleen represents a life-threatening circumstance, due to the volume of blood and functional flow of blood through this organ
   b. Splenic injuries represent 25% of all blunt abdominal injuries
   c. Peak incidence is in the age 15–35
   d. Slight male predominance, with a 3:2 ratio

2. History
   a. Presentation may be subtle to dramatic, similar to intraabdominal hepatic trauma
   b. Typical presentation involves acute onset of left upper quadrant and flank pain which may be accompanied by referred left shoulder pain (Kehr's sign)
3. Physical exam
   a. Abdominal distention and tenderness may be present in 50% of cases
   b. Hypotension may be seen in 20–30% of instances
   c. Younger patients may be able to accommodate hemodynamic losses more successfully than older patients. Thus presentation may be more subtle in younger athletes.
4. Diagnosis and treatment
   a. Conservative treatment includes diagnosis via CT scan (with IV contrast) and close inpatient monitoring with serial hematocrits and exams.
   b. Interventional treatment may include surgery, including splenectomy or ligation of splenic vasculature
      i. Postsplenectomy precautions
         (A) *H. influenza* type b, pneumococcal, and meningococcal (encapsulated bacteria) vaccinations
         (B) Those with sickle cell disease, thalassemia, or cancer—daily penicillin prophylaxis for pneumococcal infection
5. Return to play—controversial
   a. Nonoperative treatment
      i. 2–6 months based on injury severity
   b. Surgical treatment
      i. At least 6 weeks postoperative
   c. Infectious mononucleosis
      i. Splenic rupture has been reported to occur on days 4–21 postinfection
      ii. Asymptomatic athletes with a normal spleen size—gradual return to play at day 21
E. Rectus hematoma
   1. Background
      a. Relatively rare and often clinically misdiagnosed cause of abdominal pain
      b. Bleeding into the rectus sheath relates to trauma to the superior or inferior epigastric arteries or their branches or from a direct tear of the rectus musculature
      c. Mimics almost any abdominal condition
      d. The rectus sheath can accommodate a substantial amount of blood, and thus injuries can result in associated hypovolemic shock and mortality
   2. History
      a. There may be a h/o direct trauma or recurrent forceful contraction of the rectus abdominis musculature (valsalva)
      b. Patients may present with acute abdominal pain, fever, nausea, and vomiting, along with tenesmus, bladder irritability, and diarrhea
      c. Symptoms may progress to involve hypovolemic shock, confusion, and other mental status changes
      d. Patient may report pain in conjunction with a concomitant abdominal growing mass
         i. Pain may be constant, with accompanied abdominal cramping
      e. Pain is typically worse with movement
      f. Symptoms may evolve over hours
      g. Symptoms may correlate directly to the severity of peritoneal irritation.
   3. Physical exam
      a. Findings may be nonspecific and can include
         i. Abdominal pain to palpation
         ii. Abdominal mass, typically nonpulsatile, unilateral, painful and firm
      b. Low-grade fever is common; thus, assess temperature

4. Diagnosis and treatment
   a. The Fothergill sign is useful in differentiating an abdominal wall mass from an intra-abdominal mass
      i. Voluntary contraction of the rectus muscles by the patient lifting his/her head or legs while in the supine position
      ii. With this action, rectus sheath hematomas become fixed, with more pain and increased size, while intraabdominal masses become less distinct and less tender
   b. Confirmed by CT scan—with this classification scale:
      i. Type I: Intramuscular hematoma; an increase in the size of the muscle is observed
         (A) Ovoid or fusiform, with hyper-dense foci or a diffusely increased density
         (B) The hematoma is unilateral and does not dissect along the fascial planes
         (C) The patient presents with mild-to-moderate abdominal pain and typically does not require hospitalization
         (D) Type I hematomas typically resolve within 1 month
      ii. Type II: The hematoma is intramuscular (mimicking type I) but with blood between the muscle and the transversalis fascia
         (A) It may be unilateral but is usually bilateral, and no blood is observed occupying the visceral space
         (B) A fall in hematocrit may be observed. A patient may require hospitalization for close observation, but most do not require transfusions, and most are discharged within 3 days
         (C) Type II hematomas usually resolve within 2–4 months
      iii. Type III: The hematoma may or may not affect the muscle, and blood is observed between the transversalis fascia and the muscle, or within the peritoneum
         (A) Hematocrit drop is noted, and occasionally, hemoperitoneum is produced
         (B) These patients often require anti-coagulation (i.e. Warfarin)
         (C) Hospitalization and transfusion is typically required
         (D) Only rarely will patients develop hemodynamic instability that cannot be controlled with fresh frozen plasma and fluid resuscitation
         (E) Unstable patients may require surgical intervention
         (F) Type III hematomas usually resolve within 3 months
   c. Course is usually benign, requiring observation
   d. Overall mortality rate, if untreated has been reported as high as 4%, increasing to 25% if a patient is under anticoagulation therapy

F. Abdominal strains and contusions
   1. Background
      a. Strains of the abdominal wall occur in a wide variety of sports that require the use of abdominal musculature as part of sports-specific tasks and activity (tennis, lacrosse, gymnastics, baseball, jumping sports)
      b. Abdominal strains are usually due to indirect trauma rather than direct blows to the abdomen
      c. Most abdominal wall injuries involve the rectus abdominis and obliques
      d. The true incidence of such injuries is not known but thought to be quite common
      e. Injuries can be debilitating and cause prolonged periods of discomfort and prolonged withdrawal from competition
   2. History
      a. Pain is typically localized to a specific area (1–2 finger breadths), with a specific movement
      b. The most frequent sites of abdominal wall pain (in descending frequency) are the linea semilunaris, linea alba, rectus muscle, and the cartilaginous portions of the ribs
         i. Differential diagnosis may include cutaneous nerve entrapment, myofascial trigger points, athletic pubalgia with referred pain, and intraabdominal pathology

c. Mechanism of injury varies widely and may be sports specific

    i. In tennis, overloading of the abdominal musculature during the service motion can cause injury to the rectus abdominis and oblique musculature, due to force transferred via angular momentum from racket swing, accompanied by trunk rotation and flexion

    ii. Female gymnasts can develop severe bruising in the lower abdominal and ASIS by performing the beat maneuver on uneven bars, which involves hanging from the high bar and dropping the anterior pelvis and hips onto the lower bar

3. Physical exam

    a. Functional examination of the abdominal musculature during isometric, concentric, eccentric, and plyometric contraction may be warranted, as this evaluation can shed light on injury mechanism and severity, along with facilitating rehabilitation decisions and return to play

    b. There is usually tenderness of the muscle at the site of perceived pain

    c. The rectus abdominis may be isolated by asking the supine patient to lift the head and shoulders from the table

4. Diagnosis and treatment

    a. Imaging studies are not typically necessary, as diagnosis is clinical

    b. Diagnostic musculoskeletal ultrasound (U/S) can be helpful in identifying the site of injury

        i. U/S will demonstrate disruption of the normal fibrillar pattern of muscular orientation, with fluid-filled clefts and ground glass appearance of torn muscle

    c. MRI is also helpful in characterizing the injured site, identifying areas of muscular disruption on fluid weighted (T2, STIR) pulse sequences

    d. Treatment includes

        i. Abstinence from the offending activity

        ii. Cryotherapy (ice)

        iii. Five-step rehabilitation program

            (A) Initiate pain and inflammation control, primarily through rest and cryotherapy

            (B) Isometric strengthening and stretching

            (C) Concentric strengthening

            (D) Eccentric-plyometric strengthening

            (E) Maintenance phase and reinjury prevention

        iv. Mistakes in treatment typically involve early return to competition and insufficient eccentric strengthening of the abdominal musculature

G. Ischemic colitis

1. Background

    a. A set of various conditions that leads to insufficient blood supply delivered to part or all of the colon

    b. Severity is wide ranging, from transient mucosal involvement to full thickness transmural necrosis of the bowel

    c. While ischemic bowel disease is typically a condition of older age, a variety of other circumstances may cause this condition to occur in a younger athletic population, including blunt abdominal trauma, hypercoagulable state, embolic disease, hypovolemic shock, and shunting of blood away from the bowel

    d. Ischemic colitis is considered a serious complication of endurance athletic activities such as long-distance running

        i. In endurance athletes, shunting of blood away from the bowel due to splanchnic vasoconstriction, along with an accompanying hypovolemic state from exercise-related intravascular volume depletion, may be sufficient to induce this condition

        ii. Endurance runners may manifest bloody diarrhea due to transient ischemic colitis with colonic mucosal infarction

   e. Other underlying causes:
      i. Sickle cell disease
      ii. Hypercoagulable state
      iii. Thromboangitis obliterans
 2. History
   a. Patient may present with colicky abdominal pain that becomes constant, and often is accompanied by vomiting, diarrhea, and/or rectal bleeding
   b. Underlying causes (see gi5 above)
 3. Physical exam
   a. Diffuse abdominal pain on palpation, without a clearly acute abdomen
   b. Signs of hypovolemia/dehydration may present concomitantly
 4. Diagnosis and treatment
   a. Inpatient hospitalization with bowel rest, IV hydration
   b. Diagnosis can be obtained through elective flexible sigmodiscopy with biopsy, though this is rarely required
   c. Double-contrast barium enema may be helpful in identifying regions of colitis
   d. Traditionally, angiography (either CTA or MRA) is used to evaluate the splanchnic vessels to identify areas of stricture (i.e., calcified plaques)
H. Gastrointestinal bleeding
 1. Background
   a. Exercise may reduce splanchnic blood flow by up to 80%, causing transient ischemia of the colon and intestine
   b. Transient ischemia of the GI tract can cause infarction and bleeding of GI mucosa
   c. Long-distance runners, who experience both decrease in splanchnic blood flow and dehydration, may be at particular risk of GI bleeding
   d. Exercise might prompt dysfunction of the upper and lower esophageal spincters and may cause increased secretion of gastrin and pepsin
   e. In recent studies, up to 27% of recreational triathletes, 20% of marathon runners, and 87% of ultramarathoners have tested positive for stool occult blood, with overt hematochezia reported in 6% of runners completing a marathon
 2. History
   a. Presentation may vary greatly
   b. Some athletes may present with general malaise and fatigue, and laboratory work up may identify an iron-deficiency anemia
   c. Other athletes may present with GERD symptoms, nausea, and/or vomiting
 3. Physical exam
   a. Often unremarkable
   b. Rectal exam searching for hemorroids, fissure, mass, heme-occult testing
 4. Diagnosis and treatment
   a. Athletes may need to change exercise and dietary regimens
   b. Prevent dehydration during exercise to limit intestinal ischemia
   c. Avoidance of injurious drugs (NSAIDs)
   d. Trial of proton pump inhibitor for individuals suffering GERD symptoms
I. Gastroesophageal reflux disease (GERD) and peptic ulcer disease (PUD)
 1. Background
   a. GERD is one of the most common disorders in the general population and is thus a common complaint among athletes
      i. 10% of the American population report daily heartburn symptoms, with 30–40% report symptoms at least once during the month
   b. Increased exposure of food contents and acidity at the lower esophagus may produce esophageal mucosal damage and erosion

    c. Complications of GERD include peptic ulcers (2–7% of cases), hemorrhage (<2%), stricture (4–20%), and Barrett's esophagus (10–15%)

    d. Exercise (particularly endurance exercise) is a known exacerbating factor in individuals with GERD

        i. Up to 36% of healthy runners, 67% of cyclists, and 52–54% of triathletes experienced heartburn and/or chest pain consistent with GERD during exercise

        ii. Running, cycling, weight lifting, and rowing is associated with the highest risk of GERD in the athletic population

    e. Exercise may slow gastric motility and alter hydrogen ion secretion (gastric acid production increases), decrease splanchnic blood flow, increase intraabdominal pressure, change motor function of the esophagus, and may alter function of the lower esophageal sphincter, all predisposing an athlete to experiencing GERD symptoms during exercise

    f. Reflux episodes seem to be associated with the length and intensity of exercise, postprandial state, and potentially carbohydrate consumption

    g. Symptoms of GERD and PUD cross over substantially, and PUD should be suspected with recurrent episodes of "GERD" symptoms or treatment failure

2. History

    a. The athlete typically will present with symptoms of heartburn and epigastric abdominal pain, typically worse at night and with exercise, potentially meal-related pain (consider peptic or esophageal ulcer disease)

    b. The patient may report a foul acid taste in the mouth

    c. If untreated, GERD may progress to PUD

3. Physical exam

    a. Tenderness may be present in the epigastrium, though there should be no guarding, mass, or rebound tenderness

4. Diagnosis and treatment

    a. Diagnosis is typically clinical, based on history and physical findings

    b. Successful treatment directed at GERD typically involves a 2-week course of a high dose proton-pump inhibitor (PPI), which may be sufficient to solidify the diagnosis without further testing.

    c. H2 receptor antagonists are a second common medication used to treat symptoms

    d. Antacids can be used though:

        i. Those containing calcium and aluminum may cause constipation

        ii. Those containing magnesium may cause diarrhea

    e. In older patients, endoscopy may be indicated for persistent or atypical symptoms, to exclude stricture, hiatal hernia, or Barrett's esophagus, which is a precursor to esophageal adenocarcinoma

    f. Activity and diet modification are typically encouraged as adjunct treatment. Modifications include:

        i. Avoiding food consumption within 30 min from initiation of exercise

        ii. Avoiding large protein or fat intake prior to exercise

        iii. Avoiding dairy and citrus consumption

        iv. Avoidance of chocolate, coffee, or hypertonic solutions prior to exercise

    g. Should symptoms persist despite PPI treatment, consider evaluation for PUD via endoscopy with biopsy and serum *Helicobacter pylori* antigen testing

        i. Eradication of *H. pylori* requires "triple therapy (e.g., Prevpac: lansoprazole, amoxicillin, clarithromycin)" regimen, that usually involves the use of a proton pump inhibitor coupled with a penicillin and a macrolide antibiotic (substitute metronidazole for penicillin-allergic patients), for a 2-week course

J. Motility disorders

  1. Diarrhea

    a. Background

    ii. Runner's diarrhea is a common occurrence with long distance, endurance exercises (runner's trots)

    iii. Up to 26% of marathon runners have reported diarrhea, while 54% have reported fecal urgency

    iv. The mechanisms of diarrhea in exercise are not clearly understood. Mental stress, exertion, hyperthermia, dehydration, hypoglycemia, fatigue, and increased sympathetic nervous system activity, acting to shunt blood away from the viscera in favor of supplying working muscles, are all potential sources

    v. Exercising at 70% of VO_2 max may reduce blood flow to the gastrointestinal tract by 60–70%, and more intense exercise may decrease splanchnic blood flow in excess of 80%; though gastric emptying is slowed at this intensity of exercise

    vi. Worsening visceral ischemia and suppressed parasympathetic activity may manifest as intestinal mucosal dysfunction (i.e., colonic malabsorption, and hence diarrhea)

    vii. Sports drinks and gels with carbohydrate concentrations exceeding 7–10% may cause fecal urgency and diarrhea (dumping syndrome)

    viii. Gastric emptying times are decreased by:

        (A) Colder liquids

        (B) >7–10% carbohydrate solutions

        (C) Ingesting larger volumes

        (D) Exercise <70% VO_2 max

    ix. Runner's diarrhea can cause a decline in performance, due to stops required to attend to the issue, along with increased risk of dehydration, heat injury, rhabdomyolysis, and acute tubular necrosis

b. History

    i. Increase in stool frequency and volume (watery stools) with intense endurance training

    ii. Assess for concomitant bloody stool, related to mucosal ischemia, accompanying diarrhea. The physician should assess for other causes of bloody stool, including infection, inflammatory bowel disease, malignancy, and NSAID use

    iii. May be associated with diffuse, nonlocalized abdominal pain

    iv. Sense of incomplete voiding (tenesmus) present

    v. Evaluate for changes in training intensity and regimen, as well as change in diet

c. Physical exam

    i. Nonspecific, diffused abdominal pain on palpation

    ii. Assess for signs of organic pathology

d. Diagnosis and treatment

    i. Diagnosis is clinical

    ii. Treatment includes

        (A) Avoidance of food consumption 2–3 h prior to run; avoid binge eating

        (B) Decrease intake of dietary sugars (lactose, fructose), sorbitol and aspartame, avoiding high-energy, hypertonic foods and drinks during exercise,

        (C) Decrease caffeine intake and dietary fiber

        (D) Avoid use of NSAID's, EtOH, caffeine, antibiotics during exercise

        (E) Temporary decrease in duration and intensity (20–25%), with slow return to activity based on symptoms over 1–2 weeks

        (F) Antidiarrheal medications with anticholinerigic effects (Lomotil) should be used with caution due to associated risk of med-related hyperthermia (secondary to decreased sweating)

        (G) Loperamide is safer, but may have detrimental effects on athletic performance

        (H) Urinate and defecate prior to exercise.

Recommended Reading

1. Atkins JM, Taylor JC, Kane SF. Acute and overuse injuries of the abdomen and groin in athletes. *Curr Sports Med Rep.* 2010;9(2):115–120.
2. Ho GWK. Lower gastrointestinal distress in endurance athletes. *Curr Sports Med Rep.* 2009;8(2):85–91.
3. Jozkow P, Wasko-Czopnik D, Medras M, Paradowski L. Gastroesophageal reflux disease and physical activity. *Sports Med.* 2006;36(5):385–391.
4. Maquirriain J, Ghisi JP, Kokalj AM. Rectus abdominis muscle strains in tennis players. *Br J Sports Med.* 2007;41:842–848.
5. Paluska SA. Current concepts: Recognition and management of common activity-related gastrointestinal disorders. *Phys Sportsmed.* 2009;37(1):54–63.
6. Prado de Oliveira E, Burini RC. The impact of physical exercise on the gastrointestinal tract. *Curr Opin Clin Nutr Metab Care.* 2009;12:533–538.
7. Thompson JC. *Netter's Concise Atlas of Orthopaedic Anatomy,* Philadelphia: Saunders Elsevier; 2002.
8. Viola TA. Evaluation of the athlete with exertional abdominal pain. *Curr Sports Med Rep.* 2010;9(2):106–110.

36

Sports Nephrology and Urology

Cameron L. Trubey and Mark E. Lavallee

I. Exertional Rhabdomyolysis

A. Physiology

   1. Strenuous exercise elicits striated muscle cell membrane breakdown and leakage of muscle enzymes and intracellular components into the blood. Serum creatine kinase (CK) rises and myoglobinuria occurs when myoglobin in the blood exceeds 3 mg/L

   2. Myoglobin, the oxygen-carrying component of muscle, is damaging to renal tubules and may cause acute tubular necrosis

   3. During exercise, increased levels of epinephrine and norepinephrine cause arteriole vasoconstriction; blood flow to the kidneys decreases

      a. At 50% VO_2 max, renal flow decreases by 30%, at 65% VO_2 max, renal flow decreases by 75%

   4. Relative dehydration and subsequent physiologic decrease in renal perfusion further diminish clearance of muscle breakdown products

   5. Usually follows a benign course but can lead to renal failure and death

B. Symptoms

   1. Muscle pain (beginning 24–72 h after exercise), soreness, swelling; stiffness, fatigue

C. Signs

   1. Dark-colored urine ("cola-colored" or "tea-colored"), muscle swelling

D. Risk factors

   1. Eccentric muscle activity (causes extensive muscle damage)

   2. Dehydration

   3. Novel overexertion

   4. Heat stress

   5. Viral illness or infectious disease

   6. Certain drugs (e.g., stimulants, statins, anticholinergics)

   7. Sickle cell trait

   8. Underlying metabolic myopathy

E. Diagnosis

   1. History of (strenuous) exercise or muscle injury

   2. Muscle pain, weakness, swelling, or dark-colored urine

   3. Elevated serum markers: CK (≥ 5 times normal, peak 12–96 h after exercise), LDH, aldolase, AST, potassium

   4. No clear diagnostic cutoff exists for elevated CK. Elevations to 5000 and more can be seen in asymptomatic athletes with exercise

   5. Urinalysis with myoglobinuria, granular casts; no red blood cells (RBCs)

F. Treatment
  1. Aggressive hydration until urine is clear, muscle enzyme levels drop, or myoglobinuria stops. Intravenous (IV) fluids often necessary. Goal urinary output of 200–300 mL/h
  2. Bicarbonate may be added to IV fluids to maintain urine pH > 7.5
  3. Monitor electrolyte levels; watch for hyperkalemia and hyperphosphatemia. Follow BUN and creatinine to assess renal function
  4. Dialysis needed on rare occasions
  5. Return-to-play guidelines are complex, even for the low-risk athlete. Recommendations include gradually progressing intensity and volume of exercise with submaximal exertion lasting weeks

G. Potential complications of exertional rhabdomyolysis
  1. Compartment syndrome from muscle swelling
  2. Leaked intracellular potassium can trigger cardiac arrhythmias
  3. Metabolic acidosis
  4. Myoglobinuric renal failure.

II. Urine Markers

A. Hematuria
  1. More than two cells per high-power field (HPF) in centrifuged urine.
  2. Urine dipstick is very sensitive—detects 1–2 cells per HPF
     a. Myoglobin, a muscle breakdown product, will elicit false "positive" response for presence of hematuria on most dipsticks
     b. Presence of hematuria, hemoglobinuria, and myoglobinuria will all result in a "positive" urine dipstick
  3. Caused by vascular leakage into the urinary tract, most often from the lower tract, the bladder, urethra, and prostate
  4. Asymptomatic hematuria is present in 5–6% of the general population, and 4% of children
     a. Eighty percent of children and 15–20% of adults with hematuria will have no identifiable cause
  5. Potential causes
     a. Trauma—Renal—minor to severe, amount of hematuria not indicative of degree of injury
     b. Prolonged and severe exercise
        i. Mechanisms
           (A) Increased body temperature
           (B) Hemolysis
           (C) Increased production of free radicals and catecholamine
           (D) Lactic acidosis, which increases glomerular permeability, allowing the passage of erythrocytes into urine
        ii. Microscopic hematuria reported to occur in 50–70% of marathon runners.
        iii. There is a higher incidence of hematuria in events that require greater oxygen uptake
     c. Drugs
        i. Nonsteroidal anti-inflammatory drugs (NSAIDs), sulfonamides, anticoagulants
     d. Sickle cell disease, hemophilia, thrombocytopenia, and other hematologic diseases
     e. Urinary tract infections
        i. Cystitis, prostatitis, urethritis
     f. Urinary tract calculi
     g. Hypoxic nephrons
     h. Vascular malformations, malignancy, autoimmune renal diseases

B. Hemoglobinuria
  1. Presence of hemoglobin in the urine

2. Causes
   a. Intravascular hemolysis of RBCs leads to extrusion of intracellular hemoglobin into the blood
   b. If amount of hemolysis is significant enough, hemoglobin will spill into the urine (hemoglobinuria—uncommon)
      i. "March" or "foot-strike" hemolysis
         (A) Hypothesized that older RBCs are more fragile and subject to lyse with trauma → "runner's macrocytosis"
         (B) Most commonly in runners; also reported in soldiers and in many other sports
         (C) Labs will show elevated mean corpuscular volume (MCV) and reticulocyte count (to compensate for RBC losses), with a low haptoglobin (free haptoglobin bound by free hemoglobin). Peripheral smear may show fragmented RBCs (schistocytes)
      ii. Incidence of hemolysis is related to the intensity of acute exercise
      iii. Contributors to exercise hemolysis
         (A) Hardness of running surface
         (B) Increased fragility of RBC membrane
            (1) Elevated body temperature
            (2) Exertional oxidative stress
            (3) Congenital RBC fragility
            (4) Possibly increased intravascular turbulence
   c. Hematuria/hemoglobinuria/myoglobinuria can be differentiated by gross examination of centrifuged urine
      i. Hematuria → presence of RBCs
      ii. Hemoglobinuria → supernatant = pink
      iii. Myoglobinuria → supernatant = clear
C. Myoglobinuria
   1. Myoglobin is the oxygen-carrying unit of the muscle. Muscle cell membrane damage during strenuous activity causes leakage of water-soluble myoglobin into the blood and it is excreted into the urine. In high enough concentrations it is damaging to the renal tubules
D. Proteinuria
   1. Normal adults secrete 80–150 mg of protein into the urine daily
   2. Urine protein normally consists of 30% albumin, 30% serum globulins, and 40% tissue proteins. Normal concentration rarely exceeds 20 mg/dL
   3. Dipstick detection
      a. Detects protein concentration of 20–30 mg/dL
      b. Protein in urine causes pH shift that changes color on dipstick proportional to concentration.
   4. Transient proteinuria seen in response to
      a. Fever
      b. Pregnancy
      c. Emotional stress
      d. Exercise
         i. Cause of exercise-associated proteinuria
            (A) Filtration fraction doubles during exercise (despite decreases in renal plasma flow and glomerular filtration)
            (B) Exercise metabolites interfere with the glomerular barrier facilitating macromolecular filtration
            (C) Blood pH drops (increased blood lactate) alters glomerular permeability (anionic charge)

      ii. Thought to be related to muscular work intensity with intensity being more important than duration

      iii. Maximal urine-protein excretion occurs 20–30 min after strenuous exercise and persists for around 4 h.

III. Nephrolithiasis

A. Incidence

  1. Fifteen percent of White males and 6% all women (50% of individuals in each group will experience reoccurrence)

  2. Average age at occurrence

    a. Males: 45 years old (y.o.); Females: 41 y.o.

B. Types of stones

  1. 75% — calcium oxalate

  2. 20% — struvite

  3. 5% — uric acid

  4. <1% — cystine

C. Medications associated with increased stone risk

  1. Corticosteroids, vitamin C, vitamin D, vitamin B6, calcium supplementation, carbonic anhydrase inhibitors

D. Dietary risks associated with increased stone risk

  1. Low fluid intake, high sodium intake, ingestion of animal protein, low or excessive calcium diet, caffeine, low potassium intake

E. Diagnosis

  1. Identification of the presence of urologic calculi

    a. Urinalysis may show the presence of (microscopic) hematuria

    b. IV Pyelogram (Sensitivity = 64–87%; Specificity = 92–94%)

    c. Ultrasonography (sensitivity = 19%; specificity = 97%)

    d. Plain radiographs (sensitivity = 45–59%; specificity = 71–77%)

    e. Noncontrast helical computed tomography (CT) scan (sensitivity = 95–100%; specificity = 94–96%)

  2. Identify causative factors

    a. Volume status and dietary factors

    b. May require extensive workup and metabolic evaluation

F. Treatment

  1. Adequate hydration and analgesics (narcotics often required due to significant pain)

  2. Allow stone to pass

    a. <5 mm will usually pass spontaneously (98%)

    b. >1.0 cm will rarely pass (10%)

  3. Surgical intervention

    a. Depends on the type of stone present and the location

    b. Options include: Extracorporeal shockwave lithotripsy, ureteroscopy, and percutaneous nephrolithotomy.

IV. Pudendal Nerve Injury

A. Anatomy

  1. Somatic nerve (S 2,3,4) branching from the sacral plexus innervating external genitalia; provides motor component to bladder and rectal sphincter in both sexes

B. Pudendal neuropathy

  1. Increased risk with sports of prolonged perineal compression such as cycling and mountain biking

2. Symptoms
   a. Genital numbness and tingling (may only involve the distal penis/labia or may extend to the scrotum and peri-anal region depending on the level of compression)
   b. Difficulty achieving orgasm
   c. Reduced sensation of defecation
3. Epidemiology
   a. Lifetime prevalence among cyclists: 50–90%
   b. Incidence increases with increased age, increased body weight, cycling time
   c. Cycling for more than 10 years and for more than 3 h/week increase risk of occurrence

C. Etiology
   1. Potential points of nerve compression
      a. Proximally between the sacrospinal and sacrotuberous ligaments, stretching can occur during pedaling
      b. Increased friction within Alcock's canal from saddle pressure
      c. Anterior to the pelvic ring where it can be compressed in the soft tissues of the perineum by the nose of the bicycle saddle
   2. Compression may cause direct nerve compression or may impede pudendal arterial flow causing symptoms.

D. Treatment
   1. Cessation of riding until numbness completely resolves
   2. Ensure proper fitting of the bicycle and seat
   3. Saddle with central cutout has not been shown to be beneficial.

V. Scrotal Trauma

A. Penetrating trauma

B. Crush trauma
   1. Compression of the testicle against pubic arch and impacting object

C. Blunt trauma to the scrotum
   1. Seventy-five percent of testicle injuries occur from blunt trauma
   2. Blunt testis injury is bilateral 1.5% of the time
   3. Subcutaneous hematoma
      a. Blood collection between the tunica dartos and the tunica vaginalis
   4. Hematocele
      a. Liquefied hematoma or serous collection between leaves of the tunica vaginalis
   5. Epididymis/spermatic cord hematoma
      a. Epididymitis may occur after trauma
   6. Direct testicular injury
      a. Testicle rupture
         i. Tearing of the tunica albuginea with extrusion of testicular parenchyma into the scrotal sac
         ii. Usually associated with testicle laceration, fragmentation, intratesticular hematoma, or infarction
         iii. Surgical exploration is warranted if testicle injury is suspected
         iv. Ruptured testis can be salvaged in 90% of patients if repaired within 72 h, 55% after this time window
      b. Testicle contusion
      c. Testicle dislocation
         i. More common with straddle injuries where the testicle is relocated to superficial inguinal pouch; or pubic, penile, pelvic, abdominal, or perineal locations
      d. Traumatic testicular torsion

D. Physical examination
1. Often limited by pain
2. Swelling, ecchymosis are most common signs
3. Degree of scrotal hematoma is not correlative with severity of testis injury
4. Blood at the urethral meatus may indicate concomitant urethral injury

E. Imaging
1. Ultrasound of the scrotum
   a. Rapid, reliable, noninvasive
   b. May decrease the need for surgery in mild trauma cases

F. Management
1. Penetrating injuries nearly always require surgical exploration
2. Testicular rupture, large hematocele, traumatic torsion, and testicular dislocation all require surgery
3. Testicular contusions can often be managed conservatively with analgesics, bed rest, and NSAIDs.

VI. Testicular Torsion

A. Torsion of the spermatic cord (most commonly within the tunica vaginalis)

B. Most frequent cause of testicle loss in the adolescent

C. Most common in adolescents and young men one in 4,000 males < age 25

D. Will usually torse internally with anteromedial twisting of spermatic cord

E. Clinical presentation
1. Diagnosis is clinical and requires emergent surgical intervention
2. Sudden severe pain, abdominal discomfort, nausea, vomiting
3. Examination may show high-riding and tender testis, transversely oriented testis, scrotal erythema, acute hydrocele or scrotal edema, loss of cremasteric reflex (strong association with torsion)

F. Causes and risk factors
1. Abnormally mobile testis caused by lack of normal fixation of the testis and epididymis to the fascial and muscular coverings that surround the cord in the scrotum ("bell-clapper" deformity)
2. Previous, similar, transient scrotal pain (50%) is a common report
3. Can be secondary to trauma or, more commonly, occurs spontaneously

G. Treatment
1. Manual reduction should be attempted and may alleviate torsion but is not definitive treatment
   a. Attempt to rotate the testis lateral or outward to detorse
   b. A partial detorsion may alleviate symptoms but not ischemia
2. Emergent surgical exploration and fixation orchidopexy is indicated
   a. Contralateral side often fixated in same operation (prophylactic)

H. Detorsion timing—"time is testicle"
1. Younger age (<18) associated with increased delay in medical attention and subsequent increase in testicular loss.
2. Treatment within 4 h yields greater than 90% salvage rate
3. Irreversible ischemic injury to the testis occurs as soon as 4 h
4. >12 h = usual loss of the gonad

I. Imaging—consider only if it will not delay treatment.
1. Color Doppler ultrasound
   a. Assessment of anatomy, hydrocele, testicular blood flow
   b. Sensitivity = 88.9%. Specificity = 98.8%

2. Radionuclide imaging
   a. Only allows for blood flow analysis
   b. Sensitivity of 90%. Specificity of 89%.

VII. Renal Trauma

A. Causes
   1. Penetrating injury (rare in sports)
   2. Blunt trauma (most common mechanism in sports)
      a. More likely to cause renal injury in children than adults
      b. 16–30% of pediatric renal trauma is sports related
      c. Incidence of all types of abdominal trauma causing genitourinary injury is approximately 10%
   3. Sudden deceleration injury

B. Injured structures
   1. Kidney > Bladder > Urethra (Ordered by injury frequency)

C. Important indicators (absence of all three imparts very low likelihood of injury)
   1. Gross hematuria
      a. Not correlative with severity of injury
      b. May not be present initially in 25–50% of renal injuries
   2. Hypotension (only present in severe cases)
   3. Mechanism of injury (rapid deceleration or high fall)

D. Moderate indicators
   1. Flank hematoma or tenderness
   2. Rib fractures
   3. Penetrating injuries

E. Evaluation
   1. History and physical
      a. Sport and nature of injury
      b. Presence of gross hematuria
   2. Laboratory studies
      a. Urinalysis, complete blood count (CBC), electrolytes, liver function tests, creatinine, glucose, amylase, lipase, human chorionic gonadotropin (HCG)
   3. Imaging
      a. Plain films for rib fractures
      b. Bedside ultrasound
         i. Quick, portable, but suboptimal sensitivity
      c. Gold standard: contrast-enhanced computed tomography (CT) scan
         i. Threshold for ordering should be lower in children
         ii. CT findings
            (A) Medial hematoma
            (B) Medial extravasation on delayed images
            (C) Lack of parenchymal contrast on early phase

F. Management
   1. Grading (Organ Injury Severity Scale)—most sports related injuries are contusions of Grade 1. Higher injury grade is associated with increased morbidity and mortality and with the need for surgical management
      a. See Table 36.1
   2. Grade I–II: Generally observation and supportive care are adequate
      a. Bedrest, hydration, antibiotics
   3. Grade III–V: Likely needs surgical consult

Table 36.1   AAST Organ Injury Scale scores for the kidney

Grade		Injury description
I	Contusion	Microscopic or gross hematuria, urologic studies normal
	Hematoma	Subcapsular, nonexpanding without parenchymal lesion
II	Hematoma	Nonexpanding perirenal hematoma confined to renal retroperitoneum
	Laceration	<1 cm parenchymal depth of renal cortex without urinary extravasation
III	Laceration	>1 cm depth of renal cortex, without collecting system rupture or urinary extravasation
IV	Laceration	Parenchymal laceration extending through the renal cortex, medulla, and collecting system
	Vascular	Main renal artery or vein with contained hemorrhage
V	Laceration	Completely shattered kidney
	Vascular	Avulsion of renal hilum which devascularizes kidney

Advance one grade for multiple injuries to the same organ

Santucci RA, McAninch JW, Safir M, et al. Validation of the American Association for the Surgery of Trauma organ injury severity scale for the kidney. *J Trauma.* 2001;*50*(2):195–200.

4. Return to play (RTP)
   a. Wait for full resolution of hematuria
   b. Literature recommendations vary: 2–6 weeks
   c. More severe injuries necessitate longer time to RTP
      i. 6–12 months for more extensive renal injuries
G. Athletes with solitary kidney
   1. Injured solitary kidney requires urgent evaluation
   2. RTP with solitary kidney
      a. High-risk sports to be avoided
         i. Bicycling, dirt bikes, ATVs
      b. Moderate risk
         i. Skiing, snowboarding, in-line skating
      c. Contact and team sports have shown very low rate of kidney loss
      d. Full discussion with athlete/parent regarding risk is imperative
      e. Consider protective equipment/padding such as a flak jacket but no empiric evidence to support thus far.

Recommended Reading

1. Asplund C, Barkdull T, Weiss B. Genitourinary problems in bicyclists. *Curr Sports Med Rep.* 2007;6(5):333–339.
2. Bellinghieri G, Savica V, Santoro D. Renal alterations during exercise. *J Renal Nutr.* 2008;18(1):158–164.
3. Bernard JJ. Renal trauma: Evaluation, management, and return to play. *Curr Sports Med Rep.* 2009;8(2):98–103.
4. Brophy RH, Gamradt SC, Barnes RP, Powell JW, DelPizzo JJ, Rodeo SA, et al. Kidney injuries in professional American football: Implications for management of an athlete with 1 functioning kidney. *Am J Sports Med.* 2008;36(1):85–90.
5. O'Connor FG, Brennan FH Jr, Campbell W, Heled Y, Deuster P. Return to physical activity after exertional rhabdomyolysis. *Curr Sports Med Rep.* 2008;7(6):328–331.
6. Rosenberg J. Exertional rhabdomyolysis: Risk factors, presentation, and management. *Athletic Therapy Today.* 2008;13(3):11–12.
7. Styn NR, Wan J. Urologic sports injuries in children. *Curr Urol Rep.* 2010;11(2):114–121.

37

Sports Dermatology
Darryl E. Barnes

I. Mechanical Injuries

A. Abrasion
1. Trauma to epidermal layer resulting in bleeding/exudates
2. Common in contact sports
   a. Wrestling, football, baseball, sports with artificial turf
3. Clean wound with hydrogen peroxide, apply antibiotic ointment and sterile protective cover.
   a. Prevent thick crust build-up with moist dressings

B. Acne Mechanica
1. Chronic acneform eruption due to occlusive folliculitis
   a. Areas of friction and increased heat
      i. Back, chest, chin, shoulders, forehead
2. Prevent
   a. Absorbent material under padding
3. Oral antibiotic if necessary

C. Auricular Hematoma (Cauliflower ear)
1. Common in wrestlers
2. Posttraumatic hematoma between perichondrium and auricular cartilage. Interrupted blood flow results in aseptic necrosis, loss of cartilage, and deformed ear.
3. Treatment = Needle aspiration and external compression for 7–10 days

D. Black heel (Talon Noir)
1. Petechiae in upper edge of heel caused by shearing force related to stops and starts
2. Treatment not necessary
   a. May pare with scalpel to remove lesion

E. Callus
1. Epidermal hyperplasia over contact areas due to repetitive trauma
   a. May be helpful in protecting direct contact areas
2. Treatment not necessary
   a. Pumice stone, topical keratolytic agent or scalpel debridement if needed

F. Chafing
1. Erythema and ecchymosis resulting in hyperpigmentation
2. Mechanical friction between body parts or body parts and clothing
3. Treatment = lubricating agent (i.e., petroleum ointments or friction-reducing powder)

G. Corn (Clavus)
   1. Focal compact hyperkeratotic lesion located over bony prominence
   2. Treatment not necessary
      a. Pumice stone, topical keratolytic agent or scalpel debridement if needed
H. Friction blister
   1. Serous fluid collection under epidermis due to friction over contact area
   2. Treatment not necessary if it does not interfere with activity
      a. Prevent—ensure proper fitting equipment
      b. Decompress lesion if necessary
         i. Cleans area. Incise blister roof with scalpel or needle, leave collapsed dermis in place and apply ointment
I. Golfer's nails
   1. Nonblanching dark discoloration splinter hemorrhages of the nail bed
      a. Gripping club too tight
   2. Treatment—proper grip
J. Ingrown toe nail (Onychocryptosis)
   1. Lateral edge of nail grows into dermis
      a. Erythema and pain
   2. Prevent by trimming nails straight across.
   3. Treatment = Complete or partial removal of nail (matrix excision/orthonyxia)
K. Jogger's nipples
   1. Painful eroded and fissured nipples due to constant/repetitive friction
      a. Males > females
   2. Prevent with athletic bra, soft cloth wear, lubricating agent or tape
L. Piezogenic papules
   1. Skin-colored papules (2–5 mm) on medial or lateral heel
      a. Seen in heavy athletes or long-distance runners
   2. Benign—Heel cup may help if painful
M. Striae distensae (stretch marks)
   1. Lesion perpendicular to skin lines due to ruptured elastic fibers
      a. Increased muscle mass or weight gain
      b. Anterior shoulder, thigh, and low back
   2. No proven treatment.

II. Environmental-Induced Injuries

A. Chemical
   1. Chlorotrichosis (green hair) found in blonde, gray, or white-haired swimmers
      a. Exposure to copper ions from algaecides or copper pipes
      b. Treatment = 2–3% hydrogen peroxide for 30 min or Metolex
   2. Contact dermatitis—cutaneous irritation due to allergen or chemical exposure (i.e., soaps, poison ivy, latex, glue, etc.)
      a. Diagnosis = patch testing
      b. Treatment = avoid known irritating agents. Antihistamines, cool compresses, topical or oral corticosteroids
B. Weather
   1. Photoinjury (sunburn)
      a. Erythematous, swollen and painful skin
      b. Mainly caused by UVB, but UVA likely plays a role in damage
      c. Treatment
         i. Avoid sun exposure between 10 a.m. and 3 p.m.

    ii. Cover skin with proper clothing and sunscreen of at least SPF 15, 30 min prior to activity and reapply every 4 h. Hats provide only SPF of 2

    iii. For mild-to-moderate burns apply cool compresses and low-dose of topical corticosteroids

    iv. Severe burn may require oral corticosteroids

  d. Drug–solar interactions common with antibiotics (e.g., tetracycline), anti-inflammatories and antihistamines.

2. Frostnip/Frostbite

  a. Hypothermic dermal and superficial cutaneous injury

    i. Numb white patches become red, swollen and blister (necrosis if severe)

  b. Treatment = Rapid rewarming in 39–44 °C water for 20 min.

    i. Avoid friction or radiant heat

3. Pernio (chilblains)

  a. Painfully itchy erythematous lesions on extremities that may last for days or weeks

    i. More common in high-altitude cold weather sports

    ii. No freezing of tissue but rather perivascular lymphocytic infiltrate

  b. Treatment = rewarm and protect

4. Xerosis

  a. Most common cause of body pruritis during winter

  b. Dehydration of the stratum corneum

  c. Treatment = moisturizing skin products (emollient lotions)

5. Acquired cold urticaria (ACU)

  a. Urticarial plaques after cold exposure in winter athletes and swimmers

  b. Usually follows emotional stress or viral illness

    i. Diagnosis: apply ice to skin for 4–5 min and observe for 10 min

  c. Treatment = avoid cold exposures and antihistamine

6. Solar urticaria

  a. Hives/plaques after sun (UVB) exposure that clear within 1 h of exposure

  b. Allergic reaction to antigen produced by the skins interaction with sun rays. Antigen may be spread to others

  c. Treatment = avoid sun, sunscreen (at least SPF 15), antihistamine, and graded sun exposure

7. Aquagenic urticaria

  a. Plaques after 2–30 min immersion in warm or cold water

  b. Elevated histamines. It is possible that water carries epidermal antigen sensitizing the mast cell

  c. Treatment = Antihistamine

8. Exercise-Induced urticaria

  a. Cutaneous erythema, pruritis and warmth of skin with physical activity. May lead to angioedema and vascular collapse

  b. Treatment = long-acting antihistamine 1 h prior to activity. May need epinephrine if antihistamine fails. Exercise with partner.

III. Infectious Factors

A. Sea-bathers' eruption

1. Pruritic dermatosis lasting up to 6 weeks occurring under the swimsuit caused by larval stage of jellyfish and the sea anemone nematocyst triggered by entering shallow water, pressure of the swim suit, fresh water or physical activity resulting in toxin being injected into the skin

2. Seen in Florida, the Bahamas, upper Gulf region, Long Island, NY

3. Treatment = antihistamines, cool compresses, topical or oral corticosteroids, washing swimwear

B. Swimmers' Itch

   1. Itchy dermatosis lasting 10–14 days occurring on exposed areas caused by unmethodical parasitic flatworm schistosomes microscopic larvae invading unintentional human resulting in an urticarial reaction

   2. Treatment = antihistamines, cool compresses, topical or oral corticosteroids, washing swimwear

C. Swimmers' ear

   1. Gram-negative (*Pseudomonas*) or fungal external canal infection due to water-induced maceration of epithelium

   2. Swelling, maceration, erythema, and drainage

   3. Treatment = Keep ears dry (plugs), avoid abrasion, drops (EtOH/vinegar)

      a. Bacterial—Neomycin/polymyxin B/hydrocortisone 4 gtt tid-qid × 10 days. Ciprofloxacin drops alternative. Ear wick

      b. Fungal—clotrimazole 1% solution and acetic acid drops

D. Scabies

   1. *Sarcoptes scabiei*/mite burrowing/hypersensitivity reaction

   2. Wrestling, interdigital folds, wrist flexor crease, elbows, feet, penis, and intergluteal fold.

   3. Diagnosis = scrape lesions onto oiled slide to identify mite, ova, or feces

   4. Treatment = wash clothes, bedding in very hot water. Elimite/Kwell/Eurax. Treat family or room mates

E. Impetigo/Folliculitis/Furnunculosis

   1. Honey-crusted lesion/pustules/blister/boils

   2. Caused by group A beta-hemolytic streptococcus (GABHS) and/or staphylococci including methicillin-resistant *Staphylococcus aureus* (MRSA)

   3. Risk = close contact, skin damage, sharing equipment

   4. Prevention = not sharing gear or equipment, good hygiene (showering, washing clothing, etc.), cleaning gear and equipment, and treat wounds as soon as possible

   5. Treatment = topical (mupirocin ointment 2%) and/or oral (sulfamethoxazole/trimethoprim DS (commonly used but not FDA approved for use in any staphylococcal infection), tetracyclines [doxycycline or minocycline], cephalexin, amox-clavulanate, clindamycin, erythromycin) antibiotics

      a. Return to play after lesion cleared or treated (improvement seen within 24–72 h) and covered

   6. Furnunculosis or abscess may require I&D

   7. MRSA—painful skin lesion/rapidly spreading/need culture

      a. Colonized athletes = treat nasal (topical mupirocin as above) and skin surfaces (Chlorhexidine or triclosan body wash 5–7 days)

      b. Infected athletes = I&D abscess and administered antibiotics—Clindamycin, Tetracyclines, Rifampin (with another agent), Linezolid, or Trimethoprim-Sulfamethoxazole (commonly used but not FDA approved for treatment of MRSA)

         i. Fluoroquinolone and macrolides are not ideal antibiotics for MRSA = resistance is common

      c. Prevention as above

      d. Return to play after lesion cleared or treated (improvement seen within 24–72 h) and covered

F. Warts

   1. Firm elevated verrucous plaque on hands or feet

      a. Pinpoint hemorrhages

      b. Human papilloma virus

   2. Treatment = cryotherapy, topical keratolytics agents (salicylic acid), or electrocautery. Cimetidine 30–40 mg/kg/day may be helpful

G. Molluscum contagiosum

    1. 2–5 mm umblicated dome-shaped flesh-colored waxy papules

        a. Commonly found on face, trunk, and extremities

    2. Caused by poxvirus

    3. Treatment = curettage, cryosurgery, electrocautery

H. Herpes gladiatorum—Herpes simplex virus type-1 (HSV-1)

    1. Grouped vesicles on erythematous base

        a. Located on head-neck, upper extremities, trunk

        b. Recur at primary site, burning prior to lesion

        c. Reported in up to 30% of high school wrestlers

    2. Treatment = Initial episode—Acyclovir 400 mg po tid × 10 days or Valacyclovir 1 g bid × 10 days

        a. Consider prophylactic suppressive therapy for remainder of season; Acyclovir 400 mg po bid for up to 12 months or Valacyclovir 500 mg po qd (if >2 years of HSV-1)

    3. Recurrent episode—Acyclovir 400 mg po tid×5 days or Valacyclovir 500 mg po bid×3 days (alt. 1 g po qd×5 days)

    4. No participation before 120 h (5 full days) of treatment or if new lesions appear or the presence of lymphadenopathy

        a. The National Federation of State High School Association recommends any participant (i.e., athlete, coach) exposed to an epidemic (3 days or less prior to its onset) be secluded for 8 days and investigating for skin lesions before returning to play

I. Tinea Corporis (Gladiatorum)/Pedis

    1. Fungal infection—

        a. Corposis—Circinate patches with advancing rough-scaly border—*Trichophyton tonsurans*

        b. Pedis—erythematous, puritic lesions—dermatophytes

        c. Treatment = topical or oral antifungals

        d. Prophylaxis—Fluconazole 100 mg po once per week

        e. Treatment of tinea pedis—wash feet and dry (drying medicated powder).

IV. Skin Lacerations

A. Explore wound for length, depth, and complexity

B. Evaluate for involvement of nerves, muscles, tendons, bones, and/or vessels

C. Check neurovascular and functional status

D. Repair lesions >2 cm that expose underlying tissues or that easily bleed

    1. Goals—hemostasis/prevent infection/restore function/cosmetic restoration

    2. May close within 12 h if uncontaminated

    3. If >12 h place loose simple interrupted sutures or allow to heal by secondary intention

    4. Deep wounds = multiple layers (deep layer—absorbable suture)

E. Repair principles

    1. Aseptic technique

    2. Irrigate

    3. Debride

    4. Anesthesia—local, topical, or regional

        a. Avoid epinephrine in areas with end arterioles (e.g., nose, fingers, toes, etc.)

        b. Buffer solution—$NaHCO_3$ 8.4%, 1 mL/10 mL

        c. Allergy rare—ester (procaine, tetracaine) or amide (lidocaine, bupivacaine, mepivacaine)

        d. Use diphenhydramine 1% injectable as an alternative to standard local anesthetic

F. Suture—absorbable (4–8 weeks)/nonabsorbable
   1. Thickness
      a. 3-0 or 4-0 for trunk lacerations
      b. 4-0 or 5-0 for extremity or scalp lacerations
      c. 5-0 or 6-0 for facial lacerations
   2. Repair mucosal lacerations if dysfunctional or cosmetically displeasing
   3. Suture techniques—90° entry for good everted edges
      a. Multiple layer closure—deep wounds
      b. Simple interrupted—most wounds
      c. Horizontal mattress—gaping, high tension wounds
      d. Verticle mattress—max eversion, posterior neck wound
      e. Half-buried mattress—triangular wound
      f. Running "baseball"—long, low tension wounds
G. Tissue adhesives—2-octylcyanoacrylate (Dermabond)
   1. Similar results to suture repair
   2. Apply three to four layers with 5 mm overlap
   3. Low tension wounds only
   4. Sloughs in 5–10 days
   5. Do not apply to infected wounds, mucosal wounds, high moisture areas, or to immunosuppressed or diabetic patients.

Reccomended Reading

1. Adams BB. Sport dermatology. *Adolesc Med.* 2001;*12:vii:*305–322.
2. Anderson BJ. Prophylactic valacyclovir to prevent outbreaks of primary herpes gladiatorum at a 28-day wrestling camp. *Jpn J Infect Dis.* 2006;*59:*6–9.
3. Bolin DJ. Dermatologic conditions in athletes, In: McKeag DB, Moeller JL, eds. *ACSM's Primary Care Sports Medicine.* 2nd ed. Philadelphia, PA: Lippincott Williams and Wilkins; 2007.
4. Elston DM. Community-acquired methicillin-resistant *Staphylococcus aureus. J Am Acad Dermatol.* 2007;*56*(1):1–16.
5. Forsch RT. Essentials of skin laceration repair. *Am Fam Phys.* 2008;*78*(8):945–951, 952.
6. Freiman A, Barankin B, Elpern DJ. Sports dermatology part 1: Common dermatoses. *CMAJ.* 2004;*171:*851–853.
7. Helm TN, Berfeld WF. Sports dermatology. *Br J Sports Med.* 1998;*16:*159–165.
8. Herpes Gladiatorum position statement and guidelines. National Federation of State High School Association. April 2007.
9. Jones SEM, Mahendran S. Interventions for acute auricular haematoma. *Cochrane Database of Systematic Reviews.* 2004;(2). Art. No.: CD004166. doi:10.1002/14651858.CD004166.pub2

38

Sports Hematology

Irfan M. Asif and Kimberly G. Harmon

I. Anemia

A. Iron-deficiency anemia
   1. Epidemiology
      a. Most common anemia
      b. Most common nutritional deficiency in the United States
   2. Presentation
      a. Decreased aerobic performance and endurance
      b. Weakness
      c. Fatigue
      d. Shortness of breath
   3. Physical exam
      a. Pallor
      b. Severe cases may show glossitis, angular cheilitis, or koilonychia
   4. Etiology
      a. Menstruation
      b. Low iron intake
         i. Premenopausal women need 15 mg of iron daily
            (A) Women who lose more than 60 mL of blood with menstrual loss are more likely to be anemic
            (B) Average American 2,000 kcal diet has only 12 mg of elemental iron (not enough to compensate for menstrual losses)
         ii. Men and postmenopausal women need 10 mg daily
      c. Decreased gastric absorption of iron
         i. Decreased acidity of gastric fluid
            (A) H2 blockers
            (B) Proton pump inhibitors
         ii. Celiac disease
         iii. Use of other supplements concomittantly (calcium, fiber)
      d. Gastric bleeding
         i. NSAID use
         ii. Exercise-associated bowel ischemia
      e. Hemolysis
      f. Malignancy (e.g., colon cancer)
   5. Laboratory values
      a. Hgb <12 g/dL in women, Hgb <14 dL in men
      b. Microcytic, hypochromic anemia (MCV <78 fL)
      c. Low serum ferritin

      d. Low iron

      e. High total iron binding capacity

  6. Treatment

      a. Correct blood loss

      b. Iron-rich foods

         i. Heme sources of iron better absorbed than nonheme sources (red meat, poultry)

         ii. Nonheme sources less well absorbed (dark leafy green vegetables, whole grains, dried fruit, egg yolks)

      c. Need 150–200 mg of *elemental* iron daily

         i. Oral ferrous sulfate ($FeSO_4$)

            (A) More soluble than ferrous gluconate

            (B) $FeSO_4$ 325 mg po q day to tid

               (1) 325 mg of $FeSO_4$ has 65 mg of elemental iron

               (2) Can cause nausea, constipation and black stools

               (3) Consider docusate to decrease constipation

         ii. Ferrous gluconate

            (A) Better tolerated than ferrous sulfate

            (B) Not as well absorbed

            (C) Consider if $FeSO_4$ not well tolerated

         iii. Liquid iron

            (A) No better absorbed than pill forms

               (1) Ferrous sulfate elixir has 44 mg of elemental iron per 5 mL

               (2) Liquid iron has potential to stain teeth gray—may want to mix in orange juice and drink through straw

               (3) Some athletes prefer liquid iron

         iv. Best absorbed between meals

         v. Orange juice or ascorbic acid can increase absorption

         vi. May take 6–12 months to fully replenish stores

      d. IV iron

         i. Not recommended for use in athletes

         ii. Can cause anaphylactic reaction

         iii. Should be administered under supervision of hematologist

B. Sports/dilutional anemia (physiologic or pseudoanemia)

  1. Epidemiology

      a. Most common cause of anemia in athletes

      b. Not pathologic

  2. Etiology

      a. Adaptation to endurance training; thought to facilitate oxygen delivery by decreasing blood viscosity leading to increased cardiac output

      b. Occurs as a result of plasma volume expansion and hemodilution

      c. Time course

         i. Initially, volume contraction occurs immediately after strenuous exercise

            (A) Due to increase in hydrostatic pressure and insensible water losses

            (B) Causes a decrease in total plasma volume levels

         ii. 3–5 h postexercise, water levels equilibrate

         iii. >5 h postexercise, volume expansion occurs as a result of the renin–angiotensin–aldosterone system

         iv. Usually resolves within 3–5 days of discontinuing exercise

  3. Laboratory values

      a. Hemoglobin (Hgb) levels are usually 0.5–1.0 g lower in competitive athletes compared to nonathletes

       b. Hgb >13 g/dL in males, Hgb 11.5 g/dL in females

       c. Other hematologic parameters should be normal

    4. Physical exam findings

       a. No irregular findings should be present

    5. Treatment

       a. Requires no treatment

C. "Foot strike" hemolysis

    1. Etiology

       a. Mechanical—heel strike and muscle contraction can cause RBC intravascular hemolysis

       b. Elevated temperature with exercise can lead to RBC fragility and hemolysis

          i. Older microcytes are lost leading to a macrocytosis

          ii. Hemoglobinuria develops when haptoglobin becomes saturated with free hemoglobin

       c. Lactic acid can increase red blood cell fragility

       d. Not only in runners or impact sports. Also seen in nonimpact exercisers (swimmers); thus, "foot-strike" hemolysis is a misnomer

    2. Laboratory studies

       a. Urinalysis may show hemoglobinuria

       b. Often resolves 3–5 days after exercise cessation

       c. Laboratory finds

          i. Macrocytic—"runner's macrocytosis"

          ii. Reticulocytosis

          iii. Low haptoglobin

    3. Treatment

       a. Will often have higher iron needs to compensate for increased RBC production

       b. Change running shoes

       c. Exercise on softer terrain

       d. Consider decreasing training intensity.

II. Iron Deficiency Without Anemia

A. Overview

    1. Ferritin

       a. A sensitive reflection of overall iron stores

       b. A carrier protein

       c. Ferritin is an acute phase reactant so will be elevated in inflammatory states

          i. May be falsely elevated if ill or in other systemic inflammatory diseases

          ii. Could confirm if in doubt by checking simultaneous C-reactive protein or erythrocyte sedimentation rate

    2. Iron

       a. Integral part of hemoglobin molecule which transports O_2 to working muscles

       b. Also important in energy production as it is used in cytochromes in the mitochondria

    3. Impact on athletic performance is unclear

       a. Debatable whether there is an improvement in performance with iron supplementation in iron deficiency without anemia

          i. Some studies suggest any improvement is due to relative increase in Hgb (i.e., from normal to high normal)

          ii. Other studies demonstrate there is an independent positive effect on exercise to iron supplementation alone

       b. Entrenched belief with most runners that low ferritin leads to decreased athletic recovery and performance and increased fatigue

    4. Treatment

      a. Treatment regimens are anecdotal

      b. Athletes with ferritin <25 should consider iron supplementation (see section I.A.6))

        i. Laboratory cutoffs may be variable

        ii. Many labs report ferritin >10–15 in women as normal

      c. Trial of treatment should be considered in athletes with low ferritin without anemia who are symptomatic

      d. Consideration of screening female endurance athletes, athletes with a history of eating disorders, vegetarians, or other risk factors.

III. Sickle Cell Disease and Sickle Cell Trait

  A. Etiology

    1. Hgb formed by two alpha and two beta chains

      a. Hgb A is normal hemoglobin

      b. Hgb S is produced with a valine substitution for glutamic acid and is abnormal

    2. Sickle cell disease (SCD) occurs with two normal alpha chains and two Hgb S beta chains.

    3. Sickle cell trait (SCT) occurs when there are two normal alpha chains, one normal beta chain (Hgb A) and one abnormal beta chain (Hgb S)

      a. Alpha-thalassemia is protective in individuals with SCT (see section IV.D)

  B. SCD

    1. Hemoglobin S is an inherited hemoglobin that "sickles" under with deoxygenation

    2. Those with SCD are susceptible to anemia and painful crises

    3. Majority of SCD individuals do not participate in intense physical activity

  C. SCT

    1. Epidemiology

      a. Present in 7–12% of African Americans (one in 8–14)

      b. Often does not affect exercise capacity unless the athlete is placed in a stressful environment

        i. Extreme heat

        ii. High altitude

    2. Overexertion with SCT is associated with exertional collapse and sudden death

      a. Rhabdomylosis

        i. Exercise induces deoxygenation and sickling

          (A) If hypoxia is uncompensated, sickling will occur

          (B) Maximal exercise at sea level will produce mild intravascular sickling

          (C) Sickling increases with altitude

          (D) No measurable effects on exercise performance

          (E) Wide range of sickling during peak exercise (1–25%)

          (F) Athletes with SCT have varying concentration of Hgb S (30–44%)

        ii. Sickling causes vaso-occlusions and pain in the working muscles

        iii. Leads to muscle necrosis and extravasation of contents

          (A) Elevations of CK

          (B) Dark-colored urine (myoglobinuria)

          (C) Myalgia

          (D) Renal damage/failure

         iv. Typically related to exercise intensity

          (A) Usually when the athlete cannot take a break

          (B) Timed sprints

          (C) In football, occurs in conditioning

          (D) Rarely occurs during game situations when there is adequate rest time to recover

    v. Muscle pain is ischemic in rhabdomyolysis
       (A) Sometimes described as cramping
       (B) Often weak
       (C) Muscles are usually not tense or hard (as opposed to cramping)
    vi. Athlete may collapse but will be conscious (as opposed to collapse from cardiac causes)
    vii. Treatment of rhabdomyolosis in SCT athlete
       (A) Recognition
       (B) Have athlete lay down
       (C) Check vital signs
       (D) Administer supplemental oxygen
       (E) Cool the athlete if necessary
       (F) Call 911
       (G) Attach an AED
       (H) Start an IV with NS
       (I) Alert the ER doc to expect fulminant rhabdomyolysis
  b. Exertional heat stroke
    i. High core temperature increases sickling
    ii. Contributes to exertional sickling
  c. Sudden cardiac death
    i. US military study showed 28× increased risk of sudden cardiac death in SCT
    ii. Etiology in athletes with SCT is hyperkalemic arrhythmias secondary to massive rhabdomyolysis

D. Other potential risks of athletes with SCT

  1. Splenic infarction
    a. Occurs primarily at exercise with altitude
    b. Presents with LUQ pain, nausea, vomiting
  2. Hematuria
    a. Results from sickling in the renal medulla
    b. Papillary necrosis will sometimes be present
  3. Hyposthenuria (inability to concentrate urine)
    a. Cumulative effects of renal papillary necrosis
    b. May contribute to dehydration when exercising
    c. Dehydration can lead to sickling and associated sequel
    d. Athletes with SCT should be vigilant about hydration
  4. Laboratory evaluation
    a. Positive sickle cell trait test
      i. All states require neonatal screening but many athletes do not know if they are SCT positive
      ii. Required prior to participation in sports by NCAA in Division I athletes
    b. Sickle Prep Test
      i. Blood smear on a slide
      ii. Sickle-like red blood cells can be identified microscopically
      iii. Will not rule out other types of abnormal hemoglobin.
    c. Hgb Solubility Test
      i. Also called SickleDex
      ii. Can determine whether a person has sickle hemoglobin
      iii. Cannot distinguish an individual with sickle cell disease from an individual who is a sickle cell carrier
      iv. Cannot rule out or diagnose other types of abnormal hemoglobin
    d. Hgb electrophoresis
      i. Gold standard

      ii. Determine the percentage of different types of hemoglobin in a person's blood

      iii. Can distinguish an individual with a sickle cell disease from one who is a sickle cell carrier

      iv. Most individuals with abnormal Hgb will be detected with this method

    5. Treatment

      a. Training modification

        i. Acclimatize to heat and altitude

        ii. Avoid dehydration or overexertion

        iii. Gradual progression in workout intensity

        iv. Longer recovery periods between repetitions or workouts.

IV. Thalassemia

A. Epidemiology

  1. Thalessemias are inherited disorders characterized by inadequate production of alpha or beta globin chains of hemoglobin

  2. Classification is based on the absence of the globin chain

B. Etiology

  1. Hgb is composed of two alpha and two beta chains

  2. In normal Hgb, the ratio of alpha to nonalpha chains is 1.0

  3. Thalassemia refers to the spectrum of disorders characterized by reduced or absence of one or more of the globin chains

C. Beta-Thalassemia

  1. Can be either heterozygous or homozygous

  2. Leads to an underproduction of B-chains and a relative overproduction of alpha chains.

  3. Unpaired alpha chains precipitate and are toxic to cells

  4. Heterozygotes tend to be asymptomatic

    a. May be diagnosed as iron-deficiency anemia

    b. Typical pattern is Hct <30, MCV <75 and normal RDW

    c. Patients are often iron overloaded

    d. Avoid iron supplementation for presumed iron deficiency with microcytosis (i.e., check ferritin levels to confirm iron deficiency)

  5. Homozygotes have widely varying clinical pictures depending on mutation

    a. Usually exhibit some degree of alpha globin inclusion body formation, with consequent anemia, hemolysis, and varying degrees of ineffective erythropoiesis

    b. The amount of alpha globin inclusion body formation and the degree of ineffective erythropoiesis correlate best with overall severity

D. Alpha-thalassemia

  1. Due to impaired production of alpha globin chains, leading to a relative excess of beta globin chains

    a. In individuals with SCT as well as alpha-thalassemia these excess normal beta globin chains are protective

  2. Toxicity of the excess beta globin chains on the red cell membrane skeleton appears to be less than that of alpha chains

  3. There are four alpha genes, two on each chromosome (i.e., aa/aa). There are four alpha thalassemia syndromes, reflecting the loss of one, two, three, or all four of these alpha chain genes

  4. The loss of one or two alpha globin genes causes mild, usually asymptomatic microcytic anemia

    a. This should not be mistaken for iron-deficiency anemia

    b. Does not respond to iron

    c. Cannot be diagnosed with Hgb electrophoresis

5. The loss of three alpha globin genes results in a moderate degree of anemia and can be diagnosed with Hgb electrophoresis. The clinical picture is varied
6. The loss of four alpha globin genes is usually fatal *in utero*.

V. Coagulopathy

A. Factor V Leiden and prothrombin gene mutation are the most common hypercoagulable states
   1. Both are more common in Caucasians and rare in those from African or Asian descent
   2. Homozygotes are at increased risk of thrombosis
   3. Risk of thrombosis in heterozygotes depends on the amount of affected protein

B. Other potential etiologies leading to thrombosis include Protein C, Protein S, or antithrombin mutations, or antiphospholipid syndrome

C. If deep-venous thrombosis is suspected consider venous duplex ultrasound.

VI. Bleeding Disorders

A. Von Willebrand's disease
   1. Most common inherited bleeding disorder
   2. Affects 0.1–1% of the population
   3. Etiology
      a. Decreased production of von Willebrand's factor or abnormal function of von Willebrand's factor
      b. Leads to reduced platelet aggregation and lower factor VIII levels
   4. Presentation
      a. Often presents in late childhood or adolescence
      b. Varies from easy bruising to menorrhagia to heavy bleeding following minor procedures or surgeries
      c. Phenotype is heterogeneous and is dependent upon levels of normal circulating von Willebrand's factor
   5. Sports participation
      a. Increased risk of hemorrhage with contact sports
      b. Noncontact sports participation is generally acceptable

B. Hemophilia
   1. Two most prevalent hemophilias are X-linked
      a. Hemophilia A—deficiency of factor VIII
      b. Hemophilia B—deficiency of factor IX
   2. Extent of disease varies
      a. Severe disease can cause spontaneous bleeding into joints and muscles
      b. Individuals with mild disease have increased bleeding following trauma or surgery
   3. Participation in sports depends on sport demands, disease severity and should include consultation with a hematologist.

Recommended Reading

1. Beyer R, Ingerslev J, Sorensen B. Muscle bleeds in professional athletes—Diagnosis, classification, treatment and potential impact in patients with haemophilia. *Haemophilia*. 2010;16(6):858–865.
2. Eichner ER. Sickle cell trait in sports. *Curr Sports Med Rep*. 2010;9(6):347–351.
3. Friedmann B, Weller E, Mairbaurl H, Bartsch P. Effects of iron repletion on blood volume and performance capacity in young athletes. *Med Sci Sports Exercise*. 2001;33(5):741–746.
4. Garza D, Shrier I, Kohl III HW, Ford P, Brown M, Matheson GO. The clinical value of serum ferritin tests in endurance athletes. *Clin J Sports Med*. 1997;7:46–53.
5. Mercer KW, Densmore JJ. Hematologic disorders in the athlete. *Clin Sports Med*. 2005;24:599–621.

6. Robertson JA, Ray TR. Hematologic problems in athletes. In: Madden C, Putukian M, McCarty E, Young C, eds. *Netter's Sports Medicine*. Philadelphia: Elsevier, Inc.; 2010:209–211.

7. Shaskey DJ, Green GA. Sport haematology. *Sport Med*. 2000;29(1): 27–38.

8. Telford RD, Sly GJ, Hahn AG, Cunningham RB, Bryant C, Smith JA. Footstrike is the major cause of hemolysis during running. *J Appl Physiol*. 2003;94:38–42.

39

Sports Endocrinology
Darryl E. Barnes

I. Diabetes Mellitus (DM)

A. Hyperglycemia secondary to metabolic abnormality with
   1. Insulin secretion
   2. Insulin receptors

B. Type 1 DM is absolute deficiency of insulin
   1. Lack pancreatic beta cells = reliance on exogenous insulin

C. Type 2 DM most common form caused by
   1. Inadequate compensatory insulin secretory response
   2. Resistance of cell receptor to insulin

D. Diagnosis = one of the following
   1. DM symptoms and random plasma glucose of 200 mg/dL or more
   2. Two fasting glucose measurements of 126 mg/dL or more
   3. 2-h postprandial glucose measurement of 200 mg/dL or more

E. Treatments = exercise, proper diet, and medication (insulin in all type 1 DM and some type 2 DM patients and oral hypoglycemic agents type 2 DM) and monitoring hemoglobin A_{1C} (HbA_{1C}).

F. Exercise helps control hyperglycemia by
   1. Increasing glucose utilization by muscle
      a. Initial—glucose within muscle used for energy
      b. Secondary—glycogenolysis of muscle glycogen
      c. Tertiary—glucagon and other hormones stimulate liver gluconeogenesis and glycogenolysis
      d. Quaternary—Increase in the number of "slow-switch" muscle fibers, increased mitochondrial enzymes, increased muscle capillaries all result in more efficient use of glucose.
      e. Increased numbers of glucose transporters (GLUT4) on cell surfaces
         i. Type 2 DM have aberration of GLUT4 impairing glucose transport into the cell
            (A) Muscle contractions induce GLUT4 production in type 2 DM improving glucose metabolism

G. DM factors that influence the physiology of exercise
   1. Dependent on baseline cardiovascular fitness level and type of DM
   2. Medications
      a. Exogenous insulin, once given, cannot be regulated and may result in hypoglycemia
   3. Exercising in a hyperglycemic (>250 mg/dL) state may exacerbate hyperglycemia via hypoinsulinemia-induced hepatic glucose production

H. Exercise benefits in DM
   1. Mainly benefits type 2 DM measured by reduction in HbA_{1C} and decrease in dose or need of medication
      a. Regular aerobic exercise (30–60 min at 50–80% VO_2 max, 3–4/week) = 10–20% reduction in HbA_{1C}
      b. Resistance exercise 2/week = 7–13% HbA_{1C} reduction
   2. Type 1 DM still need strict control of diet and insulin therapy
I. Exercise risk in DM
   1. Hypoglycemia, hyperglycemia, peripheral vascular disease, cardiovascular disease, abnormal blood pressure response, protienuria, skin ulceration, retinal disease, and degenerative joint disease
      a. Prior to initiating an exercise program, diabetics should be evaluated for micro and macrovascular complications
   2. Hypoglycemia is the most common risk, especially in insulin-dependent DM and those taking sulfonylureas
      a. Presence of DM greater than 5 years increases the risk of poor counter-regulatory mechanism to respond to hypoglycemia
      b. Exogenous insulin placed in subcutaneous tissue of any extremity or into any muscle increases risk of hypoglycemia secondary to increased absorption rates in these tissues. However, diabetics should avoid injecting insulin into the extremity that will be involved in exercise prior to performing exercise (e.g., avoid injecting insulin into the legs before running)
      c. Delayed hypoglycemia can occur as late as 28 h postactivity as a result of the liver and muscle replenishing glycogen stores from blood glucose
         i. Prevent = consume 40 g of carbohydrate for every 30 min of intense exercise
      d. Symptoms of mild hypoglycemia (glucose 50–70 mg/dL) = headache, dizziness, and hunger
         i. Consume carbohydrate (orange juice, etc.)
         ii. Monitor symptoms and glucose level to prevent severe hypoglycemia
         iii. Glucagon 1 mg SC or IM if severe
J. Management
   1. Long duration exercise (10K runs, soccers, basketball, etc.)
      a. Do not start if glucose >250 mg/dL with ketones or >300 mg/dL (increased risk for hyperglycemia)
      b. May participate in short duration events (<10 min) if no ketones
      c. Never participate in hypoglycemic state
   2. General modifications to diabetic management regimens
      a. Low glycemic index meal 3 h before activity
      b. Small snack 1 h before activity
      c. Exercise after peak activity of insulin
         i. Reduce insulin near its peak during the exercise activity by 20–50% of their baseline dose
   3. Insulin pumps (continuous subcutaneous insulin injection system (CSII))
      a. Improve convenience and compliance by automatically delivering continuous basal rate of insulin and a premeal bolus of insulin
      b. 1 h prior to exercise reduce basal rate by 50%
         i. If low-intensity exercise just decrease premeal bolus and leave basal rate unchanged
   4. Malfunction may produce hyperglycemia
      a. Displacement of infusion set (the implanted catheter) from the implant site or heat deactivation of insulin

5. Remove unit (leave infusion set in place) with contact/collision sports if needed
   a. Activity <1 h stop 30 min prior
   b. Activity >1 h then "i." and give 50% of basal rate as injection each hour.

II. Menstrual Disorders in Athletes

A. Athletes have greater risks for menstrual disorders than nonathletes

B. Amenorrhea incidence ~50% in athletes compared to 3–5% of the general population (primarily gymnast, endurance athletes, ballet dancers, ice skaters)
   1. Primary amenorrhea = no menses by age 16
   2. Secondary amenorrhea = menses stop for >6 months

C. Athletes at risk = exercise intensely, lower body fat, abnormality in nutritional status (disordered eating), late menarche, and/or a history of menstrual irregularity.

D. Exercise alone does not cause amenorrhea and may improve dysmenorrhea

E. Diagnosis necessary in all athletes presenting with menstrual abnormalities
   1. History and physical examination
      a. Medications that produce hyperprolactinemia
         i. Amphetamines
         ii. Cannabis
         iii. Cardiovascular drugs (atenolol, verapamil)
         iv. H_2 blockers
         v. Herbal therapies (fennel, fenugreek seed)
         vi. Psychotropic drugs (selective-seretonin reuptake inhibitors, tricyclic antidepressants, buspirone)
         vii. Neurologic drugs (valproic acid, sumatriptan)
      b. Galactorrhea (hyperprolactinemia)
         i. Test prolactin level. Hyperprolactinemia is associated with 20% of amenorrhea cases in the general population.
         ii. MRI or CT of brain looking for pituitary adenoma
         iii. If prolactin is <100 ng/mL, galactorrhea probably due to medications
         iv. If prolactin is >100 ng/mL, galactorrhea probably due to pituitary adenoma
      c. Atrophic vaginal changes/dryness (hypoestrogenic state)
      d. Anatomical abnormalities associated with outlet obstruction
         i. Asherman's syndrome (hysteroscopy)
         ii. Congenital absence of the vagina and uterus
         iii. Imperforate hymen
         iv. Uterine and cervical defects
      e. Weight loss
      f. Hirsutism (polycystic ovarian syndrome)
      g. Virilization
         i. Suggests adrenal or ovarian neoplasm
      h. Visual field defect
         i. Suggests pituitary adenoma
      i. Short stature, sexual infantilism, and webbed neck = Turner's syndrome
   2. Pregnancy assessment
      a. Most common cause of secondary amenorrhea in childbearing aged women
   3. TSH
      a. If abnormal then complete thyroid cascade panel (T_3, T_4, free T_4). Hypothyroidism is rarely a cause of amenorrhea.
   4. Progestin challenge test
      a. Differentiate those with estrogen deficiency from those with normal or high estrogen levels

      b. Medroxyprogesterone acetate 10 mg by mouth once per day for 5–7 days or Norethindrone 5 mg PO once daily for 7–10 days will produce bleeding within 1 week of the final dose in those with normal estrogen levels and anovulation is the expected cause of amenorrhea. Those who do not bleed are expected to have estrogen deficiency, but outflow tract obstruction is possible

   5. Estrogen–progestin challenge test

      a. Differentiates those with outflow tract obstruction and estrogen deficiency

      b. Estrogen given for 21–25 days

      c. Progestin given for the final 5–7 days to motivate withdrawal bleeding

      d. No bleeding = outflow obstruction

      e. Bleeding = estrogen deficiency (further investigation required)

   6. Gonadotropin levels

      a. FSH >40 mIU/mL—primary ovarian failure (POF) or menopause

      b. Both FSH and LH elevated = POF

      c. LH:FSH ratio >2:1 = polycystic ovarian syndrome

      d. Low levels of LH and FSH = prepubertal state or hypothalamic and pituitary dysfunction (i.e., female athlete triad, anorexia nervosa)

   7. Androgen testing

      a. Investigate those with acne, hirsutism, and virilization.

      b. Testosterone levels >200 ng/dL probably due to ovarian source. Work-up for neoplasm.

      c. DHEAS >7 mg/dL probably due to an adrenal source. Work-up for neoplasm.

   8. Karyotyping (POF before age 30 or evidence of Turner's syndrome)

   9. In those with amenorrhea >6 months a bone density screen advised

 F. Management

   1. Four main causes of amenorrhea

      a. Hyperprolactinemic, hypogonadotropic, hypergonadotropic, normogonadotropic

         i. Hypogonadotropic is related to athletic causes of amenorrhea

   2. Treatment for hypogonadotropic amenorrhea

      a. Gain body mass and maintain intensity of exercise

      b. Maintain body mass and decrease intensity of exercise

         i. Address eating disorder if present (dietary/psychological counseling)

         ii. Take time off (2 months) or decrease training (intensity/duration/frequency) by 10%

         iii. Oral contraception for bone protection from loss until normal menses return

            (A) Avoid in patients who smoke, have HTN or history of migraine headaches

         iv. Calcium supplement 1.5 g/day and vitamin D 800 IU/day

         v. Antiresorptive therapy in those with osteoporosis who are not of childbearing age.

III. Osteoporosis/Osteopenia

 A. Diagnosis

   1. Dual energy x-ray absorptiometry (DEXA)

      a. *T*-score of ≤ −2.5 = osteoporosis

      b. *T*-score between −1.0 and −2.5 = osteopenia

 B. May be seen in athletes with large energy deficit (energy availability of <30 kcal/kg of fat-free mass per day) and hypoestrogenic state

   1. Female athlete triad (see below)

 C. Management

   1. Medications—estrogens, calitonin, biphosphonates, reloxifene, and recombinant human parathyroid hormone

   2. Cessation of smoking

3. Physical activity
   a. Weight bearing exercise
   b. Resistance exercise
   c. Impact (i.e., jumping) exercise if able
4. If due to significant energy deficits and associated with functional hypothalamic amenor-rhea then the above management will not be successful until the energy deficit is corrected.

IV. Female Athlete Triad

A. Interrelationship between
   1. Energy availability (e.g., eating disorder)
   2. Menstrual function (e.g., amenorrhea)
   3. Bone mineral density (e.g., osteoporosis)

B. Low-energy availability is the main factor in this triad
   1. Intentional, nonintentional, or pathological
   2. Need not be associated with a clinic eating disorder

C. Diagnosis
   1. Need not have all three entities present at once for diagnosis
      a. Any of the components may result in poorer performance and poorer quality health

D. Management
   1. Education
   2. Increase energy availability—eat, dietary counseling
   3. Reduce energy expenditure—decrease exercise frequency, duration, intensity, or combi-nation of these components.
   4. Estrogen supplementation (oral contraception) to protect against bone loss (see above).
   5. Psychotherapy if eating disorder is present.

Recommended Reading

1. Anish EJ, Klenck CA. Exercise as medicine: The role of exercise in treating chronic disease. In: DB McKeag, JL Moeller eds. *ACSM's Primary Care Sports Medicine*. 2nd ed. Philadelphia, PA: Lippincott Williams and Wilkins; 2007.
2. Beals KA, Meyer NL. Female athlete triad update. *Clin Sports Med*. 2007;26:69–89.
3. Colberg SR, Swain DP. Exercise and diabetes control: A winning combination. *Phys Sportsmed*. 2000;28:63–81.
4. McAuley KA, Williams SM, Mann JI, Ailsa Goulding A, Chisholm A, Wilson N, Story G, MClay RT, Harper MJ, Jones IE. Intensive lifestyle changes are necessary to improve insulin sensitivity: A randomized controlled trial. *Diabetes Care*. 2002;25:445.
5. McCulloch DK. Effects of exercise in diabetes mellitus in adults. UpToDate Online 15.3, Available: http://www.uptodate.com. 2008.
6. Nattiv A, Loucks AB, Manroe MM, Sanborn CF, Sundgot-Borgen J, Warren MP. The female athlete triad: Position stand. *Med Sci Sports Exerc*. 2007:1867–1182.
7. Report of the expert committee on the diagnosis and classification of diabetes mellitus. *Diabetes Care*. 1997;20:1183–1197.
8. Trojian TH. Endocrine. In: McKeag DB, Moeller JL, eds. *ACSM's Primary Care Sports Medicine*. 2nd ed. Philadelphia, PA: Lippincott Williams and Wilkins; 2007.
9. Warren MP, Chua AT. Exercise-induced amenorrhea and bone health in the adolescent athlete. *Ann NY Acad Sci*. 2008;1135:244–252.

40

Sports Obstetrics and Gynecology

Darryl E. Barnes

I. Pregnancy and Exercise
  A. Maternal and fetal benefits of exercise
    1. Maternal
       a. Limited weight gain during pregnancy
       b. Improved cardiovascular health
       c. Decreased musculoskeletal discomfort
       d. Decreased lower extremity edema
       e. Improved mood
       f. Control or improvement of gestational hypertension and diabetes
    2. Fetal
       a. Enhanced stress tolerance
       b. Decreased fat mass
       c. Enhance neurobehavioral maturation
       d. Some studies show possible decrease in labor times
  B. Cardiorespiratory factors
    1. Prepregnancy cardiorespiratory fitness level is maintained during pregnancy in the athlete that continues to exercise
       a. Pregnant active athletes (at rest or during submaximal exercise) are able to do more work at a given heart rate compared to sedentary controls
          i. Absolute maternal VO_2 is significantly improved compared to the nonpregnant state
          ii. Coincides with maternal weight gain
  C. Cardiovascular factors
    1. 6-8 weeks gestation - blood volume, stroke volume, and heart rate are all start to increase
    2. 16-18 weeks gestation
       a. Increased cardiac output by 30–50%
       b. Increased maternal blood volume by 40–50%
       c. Increased stroke volume
       d. Increased heart rate by 15–20 bpm
       e. Increased respiratory rate
          i. Vital lung capacity unchanged secondary to expansion of chest diameter
          ii. Decreased oxygen reserve due to decreased residual volume near end of pregnancy
          iii. Hematocrit and hemoglobin concentrations decrease

D. Energy balance factors
1. First trimester = extra 150 kcal/day
2. Second and third trimester = extra 350 kcal/day
E. Resistance exercise
1. Avoid exercise in the supine position during the second and third trimesters.

II. Fetal Health

A. Fetal birth weight
1. Some studied have demonstrated that exercise frequency is related to birth weight
   a. 5–7 days/week = lower birth weight infants than controls
   b. 3–4 days/week = higher birth weight infants than controls
   c. No evidence that reduced birth weight in this circumstance has any adverse effects on the infant
B. Acute fetal distress
1. Fetal bradycardia due to hypoxia = acute fetal distress
   a. May result from moderate to strenuous exercise
   b. Submaximal exercise = increased fetal heart rate with no adverse effects on neonatal well being = healthier baby and mother
C. Hyperthermia
1. Immersion in hot tubs = increased core body temperature = neural tube defects
2. Thermoregulatory mechanisms are intact and respond normally in appropriate environments
3. Avoid exercise in extreme (hot and humid) environments
   a. Encourage control of exercise intensity/frequency/duration and maintenance of good hydration
D. Premature delivery
1. Incompetent cervix or history of more than one preterm labor episode or miscarriage is at higher risk of recurrence and should not exercise during pregnancy
   a. If there is no history as noted above, then mild to moderate intensity exercise is OK.

III. Musculoskeletal Factors

A. Body load changes
1. Weight gain and shifts in the center of gravity (forward and upward)
   a. Increased lordosis of lumbar spine—may lead to low back pain
   b. Change in balance—modify activity to avoid injury
2. Joint laxity due to relaxin and increased estrogen
   a. Particularly susceptible joints include the knee, ankle, and sacroiliac joints, and pubic symphysis
   b. Modify activity to protect joints.

IV. Lactation Considerations

A. Breast feeding
1. May reduce weight gain associated with pregnancy faster than not breast feeding
2. Milk quality or quantity not affected significantly with exercise
   a. Intense exercise may produce increased lactic acid in milk and infant may refuse feeding
3. In general, exercise and breast feeding should be encouraged.

V. Pregnancy and Exercise Recommendations

A. Individual assessment
1. Prepregnancy fitness level and medical history

2. If healthy patient did not exercise previous to pregnancy, then start low-intensity and slow progressive exercise program
3. Safe maternal heart rate target = 140–160 bpm (70–80% maximum heart rate)
4. Athletes may continue their activity with modifications and monitoring
5. ACSM and CDC recommend exercise at least 30 min on most days of the week

B. See the tables adapted from ACOG guidelines describing absolute and relative contraindication to exercise and warning signs to stop exercise during pregnancy

C. See the table of recommendations for specific exercises during pregnancy.

VI. Pelvic Floor Dysfunction

A. Variety
   1. Urinary and anal incontinence
   2. Pelvic organ prolapse
   3. Chronic pain syndromes
   4. Sensory and functional abnormalities

B. Kegel exercises recommended postpartum to strengthening pelvic floor musculature in order to reduce pelvic floor dysfunction

C. Stress urinary incontinence (SUI) and urge urinary incontinence (UUI) have high prevalence in elite female athletes (track and field, gymnastics, and trampolining)
   1. SUI = 41%
   2. UUI = 16%
      a. If underlying eating disorder
         i. SUI = 49.5%
         ii. UUI = 20%
   3. High-impact athletes have substantial demands on the pelvic floor anatomy and function compared to nonathletes, thus requiring a stronger pelvic floor to remain asymptomatic
      a. Treat with one or a combination of the following:
         i. Behavioral—bladder training, scheduled toileting, fluid management
         ii. Nonsurgical—physical therapy, electrostimulation
         iii. Medical devices—urethral inserts, pessary
         iv. Medications—anticholinergics (use with care in athletes), topical estrogen, imipramine
         v. Interventional therapies—botulinum toxin type A, radiofrequency therapy, bulking material injection, sacral nerve stimulator
         vi. Surgeries—sling procedures, bladder neck suspensions, artificial urinary sphincter
         vii. Absorbent pads and catheters.

VII. Labial Trauma

A. Genital trauma in females is rare
   1. Cycling is the most common sport associated with female labial trauma

B. History and physical examination
   1. Inspect genitalia region and external urethra for swelling (hematoma formation), bleeding, and lacerations
   2. Look for other underlying trauma (i.e., pelvic fracture)
   3. Ice, compression, protect, and NSAIDs
   4. Repair simple laceration
      a. Refer for complex or extensive laceration
   5. Refer to specialty care if significant trauma is sustained to the pelvis/genitourinary system.

Recommended Reading

1. ACOG committee opinion. Exercise during pregnancy and the postpartum period. Number 267, January 2002. American College of Obstetricians and Gynecologists. *Int J Gynecol Obstet.* 2002;77(1):79–81.

2. American College of Sports Medicine. *ACSM's Guidelines for Exercise Testing and Prescription.* 6th ed. Philadelphia: Lippincott, Williams and Wilkins; 2000.

3. Bo K. Urinary incontinence, pelvic floor dysfunction, exercise and sport. *Sport Med.* 2004;34(7):451–464.

4. Bo K, Borgen JS, Sundgot J. Prevalence of stress and urge urinary incontinence in elite athletes and controls. *Med Sci Sports Exerc.* 2001;33(11):1797–1802.

5. Campbell MK, Mottola MF. Recreational exercise and occupational activity during pregnancy and birth weight. A case-control study. *Am J Obstet Gynecol.* 2001;184:403–408.

6. Hay-Smith EJ. Pelvic floor muscle training versus no treatment, or inactive control treatments, for urinary incontinence in women. *Cochrane Database Syst Rev.* 2006;(1):CD005654.

7. Kruger JA. Pelvic floor function in elite nulliparous athletes. *Ultrasound Obstet Gynecol.* 2007;30(1):81–85.

8. Melzer K, Schutz Y, Boulvain M, Kayser B. Physical activity and pregnancy, cardiovascular adaptations, recommendations and pregnancy outcomes. *Sports Med.* 2010;40(6):493–507.

9. Milunsky A, Ulcickas M, Rothman KJ, Willett W, Jick SS, Jick H. Maternal heat exposure and neural tube defects. *JAMA.* 1992;268:882–885.

10. Nogle SE, Monroe JS. Conditioning and training programs for athletes/nonathletes. In: McKeag DB, Moeller JL, eds. *ACSM's Primary Care Sports Medicine.* 2nd ed. Philadelphia, PA: Lippincott Williams and Wilkins; 2007:81–105.

11. Pivarnik JM, Ayres NA, Mauer MB, Cotton DB, Kirshon B, Dildy GA. Effects of maternal aerobic fitness on cardiorespiratory responses to exercise. *Med Sci Sports Exerc.* 1993;25:993–998.

12. Pivarnik JM, Perkins CD, Moyerbrailean T. Athletes and pregnancy. *Clin Obstet Gynecol.* 2003;46:403–414.

13. Wright KS, Quinn TJ, Carey GB. Infant acceptance of breast milk after maternal exercise. *Pediatrics.* 2002;109(4):585–589.

Contraindication to Aerobic Exercise During Pregnancy: Absolute and Relative

Absolute

Associated with chronic disease
Restrictive lung disease
Hemodynamically unstable heart disease

Associated with obstetrical complication
Incompetent cervix/cerclage
Multiple gestation at risk for premature labor
Persistent second- or third-trimester bleeding
Placenta previa after 26 weeks of gestation
Preeclampsia/pregnancy-induced hypertension
Premature labor during the current pregnancy
Ruptured membranes

Relative

Associated with chronic disease
Chronic bronchitis
Extreme morbid obesity
Extreme underweight (BMI < 12)
Severe anemia
Poorly controlled hypertension
Poorly controlled hyperthyroidism
Poorly controlled seizure disorder
Poorly controlled type 1 diabetes

Associated with obstetrical complication
Pregnancy with intrauterine growth restriction

Other
Heavy smoker
History of extremely sedentary lifestyle
Orthopedic limitations
Unevaluated maternal cardiac arrhythmia

Adapted from ACOG committee opinion. Exercise during pregnancy and the postpartum period. Number 267, January 2002. American College of Obstetricians and Gynecologists. *Int J Gynecol Obstet.* 2002;77(1):79–81.

Warning Signs to Terminate Exercise in Pregnancy

Associated with obstetrical complication
Amniotic fluid leakage
Decreased fetal movement
Preterm labor
Vaginal bleeding

Other
Calf pain or swelling (rule out thrombophlebitis)
Chest pain
Dizziness
Dyspnea prior to exertion
Headache
Muscle weakness

Adapted from ACOG committee opinion. Exercise during pregnancy and the postpartum period. Number 267, January 2002. American College of Obstetricians and Gynecologists. *Int J Gynecol Obstet.* 2002;77(1):79–81.

Recommendations: Pregnancy-Specific Exercises

Aerobics
* Low to moderate intensity
* Avoid supine position after 4 months gestation

Contact sports
* Avoid all collision/contact sports during pregnancy

Cycling
* OK to initiate during pregnancy—stationary bike is safer
* As pregnancy progresses, the elite cyclist can change to an upright bicycle from racing/touring bicycle

Downhill and cross-country skiing
* Educate and encourage avoidance. Experienced skiers should use extra caution.
* Novice skiers should not ski during pregnancy
* Cross-country skiing is less risky than downhill skiing

Ice skating
* Educate and encourage avoidance. Expert skaters should use extra caution
* All others should avoid skating during pregnancy

Jogging
* Do not initiate jogging during pregnancy
* Maintain same perceived level of exertion (as pregnancy progresses reduce speed and distance)

Scuba diving
* Avoid—associated increased risk of fetal decompression sickness

Swimming
* Safe to initiate during pregnancy and avoid extreme of temperatures

Weight lifting
* Encourage proper breathing techniques
* Avoid supine training

Source: Nogle SE, Monroe JS. Conditioning and training programs for athletes/nonathletes. In: McKeag DB, Moeller JL, eds. *ACSM's Primary Care Sports Medicine*, 2nd ed. Lippincott Williams and Wilkins 2007:81–105.

41

Sports Infectious Disease

John W. O'Kane Jr.

BLOOD-BORNE PATHOGENS—HIV

I. Epidemiology

A. Risk of transmission through sports felt to be exceedingly low with exception of boxing. Based on HIV prevalence in athletes, risk of percutaneous transmission, and risk of bleeding, National Football League estimates risk of transmission at less than 1 in one million games or 1 in 85 million contacts

B. Some athletes may exhibit behavior outside of competition placing them at greater risk, including injecting performance-enhancing drugs and other social high-risk behavior

C. No confirmed cases of HIV transmission in sports, one possible case in Italian soccer.

D. Guidelines from AAP and OSHA widely adopted recommending against routine testing, disclosure of HIV status, or exclusion of HIV positive athletes from participation. Adherence to universal precautions recommended and most sports organizations have rules regarding bleeding control

E. Boxing and other combat sports are the exception with many states requiring HIV testing to receive license to participate.

II. Diagnosis

A. Positive enzyme-linked immunosorbent assay (ELISA) and Western blot
   1. Standard screening, used by boxing
   2. Positive test may take 4 or more weeks from time of infection

B. Polymerase chain reaction (PCR) quantifies HIV RNA level and is positive within 11 days.

III. Treatment

A. Antiretroviral therapy is effective at reducing viral load, decreasing progression to AIDS, and decreasing opportunistic infections and death

B. Treatment facilitates sports participation through improving health and decreases risk of transmission by decreasing viral load

C. Treatment generally involves three drug regiments from two different classes. Resistance testing should precede initial drug selection. Physicians with special training in HIV drug treatment have been shown to achieve superior outcomes and should be consulted.

BLOOD-BORNE PATHOGENS–HEPATITIS B AND C

I. Epidemiology

A. HBV varies in prevalence worldwide with some areas showing >8%. Concentration of virus in blood higher than HIV and risk of transmission through percutaneous exposure 50–100 times greater than HIV. HBV transmission reported through sports exposure in wrestling and American football exposure in Japan

B. HCV prevalence in US estimated at 1.6%. HCV chronic infection most common cause of liver transplant and hepatocellular carcinoma. Risk of transmission through percutaneous exposure 10 times greater than HIV. No documented transmission through sports participation. Transmission documented between teammates sharing needles for performance-enhancing injections.

II. Diagnosis

A. Acute infection with HBV is marked by HBsAg and/or IgM to HB core Ag. Some but not all develop hepatitis clinically. Recovery and immunity is marked by absence of HBsAg and development of HBsAb. Chronic infection is marked by persistence of HBsAg and absence of HBsAb

B. Acute infection with HCV rarely causes clinical hepatitis but often results in chronic HCV infection. EIA for HCV Ab is used in screening for HCV infection and if positive, HCV RNA tests are used to confirm chronic infection and guide treatment.

III. Treatment

A. HBV vaccine universally recommended in the US and many other countries. Treatment consists of interferon and a number of antiviral medications. Professional boxing restricts participation with HBV infection and based on reports of transmission in contact sports, those with chronic HBV infection should be counseled against participation in collision and combat sports

B. Standard interferon and peginterferon alpha are current treatment options for HCV infection. Some state boxing commissions test for HCV but otherwise there are no formal recommendations for sports participation with HCV. Lack of immunization and risk of transmission warrants caution recommending participation in contact or collision sports.

FEBRILE ILLNESS

I. Epidemiology

A. Upper respiratory tract infection (URI) with picornavirus most common etiology

B. Enormous differential. In athletes, consider common infections that would be treated differently: mononucleosis, Group A strep pharyngitis, bacterial sinusitis, meningitis, pneumonia, gastrointestinal infection, pyelonephritis, systemic symptoms from disseminated bacterial skin infection.

II. Diagnosis

A. Clinical diagnosis for URI and other tests based on clinical suspicion.

III. Treatment

A. For typical URI symptoms, training can continue but should be modified for significant fatigue. Consider risk of transmission to teammates. Antipyretics, analgesics, and decongestants are helpful (certain decongestants are banned by some sports governing bodies).

B. The "neck rule" can be helpful. Symptoms below the neck (high fever, deep cough) should restrict training until resolved. Symptoms above the neck (congestion, sore throat) are compatible with continued participation.

C. Specific symptoms with contraindications to training and competition include
  1. High fever (concern for increased risk of myocarditis in setting of viremia)
  2. Vomiting and diarrhea (risk of dehydration and infection transmission)
  3. Splenomegaly (risk of splenic rupture)
  4. Contagious skin rash

5. Deep cough or wheeze with respiratory compromise/shortness of breath
6. Sinusitis in divers because of risk of barotrauma.

LYME DISEASE

I. Epidemiology

A. Tick-borne disease cause by *Borrelia burgdorferi* spread through bite of blacklegged ticks

B. Most common in US along Northeast coast with 30 cases annually per 100,000 population, next most common in upper Midwest

C. Not contagious among humans.

II. Diagnosis

A. Erythema migrans (EM) rash >5 cm diameter or common symptoms in setting of positive serology. In the US, EM occurs about 1 month after tick bite in 80% of those infected

B. Common presenting symptoms include fatigue, headache, arthralgia, myalgia, and stiff neck. Upper respiratory and gastrointestinal symptoms are uncommon

C. Serological testing is not necessary for diagnosis in setting of typical symptoms. Lyme serology often negative early in disease when patients present with EM. ELISA is the preferred screening test and Western blot is used to confirm positive screening test

D. Late manifestations if untreated include oligo-arthritis often involving knee and may include neurologic (neuropathy/encephalopathy) or cardiac abnormalities.

III. Treatment

A. EM should be treated with doxycyline 100 mg bid for 2–3 weeks

B. Amoxicillin 500 mg tid or cefuroxime 500 mg bid are alternatives or first-line treatment in children under 8 or pregnant women

C. Treatment recommendations are similar for late disease/arthritis although many recommend extending the treatment duration to 4 weeks.

INFECTIOUS MONONUCLEOSIS (IM)

I. Epidemiology

A. Most commonly caused by infection with Epstein–Barr virus (EBV), less commonly cytomegalovirus (CMV) infection

B. EBV minimally contagious
   1. <5% identify infection source, kissing vector
   2. 1–2 month incubation
   3. 15–25% of seropositive adults shed virus orally

C. EBV seroconversion generally asymptomatic
   1. 50% convert by age 5
   2. 30–50% of college students seroconverting develop IM.

II. Diagnosis

A. Presenting complaints
   1. In first week: malaise, fatigue, fever, pharyngitis, large anterior and often posterior cervical lymphadenopathy
   2. Splenomegaly occurs in 50% of cases week 2–3
      a. Splenic rupture feared complication with sports
      b. Rare, usually atraumatic, few reports after week 3 of illness
   3. Usually by 3–4 weeks systemic symptoms subsiding but significant fatigue can last 2–6 months

B. Diagnostic tests
1. WBC 10–20 K with atypical lymphocytes
2. In EBV infection, monospot (heterophile Ab) + 90% by week 3 of illness. False-negatives common in early infection
3. EBV or CMV IgM titers + 90% in first week.

III. Treatment

A. Supportive treatment and rest

B. Corticosteroids to reduce tonsillar hypertrophy compromising airway

C. No sports participation
1. For minimum 3–4 weeks from symptoms onset
2. Until systemic symptoms resolving with spleen nonpalpable

D. U/S spleen if unclear clinical exam and desire to return to collision sport before 6 weeks
1. Larger athletes may have larger spleens at baseline so mild enlargement must be interpreted cautiously

E. Gradually return as energy level allows

F. Meet with athlete weekly to follow progress
1. "Like a cold except 1 week = 1 day"
2. Symptoms except fatigue usually resolve by 1 month
3. Fatigue can persist 2–6 months and early return to training can worsen and prolong fatigue.

PROPHYLAXIS

I. Immunizations

A. Athletes are potentially at increased risk for many infections because of travel, training, and competition in close quarters, and transient immunosuppression secondary to heavy training.

B. Preparticipation exams are a good opportunity to review immunization status and initiate "catch-up" immunization if necessary. See Chapter 42 for more details. The CDC provides current guidelines for routine immunization: http://www.cdc.gov/vaccines/recs/schedules/downloads/adult/mmwr-adult-schedule.pdf

C. Immunizations with particular relevance for athletes include MMR, tetanus, influenza, varicella, meningococcal, hepatitis B, and HPV for female athletes. These are all universally recommended.

D. Hepatitis A vaccine is recommended for athletes traveling or living in endemic areas. Additional travel immunizations are recommended depending on destination and up-to-date recommendations are available from the CDC at http://www.nc.cdc.gov/travel/default.aspx.

II. Influenza

A. Influenza has received increased attention because of concerns with the H1N1 pandemic. The current annual vaccines include H1N1 protection. It is recommended that all teams receive influenza vaccine annually in the autumn months.

B. There is debate regarding the role of secondary prevention following exposure in nonimmunized individuals. Neuraminidase inhibitors (Zanamivir and Oseltamivir) can reduce the duration of influenza by 1–3 days if initiated within 48 h of symptom onset. Resistance has been more commonly reported with Oseltamivir, but Zanamivir is not recommended for those with asthma or COPD.

C. Influenza can be diagnosed clinically in those with typical symptoms in the setting of known outbreak/exposure. Otherwise, rapid antigen tests can provide in office diagnosis but the sensitivity is 40–60%. PCR testing has better sensitivity.

D. Antiviral treatment is recommended in pregnant women and others at high risk of morbidity and complications from influenza. The CDC does not recommend routine diagnostic testing or antiviral treatment for routine cases in those not at higher risk.

E. For athletes in their competitive season or nearing a big event, antiviral medication may be offered hoping to reduce the length of illness by a few days. For this strategy to be effective, athletes must be educated to report typical symptoms as quickly as possible, so treatment can be initiated and they can be quarantined from teammates.

SEPTIC JOINTS

I. Epidemiology

A. Bacterial infection of joint. Can occur by direct inoculation (bite/trauma) but most often hematogenous spread

B. Gram-positive bacterial infection most common
1. *Staphylococcus aureus* including MRSA and Strep

C. Gram-negative infection more likely following trauma, with IV drug use, in the very young and old, or otherwise immunocompromised

D. Risk factors for septic arthritis include underlying inflammatory arthritis (especially rheumatoid), diabetes, prosthetic joint or recent joint surgery, IV drug use, alcoholism, and intra-articular corticosteroid injection.

II. Diagnosis

A. Common symptoms: monoarticular swelling, stiffness, and pain often with fever

B. Knee infected most commonly. Wrist, ankle, and hip less commonly infected. Other joints rarely infected

C. Joint aspirate with high WBC count ($>100,000 \text{ mm}^3$). Gram stain generally positive for Gram + infection. Blood cultures positive in about 50% of cases.

III. Treatment

A. Intravenous antibiotics:
1. Vancomycin for Gram + stain or empiric treatment pending culture results
2. Vancomycin and third-generation cephalosporin if Gram (−) more likely based on presenting history
3. Depending on organism and severity of infection, IV treatment recommended for about 2 weeks followed by additional 2 weeks of pathogen-specific oral antibiotics

B. Joint drainage is generally recommended although studies comparing treatment with and without drainage and comparing methods of drainage (needle aspiration, arthroscopic lavage, open lavage) are lacking.

SEXUALLY TRANSMITTED DISEASES

I. Epidemiology

A. In the US, the average age of first intercourse is 16. Athletes are potentially at greater risk for STDs than the general population

B. Studies with adolescent athletes are mixed; some suggesting female athletes are at lower risk for STDs and pregnancy than their nonathlete counterparts but other studies suggest increased sexual activity and increased number of sexual partners in athletes. The social environment in certain high-profile profession sports is associated with high numbers of sexual partners.

C. Common STDs include gonorrhea, chlamydia, trichomoniasis, genital warts (primarily HPV types 6 and 11) or cervical dysplasia/carcinoma (primarily HPV types 16, 18, 52), and Herpes (HSV 2 >1 for genital lesions)

D. Adolescents engaging in early intercourse (age <16) are at particularly high risk for chlamydia and HPV with studies reporting infection rates above 30%. The highest reported rates of chlamydia are in 15–19-year-old females

E. Less common STDs include hepatitis B and C, HIV, and syphilis.

II. Diagnosis

A. Symptoms vary with the common infections. Common manifestations of STDs include vaginal or urethral discharge, warts, and ulcerations, and in women, pelvic inflammatory disease (PID).

B. Gonorrhea, trichomoniasis, and chlamydia are the most common sexually transmitted causes of discharge. Males are most likely to have symptomatic urethral discharge while women may have vaginal discharge but are more likely than men to have asymptomatic infection. Chlamydia is often asymptomatic in women but 10% of women infected will develop PID if untreated. Because of the high incidence of asymptomatic infection, CDC recommends annual screening for gonorrhea and chlamydia in all sexually active females age 25 and under.

   1. Diagnostic testing
      a. Trichomoniasis is diagnosed by identifying organisms on wet mount
      b. Gonorrhea in males can be identified by Gram stain and culture of discharge. This technique is less sensitive in females
      c. Currently, the most sensitive and specific testing for gonorrhea and chlamydia is nucleic acid amplification. Test can be performed on a urine sample or oral, vaginal, or rectal swab.

C. HSV is the most common cause of genital ulceration. Primary infection presents with prodromal itching and pain followed by the development of painful vesicles that often spontaneously rupture, resulting in ulcers. Local adenopathy and dysuria are common. Systemic symptoms including fever and myalgia occur over half the time. Lesions spontaneously resolve but viral reactivation causes clinical recurrence often with fewer vesicles recurring at the same site. Systemic symptoms are uncommon with recurrence and recurring lesions may be asymptomatic.

   1. Diagnostic testing includes viral culture of vesicle fluid during outbreak. PCR of the fluid is more sensitive. HSV serology can be used for diagnosis in patient without active lesions.

D. HPV causes genital warts and oncogenic HPV strains cause cervical and anogenital neoplasia. Genital warts appear as flat, smooth, or verrucous papules on the external genitalia, anus, or cervix. Cervical infection is asymptomatic until presentation with advanced cervical cancer. Asymptomatic infection is identified through regular cervical PAP testing, with HVP DNA testing playing a role in secondary testing and screening.

III. Treatment

A. Chlamydia is treated with azithromycin 1 g po single dose or doxycycline 100 mg po bid for 7 days. Gonorrhea is treated with cefixime 400 mg po single dose or ceftriaxone 250 mg IM. The infections often coexist and combination treatment is recommended unless infection with one is ruled out at the time of documentation of the other infection. Partners should be treated as well and intercourse should be avoided for 1 week after completion of treatment.

B. Trichomoniasis is treated with tinidazole or metronidazole 2 g po single dose. Topical metronidazole recurrence rates are 50%, possibly from urethral reinfection

C. HSV infection cannot be cured. Barrier contraceptives can decrease the likelihood of transmission and infection
   1. For primary infection, antiviral treatment within 72 h of onset can decrease length and severity of symptoms. Acyclovir 400 mg tid for 7–10 days or comparable regimen of other antiviral medication is recommended
   2. Recurring infection is treated with acyclovir 800 mg tid for 2 days started immediately at first symptom of recurrence
   3. Acyclovir 400 mg bid can be used as suppressive therapy in those with more frequent recurrences and suppressive therapy can decrease the risk of transmission.

D. HPV infection cannot be cured
   1. Warts can be destroyed or excised but may recur and infection can be transmitted in the absence of visible warts
   2. Imiquimod is a topical immunomodulator approved in the treatment of anogenital warts
   3. Two vaccines against HPV are available: Quadrivalent Gardasil (HPV 6, 11, 16, 18) covers the most common cause of genital warts (HPV 6, 11) and cervical cancer (HPV 16, 18). Cervarix is bivalent covering HPV 16 and 18. The vaccines are given in three doses and are most effective if administered prior to HPV exposure. The vaccine is generally recommended for girls starting at age 11.

UPPER RESPIRATORY TRACT INFECTION

I. Epidemiology

A. Cause by picornaviruses: Rhino, Echo, Coxsackie

B. Generally spread via secretions hand to hand or hand to face and less commonly via aerosolized droplets

C. Incubation period 2–3 days and symptoms of infection typically last 4–10 days

D. Exercise appears to influence susceptibility to URI. Moderate exercise may be protective while heavy exercise may increase susceptibility to infection
   1. High-mileage runners are twice as likely to report URI symptoms compared to lower mileage runners and studies have reported a sixfold increase in URI symptoms after running a marathon
   2. Mechanism likely combination of increased cortisol and decreased IgM, salivary IgA, and natural killer cells with high-intensity training.

II. Diagnosis

A. Diagnosis is made clinically and diagnostic testing should be reserved for symptom severity out of the ordinary, symptoms more specific for differential diagnosis listed below, or symptoms that fail to resolve in typical time course

B. Typical symptoms include congestion with secretions often becoming purulent, cough, sore throat, low-grade fever, and headache/sinus pressure

C. Common differential includes allergic rhinitis, acute bronchitis, pneumonia, bacterial sinusitis, acute otitis media, strep pharyngitis, and infectious mononucleosis.

III. Treatment

A. Antipyretics, analgesics, decongestants, and antihistamines are all effective for symptom management. Decongestants are banned by some sport governing bodies

B. Antibiotics do not shorten course or provide relief for URI or bronchitis and should be discouraged to avoid fostering the development of antibiotic resistance

C. Athletes with significant fatigue, high fever, and systemic symptoms (i.e., symptoms below the neck) should restrict training until improving (see sections on febrile illness and mononucleosis).

MRSA

I. Epidemiology

A. Methacillin-Resistant Staph Aureus (MRSA) was identified in the 1960s as a nosocomial infection. Currently, it is the most commonly community acquired skin infection in the US

B. When first identified, hospital-acquired MRSA consisted of primarily two distinct types and community-acquired MRSA represented a third type. Additional types have been described and infection with the different types is no longer limited to one setting or the other

C. Methacillin resistance is defined by an oxacillin minimum inhibitory concentration (MIC) ≥ 4 mcg/mL. MRSA is resistant to all beta-lactam antibiotics and certain types have developed rapid resistance to other antibiotics, quinolones being a prime example

D. MRSA outbreaks have been reported in athletic settings and athletes, specifically football players, are classified as an at-risk group. One large outbreak on a college football team was extensively investigated by the local health department and shared towel use was suspected in the transmission of infection. MRSA has also been cultured from surfaces and athletic equipment in the setting of outbreaks.

II. Diagnosis

A. In athletes, MRSA is most likely to present as a skin infection, most often an abscess. Other skin manifestations include cellulitis, necrotizing fasciitis, and wound infections. MRSA can also cause osteomyelitis, ear and urinary tract infection, pneumonia, endocarditis, and sepsis

B. Typical skin infections are painful, presenting with erythema, induration, and frequently an abscess that may drain pus. The initial lesion is often mistaken for a spider bite. The course varies from indolent to rapidly progressive in some individuals.

III. Treatment

A. Recommendations vary for empiric treatment of soft tissue infection. Some recommend initial coverage with cephalosporin or dicloxicillin pending culture. Others feel the prevalence of MRSA warrants empiric treatment with MRSA-sensitive antibiotic and local infection patterns should guide this decision.

B. The first-line oral treatments for MRSA are not as effective against Group A strep, so double coverage for MRSA and Group A strep is recommended by some authorities pending culture results.

C. Athletes, coaches, and athletic training staff need to be aware of early signs of infection. Often, incision and drainage (I & D) provide adequate treatment and some authorities recommend I & D without antibiotics for isolated abscess less than 5 cm in healthy individuals. Some recommend culture with sensitivities for all abscesses while others reserve culture for lesions that do not respond to initial I & D or those appearing more serious.

D. Traditional oral antibiotics that are generally effective for MRSA include trimethoprim-sulfamethoxazole (Bactrim DS) 2 tabs bid, clindamycin 300–450 mg Q 6–8 h), minocycline or doxycycline 100 mg bid. A 7–10 days course is recommended.

E. Infections not responding to the above regimes or more serious infections should be treated with vancomycin IV (15–20 mg/kg every 12 h). Linezolid is a second-line oral and IV drug with activity against strep and MRSA. There are reports of patients with MRSA developing linezolid resistance rapidly and potential toxicities require regular monitoring.

F. Athletic settings should incorporate MRSA prevention strategies including:
1. Athlete and staff education regarding the appearance of MRSA infection
2. Athlete education regarding bathing with bactericidal soap after every training session
3. Cleaning and covering any cuts or breaks in skin
4. The use of universal precautions

5. Regular cleaning of surfaces and shared equipment with antimicrobial agent effective against MRSA
6. Avoid sharing of towels and other personal hygiene items.

Recommended Reading

1. Bacon RM, Kugeler KJ, Griffith KS, Mead PS. Lyme disease—United States, 2003–2005. *MMWR Weekly.* 2007;56(23):573–576.
2. Gutierrez RL, Decker CF. Blood-borne infections and the athlete. *Dis Mon.* 2010;56:436–442.
3. King OS. Infectious disease and boxing. *Clin Sports Med.* 2009;28;545–560.
4. Kordi R, Wallace WA. Blood borne infections in sport: Risks of transmission, methods of prevention, and recommendations for hepatitis B vaccination. *Br J Sports Med.* 2004;38:678–684.
5. Luke A, d'Hemecourt P. Prevention of infectious diseases in athletes. *Clin Sports Med.* 2007;26:321–344.

42

Sports Allergy and Immunology
Joanna L. McKey and Robert J. Dimeff

I. Immunizations

A. The sports medicine physician may be the only medical doctor to provide care to an athlete. As such, this relationship can provide an opportunity to promote primary prevention with respect to immunizations.

B. Immunizations involve administration of inactivated or live, attenuated viruses to provide active immunity
   1. More side effects with live, attenuated viruses
      a. Most common side effects: local pain, hypersensitivity reaction to vaccine constituents
   2. Conditions commonly misperceived as contraindications to vaccines:
      a. Acute illness with or without fever
      b. Current antimicrobial therapy
      c. Mild or moderate local reaction to previous vaccine
      d. Recent exposure to infectious disease
      e. Allergies
      f. Family history of adverse event

C. The following considerations should be made by the sports medicine physician:
   1. Routine health maintenance
   2. Catch-up immunizations for those who fall behind or start late
   3. High-risk groups—immunocompromised, chronic cardiovascular or pulmonary disease, asplenia, sickle cell, diabetes mellitus, cirrhosis, and age over 65
   4. Close contact or recent potential exposure to infected individual
   5. Influenza vaccine is recommended for all persons with more than 6 months of age
   6. Travel planned to endemic area
      a. Ideally should plan several months in advance
      b. CDC website provides information on recommended vaccines for travel http://www.nc.cdc.gov/travel/content/vaccinations

D. CDC Vaccination Schedule (Tables 42.1 through 42.3).

II. Anaphylaxis

A. Severe, acute, potentially life-threatening systemic reaction resulting from the release of vaso-active mediators from mast cells and basophils

B. Prevalence estimated to range from 0.05 to as high as 2% in the general population

C. Asthma and atopy are risk factors for anaphylaxis

D. Signs and symptoms:
   1. Sensation of tingling or warmth, flushing, generalized pruritis, urticarial lesions typically 1–2 cm in diameter or angioedema

Table 42.1 Recommended immunization schedule for persons aged 0–6 years united states 2011

Age → Vaccine ↓	Birth	1 Month	2 Months	4 Months	6 Months	12 Months	15 Months	18 Months	19–23 Months	2–3 Years	4–6 Years
Hepatitis B	Hep B	Hep B			Hep B						
Rotavirus			RV	RV	RV						
Diphtheria, Tetanus, Pertusis			DTaP	DTaP	DTaP		DTaP				DTaP
Hemophilus Influenza Type b			Hib	Hib	Hib	HiB					
Pneumococcal			PCV	PCV	PCV	PCV					PCV catch up
Inactivated Poliovirus			IPV	IPV		IPV					IPV
Influenza						Influenza Yearly					
Measles, Mumps, Rubella						MMR					MMR
Varicella						Varicella					Varicella
Hepatitis A							Hep A (2 doses)				HepA catch up

Table 42.2   Recommended immunization schedule for persons aged 7–18 years
United States 2011

Age → Vaccine ↓	7–10 Years	11–12 Years	13–18 Years
Tetanus, Diphtheria, Pertussis		Tdap (1 dose if >5 years)	
Human Papillomavirus		HPV (3 dose series)	
Meningococcal		MCV4	
Influenza		Influenza yearly	
Pneumococcal		High-risk groups	
Hepatitis A		High-risk groups	
Hepatitis B	Hep B catch-up series		
Inactivated Poliovirus	IPV catch-up series		
Measles, Mumps, Rubella	MMR catch-up series		
Varicella	Varicella catch-up series		

2. Respiratory symptoms such as wheezing, cough, chest tightness, stridor, swelling of the mouth or airway and respiratory distress

3. Gastrointestinal (GI) symptoms such as vomiting, cramping, or diarrhea

4. Pale, diaphoresis, palpitations, chest pain, arrhythmias, hypotension

5. Pre-syncope, syncope, headache, feeling of impending doom, unconsciousness

6. Late phase or "biphasic" reactions due to slow-releasing substances

   a. Symptoms appear to resolve but return in 1–72 h (mean of 10 h) and can be more severe

   b. Occur in up to 25% of cases of fatal or near fatal anaphylaxis

E. Causes

  1. Food is the most common cause of anaphylaxis

   a. Accounts for 30% of fatal cases

   b. Commonly implicated—peanuts, tree nuts, shellfish, fish, soy, egg

  2. Drugs (penicillin), biological agents, or radiographic contrast

  3. Nonsteroidal anti-inflammatory (NSAIDS) and aspirin (second most common drug causing anaphylaxis)

  4. Insect bites or stings

  5. Natural rubber latex

   a. High-risk groups for reaction to latex: healthcare workers, workers with occupational exposure to latex, and children with spina bifida and genitourinary abnormalities

  6. Seminal fluid

  7. Allergen immunotherapy

  8. Exercise

  9. Idiopathic

F. Pathophysiology

  1. Generally thought to be IgE-mediated Type 1 hypersensitivity reaction, but may also be IgE independent, IgG dependent, or nonimmunologically mediated

  2. Exposure to allergen or other factor that activates mast cells and basophils

  3. Degranulation and release of vasoactive mediators such as histamine

  4. Production of prostaglandins, leukotrienes, platelet activating factor (PAF), cytokines (e.g., tumor necrosis factor [TNF]), chemokines

Table 42.3 Recommended vaccines for persons aged 19 years and older United States 2011

Age group → Vaccine ↓	19–26 Years	27–49 Years	50–59 Years	60–64 Years	≥65 Years
Influenza	1 dose yearly				
Tetanus, Diphtheria, Pertussis	Substitute 1 time dose of Tdap for Td booster, then boost with Td every 10 years				
Varicella	2 doses for persons who lack immunity or previous infection				
Human Papillomavirus (HPV)	3 dose series				
Zoster				1 dose	
Measles, Mumps, Rubella (MMR)	1 or 2 doses for persons who lack immunity or evidence of prior infection		1 dose if high-risk		
Pneumococcal (Polysaccharide)	1 or 2 doses if high-risk				1 dose
Meningococcal	1 or more doses if high-risk				
Hepatitis A	2 doses if high-risk				
Hepatitis B	3 doses if high-risk				

G. Diagnosis
   1. Thorough history from patient, witnesses of event and family members
      a. Characteristics of symptoms during event
      b. All medications and food consumed 4–6 h prior to episode
      c. Activities 4–6 h prior to episode (sexual activity, exercise)
      d. Any preceding bite or sting
      e. Medical history (asthma, atopy)
      f. Family medical history (asthma, atopy)
   2. Skin prick testing is more sensitive than *in vitro* specific IgE testing
      a. History may be so conclusive of a specific agent that no additional testing is needed
      b. Testing for a specific agent or potential allergen may not be available or may have a low predictive value
      c. Must consider the risk of having a severe reaction during skin testing versus the potential benefits of testing
   3. Challenge testing may be appropriate but must be performed under controlled circumstances with appropriate rescue treatment available
   4. Laboratory studies that may be helpful in diagnosing anaphylaxis
      a. Serum tryptase
         i. Level peaks in first 1–1.5 h after onset of symptoms and persists for 5–6 h
         ii. Should be drawn in first 1–2 h after onset of symptoms
         iii. May not be elevated in anaphylaxis due to food
         iv. Elevated tryptase when asymptomatic may indicate mastocytosis
      b. Plasma histamine
         i. Levels begin to increase 5–10 min after onset of symptoms and remain elevated for 30–60 min
         ii. Less helpful if not drawn within an hour after the onset of symptoms

H. Treatment of anaphylaxis
  1. Acute management
     a. Assess airway, breathing, circulation, and consciousness (unconsciousness may reflect hypoxia)
     b. Epinephrine 1:1000 dilution (1 mg/ml) 0.2–0.5 ml (0.01 mg/kg in children with max dosage 0.3 mg) intramuscular (IM) into lateral aspect of thigh, may repeat every 5 min
     c. Place patient recumbent and elevate legs
     d. Supplemental oxygen
     e. May require large volumes of intravenous (IV) colloid or cystalloid fluid
     f. Consider inhaled beta-2 agonists (e.g., albuterol metered dose inhaler [MDI] 2–6 puffs or nebulized 2.5–5 mg, repeated doses as necessary)
     g. Histamine-1 (H1) antagonist such as diphenhydramine IV or IM 25–50 mg in adults and 1–2 mg/kg in children, hydroxyzine or other H1 antagonist
     h. Histamine-2 (H2) antagonist such as ranitidine IV or IM 50 mg in adults and 12.5–50 mg (1 mg/kg) in children or cimetidine 4 mg/kg in adults (no dosage studied in children)
        i. Combination of H1 and H2 antagonist is superior to H1 antagonist alone
        ii. Should not be given in lieu of epinephrine
        iii. Glucocorticoids have the potential to prevent recurrent or protracted anaphylaxis
            (A) No conclusive evidence for prevention of biphasic reaction
  2. Prevention/lifestyle modification
     a. Identify cause if possible
     b. Immunotherapy/desensitization therapy
     c. Patient education
        i. Avoidance of known or suspected triggers
        ii. Medical alert bracelet
        iii. Epinephrine autoinjector (Epi-Pen) availability and teaching.

III. Exercise-Induced Anaphylaxis (EIA)

A. Specific form of anaphylaxis in which exercise is the only trigger
B. Can occur during vigorous exercise such as jogging, tennis, aerobics, or may occur with light activity such as walking or yard work
C. May be isolated or recurrent
   1. Most patients experience fewer and less severe attacks over time
   2. Episodes are unpredictable and occur sporadically even in the face of regularly exercise
D. 50% of patients with EIA have personal or family history of atopy
E. Cotriggers
   1. Often required for symptoms to occur
   2. In absence of exercise, cotriggers do not cause any symptoms
   3. NSAID/aspirin ingestion preceding exercise by hours to a day have been associated with EIA
   4. Alcohol ingestion 4–6 h prior to exercise
   5. Menstruation
   6. Pollen exposure in pollen-sensitive individual
F. Food-Dependent Exercise Induced Anaphylaxis (FDEIA)
   1. Ingestion of specific food or a meal consumed within 4–6 h of exercise leads to symptoms
   2. Ingestion of food alone does not cause symptoms
   3. Most common food implicated is wheat, specifically water-insoluble gliadins
      a. Other foods: shellfish, tree nuts, peanuts, vegetables (celery), fruits, cow's milk and eggs

G. Variant Type Exercise-Induced Anaphylaxis (VTEIA)
  1. About 10% of cases
  2. Combination of features of EIA and cholinergic urticaria (CU)
    a. Punctate (2–4 mm) urticaria as seen in CU and can progress to complete vascular collapse as seen in EIA
  3. Precipitated only by exercise and not by passive warming

H. Symptoms
  1. Feeling of warmth, flushing, fatigue, malaise, pruritus, and urticaria
    a. May progress to angioedema, respiratory distress and laryngeoedema, GI symptoms, hypotension, and cardiovascular collapse
  2. Headache that can persist for several days
  3. Symptoms frequently abate over several hours with cessation of exercise

I. Pathophysiology of EIA
  1. Not well understood, likely mast cell mediated
  2. Exact mechanism leading to mast cell activation has not been elucidated

J. Diagnosis
  1. Thorough clinical history, including detailed dietary recall and medications to identify any cotriggers
  2. Skin or *in vitro* allergen testing
  3. Exercise treadmill testing
  4. Food challenge with exercise treadmill testing

K. Differential diagnosis
  1. Exercise-induced asthma, cholinergic urticaria, exercise-associated gastroesophageal reflux, arrhythmias
  2. Cholinergic urticaria can usually be differentiated by smaller 1–3 mm punctuate wheals and symptoms can be elicited by passively increasing body temperature

L. Treatment of EIA
  1. Immediate cessation of exercise at onset of symptoms
  2. Acute treatment as in anaphylaxis of any cause
  3. Patient education/lifestyle modification
    a. Avoid exercise 4–6 h after eating
    b. Avoid foods known to trigger FDEIA
    c. Avoid aspirin and other NSAIDS before exercise
    d. Refrain from exercise around menses
    e. May need to avoid exercise on warm/humid days or reduce intensity
    f. Epinephrine availability at all times and proper training on use
    g. Exercise with a partner who is aware of medical condition and epinephrine use
    h. Cease exercise immediately at first signs or symptoms
      i. Impending anaphylactic reaction may abate spontaneously
      ii. Seek immediate medical assistance if symptoms occur

M. Prophylactic medications
  1. Controversial, not effective in majority of patients with EIA
  2. Small subset of patients may benefit from daily use of antihistamine
  3. H1 antagonists can be used to treat dermatologic symptoms
    a. Hydroxyzine 25–50 mg four times daily
    b. Other nonsedating H1 antagonists (cetirizine, loratadine, fexofenadine) may have similar effects and should not impair athletic performance
    c. H2 antagonists (famotidine, ranitidine) can be added for refractory symptoms

4. Cromolyn, a mast cell stabilizer that prevents degranulation and release of plasma histamine and other inflammatory mediators, has had inconclusive results in prophylactic treatment of EIA

5. Other medications such as leukotreine modifying agents (montelukast, zafirlukast, zileuton) to date have not been studied for the management of EIA.

IV. Urticaria

A. Circumscribed, raised, erythematous evanescent areas of edema involving superficial portion of dermis
   1. Usually highly pruritic and arises suddenly
   2. Rarely persists more than 24–48 h
   3. Acutely affects 20% of the population

B. Angioedema occurs when edematous process extends into the deep dermis and/or subcutaneous and submucosal layers
   1. Commonly affects face, neck, and part of extremity
   2. Can be painful but usually not pruritic
   3. Can persists for 72 h
   4. Adults more likely to experience angioedema with urticaria

C. Classification
   1. Acute urticaria <6 weeks
      a. Causes include drugs, foods, viral upper respiratory tract infections
   2. Chronic urticaria >6 weeks duration
      a. Causes include autoimmune, idiopathic, physical (e.g., pressure, cold, solar), infections, paraneoplastic, enzymatic defects (hereditary angioedema)

D. Physical urticarias
   1. Dermographism
      a. Exaggerated response in which stroking of the skin produces an initial red line followed by broadening erythema and formation of a linear wheal
   2. Cold urticaria/angioedema
      a. Occurs within minutes of exposure to changes in ambient temperature or direct contact with cold objects or air
      b. Can be associated with headache, hypotension, syncope, wheezing, shortness of breath, palpitations, GI symptoms
      c. Can affect inside of the mouth and tongue in 25% of patients
      d. Wheal elicited after application of ice is diagnostic (cold contact test)
      e. Can be lethal if hypotension and syncope occur when entire body is cooled (e.g., swimming)
      f. Can be associated with infectious diseases (syphilis, measles, hepatitis, human immunodeficiency virus, and mononucleosis)
      g. Frequently associated with cholinergic urticaria
      h. Cyproheptadine is drug of choice for cold-induced urticaria
   3. Cholinergic urticaria (CU)
      a. Develops after increase in core body temperature of 0.5–1.5 °C or 0.9–2.7 °F
      b. During exercise, warm bath, stress, emotions, spicy foods
      c. Predominately in 20–30-year-old patients
      d. Associated with increased prevalence of atopy
      e. Pruritic, punctate wheals often surrounded by erythematous halo
      f. Lesions can become confluent and angioedema may develop
      g. Typically begins on neck and upper trunk but may spread to entire body
      h. Can be associated with systemic symptoms but rarely with vascular collapse/shock
      i. Lesions usually resolve within 20 min, multiple lesions may persist hours

    j. Diagnosis
      i. Intradermal injection of methacholine produces a nonfollicular distribution of characteristic wheals in one third of patients
    k. Frequently occurs with cold urticaria
    l. May also have cold-induced cholinergic urticaria
  4. Solar urticaria
    a. Erythema, wheals, pruritus, and occasionally angioedema occur within minutes after exposure to sun or artificial light sources
    b. Can be associated with systemic symptoms
    c. Usually occurs in the third decade of life
    d. Diagnosis
      i. Irradiation with UV solar stimulator or visible light produces characteristic wheals
  5. Aquagenic urticaria
    a. Contact with water produces wheals
  6. Delayed pressure urticaria
    a. Lesions are typically deep, painful swellings that develop 4–8 h after applied pressure
    b. Frequently involve buttocks, palms, soles
  7. Contact urticaria
    a. Eruption appears within minutes of exposure
    b. Most commonly nonimmunologically mediated
    c. IgE mediated may be associated with systemic symptoms
    d. Most frequent allergen = latex, cross-reactivity frequently seen (banana, avocado, kiwi)
    e. High-risk groups for reaction to latex: healthcare workers, workers with occupational exposure to latex, and children with spina bifida and genitourinary abnormalities
    f. Associated manifestations include allergic rhinitis, conjunctivitis, and respiratory symptoms
    g. Rarely associated with shock
    h. Diagnosis with skin prick testing or IgE-specific *in vitro* assays when indicated
  E. Treatment
    1. General management
      a. Avoidance of identified triggers
      b. Treatment of any coexisting infections
    2. Pharmacotherapy (see Table 42.4).

V. Allergic Rhinitis (AR)

  A. Caused by allergen-induced inflammation of the nasal mucosa
  B. Affects 10–20% of the population
  C. Signs and symptoms
    1. Watery rhinorrhea, sneezing, itching of nose, throat or eyes, nasal congestion, mouth breathing, snoring, nasal voice, sniffing, postnasal drainage, and occasionally cough
    2. Systemic symptoms can include headache, fatigue, decreased concentration, reduced productivity, difficulty in sleeping
    3. Can have negative effect on quality of life and impair athletic performance
  D. Diagnosis
    1. Not necessary to identify exact offending allergen
    2. Time of year and circumstances of symptoms can provide clues
    3. Nasal smear with >4% eosinophilia may be suggestive
    4. Specific IgE *in vitro* assays such as radioallergosorbent testing or skin prick testing can help identify specific allergen
  E. Treatment

Table 42.4 Medications to Treat Urticaria

H1 blocking antihistamines	Non-Sedating Cetirizine Levoceterizine Loratadine Desloratadine Fexofenadine	First-line treatment for acute and chronic urticaria. Start with non-sedating antihistamines Treat 4–6 weeks then may try tapering off
H1 blocking antihistamines	Sedating Doxepin Hydroxyzine Diphenhydramine Cyproheptadine	Added if symptoms uncontrolled after 1–2 weeks of non-sedating H1 blocker. Anticholinergic side effects- dry mouth, urinary retention, cognitive impairment Sedative effect is variable and medication should be taken before bedtime. Avoid alcohol, hypnotics, opioids and mood-elevating drugs. Doxpein is a tricyclic antidepressive with H1 and H2 antagonist. Cyproheptadine beneficial for cold induced urticaria.
H2 Antagonists	Ranitidine Cimetidine	Can be added to H1 blocker to achieve better control
Corticosteroids	Prednisone Dexamethasone	Short course can be helpful in reducing duration of symptoms if severe episode. Refer to specialists if unable to stop because of recurrence of urticaria
Leukotriene Receptor Antagonist	Montelukast Zafirlukast	Second – line treatment Efficacy not well established
Immunomodulatory Agents/ Anti-inflammatory Agents	Cyclosporine Methotrexate Hydroxychloroquine Dapsone Sulfasalazine Cyclophosphamide Cyclophosphamide	Significant potential side effects Should be monitored by specialist Sulfasalazine may be beneficial in delayed-pressure urticaria

1. Allergy avoidance/limit exposure: avoid peak pollen times (5 a.m. to 10 a.m.), keep air conditioning on during pollen seasons
2. Antihistamines
   a. Oral: second- or third-generation H1 blocking antihistamines (ceterizine, loratadine, fexofenadine) have little sedation and less anticholinergic side effects
   b. Intranasal: azelastine is a fast-acting spray good for acute allergy management without adverse effects of sedation
3. Intranasal corticosteroids (INS)

    a. INS (beclomethasone dipropionate, flunisolide, budesonide) should be used as first-line therapy

    b. Onset of action as soon as 12 h and can be taken on an as-needed basis

    c. Do not compromise eligibility to participate in sports

    d. Few side effects other than local irritation

  4. Oral leukotriene receptor antagonists (LTRA)

    a. LTRA (montelukast, zafirlukast) improve symptoms

  5. Intranasal decongestants

    a. Oxymetazoline (long acting alpha-1 and 2a agonist)

    b. Phenylepherine (alph-1 agonist)

    c. Very effective for treatment of nasal obstruction

    d. Risk of rebound vasodilation and rhinitis medicamentosa with prolonged use

  6. Oral decongestants

    a. Pseudoephedrine (alpha and beta agonist properties)

    b. More systemic side effects, longer acting than topical

    c. May require a therapeutic use exemption for use during competition season.

Recommended Reading

1. Beaudouin E, Renaudin JM, Morisset M, Codreanu F, Kanny G, Moneret-Vautrin DA. Food-dependent exercise-induced anaphylaxis—update and current data. *Eur Ann Aller Clin Immunol.* 2006;*38*(2):45–51.
2. Dice J. Physical urticaria. *Immunol Aller Clin North Am.* 2004;*24*(2):225–246.
3. Frigas E, Park M. Acute urticaria and angioedema—diagnostic and treatment considerations. *Am J Clin Dermatol.* 2009;*10*(4):239–250.
4. Hosey R, Carek P, Goo A. Exercise-induced anaphylaxis and urticaria. *Am Fam Physician.* 2001;*64*(8):1367–1372.
5. Lieberman P, Nicklas R, Oppenheimer J, Kemp S, Lang D. The diagnosis and management of anaphylaxis practice parameter: 2010 update. *J Aller Clin Immunol.* 2010;*126*(3):477–480.e1-42.
6. MacKnight J, Mistry D. Allergic disorders in the athlete. *Clin Sports Med.* 2005;*24*(3):507–523.
7. Mahr T, Sheth K. Update on allergic rhinitis. *Pediatr Rev.* 2005;*26*(8):284–289.
8. Robson-Ansley P, Toit G. Pathophysiology, diagnosis and management of exercise-induced anaphylaxis. *Curr Opin Aller Clin Immunol.* 2010;*10*(4):312–317.
9. Schwartz L, Delgado L, Bonini S, et al. Exercise-induced hypersensitivity syndromes in recreational and competitive athletes: A PRACTALL consensus report (what the general practitioner should know about sports and allergy). *Allergy.* 2008;*63*(8):953–961.

43

Sports Rheumatology

Ryan Foreman, Bryan Mason, and Mark E. Lavallee

I. General

A. Arthritis and rheumatism are the most common causes of disability in the United States, and affected persons have a substantially lower health-related quality of life

B. There is no "cure" and they require ongoing management, including activity modifications, rehabilitation to correct biomechanical deficits, judicious use of braces and assistive devices, and medical therapy to decrease inflammation and slow joint destruction (e.g., disease-modifying antirheumatic drugs [DMARDs], monoclonal antibodies).

II. Rheumatoid Arthritis (RA)

A. Prevalence
  1. Affects nearly 1% of adults over 35 years in the United States
  2. Nearly twice as common in females
  3. Currently, a decline in the incidence of the disease

B. Pathogenesis
  1. Joint destruction begins with inflammatory cell invasion
  2. A viscous cycle of inflammatory cell invasion and irregular tissue growth
  3. Chronic destructive synovitis
  4. Inflammatory burden can also affect other organs and organ systems leading to systemic complications

C. Physical findings
  1. Patients commonly present with joint swelling, pain, and stiffness
  2. One should consider workup in patient with even a single joint with unexplained synovitis
  3. Joints of the wrist and hand often involved
     a. Metacarpophalangeal
     b. Interphalangeal
  4. Joints are often boggy, tender, and warm

D. Diagnostic guidelines (2010)
  1. Intended to help physicians diagnose RA earlier in the disease course
  2. Target population for workup
     a. Synovitis (swelling) of one or more joints
     b. Synovitis not explained by another disease/cause
  3. Classification criteria (see *2010 Rheumatoid Arthritis Classification Criteria; Arthritis and Rheumatism 2010* for details). Score of 6 or greater is diagnostic of rheumatoid arthritis
     a. Joint involvement
        i. 2–10 *large joints (1 point)
        ii. 1–3 **small joints (2 points)

      iii. 4–10 **small joints (3 points)

      iv. >10 joints, with at least 1 small joint (5 points)

      *Large joints: shoulder, elbow, hip, knee, and ankle

      **Small joints: metacarpophalangeal (MCP), proximal interphalangeal (PIP), second through fifth metatarsophalangeal (MTP) joints, thumb interphalangeal (IP) joints, and wrist

   b. Serology (rheumatoid factor [RF] and anticitrullinated protein antibody [ACPA])

      i. Low positive (<3 times the upper limit of normal) RF or ACPA (1 point)

      ii. High positive (>3 times the upper limit of normal) RF or ACPA (2 points)

   c. Elevated ESR or CRP (1 point)

   d. Symptoms lasting >6 weeks (1 point)

E. Treatment

   1. Early initiation of DMARDs intended to slow progression of disease

      a. Methotrexate (first-line therapy in most cases)

      b. Sulfasalazine, leflunomide, minocycline, and injectable gold salts (can be used as first-line therapy for mild disease or in patients who cannot tolerate methotrexate)

      c. Biological agents should be added when inadequate response to first-line therapy. They include tumor necrosis factor antagonists, etanercept, infliximab, adalimumab, rituximab, anakinra, azathioprine

      d. 30%–40% remission rates have been reported with use of DMARDs

   2. Other pharmacological agents for symptom management

      a. Nonsteroidal anti-inflammatory drugs (NSAIDs)

      b. Low dose oral or intra-articular glucocorticoids

   3. Nonpharmacological therapies

      a. Essential fatty acid supplements

      b. Regular exercise with an activity prescription tailored to disease severity

      c. Joint replacement surgery (knee, hips, MCP)

F. Prognosis

   1. Factors that negatively affect prognosis

      a. Early involvement of multiple joints

      b. Strong family history

      c. Marked elevation of acute-phase reactants (ESR and CRP) at time of diagnosis

      d. Radiographic changes early in the disease process

      e. Presence of other autoimmune conditions (sjorgen's, lupus, scleroderma, etc.)

      f. Those with severe disease less likely to respond to DMARD therapy

G. Rheumatoid arthritis and exercise

   1. Avoid combative/collision/contact sports, especially during the early phases of the condition when DMARDs are starting to work or if there is evidence of atlanto-axial instability

   2. Activity based on severity of disease

      a. Disease state is quiescent with complete functional recovery: moderate to vigorous activity as tolerated (e.g., running, weight lifting)

      b. Disease state is quiescent with minimal to moderate impairment: mild to moderate activity (e.g., swimming, cycling)

      c. Symptomatic with effusions and synovial changes in weight bearing joints: mild activity with participation at own tolerance (e.g., walking, water aerobics)

   3. Low-impact aerobic activity (e.g., swimming, cycling) can be beneficial without increasing pain or compromising function. Exercise should be modified to the individual as needed to be safe and not damaging to joint or muscle tissue

H. Osteoarthritis and exercise

   1. Physical activity as tolerated by pain and mechanical defect is a crucial aspect of arthritis management

   2. Long-term impact of overloading affected joint(s) may advance disease more quickly

3. Range of motion, balance exercises, low-impact aerobic activity, and strength training are preferred forms of exercise
4. A variety of exercise protocols have been developed specifically for persons with arthritis that emphasize:
   a. Reducing biomechanical stress on joints
   b. Reducing impact overloading through use of shock-absorbing footwear or alternating weight-bearing/non-weight-bearing activities
   c. Reducing compressive forces at hip and knee by limiting running/jumping
   d. Controlled, static stretching to avoid hypermobility
   e. Avoiding high-repetition exercises by modifying mode of exercise, no more than 15 repetitions for weight-bearing activities
   f. Modifying mode of exercise to adapt to changes in disease status.

III. Systemic Lupus Erythematosus

A. Overview: Lupus is a chronic multisystem inflammatory condition
B. Prevalence: Estimated to affect 40–50 per 100,000 persons in the United States
   1. 10 per 100,000 in white males
   2. 400 per 100,000 in black females
C. Presentation and diagnosis
   1. Suspect in persons with:
      a. Unexplained symptoms of two or more organ systems
      b. Unexplained fevers
   2. Screen with antinuclear antibody (ANA) testing
      a. Titer greater than or equal to 1:40, full SLE workup indicated
      b. Titer less than or equal to 1:40, exclude other diagnosis prior to workup
   3. Diagnosis made by presence of at least 4 of the following 11 criteria
      a. Malar "butterfly" rash
      b. Discoid lesions
      c. Photosensitivity
      d. Oral ulcers
      e. Arthritis
      f. Pleuritis or pericarditis
      g. Proteinuria or cellular casts
      h. Psychosis or seizures
      i. Hemolytic anemia, leucopenia, lymphopenia, or thrombocytopenia
      j. Antinuclear antibodies
      k. Immunologic disorder
         i. Anti-dsDNA
         ii. Anti-Sm
         iii. Anti-LA
         iv. Anti-RO
         v. Antiphospholipid antibody (abnormal serum level of IgG or IgM anticardiolipin antibodies)
         vi. Lupus anticoagulant
         vii. Positive serologic syphilis test with negative *Treponema pallidum* test
D. Treatments
   1. Symptomatic treatment for fever, rash, and arthralgias
      a. NSAIDs (caution with renal disease)
      b. Hydroxychloroquine (possibly improves survival)
      c. Acetaminophen (caution with hepatic disease)
      d. Low-dose corticosteroids

     3. Cyclophosphamide (used for severe disease)

     4. Prednisone (used for acute exacerbations)

  E. Prognosis

     1. Progressive organ damage

     2. Common for disease to be in remission with periodic flares

     3. SLE-associated death due to

       a. Infections

       b. Cardiovascular disease

       c. Pulmonary disease

       d. Central nervous system disease

     4. Worse prognosis if diagnosed as a child

  F. Systemic lupus erythematosus and exercise

     1. Protect from sun exposure as it may worsen dermatologic manifestations

     2. Evaluate for possible renal involvement prior to participation if patient suffers flare

     3. Obtain baseline echocardiogram to rule out pericarditis and follow-up echocardiograms prior to clearance for moderate- to high-intensity exercise

     4. Discourage from participation during flares that include fever due to increased risk of endocarditis, vasculitis, and worsening synovitis

     5. Patients starting a new regime after a long history of SLE should be screened for coronary artery disease

     6. Caution is warranted during times of stress, surgery, or pregnancy as these are known triggers for relapses.

IV. Spondylarthropathies (Ankylosing Spondylitis, Reactive Arthritis, and Psoriatic Arthritis)

  A. Overview: A group of inflammatory conditions associated with the HLA-B27 gene (present in up to 90% of cases)

  B. Ankylosing spondylitis

     1. Prevalence

       a. 0.1%–0.2% of U.S. population

       b. Predominance in white males

     2. Presentation

       a. Back pain

         i. Radiates to the gluteal regions

         ii. Worse in the morning (stiffness lasting >1 h), relieved with activity

       b. Enthesitis (inflammation at attachment site of tendon, ligament, and joint capsule to bone)

         i. Achilles tendon

         ii. Plantar fascia calcaneal insertion

       c. Uveitis

     3. Diagnosis

       a. Positive Schober test (less then 5 cm increase with forward flexion) (see Figure 43.1)

       b. Negative RF

       c. Elevation of acute-phase reactants (erythrocyte sedimentation rate [ESR] and c-reactive protein [CRP])

       d. Imaging

         i. Bilateral sacroiliitis seen on radiographs and magnetic resonance imaging (MRI)

         ii. Vertebral syndesmophytes causing squaring of the vertebral bodies, "Bamboo spine" seen on radiograph (find picture)

     4. Treatments

       a. NSAIDs (first line)

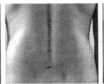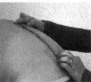

FIGURE 43.1   Schober's test: A mark is made over the spinous process of L5 (at the level of the superior iliac crest). A second mark is made 5 cm below the first mark, and a third mark is made 10 cm above the first mark. The patient is then asked to perform maximal forward flexion. The test is positive if the distance between the second and third marks (15 cm while standing) does not increase by at least 5 cm (20 cm between second and third marks with forward flexion). Photos courtesy of Natalie M. Mason

      b. Sulfasalazine
      c. Methotrexate
      d. Tumor necrosis factor-alpha inhibitors
         i. Etanercept
         ii. Infliximab
      e. Intra-articular steroid injections
      f. Physical therapy and home exercise programs
   5. Ankylosing spondylitis and exercise
      a. Continuous flexibility training (focusing on thoracic and hip flexors) and core strengthening with mild to moderate exercise within limits of disease activity
      b. Aerobic exercise with full expansion of breathing muscles that helps maintain opens airways
      c. Swimming preferred as it avoids high impact to the spine. Avoid contact sports due to risk of fracture. Can participate in carefully chosen aerobic sports when disease inactive
C. Reactive arthritis
   1. Prevalence and pathogenesis
      a. 0.1% of U.S. population
      b. Triggered by an extra-articular infection
         i. Gastrointestinal (*Shigella, Salmonella, Yersinia, Campylobacter*)
         ii. Genitourinary (*Chlamydia, Ureaplasma*)
   2. Presentation
      a. Reiter's syndrome (a classic reactive arthritis syndrome)
         i. Conjunctivitis (cannot see)
         ii. Urethritis (cannot pee)
         iii. Arthritis (cannot climb a tree)
      b. Arthritis begins 1–4 weeks following infection
      c. Asymmetric arthritis (more common in lower extremities)
      d. Back pain
   3. Diagnosis
      a. Primarily a clinical diagnosis
      b. Elevated ESR and/or CRP that returns to normal with resolution of inflammation
      c. Bacterial cultures from the throat, stool, or urogenital tract occasionally identify the causative organism
   4. Treatment
      a. NSAIDs
      b. Sulfasalazine for chronic symptoms

      c. Intra-articular steroid injections

      d. Antibiotics are not effective

   5. Prognosis

      a. Frequently self-limited (resolves in 3 months to a year)

      b. 15%–30% develop chronic arthritis

D. Psoriatic arthritis

   1. Presentation

      a. Skin manifestations typically precede the arthritis

      b. Asymmetric arthritis commonly found in distal joints

      c. Uveitis

      d. Severity of arthritis does not necessarily correlate with severity of skin manifestations

   2. Diagnosis

      a. Presence of psoriatic lesions on the skin or nails

      b. Elevated ESR and/or CRP

      c. Radiographic evidence of erosive arthritis, commonly seen at the DIP joints

   3. Treatment

      a. Joint therapies

         i. NSAIDs (first line)

         ii. Oral corticosteroids

         iii. Intra-articular steroid injections

         iv. Sulfasalazine, methotrexate, cyclosporine, and TNF antagonists (second line)

      b. Topical therapies

         i. UV light therapy

         ii. Topical corticosteroids

         iii. Topical retinoids

   4. Exercise for reactive arthritis (Reiter's syndrome) and psoriatic arthritis

      a. Same protocols as osteoarthritis in addition to increased emphasis on

         i. Maintaining range of motion

         ii. Avoiding impact to joint when effusion present

         iii. Strength training to stabilize joints.

Recommended Reading

1. Aletaha D, Neogi T, Silma AJ, Funovits J, et al. 2010 rheumatoid arthritis classification criteria. *Arthritis Rheum.* 2010;*62*(9):2569–2581.
2. Clark BM. Rheumatology: Physical and occupational therapy in the management of arthritis. *CMAJ.* 2000;*163*(8):999–1005.
3. Clinical Update in Musculoskeletal Medicine. Rheumatology update: New approaches to diagnosis and treatment. *J Musculoskeletal Med.* 2005;*22*(12):650, 653–654.
4. Gill JM, Quisel AM, Rocca PV, Walters DT. Diagnosis of systemic lupus erythematous. *Am Fam Physician.* 2003;*68*(11):2179–2186.
5. Kataria RK, Brent LH. Spondyloarthropathies. *Am Fam Physician.* 2004;*69*(12):2853–2860.
6. Keysor JJ, Currey SS, Callahan LF. Behavioral aspects of arthritis and rheumatic disease self-management. *Dis Manage Health Outcomes.* 2001;*9*(2):89–98.
7. Labowitz RJ, Challman J, Palmeri S. Aerobic exercise in the management of rheumatic diseases. *Del Med J.* 1988;*60*(11):659–662.
8. Lavallee ME. Connective tissue and rheumatologic conditions in sports. In: O'Grady E. (ed.), *Netter's Sports Medicine: The Team Physician's Handbook.* Chapter 35. Philadelphia, PA: Saunders; 2010:285–295.
9. Minor MA. Physical activity and management of arthritis. *Ann Behav Med.* 1990;*13*:117–24.
10. Rindfleisch JA, Muller D. Diagnosis and management of rheumatoid arthritis. *Am Fam Physician.* 2005;*72*(6):1037–1047, 1049–1050.
11. Speed CA. Sports and exercise medicine and rheumatology. *Rheumatology (Oxford).* 2005;*44*(2):143–144.
12. United States Bone and Joint Decade. *The Burden of Musculoskeletal Diseases in the United States* 2008:71–96.

44

Sports Neurology

Jeffrey S. Kutcher and Kerry L. Hulsing

SEIZURE DISORDERS

I. Seizure

A. Transient occurrence of signs or symptoms due to abnormal excessive or synchronous neuronal activity in the brain

B. Usually self-limited, lasting 1–2 min

C. Followed by a "post-ictal" state of decreased cerebral activity

D. Can be induced by preexisting intrinsic brain pathology or from acute provocation
   1. Common provocations include metabolic derangements, substance use, and head trauma
   2. Provoked seizures are not necessarily associated with epilepsy

E. Classification
   1. Partial (localization related)—involving a particular region of cortex
      a. Simple partial—no alteration in mental status
         i. Motor signs
         ii. Somatosensory or special sensory signs
         iii. Autonomic signs
         iv. Psychic symptoms (i.e., déjà vu)
      b. Complex partial—with alteration in mental status
         i. Typically a transient state of confusion
         ii. May involve automatic behavior (automatisms)
   2. Generalized—involving both hemispheres of the brain synchronously
      a. Absence—lapse in consciousness
      b. Myoclonic—brief, sudden, bilateral, synchronous muscle jerks without alteration in mental status
      c. Tonic—increase in tone, rigidity
      d. Clonic—rapidly alternating muscular contraction and relaxation
      e. Tonic–Clonic (GTC)—Period of tonic posturing followed by clonic activity

F. Seizures can evolve from simple partial to complex partial, and from either to a generalized seizure, termed a "secondarily generalized" seizure.

II. Epilepsy

A. Chronic condition of recurrent unprovoked seizures
   1. Localization related—focal or partial onset
      a. Idiopathic—inherited primary cerebral dysfunction
      b. Symptomatic—secondary to structural lesion (i.e., cerebral hemorrhage)
      c. Cryptogenic—no etiology identified

    2. Generalized

      a. Idiopathic—inherited primary cerebral dysfunction (i.e., Juvenile Myoclonic Epilepsy)

      b. Symptomatic—secondary to diffuse or multiregional structural pathology

      c. Cryptogenic—no etiology identified

B. Epidemiology

    1. United States prevalence is 5–10/1000

    2. Unites States incidence is approximately 50/100,000

    3. Bimodal age of presentation with diagnoses made more commonly in the pediatric and geriatric populations

C. Diagnosis

    1. If possible, try to determine from the history the presence or absence of signs that support the diagnosis of seizure

      a. Increased muscle tone during the event

      b. Witnessed convulsive movements

      c. Post-ictal state of confusion, especially if lasting longer than 1 h

      d. Oral trauma from tonic jaw contraction

    2. Consider possible nonseizure causes of the ictal event

      a. Syncope

        i. May be preceded by "presyncopal" symptoms

        ii. Typically eyes are closed and muscle tone is decreased

        iii. Loss of consciousness is typically less than 30 s

        iv. Minimal postevent confusion

      b. Sleep behaviors—parasomnias can mimic seizures because of symptoms such as confusion or limb jerking

      c. Paroxysmal dyskinesias—involuntary movements involving various regions of the body

      d. Migraine headache—visual or other neurological signs or symptoms can occur as part of a migrainous event, even in the absence of headache

      e. Nonepileptic (psychogenic) spell

        i. Transient alteration or appearance of alteration of consciousness

        ii. Can have hyper- or hypomotor features

        iii. Often as the result of psychological trauma

    3. Evaluate for evidence of pathology

      a. Noncontrast head CT—in emergency setting to evaluate for pathology requiring immediate attention (i.e., hemorrhage)

      b. EEG—may show electrographic changes suggestive of an increased risk of unprovoked seizures or neuronal dysfunction but is not sufficiently sensitive to rule out epilepsy

      c. MRI—preferably "epilepsy protocol"

        i. Evaluation for structural pathology as an etiology for seizures

        ii. More sensitive than CT for identifying structural abnormalities

D. Treatment

    1. If a single unprovoked seizure occurs and the evaluation is unremarkable, medication may not be needed

    2. Typically, medical therapy will need to be initiated if a second unprovoked seizure occurs or if studies suggest an increased risk of seizure recurrence

    3. Start with one medicine and titrate the dose up until seizures are under control or adverse side effects occur

    4. Most cases of epilepsy can be managed with monotherapy

    5. Second-generation antiepileptic medications such as levatiracetam and lamotrigine have fewer potential side effects as compared to first-generation medications such as phenytoin and valproate

E. Implications for participation in sports
  1. In most cases, well-controlled epilepsy should not limit sports participation
  2. Standard seizure precautions should be followed, including avoiding swimming alone and adhering to local motor vehicle laws
  3. Teammates and coaches should learn prodromal symptoms and basic acute management.

III. Convulsive syncope

  A. A common variant of syncope that presents with tonic or myoclonic activity
  B. The convulsion is usually less than 1 min, arrhythmic, and multifocal
  C. Duration of postevent confusion is typically short
  D. Convulsive syncope is not an indication of an increased risk of epilepsy.

HEADACHE

I. Exertional headache

  A. Headache precipitated by any form of exercise, often called "benign exertional headache"
  1. Symptoms similar to migraine headache, including nausea and photophobia
  2. Unilateral or bilateral
  3. Pulsating pain
  4. Typically occurs during the peak of exertion

  B. Epidemiology
  1. More common in males
  2. Occurs in both trained and untrained individuals
  3. Lifetime prevalence is ~1%
  4. More common with activities that double the resting pulse for at least 10 s
  5. Most patients also have a personal or family history of migraine headache

  C. Diagnosis
  1. Establish a pattern of headache precipitated by exercise, occurring either during or shortly after significant exertion
  2. Pulsating headache
  3. Lasting 5 min to 48 h
  4. Not attributed to another disorder
      a. Consider brain MRI for mass lesion
      b. Consider MRA for aneurysm

  D. Treatment
  1. Nonpharmaceutical prevention
      a. Improve overall physical condition
      b. Careful warm-up period with graded titration of exertion
      c. Use objective data such as pulse or watts to uncover any predictable threshold for headache generation, and adjust the workout as able
  2. Pharmacotherapy
      a. Indomethacin, 25–100 mg/day, or triptan medications can be used prophylactically or therapeutically
      b. Migraine prevention medications may also be used
          i. Topiramate—start at 25 mg/day and titrate up to 50 mg po/bid by adding 25 mg/day/week
          ii. Amitriptyline or nortriptyline up to 100 mg po/qhs as tolerated.

II. Posttraumatic headache

  A. Headache is the most common symptom following head injury
  1. Acute posttraumatic headache—develops within 7 days of trauma and resolves within 3 months
  2. Chronic posttraumatic headache—lasts beyond 3 months after trauma

B. Commonly occurs as part of a postconcussion syndrome

C. Heterogeneous presentations

1. Throbbing or squeezing pain quality
2. Focal or diffuse location
3. Occasional or daily episodes

D. Epidemiology

1. Estimated to occur in 30–80% of cases of head trauma
2. Up to 60% estimated to have chronic headache, lasting greater than 3 months
3. Pediatric prevalence estimated at 3–7%

E. Diagnosis

1. Historical verification of inciting traumatic event
2. Headache symptoms begin within 7 days following head trauma
3. Differential diagnosis
   a. Primary headache disorder—head trauma will often exacerbate a primary headache disorder
   b. Subdural or epidural hematoma—consider neuroimaging if any focal neurological process is suspected based on history or physical examination
   c. Carotid or vertebral artery dissection—consider CTA of the head and neck, especially if neck pain is present, or any focal neurological deficit
   d. Medication overuse headache—carefully document symptom timing and limit the use of daily analgesics as tolerated

F. Treatment

1. Management should be individualized and multidisciplinary
   a. Pharmacotherapy
      i. No evidence-based options
      ii. Tailor medication treatment to be consistent with the primary headache disorder most similar to the presentation
   b. Physical therapy
   c. Biofeedback
   d. Manual therapy
   e. Cognitive therapy
   f. Psychiatric consultation may be warranted for depression or anxiety.

COMPLEX REGIONAL PAIN SYNDROME (CRPS)

I. Definition and pathophysiology

A. Clinically diagnosed neuropathic pain syndrome

B. May begin following a mechanical injury or surgical procedure

C. Symptoms disproportionate in time and severity to any known trauma

D. Hyperalgesia, allodynia, vasomotor, motor, and trophic symptoms

E. Symptoms are regional, as opposed to being in a specific dermatome or peripheral nerve distribution

F. Specific pathophysiology is unclear but likely includes several mechanisms

1. Small-fiber neuropathy
2. Sympathetic nervous system dysfunction
   a. Sympathetic nervous system overactivity
   b. Sympathetic-afferent fiber coupling
   c. End-organ norepinepherine hypersensitivity
3. Central and peripheral nervous system inflammation

    4. Central nervous system sensitization

        a. Nociceptive pathway enhancement

        b. Increased neuronal membrane excitability

        c. Reduced pathway inhibition.

II. Epidemiology

    a. Most commonly seen after sprains, fractures, or surgical procedures that result in immobilization

    b. Median age of onset in the fifth decade of life

    c. Rare in children or the elderly

    d. Estimated annual incidence: between 5 and 25/100,000

    e. Female to male ratio: 3/1.

III. Diagnosis

    A. No confirmatory diagnostic tests exist

    B. Four criteria must be met for clinical diagnosis:

        1. Continuing pain disproportionate to any inciting event

        2. Must report one symptom in three out of four categories:

            a. Sensory: hyperesthesia or allodynia

            b. Vasomotor: temperature asymmetry, skin color change or asymmetry

            c. Sudomotor: edema, sweating changes or asymmetry

            d. Motor/trophic: decreased range of motion, weakness, tremor, dystonia, or trophic changes in skin, hair, or nails

        3. Must display one sign at the time of evaluation in two or more categories:

            a. Sensory: hyperalgesia or allodynia

            b. Vasomotor: temperature asymmetry

            c. Sudomotor: edema, sweating changes or asymmetry

            d. Motor/trophic: decreased range of motion, weakness, tremor, dystonia, or trophic changes in skin, hair, or nails

        4. There is no other diagnosis that better explains the signs or symptoms

    C. Clinical tests can be used to help confirm the presence of pathology or diagnose other causes of signs or symptoms

        1. Punch skin biopsy is the best diagnostic test for small-fiber polyneuropathy

        2. Quantitative sensory testing can provide subjective data on sensory function

        3. EMG can be used to document peripheral nerve damage but a normal study does not rule out CRPS

        4. Sympathetic block can be used to determine the amount of sympathetic nervous system involvement.

IV. Treatment

    A. Physiotherapy

        1. Graded motor imagery

        2. Desensitization

        3. Mirror therapy

    B. Pharmacotherapy for pain

        1. Five classes of medications are useful for neuropathic pain in general, with none specifically shown to treat CRPS in a randomized clinical trial

            a. Tricyclics and serotonin–norepinephrine reuptake inhibitors (SNRIs)

            b. Gabapentinoids

            c. Opiods

            d. Topical or local anesthetics

            e. Corticosteroids

2. Start with one medication from one class and titrate to maximum dose
3. If symptoms persist, switch to one medication from a different class
4. If no class provides benefit alone, then consider using more than one class
5. Most patient with CRPS will require polypharmacy.

Recommended Reading

1. Bruehl S. An update on the pathophysiology of complex regional pain syndrome. *Anesthesiology.* 2010;113(3):713–725.

2. Chen SP, Fuh JL, Lu SR, Wang SJ. Exertional headache—A survey of 1963 adolescents. *Cephalalgia.* 2009;29(4):401–407.

3. Fisher RS, van Emde Boas W, Blume W, Elger C, Genton P, Lee P, Engel J. Jr. Epileptic seizures and epilepsy: Definitions proposed by the International League Against Epilepsy (ILAE) and the International Bureau for Epilepsy (IBE). *Epilepsia.* 2005;46(4):470–472.

4. French JK, Pedley TA. Clinical practice: Initial management of epilepsy. *N Engl J Med.* 2008;359:166–176.

5. Harden RN, Bruehl S, Stanton-Hicks M, Wilson PR. Proposed new diagnostic criteria for complex regional pain syndrome. *Pain Med.* 2007;8(4):326–331.

6. Lambert RW, Burnet DL. Prevention of exercise-induced migraine by quantitative warm-up. *Headache.* 1985;25(6):317–319.

7. Latremoliere A, Wolf CJ. Central sensitization: A generator of pain hypersensitivity by central neural plasticity. *J Pain.* 2009;10(9):895–926.

8. Lew HL, Lin PH, Fuh JL, Wang SJ, Clark DJ, Walker WC. Characteristics and treatment of headache after traumatic brain injury: A focused review. *Am J Phys Med Rehabil.* 2006;85(7):619–627.

9. de Mos M, Sturkenboom MC, Huygen FJ. Current understandings on complex regional pain syndrome. *Pain Pract.* 2009;9(2):86–99.

10. Shorvan SD, Perucca E, Engel J Jr, eds. *The Treatment of Epilepsy.* 3rd ed. New York, NY: Blackwell Publishing; 2009.

11. Zafonte RD, Horn LJ. Clinical assessment of posttraumatic headaches. *J Head Trauma Rehabil.* 1999;14(1):22–33.

Sports Concussion and Traumatic Brain Injury

Scott R. Laker

I. Introduction and Definitions

A. Brain injuries are noncongenital insults to the brain arising from an external force. They are classified as mild, moderate, and severe. Symptoms can be temporary to permanent. Severe brain injuries can result in death and varying degrees of disability. The overwhelming majority of brain injuries in sports are mild and do not result in permanent morbidity

   1. Definitions of moderate and severe brain injury vary but are based on multiple factors, including intracranial bleeding, skull fracture, Glasgow Coma Scale, Rancho Los Amigos scale, and length of hospital stay

   2. Moderate and severe brain injuries are relatively rare in sports but are more commonly seen in

      a. High-velocity sports like alpine sports, cycling, motorsports, bull-riding, boxing, and martial arts

      b. Contact and collision sports like football, basketball, soccer, and hockey

B. Concussions are mild brain injuries and as many as 3.8 million sports-related concussions occur in the United States every year. Concussion is defined as a complex pathophysiologic process affecting the brain, induced by traumatic biomechanical forces. Common features include

   1. Direct blow to the head or neck, or an "impulsive" force transmitted to the head

   2. Rapid onset of short-lived neurologic dysfunction that resolves spontaneously

   3. Represents a functional disturbance, not a structural one

   4. Results in a graded set of symptoms that may or may not involve loss of consciousness. Resolution follows a sequential course but may be prolonged in postconcussion syndrome. 80–90% resolve within 7–10 days

   5. No abnormalities are seen on MRI or CT.

II. Concussions

A. Epidemiology:

   1. NCAA overall rate is 0.43 concussions per 1000 athletic exposures

   2. High school rate is 0.23 concussions per 1000 athletic exposures

   3. The largest number of concussions occur in men's football

   4. The highest rate is found in women's ice hockey

   5. Concussions occur at a higher rate during competition as compared to practice

   6. Within a given sport, female athletes have a higher rate of concussion. For example, men's basketball overall rate is 0.07 per 1000 exposures, women's basketball overall rate is 0.21 per 1000 exposures

      a. Gender-specific reporting differences may play a role, but it is widely felt that there is an objective difference in concussions in females and males. The differences are multifactorial, including differences in head–neck geometry, body mass, neck strength, style of play, and hormonal influences

    b. Cultural issues: differences in reporting patterns between male and female athletes and differences in provider responses based on sex of the athlete

B. Pathophysiology

    1. Moderate and severe brain injuries involve structural damage, including intrinsic brain tissue damage and intracranial bleeding

    2. Concussions do not involve structural abnormalities but are thought to occur secondary to the neurometabolic cascade theory:

        a. Axonal stretch

        b. Release of excitatory amino acids

        c. Cellular depolarization

        d. Calcium (Ca^{2+}) influx into the mitochondria

            i. Decreases ATP production and initiates apoptosis

        e. Cellular membrane disruption creates intracellular ionic shift

            i. Na^+/K^+ ATP-dependent pump works to regain ionic balance. Hyperglycolysis leads to lactate accumulation

        f. Axolemmnal disruption, neurofilament compaction, microtubule disruption, axonal swelling, and axonotmesis

C. Biomechanics: There is no proven concussion "threshold" (i.e., concussions can occur with small forces and may not occur with large forces). Linear and angular acceleration are equally important. The magnitude of impact does not predict outcome, severity, or presentation

D. Symptoms

    1. Wide range of nonspecific symptoms

        a. Cognitive: confusion, posttraumatic amnesia, retrograde, amnesia, loss of consciousness, feeling "in a fog," vacant stare, delayed motor and verbal responses, slurred speech

            i. Posttraumatic amnesia is defined as confusion or loss of memory immediately following the injury

            ii. Retrograde amnesia is defined as loss of memories that occurred shortly before the injury

            iii. Amnestic athletes may be able to complete complex mental and physical tasks but have no recollection of the events that took place immediately after the injury

        b. Somatic: headache (most common symptom), fatigue, photophobia, phonophobia, balance problems, nausea, vomiting

        c. Affective: emotional lability, irritability

        d. Sleep: drowsiness, sleeping less, sleeping more, trouble falling asleep

    2. Loss of consciousness (LOC) occurs in less than 10% of cases and is not predictive of severity

    3. Seizure activity is rare and not predictive of severity and does not imply an underlying seizure disorder

E. Sideline management of concussion

    1. Any athlete with a suspected concussion should be immediately removed from play

    2. Evaluate with the Sport Concussion Assessment Tool 2 (SCAT2) or similar tool (see Section II.F.)

    3. The athlete should be monitored for progression of symptoms and should not be left alone

    4. Appropriate disposition and instructions should be provided to the athlete and parents, if applicable

        a. Athletes with prolonged LOC, vomiting, neurologic signs, severe neck pain (concern for concomitant spinal injury in a brain-injured athlete), or worsening mental status should be sent to the emergency department via ambulance for evaluation

        b. Appropriate instructions include a discussion of "red flag" symptoms, including decreasing levels of consciousness, neurologic signs (weakness, increasing disorientation, severe headache)

   c. The athlete and parents/guardians should be instructed that no RTP or sport/exercise involvement can begin until symptoms have resolved

   d. Many clinicians recommend avoidance of excessive mental exertion, including video games, text messaging, computer use, and homework temporarily

F. Diagnosis: largely clinical, based on context but several testing paradigms have been suggested

  1. SCAT2 is recommended by the most recent consensus statement

   a. The SCAT2 includes a symptom score, neurologic signs report, and a Glasgow Coma Scale score. It also tests orientation, concentration, coordination, balance, and immediate and delayed memory. It is recommended for athletes 10 years old and above. It combines the Standardized Assessment of Concussion (SAC) and the Balance Error Scoring System (BESS). See below

  2. Standardized Assessment of Concussion

   a. Consists of orientation, immediate memory, delayed memory, concentration, and neurologic screening (exam and report of LOC or amnesia). No balance testing or symptom inventory

  3. Balance Error Scoring System

   a. Consists of testing an athlete in double-leg stance, single-leg stance, and tandem stance. Each test lasts for 20 s and the number of errors is recorded

G. Imaging

  1. By definition, concussions do not result in intracranial bleeding or imaging abnormalities on standard MRI and CT

  2. CT is used in emergency settings to quickly evaluate for intracranial bleeding. Given the radiation involved, CT should not be used unless the situation is emergent

  3. MRI offers better soft tissue differentiation but rarely reveals abnormalities. Reserved for athletes with prolonged or severe symptoms, when evaluating for alternative diagnoses

  4. Experimental imaging modalities: not part of typical concussion diagnosis and management. The goal of imaging in concussion is to more accurately diagnose the condition, to prognose improvement, and to determine safe RTP. Currently, no diagnostic imaging tool is available for concussion

   a. Functional MRI is the most studied of the experimental concussion imaging modalities. It creates images based on blood oxygenation changes observed as the patient performs a task. Most studies have focused on motor or cognitive tasks in their design

   b. Diffusion tensor imaging (DTI) allows for assessment of the integrity of white and gray matter tracts in the brain. This is based on water molecule diffusion properties. Several studies are using DTI in their research protocols

   c. MRI spectroscopy combines MRI image quality with the ability to detect chemical signature abnormalities in neurometabolites like N-acetylaspartate, creatine, choline, myoinositol, and lactate. Still considered a research protocol

   d. fMRI and DTI hold the most promise but are expensive and are currently difficult to obtain

H. Neuropsychological (NP) testing

  1. A criterion standard for NP testing in concussion does not currently exist

  2. NP testing is design to add depth to the understanding of a concussed athlete's processing speed, memory, and overall cognitive function

  3. Computerized testing (imPact™, CogSport™, Automated Neuropsychological Assessment Metrics™, Headminders™)

   a. Performed during the preseason to create a "baseline" and repeated postconcussion to document improvement

   b. Relatively inexpensive, easy to mass-administer, retests are convenient

   c. Scope of practice issues surround interpretation of these tests. Neuropsychologists are most experienced in interpreting these tests. A provider is wise to carefully consider making clinical decisions based on the interpretation of these tests

    4. Formal pencil-and-paper neuropsychological testing

      a. More of a panel of possible tests than one universally accepted protocol

      b. Multiple tests are typically administered during a visit. Some of the most commonly used tests include the Hopkins verbal learning test, Trailmaking test Parts A and B, digit span, Stroop color word, and digit symbol test

      c. Main limitation is limited access and expense

    5. Regardless of documented improvement on NP testing, no symptomatic athlete may be returned to play

I. Biomarkers

    1. Specific substances are released by injured brain tissue and cross the blood–brain barrier into the peripheral blood supply, where they can be more easily accessed. None of the biomarkers are completely specific for injured brain tissue

    2. Still in the research phase for all biomarkers. Examples most commonly include S100B protein, neuron-specific enolase, and cleaved Tau protein

J. Modifying factors: certain intrinsic and extrinsic factors are associated with increased risk of future concussion, prolonged postconcussion symptoms, and severity of overall presentation. These should be discussed with each athlete

    1. Overall number of previous concussions

    2. Decreasing force threshold (i.e., each subsequent concussion is requiring smaller and smaller blows to the head)

    3. Severity of symptoms

    4. Increasing number of symptoms

    5. Duration of symptoms (>10 days)

    6. Gender

      a. Females have higher rates than males

    7. Younger age

      a. Children and adolescents have longer recovery times than adults. Limited data exist regarding athletes under 10 years of age

    8. Personal or family history of attention-deficit disorder, headache disorder, migraines, psychiatric disease, learning disability

    9. Medications

      a. Psychoactive medications

      b. Anticoagulants

    10. Style of play

      a. Aggressive, dangerous play

      b. Poor technique

    11. Level of play (adult professional, adult amateur, college, high school, junior, peewee)

    12. Sport of choice

    13. Apolipoprotein E (ApoE) polymorphisms are associated with increased brain injury risk. ApoE testing has not been integrated into clinical practice to date and does not need to be routinely discussed with concussed athletes

K. Return-to-play (RTP)

    1. Same-day RTP

      a. No same-day RTP for athletes <18 years old or collegiate athletes

      b. Consideration can be given to a professional athlete returning to play if symptoms resolve before the end of that competition

      c. If covering an event, be up to date on your league's policy regarding same-day RTP and have a plan for athlete disposition

    2. RTP determination

      a. RTP is a medically supervised, stepwise approach to returning to full competition

      b. RTP is a medical decision

      c. All RTP is individualized

    d. Athletes should be asymptomatic before considering RTP

    e. Consensus agreement suggests at least a 5-day protocol. An athlete should be asymptomatic for 24 h before proceeding to the next step (see Table 45.1)

      i. This outline is not comprehensive; some athletes may take weeks to months before being able to fully return to competition

      ii. The risk for repeat concussion is limited but increases once the potential for contact resumes

      iii. Other nonorganic factors should be considered when returning athletes to full contact. These include fear of repeat injury, concern about future disability, and performance anxiety

      iv. Athletes that have been sidelined for prolonged periods must regain their cardiovascular fitness, strength, and flexibility to prevent other injuries once they return

  3. Subdural and epidural hematomas and RTP

    a. Expert opinion differs between 6 and 12 month periods of rest before return to sport

    b. The hematoma needs to be completely resolved, with no residual hygroma

    c. Intrinsic risk factors must be explored (coagulopathy, arteriovenous malformation, aneurysm, etc.)

    d. Return to contact sports after craniotomy is considered on an individual basis after consulting with the athlete, primary care physician, and neurosurgeon

  4. Consider retirement from collision or contact sports in the setting of

    a. Multiple concussions

    b. Increasing severity and duration of symptoms with successive concussions

    c. Decreasing impacts leading to concussion

    d. Fixed neuropsychological testing abnormalities.

III. Second Impact Syndrome

Catastrophic brain swelling resulting from a second trauma while the patient is still symptomatic from a previous concussion. The second trauma is typically much smaller than the first and results in rapid neurologic deterioration and cerebral herniation within minutes

  A. Pathophysiology is thought to be due to cerebral dysautoregulation and posttraumatic catecholamine release

  B. Extraordinarily rare, true incidence and prevalence are not known but at least 17 autopsy-confirmed cases exist in the literature, though a larger number of similar "unconfirmed" cases have been reported

Table 45.1   Return-to-Play Protocol

	Functional Task	Goal
Step One	Rest until asymptomatic	Symptom management and recovery
Step Two	Light aerobic exercise example walking, stationary bike, elliptical trainer	Increase heart rate
Step Three	Sport-specific exercise example shoot around drills, soccer juggling, baseball long-toss	Adding motion and coordination, increased aerobic challenge
Step Four	Noncontact training drills example running drills, cutting drills, pass patterns	Coordination, cognitive challenge, increased aerobic challenge
Step Five	Full-contact practice	Assess readiness for play, return to full-speed participation
Step Six	Return to competition	

C. More commonly seen in adolescents, but has been reported in college-age athletes

D. By definition, no intracranial bleed is present, although this is increasingly called into question. Several reported cases involve massive cerebral edema with small subdural hematomas that would not explain the amount of mass effect or cerebral herniation.

IV. Long-Term Sequelae of Multiple Concussions

A. Cognitive impairment and executive function impairments have been found on NP testing when athletes with a history of multiple concussions are compared to nonconcussed controls

B. Headache disorders

C. Decreased perceived health-related quality of life measures

D. Psychiatric: athletes with multiple concussions may be at increased risk of depression

E. Dementia pugilistica: dementia associated with retired professional boxers.

V. Chronic Traumatic Encephalopathy (CTE)

A. Currently diagnosed upon autopsy and microscopic evaluation of brain tissue. Impossible to premorbidly differentiate from other dementias prior to autopsy and evaluation for Tau protein deposition patterns. Increasing numbers of professional athletes are donating their brain tissue to evaluate for CTE

B. True incidence unknown but at least 50 cases have been reported to date

C. Pathologic findings: distinguished from other tauopathies by the predominant involvement of the superficial cortical layers, the distribution patterns in the frontal and temporal cortices, and the accumulation of tau-immunoreactive astrocytes as well as
   1. Atrophy of cerebral hemispheres, medial temporal lobe, thalamus, mammillary bodies, and brainstem
   2. Ventricular dilatation
   3. Widespread deposition of tau-immunoreactive neurofibrillary tangles, astrocytic tangles, and neuritis throughout the brain

D. Clinical syndrome associated with subconcussive blows rather than multiple frank concussions
   1. Insidious and progressive cognitive decline, confusion, disorientation, and behavioral changes
   2. Physically, patients may present with Parkinonian features (shuffling gait, masked facies, and tremor)
   3. Psychotic features, homicidality, suicidality, and parasuicidality.

VI. Concussion Prevention

A. Rule changes to prevent head-to-head contact, dangerous play, and enforcing rules that support fair play and unnecessary violence have proven helpful

B. Use of padded goal posts in soccer and field-goal markers in football

C. There is no convincing evidence that new helmet technology, mouthpieces, or protective headgear prevent concussions

D. Helmets in alpine sports, cycling, equestrian, bull-riding, football, and motorsports help prevent moderate and severe TBI.

Recommended Reading

1. Barkhoudarian G, Hovda DA, Giza CC. The molecular pathophysiology of concussive brain injury. *Clin Sports Med.* 2010;30:34–48.
2. Benson BW, Hamilton GM, Meeuwisse WH, et al. Is protective equipment useful in preventing concussion? A systematic review of the literature. *Br J Sports Med.* 2009;43(Suppl 1):i56.

3. Cantu RC, Gean AD. Second-impact syndrome and a small subdural hematoma: An uncommon catastrophic result of repetitive head injury with a characteristic imaging appearance. *J Neurotrauma.* 2010;27:1557.

4. Davis G, Marion DW, Le Roux P, et al. Clinics in neurology and neurosurgery—Extradural and subdural haematoma. *Br J Sports Med.* 2010;44:1139.

5. Dick RW. Is there a gender difference in concussion incidence and outcomes? *Br J Sports Med.* 2009; 43(Suppl 1):i46.

6. Difiori JP, Giza CC. New techniques in concussion imaging. *Curr Sports Med Rep.* 2010;9:35.

7. Guskiewicz KM, Mihalik JP Biomechanics of sport concussion: Quest for the elusive injury threshold. *Exerc Sport Sci Rev.* 2011;39:4.

8. McCrory P, Meeuwisse W, Johnston K, et al. Consensus Statement on Concussion in Sport: the 3rd International Conference on Concussion in Sport held in Zurich, November 2008. *Br J Sports Med.* 2009;43(Suppl 1):i76.

9. McKee AC, Cantu RC, Nowinski CJ, et al. Chronic traumatic encephalopathy in athletes: Progressive tauopathy after repetitive head injury. *J Neuropathol Exp Neurol.* 2009;68:709.

10. Nowak LA, Smith GG, Reyes PF. Dementia in a retired world boxing champion: Case report and literature review. *Clin Neuropathol.* 2009;28:275.

11. Tierney RT, Mansell JL, Higgins M, et al. Apolipoprotein e genotype and concussion in college athletes. *Clin J Sport Med.* 2010;20:464.

12. Wetjen NM, Pichelmann MA, Atkinson JL. Second impact syndrome: Concussion and second injury brain complications. *J Am Coll Surg.* 2010;211:553.

46

Neurovascular Injuries of the Upper and Lower Limbs

Jason Friedrich and Venu Akuthota

I. Principles of Nerve Injury Evaluation and Management

A. Peripheral nerve anatomy
   1. Includes afferant sensory and efferent motor pathways
   2. Sensory pathway = cutaneous receptors → sensory axons → pure sensory or mixed nerves → nerve plexus (e.g., brachial plexus, lumbosacral plexus) → cell bodies in the dorsal root ganglion → dorsal roots synapse in the dorsolateral spinal cord
   3. Motor pathway = anterior horn cell (spinal cord) → spinal nerves, subsequently dividing into ventral and dorsal rami. Ventral rami → nerve plexus → peripheral motor nerve → neuromuscular junction → muscle fibers
   4. Motor unit = an alpha motor neuron, its axon, neuromuscular junction and all the muscle fibers it innervates
   5. Support structures
      a. Fascicle = bundle of axons running together
      b. Endoneurium = connective tissue surrounding axons within a fascicle
      c. Perineurium = connective tissue surrounding each fascicle
      d. Epineurium = connective tissue binding fascicles into a nerve trunk
      e. Myelin = axon insulation (from Schwann cells)
         i. Myelinated fibers conduct rapidly by way of saltatory ("jumping") conduction; depolarization occurs only at interspersed nodes of Ranvier
   6. Nerve fiber types: classical (and modern) classifications
      a. Ia (A-alpha) = motor, muscles/muscle spindles
      b. Ib (A-alpha) = motor, Golgi tendon organs
      c. II (A-beta) = sensory, pressure/touch
      d. III (A-delta) = sensory, pain/temperature/touch
      e. IV (C) = pain and other receptors

B. Pathophysiology of peripheral nerve injury
   1. Seddon classification
      a. Neurapraxia = partial injury affecting the myelin, but intact axon. Conduction block occurs
      b. Axonotmesis = interruption of axons and myelin sheath, but intact nerve stroma. Wallerian degeneration occurs
      c. Neurotmesis = complete disruption of the axon and enveloping nerve sheath. Regeneration without surgical intervention is not possible

   2. Mixed axonal and myelin injury
      a. Most athletic nerve injuries produce a neurapraxic lesion (injury to myelin) and also often display axonal involvement
      b. Electrodiagnostic (EDX) testing can help classify nerve injuries as primarily axonal, demyelinating, or mixed type
C. Mechanisms of athletic nerve injury (can be acute or chronic)
   1. Compression (pressure)
      a. Causes motor and/or sensory deficits
      b. Secondary effects of chronic compression can also include edema, hemorrhage, and neural fibrosis
   2. Ischemia (hypoxia)
      a. Rarely the sole cause of athletic nerve injury
      b. Important secondary cause of nerve injury in situations of sustained compression or compartment syndrome
      c. *Rapidly reversible physiologic block of conduction* = rapid restoration of nerve conduction with reperfusion (if less than 6 h of ischemia)
      d. Causes pain and paresthesias
   3. Traction (stretch, angulation)
      a. Most nerves can stretch 10–20% without significant damage
      b. Nerves can adapt to slow chronic stretch better than acute tension
      c. Examples of athletic nerve stretch injuries
         i. 15% of all grade II and III lateral ankle sprains have damage to the peroneal nerve on EDX studies
         ii. *Burner or stinger* = acute tension on the superior trunk (C5 and C6) of the brachial plexus, with contralateral deviation of the neck and ipsilateral shoulder depression
   4. Laceration
      a. Rare traumatic event in sports
      b. Immediate surgical repair of nerve may reduce neuronal loss
D. Evaluation of athletic nerve injury
   1. History: clearly define symptom perception and time course
      a. Neuropathic pain = pain originating from nervous system
      b. Paresthesia = any abnormal sensation on the skin
      c. Dysesthesia = unpleasant abnormal sensation
      d. Numbness = lacking sensation
   2. Neurologic examination
      a. Strength = manual muscle testing and functional strength testing
      b. Reflexes = abnormalities rarely seen in athletic peripheral nerve injuries, except in cases of radiculopathy and significant motor nerve injury
      c. Sensation = fine touch/vibration/proprioception (dorsal column/medial lemniscus pathway) and pain/temperature (anterolateral pathway)
      d. Provocative maneuvers
         i. Neural tension tests (numerous variations exist)
            (A) Upper limb tension testing (ULTT) (see Figure 46.1)
            (B) Straight-leg raise
            (C) Sit-slump test
            (D) Femoral stretch test
         ii. Direct nerve compression or percussion
   3. Electrodiagnostic (EDX) testing
      a. Evaluates the physiology and function of a nerve, which can complement structural abnormalities found on imaging
      b. Localizes and characterizes nerve injury
      c. Can differentiate neurapraxia from axonotmesis (important for prognosis)

d. Consists of nerve conduction studies (NCS) and needle electromyography (nEMG)
e. NCS = evaluate motor and sensory nerves and provide data about the integrity of the myelin and the number of functioning axons
f. nEMG = evaluates the motor unit (lower motor neuron pathway), but not the sensory pathway and assesses for muscle denervation from axonal injury
4. Imaging
a. Magnetic resonance neurography = specific MRI sequences for optimal visualization of peripheral nerves

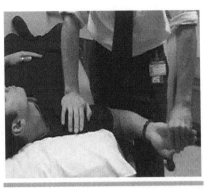

Figure 46.1 Upper limb tension test, with median nerve bias. Positioning includes shoulder abduction with scapular depression; increasing elbow extension, forearm supination, wrist and finger extension; and cervical spine contralateral flexion.

   i. On T2 sequences, normal nerves appear uniform in size, intermediate in signal, and often slightly hyperintense compared to adjacent muscle
   ii. Enlargement and/or hyperintense T2 signal in a nerve are abnormal findings (see Figure 46.2)
   iii. Allows visualization of space-occupying lesions compressing the nerve
   iv. Can complement EDX findings for localization of nerve injury
   v. MR signal patterns in muscle can identify acute and chronic denervation
      (A) Acute denervation = increased T2 STIR signal
      (B) Chronic denervation = decreased volume/ fatty infiltration on T1
b. Musculoskeletal ultrasound
   i. Focal peripheral nerve entrapments can often be visualized by ultrasound
   ii. In longitudinal view, normal peripheral nerves have a fascicular appearance with hypoechoic fascicles surrounded by hyperechoic connective tissue
   iii. In transverse view, nerves display a honeycomb or speckled appearance (see Figure 46.3)
   iv. Hypoechoic swelling of a nerve can be seen just proximal to the site of nerve compression
   v. Transducer pressure on the nerve can elicit symptoms

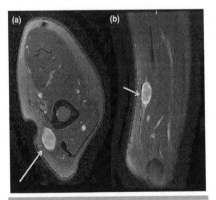

Figure 46.2 MR neurogram of left ulnar nerve demonstrating well-circumscribed T2 hyperintense lesion intimately associated with the ulnar nerve, consistent with a schwannoma (arrows). (a) Axial view. (b) Coronal view. Courtesy of Dr. Colin Strickland, University of Colorado

E. Management of athletic nerve injury
  1. Nerve recovery
    a. Capacity for regeneration persists for at least 1 year (but survival of neuron not ensured after severe injury)
    b. Order of recovery in mixed lesions
      i. Resolution of conduction block
      ii. Distal axon sprouting of spared axons
      iii. Muscle fiber hypertrophy
      iv. Redistribution of sensory function
      v. Axonal regeneration of injured axons
    c. Timeline for nerve recovery
      i. Ischemia-producing conduction block: reversal is rapid, often minutes to hours
      ii. Compression-induced conduction block (neurapraxia): recovery over several months

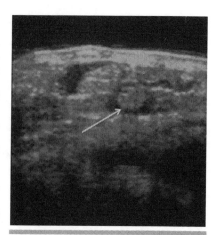

Figure 46.3 Axial (or transverse) ultrasound image of volar wrist, including median nerve (arrow). Courtesy of Dr. John Hill, University of Colorado

      iii. Axonal injury (axonotmesis): axon regrowth 1 mm/day, 1 cm/week, 1 inch/month
        (A) Denervated muscle fibers are viable for only 18–24 months after injury
        (B) Excessive scar tissue or injury to neural tubes reduces the potential for functional regeneration
  2. Nonoperative treatment
    a. Rehabilitation
      i. Activity modification = a period of relative rest (including temporary avoidance of the aggravating activity) and an emphasis on cross-training
      ii. Bracing may be necessary for protection of joints, tendons, and ligaments
      iii. Pads may be useful over hypersensitive regions
      iv. Kinetic chain rehabilitation
        (A) Formulate biomechanical diagnosis that led to the nerve injury
        (B) Evaluate entire kinetic chain for proximal deficits that predispose to more distal injury
        (C) Correct biomechanical faults within the kinetic chain, optimizing flexibility, endurance, strength, and power
        (D) Strengthening through closed kinetic chain training is emphasized to restore coordination, proprioception, and functional sequential muscle activation patterns
        (E) Careful adaptive strengthening of compensatory muscles may help maintain function while a nerve recovers
      v. Neuromobilization = nerve glides (often akin to flossing) and nerve mobilization (avoiding end range) may help with nerve healing, nerve pain, and reduction of nerve scarring
    b. Nonpharmacologic pain relief = considerations include ice, heat, transcutaneous electrical stimulation (TENS), acupuncture
    c. Medications
      i. Minimal efficacy data for medication use for athletic peripheral nerve injuries

      ii. Initial considerations for symptom control include topical lidocaine gel or patches, nonsteroidal anti-inflammatory gel/patches/oral agents, acetaminophen, low-dose tricyclics, or anticonvulsants

   d. Injections = rarely indicated for peripheral nerve injury

      i. Exception = corticosteroid injection for carpal tunnel syndrome

  3. Surgery

   a. Open or endoscopic surgical release and/or decompression may be indicated for severe or refractory peripheral nerve entrapments

   b. Traumatic nerve lacerations may be treated by direct repair or grafting

   c. Salvage procedures, including muscle transfers, may be necessary for restoration of basic function in setting of severe chronic nerve injury and weakness

  4. Return to play

   a. The best determination for return to play remains the athlete's functional performance in simulated sports activities

   b. EDX or imaging studies may lag behind clinical recovery.

II. Peripheral Nerve Entrapments and Injuries

Upper Limb Nerve Injuries

A. Neurogenic thoracic outlet syndrome (N-TOS)

  1. Neurovascular entrapment syndrome of the upper extremity, separated into N-TOS and vascular TOS (V-TOS) depending on which components of the neurovascular bundle are thought to be entrapped (see also section on V-TOS below)

  2. N-TOS is a controversial diagnosis

  3. Definitive (true) N-TOS = objective neurological deficit (most often lower trunk, C8-T1 roots)

   a. Very rare (~1/1 million cases of N-TOS)

   b. Often requires surgery

  4. Disputed N-TOS = no objective neurological deficit (pain predominates)

   a. More common and more controversial

   b. Generally managed conservatively

  5. Three potential sites of compression of neurologic structures

   a. Scalene triangle (most common)

   b. Costoclavicular space

   c. Retropectoralis minor space

  6. Common etiology = anatomic variant + cumulative trauma (i.e., repetitive overhead motion)

   a. Anatomic variants

     i. Cervical rib (<1% of general population) or elongated C7 transverse process

     ii. Anterior or middle scalene hypertrophy (weight lifters)

     iii. Pectoralis minor hypertrophy (swimmers)

     iv. Subclavius hypertrophy (figure skaters)

     v. Anomalous fibrous band(s)

  7. Clinical presentation = highly variable

   a. Ranges from pain/paresthesia (often medial forearm/hand) to weakness/atrophy (hand intrinsics)

   b. Often worse with overhead activity

  8. EDX studies = usually normal

   a. May see abnormal medial antebrachial cutaneous nerve and rarely abnormalities on needle EMG in the C8/T1 pathways

   b. Generally better for ruling out more common neurologic diagnoses (i.e., carpal tunnel syndrome, ulnar neuropathy, cervical radiculopathy) that may mimic TOS symptoms

9. Imaging
   a. Chest x-ray with apical lordotic view evaluates for cervical rib or elongated transverse process
   b. MRI of brachial plexus assesses for mass effect on neurological structures
10. Diagnostic anterior scalene block (with local anesthetic)
    a. May help predict surgical response
11. Treatment
    a. Nonoperative treatment considerations
       i. Individualized, depending on suspected etiology of N-TOS
       ii. Most patients can be managed conservatively
       iii. Activity modification/relative rest
       iv. Therapy: PT for postural reeducation, improving biomechanics for overhead activities, stretching pectoralis minor and scalenes, strengthening scapular stabilizers
       v. Medications (see Management section above)
       vi. Injections (minimal efficacy data)
          (A) Trigger point injections
          (B) Botulinum toxin injections
          (C) Scalene local anesthetic blocks
    b. Surgical treatment
       i. Supraclavicular approach: anterior and middle scalenectomy +/− cervical and first rib resection
       ii. Transaxillary approach: resection of first rib, partial resection of anterior scalene, removal of other anomalous structures
       iii. Outcomes vary depending on etiology, approach, duration of symptoms, premorbid disability, and other factors
       iv. Complications: pneumothorax, nerve injury
B. Parsonage–Turner syndrome
   1. Also known as (idiopathic) brachial neuritis (or plexitis) and neuralgic amyotrophy
   2. Propensity for upper brachial plexus and pure motor nerves
      a. Suprascapular, long thoracic and/or anterior interosseus nerves commonly affected
   3. Etiology = usually idiopathic (possibly viral)
   4. Clinical presentation
      a. Exquisite pain around the medial scapula occurs before weakness
      b. Pain lasts 10 days, followed by weakness sometimes for months
      c. Bilateral in 1/3 of cases
   5. EDX testing indicated to confirm diagnosis
   6. Imaging usually not necessary unless concern for compressive plexus lesion
   7. Treatment = nonoperative
      a. Spontaneous remission over time
      b. Rehabilitation to prevent contractures and secondary shoulder problems due to altered mechanics from weakness
C. Suprascapular nerve injury
   1. Relatively common upper limb peripheral nerve injury in athletes
   2. 1–2% of all shoulder disorders that cause pain
   3. Most common in overhead athletes under the age of 40
      a. Example: service-arm in volleyball players
   4. Etiology = shoulder instability, compression (e.g., backpack), traction, repetitive microtrauma, direct trauma, idiopathic brachial neuritis, complication of distal clavicle resection, rotator cuff surgery, or positioning during spine surgery

    a. Injury at suprascapular notch = compression by overlying transverse scapular ligament causing weakness in both *supraspinatus* and *infraspinatus*

    b. Injury at spinoglenoid notch = most common site in athletes

        i. Isolated *infraspinatus* weakness

        ii. Often caused by ganglion cyst near labral tear or traction/microtrauma along lateral scapular spine

  5. Clinical presentation = posterior–lateral shoulder ache, weakness on shoulder external rotation +/− atrophy of affected muscles

  6. EDX testing may localize abnormality and rule out C5/6 radiculopathy

  7. Imaging

    a. X-rays: usually normal; may visualize calcified transverse scapular ligament on Stryker notch view

    b. MRI may show ganglion or labral cyst, other space-occupying lesion, other shoulder pathology, or denervated muscle changes

  8. Suprascapular nerve block: considered positive if relief of shoulder pain after injection at the suprascapular notch

  9. Treatment = usually nonoperative

    a. PT to maintain shoulder ROM (especially posterior capsule), scapular stabilization and compensatory muscle strengthening

    b. Usually resolves completely within 6–12 months

    c. Surgery if confirmed space-occupying lesion (e.g., ganglion cyst) and weakness/atrophy or failure to improve over 6–12 months

        i. Shoulder arthroscopy to treat associated labral tear

        ii. May also involve release of transverse scapular ligament

        iii. Return to sport is anticipated postoperatively

D. Long thoracic nerve injury

  1. Uncommon in sports, but disabling when present

  2. Etiology = repetitive microtrauma from stretching or traction (e.g., tennis serve), direct trauma, compression, idiopathic brachial neuritis

  3. Clinical presentation

    a. Dull periscapular pain, often worse with overhead activity

    b. Insidious onset shoulder weakness or loss of throwing power

    c. Scapulohumeral dyskinesis and medial scapular winging (*serratus anterior* weakness)

  4. Imaging not usually helpful

  5. EDX testing may show needle abnormalities isolated to the *serratus anterior*, if axonal injury is present

    a. Differentiates from other causes of winging (dorsal scapular nerve injury [rhomboids] or spinal accessory nerve injury [trapezius])

  6. Treatment = usually nonoperative

    a. PT = prevent shoulder contracture with ROM, strengthen along kinetic chain, including other periscapular muscles

        i. Muscular compensation difficult with *serratus* injury—no good substitutes

    b. Improvement by 6–9 months, but recovery takes 1–2 years

    c. Surgical indication = symptoms persisting beyond 1–2 years and no improvement on EDX testing

    d. Surgical options = muscle transfer, fascial sling, scapulothoracic fusion, nerve transfer

        i. Return to sport unlikely if surgery required

E. Axillary nerve injury

  1. Third most common mononeuropathy in sports

  2. Etiology = blunt shoulder trauma, glenohumeral dislocation, humeral fracture, idiopathic brachial neuritis, quadrilateral space syndrome

3. Quadrilateral space syndrome = fibrous bands or hypertrophied muscles causing chronic compression of posterior humeral circumflex artery, accompanied by axillary nerve entrapment
   a. Nebulous, controversial, and rare
   b. May be seen in throwing athletes
4. Quadrilateral space borders = *teres minor* (superior), *teres major/lat* (inferior), *long-head triceps* (medial), *subscapularis* (anterior), humeral shaft (lateral)
5. Clinical presentation of axillary neuropathy = lateral shoulder numbness and/or deltoid weakness (one or all regions) and/or teres minor weakness
6. EDX testing is indicated for diagnosis and prognosis
7. Imaging
   a. X-rays assess for proximal humerus fracture, dislocation
   b. MRI assesses for nerve compression, denervation/atrophy in deltoid or teres minor
8. Treatment = initially nonoperative (relative rest, observation, PT)
   a. PT = maintain shoulder ROM and strengthen proximal to distal
   b. Surgical exploration if no evidence of recovery within 3–6 months

F. Radial nerve injuries
1. Proximal radial nerve entrapment
   a. Etiology = compression in spiral groove (honeymooner's palsy, muscular effort compression by triceps)
      i. Runner's radial palsy = dorsal hand numbness in runners who keep elbows acutely flexed; resolves with correction of running form
   b. Clinical presentation = wrist/MCP finger extension weakness and/or sensory changes +/− mild elbow flexion weakness (*brachioradialis*)
      i. Triceps/anconeus may be spared
   c. EDX studies confirm diagnosis and better localize lesion
   d. Treatment = usually nonoperative, with spontaneous recovery in 4–5 months
2. Radial tunnel syndrome = controversial syndrome of forearm radial nerve entrapment causing persistent lateral elbow pain, often without objective motor or sensory loss
   a. Tenderness of extensor forearm muscle mass (a few cm distal to lateral epicondyle)
   b. Forearm pain with resisted supination
   c. Lateral elbow pain with resisted elbow, wrist, long-finger extension
   d. In athletes with repetitive pronation/supination
   e. EDX studies usually normal
   f. Treatment is usually nonoperative
3. Posterior interosseus nerve syndrome (PINS) = painless weakness of wrist/finger extensors without sensory impairment
   a. Entrapment sites = fibrous bands in front of radial head, recurrent radial vessels, Arcade of Frohse, tendinous margin of extensor carpi radialis brevis muscle
   b. EDX studies (nEMG) often abnormal (sparing of *brachioradialis*)
   c. Surgery often necessary

G. Ulnar neuropathy at the elbow
1. Commonly referred to as cubital tunnel syndrome (but injury can occur more proximally at the retrocondylar groove)
2. Cubital tunnel = just distal to the medial epicondyle, between the two heads of the FCU, beneath the humeroulnar aponeurotic arcade, with underlying bone and ligaments
3. Etiology = Second most common entrapment neuropathy, traction or compression (especially during repetitive elbow flexion), or direct trauma
   a. Most common in throwers (cocking phase)
   b. Also described in skiing (poling), weight lifting, and racquet sports
4. Clinical presentation = sensory disturbance in the ulnar digits, hypothenar region and dorsal ulnar hand (spares the forearm) +/− ulnar intrinsic hand weakness

a. Tinels sign present at elbow in 80% of asymptomatic people
b. Wartenberg sign = little finger adduction weakness causes it to get caught on edge of pants pocket as it rests in slight extension
c. Froment sign = adductor pollicis weakness causes decreased pinch between thumb and index finger (substitution with median innervated FPL causes flexion at the IP joint) (see Figure 46.4)

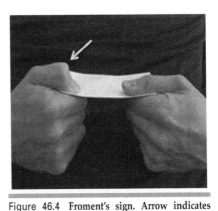

Figure 46.4 Froment's sign. Arrow indicates flexion of the IP joint of the thumb, indicating weakness of the ulnar innervated adductor pollicis muscle, with compensation by the flexor pollicis longus (innervated by the anterior interosseus branch of the median nerve).

5. EDX testing can confirm diagnosis and rule out C8/T1 radiculopathy, lower trunk plexopathy, carpal tunnel syndrome
6. Imaging = usually not necessary
   a. Plain films: usually normal
   b. MRI: mainly for surgical planning or evaluating for other pathology; may see focal increased signal at site of injury (though some asymptomatic individuals may also show this at the elbow)
   c. Ultrasound: may show focal increased swelling just proximal to site of compression and may be able to visualize compression in dynamic flexion
7. Treatment = usually nonoperative
   a. Bracing often helpful (elbow pad or splint to prevent full flexion)
   b. Surgery for recalcitrant cases
      i. May include decompression +/ − transposition
      ii. In athletes, surgery often accompanied by repair of injured ulnar collateral ligament

H. Ulnar neuropathy at the wrist
   1. Uncommon (compared to elbow)
   2. Also known as "handlebar palsy"
   3. Entrapment at Guyon's canal = ulnar tunnel = between the pisiform medially and hook of hamate laterally
      a. Contents include the ulnar nerve, ulnar artery, and associated veins
   4. Etiology = compression (e.g., pressure from handlebars in cyclists), ganglion cysts, ulnar artery thrombosis, carpal fractures, anomalous muscles, or fibrous bands
   5. Hypothenar hammer syndrome = vascular syndrome with similar presentation (see vascular injury section below)
   6. Classification: Shea's system
      a. Type I: All parts involved (deep motor branch, including hypothenar muscles, and sensory)
      b. Type II: Involves only the deep motor branch (*palmaris brevis* always spared and hypothenar muscles may be spared)
      c. Type III: Involves only the superficial sensory branch
   7. Clinical presentation = motor and sensory symptoms depend on specific branch affected
      a. Dorsal ulnar hand sensation always spared (supplied by dorsal ulnar cutaneous nerve that originates proximal to wrist)
      b. Palmaris brevis sign = intact or excessive contraction of the palmaris brevis (wrinkling of hypothenar skin with little finger abduction/flexion) implicates Guyon's canal as the

      8. EDX testing often confirms diagnosis and rules out carpal tunnel syndrome

      9. Imaging = usually not necessary unless trauma or suspicion of cyst

     10. Treatment = usually nonoperative

        a. Padded bicycling gloves and activity modification

        b. Surgical decompression rarely needed

I. Pronator syndrome

    1. Proximal median neuropathy causing diffuse forearm pain with paresthesia in the distal median nerve distribution

    2. Sites of compression = between heads of pronator teres, at Lacertus Fibrosis (biceps aponeurosis), or under sublimus bridge

    3. Clinical presentation = athletes who require repetitive forceful pronation or gripping (throwers, tennis, archery, arm wrestling, weight lifting, rowers)

    4. EDX testing = conduction abnormal across forearm segment and/or nEMG abnormalities in median innervated muscles (pronator teres may be spared)

    5. Treatment = rest, splinting, technique modification, and rarely surgical release

J. Carpal tunnel syndrome

    1. Median neuropathy at the wrist

    2. Most common peripheral nerve entrapment in general population

    3. Common in wheelchair athletes, gymnastics, cycling, and rowing

    4. Carpal tunnel = osseofibrous canal with carpal bones making up floor and sides and transverse carpal ligament as roof

    5. Carpal tunnel contents = 10 structures (4 tendons of *flexor digitorum profundus*, 4 tendons of *flexor digitorum superficialis*, *flexor pollicis longus tendon*, and median nerve)

    6. Etiology = compression of median nerve from anything that decreases canal size (e.g., flexor retinaculum thickening) or increases volume of contents (e.g., tendonitis)

    7. Clinical presentation = paresthesias affecting thumb, index and long fingers, often increased at night and with activity; clumsiness with fine motor skills (e.g., buttons); $+/-$ sensory and/or motor loss in median distribution (e.g., *abductor pollicis brevis* weakness), thenar atrophy in severe cases

    8. Provocative tests: Tinels, Phalens, carpal compression test

    9. EDX testing confirms diagnosis

   10. Imaging = usually not necessary

   11. Treatment = conservative or surgical depending on severity

      a. Stretching, avoidance of repetitive flexion/extension, improve ergonomics/technique

      b. Neutral wrist splints (effective in ~30%)

      c. Carpal tunnel injection with steroid (often temporary; 50% relapse by 1 year)

      d. Surgical release (curative in 75%).

Lower Limb Nerve Injuries

K. Obturator nerve injury

    1. Etiology: Direct pelvic trauma, obturator hernia, fascial band at outlet of obturator canal (described in rugby players)

      a. Rare in sports

    2. Clinical presentation = hip adduction weakness and altered sensation over medial thigh

    3. EDX testing = abnormal nEMG if axonal injury

    4. Treatment = correction of underlying cause

      a. Surgical correction of hernia or obturator neurolysis if compressed by fascial band

L. Meralgia paresthetica

    1. Lateral femoral cutaneous nerve injury

    2. Etiology = usually compression or trauma of nerve near inguinal ligament (e.g., gymnast on uneven bars, scuba diver with weighted belt, long-distance backpackers)

3. Clinical presentation = pure sensory syndrome, including pain, paresthesia over antero-lateral thigh, often worse with hip extension
4. EDX testing primarily used to rule out other conditions
5. Treatment = nonoperative
   a. Most cases resolve with relative rest
   b. Surgical exploration for resistant cases
M. Saphenous nerve injury
   1. Supplies cutaneous sensation to anteromedial leg and medial ankle
   2. Etiology = most often injured at distal portion of Hunter's canal as it pierces dense fascia (distal 1/3rd of thigh)
      a. Possible injury with local muscle contraction/hypertrophy (e.g., bodybuilders), patellar dislocation, swollen local structure (e.g., pes anserine bursa), iatrogenic (e.g., knee or ankle arthroscopy)
      b. Rare in athletes
   3. Clinical presentation = pain +/− paresthesias in the medial knee, leg, or ankle, possibly worse with femoral stretch test. No weakness
   4. EDX testing helps exclude other causes of medial leg pain (e.g., L4 radiculopathy, lumbar plexopathy, femoral neuropathy)
   5. Treatment = usually nonoperative
      a. May include simple reassurance, adjusting tight equipment, avoidance of provocative factors, local anesthetic/steroid injection
      b. Surgical release rarely needed (e.g., excision of neuroma)
N. Fibular nerve injuries
   1. Common fibular nerve injury
      a. Most common lower limb nerve injury in sports
      b. Etiology = compression (direct blow, accessory sesamoid in the lateral gastrocnemius tendon, tight fascial band at the edge of fibularis longus), hypermobility of fibular head, and stretch injuries at the fibular neck (proximal tibiofibular dislocation, varus stress injuries at knee or ankle), or iatrogenic (knee surgeries)
      c. Clinical presentation = combination of the findings for both the superficial and deep fibular nerve injuries
   2. Superficial fibular nerve injury
      a. Etiology = lateral compartment syndrome, compression to anterolateral lower leg, iatrogenic (ankle surgeries)
      b. Clinical presentation = proximal injury causes weakness of ankle everters (possible recurrent ankle sprains) and numbness over dorsal ankle/foot
   3. Deep fibular nerve injury
      a. Etiology = anterior compartment syndrome, entrapment at septum between lateral and anterior compartments, compression beneath inferior extensor retinaculum (e.g., tight ski boots), traction at anterior ankle (e.g., ballet), compression by tarsal bone osteophytes
      b. Clinical presentation = proximal injury causes foot drop (weakness of *tibialis anterior*) and sensory changes at first web space; injury at anterior tarsal tunnel may cause atrophy of *extensor digitorum brevis* and sensory changes at the first web space
   4. EDX testing helps localize the lesion and rules out more proximal nerve injury (e.g., sciatic nerve injury, L5 radiculopathy)
   5. Imaging = x-rays indicated if history of trauma to evaluate for fibular injury
   6. Treatment = depends on severity and etiology
      a. Consider surgery for intrinsic compression (fascial band, perineural cyst, abnormal bony prominence), severe injury (complete or nearly complete disruption of axons)

    b. Nonoperative treatment and observation for mild, partial injuries
      i. Bracing or splinting and proprioceptive training to decrease risk of ankle sprain

O. Tarsal tunnel syndrome

1. Tarsal tunnel = at medial ankle, tibial nerve travels underneath the flexor retinaculum (which extends from medial malleolus to medial calcaneus)
2. Contents (anterior to posterior) = *tibialis posterior, flexor digitorum longus*, posterior tibial artery/vein, tibial nerve, *flexor hallucis longus*
3. Etiology = space-occupying lesions (accessory calf muscles, ganglion cysts, tumors, bone fragments, scar tissue), tenosynovitis of tendons within the tunnel, external compression (tight ski boots or ankle orthoses), stretch injury from abnormal ankle/foot biomechanics (overpronation in running)
4. Clinical presentation = pain +/− dysesthesias in medial ankle, heel and/or foot, often worse at night
    a. Atrophy of intrinsic foot muscles is rare, but possible with severe cases
5. Differential diagnosis
    a. Tarsal tunnel syndrome causing neuropathy is rare
    b. Other considerations may include plantar fasciitis, calcaneal fat pad atrophy, calcaneal or navicular stress fracture, osteochondritis of talus, sinus tarsi syndrome, synovial impingement, and tenosynovitis
6. EDX testing often normal, unless a space-occupying lesion in the tarsal tunnel
7. Imaging = MRI may be used to rule out space-occupying lesion or when evaluating for other pathology
8. Treatment = usually nonoperative
    a. Conservative treatment = relative rest (may include walking boot or other AFO), correct overpronation, anesthetic/steroid injection, hip abductor strengthening (helps mitigate overpronation)
    b. Surgical release sometimes needed

P. Morton's interdigital neuroma

1. Etiology = compressive neuropathy of interdigital nerve (second or third web space most commonly affected), from recurrent impingement under intermetatarsal ligament, MTP joint synovitis/capsular swelling, hypermobility of metatarsals (e.g., fourth metatarsal in overpronation), tight-fitting or high-healed shoes
2. Clinical presentation
    a. Symptoms: plantar foot pain +/− radiation and/or paresthesias to the affected toes, often worse in tight shoes or walking on uneven ground
    b. Signs: Positive compression test (of the web spaces), Mulder's click (squeeze test causing palpable click as the neuroma is squeezed between MT heads), and/or decreased sensation to pinprick in affected toes
3. Differential diagnosis = more proximal nerve entrapment (e.g., tarsal tunnel, peripheral neuropathy, lumbosacral radiculopathy), metatarsalgia, MTP joint synovitis or subluxation, MT stress fracture, Freiberg's infarction (AVN causing painful collapse of second MT head), and soft tissue or bony tumor of forefoot
4. EDX testing can rule out more proximal neuropathies, but unable to specifically rule in interdigital neuroma
5. Imaging = usually not necessary, but MRI or U/S may demonstrate neuroma
6. Interdigital block = diagnostic local anesthetic injection may help confirm diagnosis
7. Treatment = both nonoperative and surgical options
    a. Appropriate footwear (cushioned, wide toe box, low heel, +/− metatarsal pad), trial one-time steroid injection (repeat injections not recommended)
    b. Surgical = dorsal incision for partial resection of intermetatarsal ligament and nerve resection.

III. Principles of Vascular Injury Evaluation and Management
  A. Types of vascular injuries in sports
    1. Complete occlusion is rare
      a. Emergent treatment required within 6 h
    2. Nonocclusive injury is more common
      a. Dissection, aneurysm, direct injury, intermittent compression/entrapment, stenosis, thrombosis
      b. Most common venous injury in sports = subclavian vein thrombosis (Paget–von Schroetter syndrome)
      c. Most common arterial injuries in sports = axillary and popliteal artery entrapments
      d. Allows time for evaluation with vascular diagnostic testing
  B. Evaluation of athletic vascular injury
    1. High index of suspicion is most important
      a. Physical exam may be normal with exercise-induced symptoms
      b. Pain, paresthesias or paralysis and coolness, swelling, asymmetric pulses, fatigue, pallor, and/or prolonged capillary refill
    2. Vascular diagnostic tests
      a. Ankle brachial index (ABI) (aka ankle arm index [AAI])
        i. In athletes, postexercise measurements and side-to-side comparison may be useful as a screening test
      b. Duplex ultrasonography
        i. Useful for identification of thrombi, stenosis, vessel wall thickening
        ii. Modality of choice for diagnosis of deep venous thrombosis
        iii. If testing equivocal, venography may be necessary
      c. Angiography (or arteriography)
        i. Gold standard for diagnosis of arterial disease
        ii. Advantages = excellent visualization of arterial tree
        iii. Disadvantages = invasive test with complications including cost, bleeding, thrombosis, AV fistula, pseudoaneurysms, allergic reaction or nephrotoxicity to contrast, 5% false positives
        iv. Rarely needed in sports-related injuries
      d. Advanced imaging angiography
        i. Includes computed tomography angiography (CTA) and magnetic resonance angiography (MRA)
        ii. MRA and CTA allow simultaneous visualization of vasculature and any surrounding anatomic abnormalities
        iii. MRA increasingly being used for thoracic outlet syndrome (most sensitive with arms abducted)
        iv. Side effect profile better than with conventional angiography
      e. MRI
        i. Can be useful in vascular injuries/compression, compartment syndrome, and thoracic outlet syndrome
        ii. In compartment syndrome, MRI may show edema, hemorrhage, hematoma, vessel injury, and/or inflammation
  C. Principles of management of athletic vascular injury
    1. Vascular surgery referral for acute vascular compromise or refractory vascular insufficiency symptoms
    2. Activity modification = reduce or eliminate the aggravating activity and emphasize cross-training
    3. Therapeutic exercise = optimize biomechanics with goal of eliminating functional vascular compression/microtrauma (kinetic chain concepts still apply)
    4. Smoking cessation.

IV. Peripheral Venous Entrapments and Injuries

A. Effort thrombosis

   1. Spontaneous thrombosis of axillary or subclavian vein (aka Paget–von Schroetter syndrome)

   2. Rare, but potentially disastrous syndrome

   3. May follow strenuous upper limb activity or trauma

   4. Pulmonary embolism in 36% of patients

   5. Clinical presentation

     a. Chronic low-grade compression = dull pain in upper limb $+/-$ arm/hand swelling $+/-$ collateral vessel formation; distal pulses usually intact

     b. Acute thrombosis = rapid onset of nonpitting edema, cyanosis and pain; distal pulses generally intact unless thrombosis is massive/acute

   6. Diagnosis = Doppler ultrasonography

   7. Treatment = emergent thrombolysis/confirmatory venography, often followed by decompression of the thoracic inlet and usually 8 weeks of anticoagulation

     a. Return to play = 3.5 months on average.

V. Peripheral Arterial Entrapments and Injuries

A. Quadrilateral space syndrome (see Axillary nerve injury section above)

   1. Posterior humeral circumflex artery may get entrapped with the axillary nerve

B. Vascular thoracic outlet syndrome (V-TOS)

   1. Focal vascular compressive trauma from bony abnormalities near the thoracic inlet leading to stenosis of vessels or acute thrombosis

   2. Less controversial and better defined than N-TOS (see also N-TOS section above)

   3. Paget–von Schroetter syndrome is a venous type of V-TOS seen in athletes

   4. Etiology = most commonly acute or cumulative trauma to neurovascular bundle + anatomic predisposition (*as in N-TOS*)

     a. Clavicle and first rib fractures can impinge neurovascular bundle

     b. Cervical ribs are common in surgical TOS patients

   5. Clinical presentation = may include variable degrees of ischemia, including pallor, numbness, Raynaud's phenomena, digit ulceration, gangrene, pulse deficit, or subclavian steal syndrome

     a. Exam may reveal unilateral scalene tenderness or supraclavicular fossa bruits

     b. Dynamic positioning provocative tests for V-TOS

       i. Roos test (aka elevated arm stress test (EAST)) = Reproduction of symptoms with abduction/external rotation of arms and opening and closing fists for 3 min (*sensitivity = 84%; specificity = 30%*)

       ii. Wright test = loss of radial pulse or reproduction of symptoms with arm in 90° abduction/external rotation position (*sensitivity = 90%; specificity 29%*)

       iii. Adson maneuver = loss of radial pulse during deep inspiration with the arms in anatomic position and the neck actively rotated toward the affected side (*sensitivity = 79%; specificity = 76%*)

       iv. Halstead (costoclavicular) maneuver (aka military position test) = loss of radial pulse or reproduction of symptoms with scapular retraction and depression (*sensitivity = 84%; specificity = 47%*)

   6. Diagnosis

     a. Plain radiography, including apical lordotic view to evaluate for bony abnormalities (such as cervical rib)

     b. Doppler ultrasonography can evaluate for aneurysm or thrombosis

     c. MRA or CTA may be helpful to diagnose both vascular and bony abnormalities

     d. Angiography remains the gold standard for V-TOS

7. Treatment = Prompt vascular surgery referral is indicated when V-TOS is suspected
   a. If true vascular compromise is ruled out, an initial trial of nonsurgical treatment may be pursued
   b. Surgical options vary depending on specific pathology (see N-TOS section above for common surgical approaches)
C. Hypothenar hammer syndrome
   1. Repeated blunt trauma to the hypothenar portion of the hand leading to ulnar artery damage against hook of hamate, potentially causing digital ischemia
   2. Etiology = most commonly described in manual laborers (where hypothenar region is used as a tool to hammer, push, or squeeze objects) or vibration-exposed workers
      a. Reported in a variety of athletes (baseball, karate, badminton, biking, golf, tennis, handball, softball, weight lifting, break dancing, hockey)
   3. Clinical presentation = variable depending on severity
      a. Usually unilateral
      b. Symptoms may include digital pain, paresthesias, cold sensitivity, blanching or discoloration of fingertips, finger claudication, or hypothenar pain
      c. Signs may include hypothenar callus/tenderness or pulsatile mass (aneurysm), discoloration of fingertips, coldness, splinter hemorrhages, ulceration, or gangrene
      d. Allen test = attempts to assess patency of superficial palmar arch
   4. Diagnosis
      a. Angiography is the gold standard
      b. CTA can show vascular anatomy and evaluate for hamate fracture
      c. MRA can identify ulnar artery trauma from soft tissue structures, such as accessory muscles
   5. Treatment = controversial due to limited studies
      a. Trial of conservative treatment is reasonable unless acute ischemia
      b. Conservative treatments may include smoking cessation, avoidance of inciting repetitive trauma, padded gloves, cold avoidance, calcium channel blockers (nifedipine, diltiazem), antiplatelet agents or anticoagulation, pentoxifylline to reduce blood viscosity
      c. Various surgical options exist
D. Subclavian steal syndrome
   1. Proximal stenosis or occlusion of the subclavian artery leading to reversal of blood flow down ipsilateral vertebral artery to supply the arm (at the expense of the vertebrobasilar circulation)
   2. Etiology
      a. In athletes, causes are similar to vascular TOS + vigorous exercise in the affected arm
      b. Atherosclerosis is the most common cause in the general population
   3. Clinical presentation = vertebrobasilar insufficiency (presyncope, syncope, CNS deficits); subclavian insufficiency (arm weakness, paresthesias, exertional claudication)
   4. Provocative maneuver = vigorous exercise of affected arm causes symptoms or loss of radial pulse
   5. Diagnosis
      a. Clinical = blood pressure difference >20 mmHg between arms, subclavian bruit, diminished pulses
      b. Imaging = duplex ultrasonography, MRA, CTA, angiography (gold standard)
   6. Treatment = vascular surgery referral (options may be similar to TOS in mild cases or require angioplasty, stenting or bypass in severe cases)
E. External iliac artery endofibrosis (EIAE)
   1. Etiology = mechanical stress on the vessel (e.g., hip flexion) coupled with shear stress from high blood-flow during intense exertion (+/− arterial kinking and compression from hypertrophied psoas muscle and from inguinal ligament) → smooth muscle hyperplasia, collagen deposition in the intima → arterial stenosis

    a. Elite cyclists, age 20–30 years, are the most common athletes affected

    b. Risk increases with distance traveled

    c. Also described in cross-country skiers, runners, weight lifters, and rugby

    d. No association with atherosclerotic disease

  2. Clinical presentation = unilateral limb pain and lack of power during intense exercise +/− subjective sense of thigh edema, paresthesias, and progressive worsening over time

    a. 15% have bilateral symptoms

    b. Physical exam usually normal (some patients may have bruit if checked following exertion or in extreme hip flexion

  3. Diagnosis

    a. Tests may include ABI, duplex ultrasonography, MRA, and angiography

    b. Postexertional testing improves the sensitivity of both ABI and duplex U/S

    c. MRA with gadolinium can identify kinking and luminal stenosis

    d. Angiography is the most useful confirmatory test

  4. Treatments = little consensus

    a. Nonoperative treatment, including activity modification, may lead to some improvement in flow limitations over time

    b. Minimally invasive, percutaneous transluminal balloon angioplasty (PTBA) has been successful, but risks include arterial dissection with angioplasty

    c. Other more invasive surgical options include release of kinked vessel, arterial resection and saphenous vein graft, or endarterectomy

    d. Medical therapy with antiplatelet agents or statins is not effective

F. Popliteal artery entrapment (PAE)

  1. Congenital type: fibromuscular anomalies in the popliteal fossa causing extrinsic compression of the neurovascular bundle

    a. Type I: artery is displaced medially (variant arterial course)

    b. Type II: medial head of gastrocnemius arises from an abnormal lateral origin

    c. Type III: accessory muscle slip arising from the gastrocnemius head caused the compression

    d. Type IV: fibrous band from the popliteus causes the compression

    e. Type V: popliteal vein is also compressed

  2. Functional type: physiologic impingement of the popliteal artery caused by exercise-induced increased blood flow and muscle hypertrophy of *gastrocnemius, soleus, plantaris,* or *semimembranosus*

    a. Most commonly in young healthy athletes participating in sports requiring overuse of the lower limbs

  3. Clinical presentation = calf claudication, paresthesias, exertional calf muscle fatigue

    a. Symptoms typically not present at rest

    b. Usually unilateral (25% bilateral)

    c. Physical examination usually normal (+/− postexercise popliteal bruit)

    d. Decreased peripheral pulses can be seen with active ankle dorsiflexion/plantarflexion and knee extension (although this may also occur in asymptomatic people)

  4. Diagnosis = tests may include postexertional ABI, arterial Doppler segmental pressures, CT, MRI, or arteriography

    a. Most sensitive test for functional PAE = photoplethysmography (high false-positive rate (50–60%))

  5. Treatment

    a. Functional PAE may be initially treated conservatively (relative rest, compression stockings, stretching, lower limb elevation)

    b. Congenital or refractory PAE is usually treated with surgical exploration for release of fascial or myotendinous band compressing the artery +/− vascular grafting if vessel

Recommended Reading

1. Ablett CT, Hackett LA. Hypothenar hammer syndrome: Case reports and brief review. *Clin Med Res.* 2008;6(1):3–8.
2. Akuthota V, Herring SA, eds. *Nerve and Vascular Injuries in Sports Medicine.* New York, NY: Springer; 2009.
3. Chan-Tack KM. Subclavian steal syndrome: A rare but important cause of syncope. *South Med J.* 2001;94(4):445–447.
4. Dumitru D, Zwarts MJ, Amato AA. Peripheral nervous system's reaction to injury. In: Dumitru D, Amato AA, Zwarts MJ, eds. *Electrodiagnostic Medicine.* 2nd ed. Philadelphia: Hanley and Belfus; 2002:115–156.
5. Zimmerman NB. Occlusive vascular disorders of the upper extremity. *Hand Clin.* 1993;9(1):139–150.

47

Sport Psychology
Nicole Detling Miller

I. Depression (Major Depressive Disorder)

A. One of most prevalent psychiatric disorders
   1. 16.2% of people meet criteria at some point in their lives
   2. Two times more common in women than men
   3. Median age of onset is late teens to early twenties

B. Sad mood and/or loss of pleasure in usual activities plus at least four of the following:
   1. Sleep disturbances (difficulty falling asleep, staying asleep, not returning to sleep, or prolonged duration of sleep)
   2. Psychomotor retardation or agitation
   3. Poor appetite and weight loss, or increased appetite and weight gain
   4. Loss of energy
   5. Feelings of worthlessness
   6. Difficulty in concentration, thinking, or making decisions
   7. Recurrent thoughts of death or suicide
      a. Symptoms must be present nearly every day, most of the day, for at least two weeks
      b. Symptoms cause significant distress or functional impairment
      c. Symptoms not due to normal bereavement

C. Biological treatment
   1. Medications
      a. Monoamine oxidase (MAO) inhibitors
      b. Tricyclic antidepressants
      c. Selective serotonin reuptake inhibitors (SSRIs)
         i. SSRIs have been linked to an increased risk of suicide in patients less than 24 years of age and should be used in this population with caution
   2. Electroconvulsive therapy (ECT)

D. Psychological treatment
   1. Exercise
      a. Both aerobic and anaerobic exercise reduces depression
   2. Interpersonal therapy (IPT)
      a. Focus is on current interpersonal problems (e.g., role transitions, conflicts, bereavement, isolation) rather than repressed issues from childhood
   3. Cognitive therapy
      a. Aim is to alter maladaptive thought processes by examining and contradicting negative self-beliefs
   4. Social skills training
      a. Behavioral treatment designed to improve social interactions

5. Behavioral activation therapy
  a. Focuses on increasing participation in positively rewarding activities
6. Behavioral marital therapy
  a. Aim is to improve communication and satisfaction within marriage.

II. Eating Disorders/Disordered Eating

A. Anorexia nervosa
  1. Typically begins mid- to late adolescence (14–18 years)
    a. Onset may be associated with stressful life event
  2. Four diagnostic criteria
    a. Maintains body weight below minimally normal level for age and height
      i. Less than 85% normal for age and height
      ii. BMI $\leq$ 17.5 kg/m^2
    b. Intense fear of gaining weight or becoming fat
    c. Perception of body weight and shape is distorted
    d. Amenorrhea in postmenarcheal females (i.e., absence of at least three consecutive periods)
  3. Types
    a. Restricting
      i. Weight loss accomplished by dieting, fasting, or excessive exercise
    b. Binge eating/purging
      i. Regular engagement in binge eating, purging, or both
B. Bulimia nervosa
  1. Usually begins in late adolescence or early adult life
    a. Binge eating frequently begins during or after dieting episode
  2. Five diagnostic criteria
    a. Recurrent episodes of binge eating
      i. Eating a larger amount of food during a discrete time period than most people
      ii. Perception of lack of control overeating during episode
    b. Recurrent inappropriate compensatory behavior to prevent weight gain (i.e., self-induced vomiting, fasting, excessive exercise, laxatives, diuretics)
    c. Average occurrence of binge eating and compensatory behaviors is at least twice a week for three months
    d. Self-evaluation largely dependent on body shape and weight
    e. Does not occur exclusively during episodes of anorexia nervosa
  3. Types
    a. Purging
      i. Regularly engaging in self-induced vomiting or misuse of laxatives, diuretics, or enemas
    b. Nonpurging
      i. Other inappropriate compensatory behaviors (i.e., fasting or excessive exercise) but has not regularly engaged in purging
C. Treatment
  1. Hospitalization may be required to restore weight and to address imbalances in fluids and electrolytes
  2. Antidepressants (e.g., SSRIs)
  3. Operant conditioning behavior therapy
    a. Rewarding eating behaviors helps immediate goal of gaining weight in patients with anorexia nervosa
  4. Cognitive behavior therapy
    a. Best validated and current standard for treating bulimia nervosa
    b. Patients encouraged to evaluate societal ideas of physical attractiveness and educate

III. Sport Psychology

A. The scientific study of people in sports and the implementation of that knowledge with athletes and exercisers

B. Specialties
1. Educational sport psychology specialists
   a. Graduate degree in sport and exercise science, physical education, or kinesiology; with an emphasis in sport psychology should also have training in psychology
   b. Mental coach approach
   c. Focus is on performance enhancement
2. Clinical sport psychologists
   a. Graduate degree in psychology; should also have training in sport and exercise
   b. Licensed by state boards
   c. Focus is on treating emotional disorders (e.g., eating disorders, substance abuse)

C. Current recognized field-specific certification is offered through the Association for Applied Sport Psychology (AASP); to be given the CC-AASP designation, individuals must have the following:
1. Masters or doctorate degree (as either educational sport psychology specialist or clinical sport psychologist)
2. Specific coursework encompassing both sport science and psychology courses
3. Practicum training in performance enhancement supervised by a CC-AASP
   a. 400 h for doctorate degree
   b. 700 h for masters degree.

IV. Performance Enhancement

A. Mental skills training with primary purpose to improve performance of individuals and/or teams
1. Athletes, coaches, parents, exercisers, performers (dance, music, etc.), businesses

B. Sample mental skills training
1. Anxiety control
   a. Relaxation strategies specific to type of anxiety: state, trait, cognitive, and/or somatic
2. Arousal regulation
   a. Strategies that either increase or decrease physiological activation
3. Concentration training
   a. Specific skills to train each type of attention: broad internal, broad external, narrow internal, narrow external, and transitional
4. Confidence training
   a. Strategies specific to building and maintaining confidence levels in a variety of situations
5. Team building, team cohesion
   a. Skills used to develop unity among teams
6. Imagery
   a. Uses all the senses (e.g., visual, auditory, gustatory, olfactory, kinesthetic) to program the muscles for action
7. Self-talk training
   a. Strategies that ensure the individual's internal dialogue is productive
8. Composure training
   a. Specific interventions that can be used to deal with adversity and mistakes made while performing
9. Anger control
   a. Proper and appropriate outlets are taught for dealing with anger

10. Identity awareness
   a. Understanding how the individual's identity is connected with performance
11. Development of preperformance routines
   a. Used as a mental warm-up, similar to a physical warm-up, that ensures competition readiness
12. Leadership training
   a. Can be used with coaches, captains, business executives, etc.
13. Communication
   a. Facilitation techniques for coach–coach, coach–athlete, athlete–athlete, and other relationships.

V. Performance Anxiety

A. Immediate negative emotional state, prior to performance, characterized by apprehension, fear, tension, and an increase in physiological arousal; anxiety disappears within 24 h following performance
   1. Primary antecedents
      a. Fear of failure
      b. Fear of negative social evaluation
      c. Fear of physical harm
      d. Situation ambiguity
      e. Disruption of well-learned routine
   2. Multidimensional
      a. Cognitive
         i. Mental component of anxiety (e.g., fear of negative social evaluation, fear of failure, loss of self-esteem)
      b. Somatic
         i. Physical component of anxiety (e.g., increased heart rate, respiration, and muscular tension)
B. Psychological treatment (primary method)
   1. Cognitive behavioral therapy
   2. Relaxation training
   3. Imagery
   4. Self-talk training
   5. Hypnosis
   6. Confidence training
C. Biological treatment (secondary method)
   1. Benzodiazepines
   2. Antidepressants (tricyclic antidepressants and SSRIs).

VI. Coping with Injury

A. Poor psychological adjustment to injury
   1. Abnormally high anger and confusion
   2. Obsession with "when can I play again"
   3. Denial
   4. Repeatedly going back to sport too soon resulting in reinjury
   5. Exaggerated bragging about accomplishments
   6. Dwelling on minor physical complaints
   7. Increased sense of guilt
   8. Withdrawal from significant others
   9. Rapid mood swings
   10. Apathy
   11. Malingering

B. Treatment
   1. Cognitive restructuring
   2. Confidence training
   3. Imagery
   4. Coping skills
   5. Panic mitigation
   6. Positive self-talk
   7. Rational emotive therapy
   8. Relaxation skills
   9. Systematic desensitization.

VII. Burnout

A. Response to chronic stress, it is a psychological syndrome of emotional and physical exhaustion brought on by the persistent devotion toward a goal; athlete no longer receives physical benefits of exercise
   1. Physiological symptoms
      a. Increased resting and exercise heart rate
      b. Increased resting systolic blood pressure
      c. Increased muscle soreness and chronic muscle fatigue
      d. Increased presence of biochemical indicators of stress in the blood
      e. Increased sleep loss
      f. Increased colds and respiratory infections
      g. Decreased body weight
      h. Decreased maximal aerobic power
      i. Decreased muscle glycogen
      j. Decreased libido and appetite
   2. Psychological symptoms
      a. Increased mood disturbances
      b. Increased perception of physical, mental, and emotional exhaustion
      c. Decreased self-esteem
      d. Negative change in the quality of personal interaction with others (cynicism, lack of feeling, impersonal relating)
      e. Negative cumulative reaction to chronic everyday stress as opposed to acute doses of stress

B. Treatment
   1. Relaxation training
   2. Take time off
   3. Reestablish goals
   4. Mental reprogramming (self-talk)
   5. Imagery
   6. Time management skills
   7. Learn to walk away from imperfection
   8. Communicate needs to significant others
   9. Discussion of motivation
   10. Re-evaluation of physical training program.

Recommended Reading

1. American Psychiatric Association. *Diagnostic and Statistical Manual of Mental Disorders.* 4th ed. Text Revision (DSM-IV-TR). Arlington, VA: American Psychiatric Association; 2000.
2. Cox RH. *Sport Psychology: Concepts and Applications.* 6th ed. Boston, MA: McGraw Hill; 2007.
3. Davis MD, Eshelman ER, McKay M. *The Relaxation and Stress Reduction Workbook.* 6th ed. Oakland, CA: New Harbinger Publications, Inc.; 2008.

4. Feltz DL, Landers DM. The effects of mental practice on motor skills learning and performance: A meta-analysis. In: Smith D, Bar-Eli M, eds. *Essential Readings in Sport and Exercise Psychology.* 2007:219–229. Champaign, IL: Human Kinetics.

5. Gould D, Eklund RC. The application of sport psychology for performance optimization. In: Smith D, Bar-Eli M, eds. *Essential Readings in Sport and Exercise Psychology.* 2007: 231–240. Champaign, IL: Human Kinetics.

6. Kring AM, Davison GC, Neale JM, Johnson SL. *Abnormal Psychology.* 10th ed. Hoboken, NJ: John Wiley & Sons; 2007.

7. Weinberg RS, Gould DG. *Foundations of Sport & Exercise Psychology.* 4th ed. Champaign, IL: Human Kinetics; 2010.

48

The Master Athlete

Christopher J. Visco and Marni G. Hillinger

I. The Master Athlete Defined

A. "There are various definitions of master athletes. For the purpose of this chapter, master athletes will be defined as active individuals aged 50 years or older."—ACSM.

II. Effects of Age on Performance

A. Physiologic changes should be differentiated from pathologic changes (i.e., disease, injury, etc). Similar rate of change in both genders. See Table 48.1 for a summary of functional changes. The following are common age-related changes:

1. Cardiopulmonary changes:
   a. Increased:
      i. Risk of sudden death primarily at the onset of exercise and with vigorous exercise
   b. Decreased:
      i. Cardiac output
      ii. Stroke volume
      iii. Maximal heart rate (by 10 beats/min/decade)
      iv. Blood vessel and pulmonary compliance
      v. Vital capacity
         (A) 9–10%/decade after age 25
      vi. Expiratory flow
2. Altered fluid requirements
   a. Decreased thirst mechanism combined with increased kidney output leads to faster dehydration
   b. Recommended fluid intake is two cups prior to exercise followed by 200–400 ml water every 20–30 min of activity
3. Tissue changes
   a. Increase in tissue stiffness and decrease in overall flexibility
   b. Decreased tendon, cartilage, and soft tissue compliance
   c. Decreased quantity of capillaries supplying tendons
   d. Sarcopenia
      i. Decreased muscle mass and cross-sectional area
      ii. Fatty infiltration
4. Exercise performance changes include decreases in:
   a. Endurance
   b. Reaction and performance
      i. Decrease in overall performance occurs at a steady and slow rate from 50–75 years, 1–3% per year
      ii. After age 75 there is a sharp decline of 4–10%

Table 48.1   Functional changes with aging

Variable	Physiologic change	Functional change
Muscle mass	↓ Total muscle mass ↓ Fiber number and size	↓ Speed ↓ Power ↓ Strength
Body fat	↑ Body fat in 3rd–5th decade ↓ Body fat after age 70	Fat ↑ rates of cardiovascular and metabolic disease
Metabolism	↓ V_{O2max} by 9–10% per decade	↓ Functional reserve early fatigue
Motor control	↓ Walking speed ↓ Reaction time ↑ Injury risk	↑ Fall risk ↑ Injury risk
Cardiovascular	↓ Total plasma volume ↓ Thirst sensation ↑ Arterial stiffness ↑ Injury risk	↑ Dehydration risk ↑ Work of heart ↑ Cardiac disease risk

   c. Running stride length
      i. A shorter stride length results in decreased exercise economy (more effort to cover the same distance)
   d. Balance and proprioception
   5. Metabolic changes include:
      a. Decreased metabolic rate and glucose tolerance
      b. Decreased lactate threshold
      c. Bone loss, osteopenia, and osteoporosis
  B. Strength
   1. Muscle mass decreases 1.25% per year after age 35
      a. Regular resistance training may decrease the rate of loss by as much as half. Prolonged periods of inactivity should be avoided
      b. Decreases occur in myofibril size, number, and ratio of type II to type I fibers. Overall this decreases strength
      c. Strength of each muscle fiber remains the same; however, the overall body strength diminishes due to smaller cross-sectional area of each muscle group.

III. Effects of Age on Injuries

  A. A delay in diagnosis of musculoskeletal problems is common in master athletes compared to younger counterparts
  B. Generally injuries in master athletes should be treated similarly to those that are younger with the caveat that recovery period may be prolonged
  C. Recovery after exercise
   1. Muscle demonstrates a slower return to contractile functioning after endurance exercise
   2. Tendon demonstrates an slower recovery to original dimension after distension
  D. Degenerative changes involving articular surfaces and tendons are common
   1. Collagen changes include decreased quantity, increased cross-linking, increased stiffness, and decreased resilience
   2. Arthritis and tendinopathy may lead to chronic exacerbations of symptoms which should be treated to maintain and support activity.

IV. Exercise with Chronic Disease

A. Physiologic changes occur with chronic disease, including osteoarthritis, cardiopulmonary disease, peripheral vascular disease, and diabetes
   1. Regular exercise decreases the long-term effects of chronic disease
   2. Maintain caution with polypharmacy. Multiple medication use is common in older adults and can affect performance and lead to adverse events

B. Osteoarthritis
   1. The most common cause of pain and disability
   2. Prevalence of radiographic evidence >65 years is 70% at hip/knee
   3. Shearing and repetitive articular cartilage or meniscal injuries can culminate in degenerative joint surfaces beginning with fibrillation of the articular surface and micro tears
   4. Posttraumatic or postsurgical arthritic changes are common
   5. Treatment is multimodal and includes
      a. Analgesics
      b. Physical therapy, including strengthening
      c. Unloader braces used during sport
      d. Activity modification
      e. Injections, including steroid or viscosupplementation
      f. Surgery, including arthroscopy, osteotomy, and arthroplasty
   6. Effect of osteoarthritis on exercise performance
      a. Pain with joint movement → pain with rest → joint swelling → activity restricted → decrease in strength and mobility
      b. Improvements occur in pain scores and increased independence of activities of daily livings (ADLs) with exercise training
   7. Exercise recommendations and considerations
      a. 10 min warm-up prior to strengthening
      b. Goal is to enhance muscle strength around an affected joint
      c. Focus on strength and coordination
      d. Pain and function better for land-based activities versus aquatic
      e. Benefit is also shown with tai-chi
      f. Ideally, exercise program is supervised for the first 3 months
   8. Contraindications
      a. Acute joint inflammation—rest until inflammation is reduced
      b. Modify or hold regimen if pain after exercises
      c. Caution with sports that cause both compression and twisting: for example, basketball, football, volleyball, and soccer

C. Spine
   1. Spondylotic disease
      a. Degenerative changes at the zygapophysial joints (facet joints) decreases lumbar range of motion in extension
      b. Stiffness and pain are common complaints
      c. Thoracolumbar junction is susceptible to injury
   2. Spinal stenosis
      a. Neurogenic claudication, pain, and paresthesias with prolonged walking and standing
      b. Onset is common in fifth or sixth decade
      c. Can occur in central canal versus lateral/foraminal/subarticular
      d. Men are twice as likely to develop stenosis than women

D. Cardiopulmonary disease
   1. Contraindications to exercise include
      a. Severe coronary heart disease
      b. Severe aortic or carotid stenosis

    c. Exacerbation of congestive heart failure

    d. Uncontrolled arrhythmia or hypertension

    e. Cardiomyopathy, myocarditis

    f. Patients on anticoagulation therapy should be advised of the risk of contact sports

2. Congestive heart failure (CHF)

    a. Effect of CHF on exercise performance

        i. V_{O2max} is reduced, leads to more rapid exhaustion

        ii. Muscle atrophy and decreased strength

    b. Exercise improves

        i. V_{O2max}, resting pulse, systolic blood pressure (SBP), and ventilation

        ii. Independence of ADLs and quality of life (QoL)

    c. Recommendations

        i. Aerobic training—cycling, walking, and jogging

           (A) Gradual interval training

           (B) Preferably supervised

        ii. Strength training—sequential training of small groups of muscles to minimize cardiovascular stress

    d. Precaution with angina pectoris—decrease pace or take frequent breaks

3. Chronic obstructive pulmonary disease (COPD)

    a. Irreversible reduction in pulmonary function

        i. Severe disease leads to decrease in functional level which can further worsen dyspnea

        ii. At least 4 weeks of endurance training improves quality of life, including less fatigue and dyspnea, *but* does not improve lung function

    b. Recommendations:

        i. Moderate-intensity endurance training, walking, or cycling, gradually increasing distance/time

        ii. Targeted Inspiratory Muscle Training may improve inspiratory strength, endurance, exercise capacity, and quality of life

E. Peripheral vascular disease (PVD)

1. Effect of PVD on exercise performance

    a. Those with intermittent claudication take 26% fewer strides and spend 15% less time ambulating versus controls

    b. 12% slower ambulation and ambulate discontinuously

    c. Decreased cadence

2. PVD → insufficient tissue perfusion

    a. PVD cycle: Increasing severity of disease → decreased function and mobility → more sedentary lifestyle → muscle atrophy → progression of atherosclerotic disease

    b. Physical activity improves fitness, strength, pain tolerance, and psychological impact of pain

    c. Regular exercise increases walking distance to the onset of pain by 179% and maximum walking distance by 122%

        i. Possible mechanisms: training → muscle contraction during ischemia → increased vascular endothelial growth factor (VEGF) → induces formation of collaterals

3. Recommendations

    a. Begin a walking protocol

        i. 3 × /week for 30 min, preferably supervised for first 6 months → continued lifelong

    b. Walking should be pushed beyond onset of pain, followed by rest until pain dissipated → increases walking tolerance

        i. May help to add bursts of rapid ambulation

F. Diabetes

    1. General

        a. Often coexists with hypertension, obesity, and dyslipidemia

        b. Mortality is 2 to 4× general population

          i. Poor fitness is an independent prognostic factor for mortality in type 2 diabetics

        c. Physical activity can improve glycemic control, decrease hypertension, and increase V_{O2max}, muscle strength, and motivation

    2. Precautions

        a. Consume carbohydrates (10–20 g) prior to exercise initiation to prevent hypoglycemia

        b. Monitor blood glucose during and after exercise

          i. Consider decreasing hypoglycemic agents

        c. Cushioned footwear may help symptomatic neuropathy or foot arthritis

        d. Avoid valsalva if known history of hypertension or retinopathy

        e. Caution with excessive weight bearing if foot ulcers are present.

V. Exercise Status Post-Joint Arthroplasty

    A. Joint replacement is a cost-effective treatment which has been shown to improve quality of life.

        1. Improves pain, function, mobility, and psychological well-being

        2. Between 2005 and 2030, rate of total hip arthroplasty (THA) expected to increase by 174%, and total knee arthroplasty (TKA) by 673%

    B. Common goals include functional improvement and return to athletic activity

        1. A high activity level presurgery predicts a return to sports post-op

    C. Few prospective randomized trials look at athletics post-replacement

        1. Most surgeons recommend low-impact activities

        2. Recent trend is to allow for more athletic activity and less restrictions

    D. Postsurgical considerations for exercise

        1. Force across the reconstructed joint (load and moments)

          a. Variable—based on activity level and activity type

          b. Normal joint loads:

              i. Daily activity—3–4× body weight

              ii. Sports—5–10× body weight

              iii. For endurance activities, load is speed dependent

          c. TKA may wear more quickly than THA for high load activities

        2. Stress at bone–implant interface should be considered, including the type of prosthesis fixation

        3. Balance between too little activity (less wear and prosthesis but risk of decreased bone density and early loosening) and too much activity (increased wear and late loosening)

          a. Presurgical experience with a particular sport also matters

          b. Not recommended to take up new high-impact sport post-surgery

          c. Beginners experience higher joint loads versus experienced

          d. Efforts should be taken to decrease load (e.g., using ski poles to assist with hiking)

    E. Lifetime sports post-joint arthroplasty

        1. No definite guideline for return to sport following a THA or TKA

        2. Tennis

          a. High-impact loading and twisting across joint may accelerate wear of the prosthetic joint

          b. Unclear whether patients should return to high-level tennis post-joint replacement

          c. Many recommend doubles tennis due to decreased joint stress

          d. Following THA or TKA, patients experience increased court mobility and decreased court speed. Pain relief demonstrated post-THA

        3. Golf

          a. Many surgeons encourage golf after total joint replacement

   b. Decreased pain while playing and after playing post-replacement
   c. Following THA—average handicap increased by 1.1 strokes and average drive length increased by 3.3 yards
   d. Following TKA—average handicap increased by 1.9 strokes but average drive length decreased by 12 yards.

Recommended Reading

1. ACSM Consensus Statement. Selected issues for the master athlete and the team physician. *Med Sci Sports Exerc.* 2010;42(4):820–833.
2. Chodzko-Zajko WJ, Proctor DN, Fiatarone Singh MA, Minson CT, Nigg CR, Salem GJ, Skinner JS. Exercise and physical activity for older adults. *Med Sci Sports Exerc.* 2009;41(7):1510–1530.
3. Evans WJ. Protein nutrition, exercise and aging. *J Am Coll Nutr.* 2004;23(Suppl_6):601S–609.
4. Faulkner JA, Davis CS, Mendias CL, Brooks SV. The aging of elite male athletes: Age-related changes in performance and skeletal muscle structure and function. *Clin J Sport Med.* 2008;18(6):501–507.
5. Kuster M. Exercise recommendations after total joint replacement: A review of the current literature and proposal of scientifically based guidelines. *Sports Med.* 2002;32(7):433–445.
6. Leyk D, Rüther T, Wunderlich M, Sievert A, Eßfeld D, Witzki A, Erley O, Küchmeister G, Piekarski C, Löllgen H. Physical performance in middle age and old age. *Dtsch Arztebl Int.* 2010;107(46):809–816.
7. Maharam LG, Bauman PA, Kalman D, Skolnik H, Perle SM. Masters athletes: Factors affecting performance. *Sports Med.* 1999;28(4):273–285.
8. Marcell TJ, Hawkins SA, Wiswell RA. Exercise and the master athlete—A model of successful aging? *J Gerontol.* 2003;58A(11):1009.
9. Petrella RJ, Chudyk A. Exercise prescription in the older athlete as it applies to muscle, tendon, and arthroplasty. *Clin J Sport Med.* 2008;18(6):522–530.
10. Wright VJ, Perricelli BC. Age-related rates of decline in performance among elite senior athletes. *Am J Sports Med.* 2007;36(3):443–450.

49

The Pediatric Athlete

Holly J. Benjamin and David Jewison

I. The pediatric athlete is defined as a child or adolescent usually under the age of 18 that participates regularly in sports activities. An estimated 20–45 million youth 6–18 years of age participate in athletics (two-thirds in organized sports, one-third recreational). It is important for the sports medicine physician to be aware of the varying levels of sport, skill level, and motivations for participation.

II. **Common reasons for the pediatric athlete's participation in sports**

   A. To have fun, to socialize, to attain self-confidence, to further life goals, and to become physically fit.

III. **Benefits of participation in sports and regular physical activity**

   A. Causes weight reduction and decreased insulin sensitivity in youth with Type 2 Diabetes Mellitus

   B. Reduces systolic and diastolic blood pressure in hypertensive adolescents

   C. Beneficial psychologically for all youth regardless of weight to increase self-esteem and self-concept and to decrease risks of anxiety and depression

   D. Asthma is not a barrier to sport participation with proper precautions.

IV. **Growth and development**

   A. Boys and girls grow at approximately the same rate during childhood
      1. Growth spurt in girls occurs ages 10–13, usually ending growth at ages 15–16; or more specifically ~2 years after the onset of menses
         a. Girls develop 2/3 the amount of muscle as boys and twice as much body fat
         b. Physiologic differences are small between girls and boys in the preadolescent growth phases
      2. Growth spurt in boys occurs ages 12–15, stopping growth at age 18–19
      3. Tanner stages are used to standardize development for males and females (see Table 49.1)

   B. Bone growth
      1. Bone lengthens before and more rapidly than muscles and tendons which is a risk factor for overuse injuries
      2. Articular cartilage of growing bone is thicker than in adult bone and is able to remodel more easily
      3. Junction of epiphysis and metaphysis is vulnerable to disruption
      4. Apophyses (growth plates at which tendon attaches to bone) are at risk for avulsion injuries
      5. Metaphyseal injuries in children include incomplete fractures (i.e., greenstick) due to thickened periosteum.

Table 49.1 Tanner stages of pubertal development

Stages	Pubic hair	Breasts (Female)	Genitals (Male)
Tanner 1	None	No glandular tissue	No enlargement
Tanner 2	Minimal hair	Breast buds	Testicular enlargement and thinning of scrotal skin
Tanner 3	Hair becomes curly	Enlargement of breasts	Penile enlargement and increased testicular size
Tanner 4	Curly hair, diffuse, sparing thighs	Increased size of areola	Enlargement of penis and testicles
Tanner 5	Hair covers medial thighs	Full adult size, areola contours with breast	Adult penis and testicular size

V. Physiological differences in the child athlete versus the adult

 A. Regular exercise, including high-intensity and prolonged exercise, does not appear to have adverse effects on growth and development in the presence of adequate nutrition

 B. Aerobic capacity

  1. Preadolescent aerobic capacity is close to adult levels, and can only be increased by conditioning at puberty and into adulthood

  2. Aerobic capacity increases with age in general until physiologic maturity is reached

 C. Anaerobic performance in children is much lower than in adolescents and adults, and training may not improve this because of immaturity

 D. Strength gains are seen steadily in children as they grow. Strength training can result in strength gains above and beyond growth-related gains

  1. Strength gains occur through neuromuscular adaptation in the prepubescent athlete. Muscle hypertrophy is not seen until after puberty

  2. Deconditioning is seen in youth athletes if strength training is discontinued

 E. Metabolic costs of body movement during physical activity are higher in children due to shorter stride length during running and greater inflexibility of antagonist muscle groups during contraction

 F. Speed, power, and mass are lower in children due to lower levels of circulating androgens. Gender differences are virtually nonexistent in the prepubescent athlete

 G. Thermoregulation

  1. Historically, pediatric athletes were considered to be an at-risk group for exertional heat illness (EHI) with an impaired thermoregulatory response to exercise in hot environments due to:

   a. Higher body surface area to mass ratio, which increases their heat absorption rate in hot environments

   b. Decreased sweating capacity, and thus, an impaired cooling mechanism

   c. Lower cardiac output and higher metabolic (heat production) rate at the same work load

  2. Recent research has demonstrated that any increased risk of EHI in children is related primarily to excessive physical exertion, improper clothing in extremely hot, humid environments, dehydration, and insufficient recovery time between repeated bouts of exertion

  3. Children are no longer believed to have less effective thermoregulatory abilities, lower exercise tolerance, or insufficient cardiovascular capacities than adults when hydration status is maintained and excessive exertion is avoided

Table 49.2 Risk factors for Exertional Heat Illness in children

1. High heat and humid environment

2. Dehydration

3. Lack of proper rehydration due to insufficient time or lack of access to fluids

4. Deconditioned state of fitness or lack of acclimatization

5. Extreme physical exertion

6. Chronic disease

7. Medications

8. Insufficient recovery time between bouts of exertion

4. Certain acute and chronic illnesses and medications are known to increase the risk of EHI in children who exercise as exemplified by the following (see Table 49.2)
   a. Gastrointestinal illnesses, dehydration, and fever
   b. Chronic illnesses such as diabetes mellitus, cystic fibrosis and chronic lung disease, juvenile hypothyroidism, obesity, and sickle cell trait (also associated with exertional rhabdomyolysis)
   c. Anticholinergic drugs, diuretics, and certain stimulant medications (e.g., ADHD medications)
5. Table 49.3 lists preventive strategies for EHI in children.

H. Nutrition
   1. Minerals such as calcium, phosphorus, and magnesium play a prominent role in forming the skeleton; therefore, adequate amounts should be included in the growing athlete's diet as 25% of peak bone mass is formed during growth spurt
   2. Onset of menses is a risk factor for the development of iron deficiency anemia in preadolescent and adolescent females
   3. Food of poor nutritional value and inadequate energy intake negatively affects growth and maturation even when other nutrient requirements are met
   4. Frequent causes of energy imbalances in young athletes
      a. Inadequate energy intake relative to the amount, intensity, and frequency of exercise
      b. Increased metabolic demands in a growing child.

Table 49.3 Preventive strategies for Exertional Heat Illness in children

1. Gradual acclimatization

2. Unlimited access to water with frequent breaks

3. For prolonged, vigorous exercise consume carbohydrate-electrolyte drinks in addition to water

4. In excessively hot and humid environments exercise time should be shortened, intensity lessened, and schedule more frequent breaks

5. Children who are ill with systemic symptoms should limit participation

6. Children with chronic disease should be monitored for possible activity modification and may require prolonged time for acclimatization early in sport seasons

7. Provide education for coaches, parents, and school personnel to recognize early signs of heat illness

8. Ensure children wear proper uniforms and attire for exercising in a hot, humid environment

VI. Age-appropriate physical activity and sports participation

A. Infants and toddlers (0–2 years)
   1. Motor skills rely on reflexes, training is difficult and not remembered, vision is farsighted, supervised free-play recommended
B. Early childhood (3–5 years)
   1. Fundamental skills (running, throwing, swimming, tumbling) and balance skills are limited, short attention span, response to training limited, vision is farsighted, avoid competition, demonstrate sports. Sports that only entail the fundamental skills are reasonable at this age: walking, running, throwing, and swimming.
C. Childhood (6–9 years)
   1. Improvements in fundamental skills, balance, coordination, vision, and tracking are seen. Ability to understand rules of competition and follow basic commands is emerging. Emphasis is on sport-specific skills and fun over winning. Simple rules and minimal instruction time recommended. Swimming, running, gymnastics, beginner soccer, and baseball are common sports.
D. Late childhood/early adolescence (10–12 years)
   1. Transitional skills (varied combinations of the fundamental skills) improved, balance worsens during puberty and times of rapid growth spurts, selective attention span, vision patterns near/at adult levels, increase exposure to competition can start entry-level contact sports.

VII. Effects of physical activity and participation in athletics

A. No adverse effects on growth and development noted in the presence of adequate nutrition
B. Young female athletes participating in sports with emphasis on low body weight such as gymnastics and figure skating often show signs of late sexual maturation and tend to have a lower average height and weight as compared with sedentary females of the same age or female athletes in sports that do not emphasize the same physical appearance and preadolescent body build.
C. There is evidence that intense, high-volume training can adversely affect growth, but if training is decreased, then growth can catch up when training levels decrease.

VIII. Strength and resistance training in children and adolescents

A. When properly supervised and performed with good technique within recommended guidelines, it is considered safe and efficacious
B. Growth in height and weight are not influenced by resistance training
C. Strength training can improve cardiovascular fitness, body composition, bone mineral density, blood lipid profiles, and mental health in children
D. Can increase muscle strength significantly primarily through neuromuscular adaptation in preadolescents, and through muscle hypertrophy in postpubertal adolescents
E. Strength training programs have not been consistently correlated in scientific studies to injury prevention or enhanced sport performance; however, they are useful adjuncts to a comprehensive sport training program
F. Children should avoid power lifting, body building, and maximal lifts until physical and skeletal maturity is reached.

IX. Risk of injury in the pediatric athlete

A. Use of appropriate and properly sized equipment is essential for the pediatric athlete
   1. Equipment should be properly sized for the athlete and in good condition, which can be difficult due to the varying rates of growth within age groups

2. Both protective equipment and weight training equipment is made in children's sizes

3. Mouthguards should be encouraged for use in all contact sports

B. Participation in multiple sports and year-round participation can lead to burnout and overuse injuries, therefore it is important to assess the nature and level of sports participation in the young athlete in the context of their chronological age, developmental stage, and physical maturity

1. Risks of overuse injuries

a. Extrinsic factors

i. Training errors, environment, and equipment

b. Intrinsic factors

i. Growth, anatomic alignment, muscle–tendon imbalance, flexibility, and conditioning

c. Recommendations for overuse injury prevention

i. Limit one sporting activity to 5 days per week

ii. At least 1 day of rest from organized activity

iii. 2 to 3 months off per year from a single sport

iv. Focus on wellness, fun, and sportsmanship.

X. Rehabilitation of the young athlete

A. Muscles imbalances, flexibility differences, and sport biomechanics are emphasized in both injury prevention and successful rehabilitation of an injured youth athlete

B. Proper supervision is required at all times

C. Use of appropriately sized equipment is necessary

D. Activity modification and relative rest to allow healing, avoid overstress and promote strength gains are combined in successful rehabilitation programs

E. The use of topical, oral, or injectable anesthetics prior to activity that may mask injury symptoms is strongly discouraged.

XI. Select medical conditions in the pediatric athlete (see Chapter 8 for more details)

A. Hypertension evaluation

1. Prehypertension is 90th to 95th percentile systolic or diastolic blood pressure for age

2. Stage 1 Hypertension is 95th to 99th percentile plus 5 mm Hg systolic or diastolic blood pressure for age

3. Stage 2 Hypertension is greater than 99th percentile plus 5 mm Hg systolic or diastolic blood pressure for age

B. Asthma classification

1. Mild intermittent: symptoms up to two times per week

2. Mild persistent: symptoms more than two times per week, not daily

3. Moderate persistent: symptoms daily

4. Severe persistent: continual symptoms

5. Exercise-induced asthma: symptoms only occur with physical activity

C. Eating disorders

1. Recognition is difficult: highest prevalence in sports that promote a lean body image or where leanness is equated with optimal performance (gymnastics, figure skating, distance running, swimming, diving) or where "cutting weight" is a part of the sport (wrestling, boxing, weight lifting, and martial arts)

a. Anorexia and bulimia most common eating disorders

b. Girls experience eating disorders more (9:1) than boys (see Chapter 50 for more details)

c. Many athletes have disordered eating rather than a diagnosed eating disorder.

Recommended Reading

1. Agosta J. The young athlete. In: Brukner P, Khan K, eds. *Clinical Sports Medicine.* 2nd ed., Australia: McGraw-Hill Book Company; 2002:43–83.

2. Benjamin H. The pediatric athlete. In: Madden C, Putukian M, McCarthy E, Young C, eds. *Netter's Sports Medicine.* Philadelphia, PA: Saunders/Elsevier; 2010: Chapter 8.

3. Brenner JS and the Council on Sports Medicine and Fitness. Overuse injuries, overtraining, and burnout in child and adolescent athletes. *Pediatrics.* 1997;*119*(6);1242–1245.

4. Council on Sports Medicine and Fitness. Strength training by children and adolescents. *Pediatrics.* 2008;*121*(4):835–840.

5. IAAF Medical Manual: Specific Considerations for the Child and Adolescent Athlete. Retrieved from: http://www.iaaf.org/medical/manual/index.html

6. Luke AC, Bergeron MF, Robert WO. Heat injury prevention practices in high school football. *Clin J Sports Med.* 2007;*17*(6):488–493.

7. Rice SG and the Council on Sports Medicine and Fitness. Medical conditions affecting sports participation. *Pediatrics.* 2008;*121*(4):841–848.

8. Rowland T. Thermoregulation during exercise in the heat in children: Old concepts revisited. *J Appl Physiol.* 2008;*105*(2):718–724.

50

The Female Athlete

Megan L. Noon and Anne Z. Hoch

I. Anterior cruciate ligament (ACL) injuries—gender difference

A. Women have a 2.3–9.7 times higher risk of ACL rupture than men

B. Most common ACL injury mechanisms: noncontact plant-and-cut movement and landing from a jump
   1. Injuries occur during early deceleration phase of cutting or landing
   2. External tibial rotation (5–13°) with valgus (8°) leads to ACL impingement—rupture when knee is near full extension to moderate flexion

C. Poor biomechanical and neuromuscular control of the lower limb are thought to be major risk factors of an ACL injury in women
   1. Reported that women have greater dynamic lower extremity malalignment (valgus with hip adduction and internal rotation, knee valgus, tibial external rotation, and forefoot pronation) and land from jumps with less knee flexion increasing anterior tibial shearing forces (Figure 50.1)
   2. The 2010 literature review of gender differences in ACL injuries did not find significant differences in knee kinetics or kinematics, although there were differences in neuromuscular control—women had less activity of the vastus medialis and less activity with earlier timing of activation of the biceps femoris
   3. Hewett et al. in 2005 reported lower gluteal activity and increased quadriceps activation in women compared to men
   4. Zebis et al. in 2009 reported higher ACL injury risk in women with preactivity of the semitendinosus and vastus lateralis during side cutting activities

D. Other considerations:
   1. Notch width—smaller in women, may contribute to stenosis and impingement
   2. ACL size—thinner at mid-substance, correlates with smaller notch width
      a. On average, women have 40–50% smaller ACL cross-sectional area than men
   3. Hormonal influences
      a. No definite conclusion can be made on the effects of menstrual cycle and sex steroid hormones on ACL injury risk
      b. Studies have found increased incidence of ACL injuries both at time of ovulation (high concentration of estradiol) and during follicular phase (low concentrations of estradiol and progesterone)

E. Evaluation and treatment—see Chapter 25 (II.E.i.)

F. Neuromuscular training prevention programs
   1. 24–82% reduction of ACL injury; 50% reduction in ACL injury risk

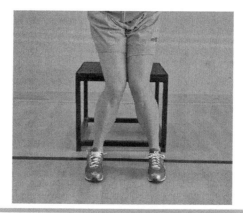

Figure 50.1   Increased dynamic valgus of the knee on landing a jump

2. Goal: correct neuromuscular imbalances more commonly found in women
   a. Ligament dominance—when absorbing ground forces, women allow stress on ligaments before initiating muscular activation
   b. Quadriceps dominance—when stabilizing the knee during movements the knee extensors are activated more than knee flexors
   c. Leg dominance—one limb will have greater strength and coordination
   d. Trunk dominance—to compensate for poor neuromuscular control there is increased motion of the body's center of mass
3. Training programs include a warm-up, plyometric training with emphasis on body posture and control, core and lower limb strength training, and sport-specific aerobic/skill components (e.g., landing drills in basketball)
4. After participating in a prevention program the athlete has learned strategies to avoid vulnerable positions, improved strength and flexibility, and improved proprioception.

II. Female athlete triad (Triad)

A. American College of Sports Medicine (ACSM) redefined the Triad in 2007 as a spectrum of three components:
   1. Low energy availability (with or without eating disorders)
   2. Menstrual dysfunction
   3. Low bone mineral density
B. Each clinical condition is now understood to comprise the pathological end of a spectrum of interrelated subclinical conditions between health and disease (Figure 50.2)
C. Low energy availability
   1. "Spectrum" ranges from optimal energy availability to low energy availability with an eating disorder
   2. Disordered eating spectrum may range from inadvertent calorie restriction to anorexia nervosa or bulimia nervosa
   3. "Energy availability"—amount of energy remaining for all other bodily functions such as cellular maintenance, thermoregulation, growth, and reproduction
      a. Energy availability (kcal/kg/lean body mass) = dietary energy intake-exercise energy expenditure
      b. Positive energy balance is $\geq$45 kcal/kg/Lean Body Mass (LMB)
      c. $\leq$30 kcal/kg/LBM is associated with amenorrhea

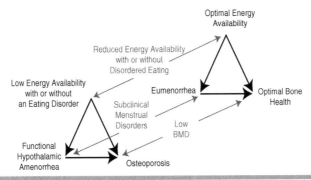

Figure 50.2   From ACSM 2007 position stand: The female athlete triad. Reprinted from Nattiv A, Loucks AB, Manore MM, Sanborn CF, Sundgot-Borgen J, Warren MP. American College of Sports Medicine position stand. The female athlete triad. *Med Sci Sports Exerc.* 2007;39(10):1867–1882

4. Energy deficit may be secondary to:
   a. Increased total output—increased exercise (kcal)
   b. Reduced total energy intake—calorie restriction, fasting, binge eating, and purging, use of diet pills and laxatives
   c. Combination of increased output and reduced intake
5. An athlete can still be at a stable body weight while energy availability is low by compensatory mechanisms to restore energy balance:
   a. Reducing metabolism
   b. Decreasing energy available for reproduction
   c. Decreasing energy available for cellular maintenance
6. Risk factors for disordered eating:
   a. Body image dissatisfaction
   b. Drive for thinness
   c. Preoccupation with weight
   d. Participation in sports with an aesthetic component
   e. Pressure from parents, coaches, judges, and peers
   f. Low self-esteem
   g. Depression

D. Menstrual dysfunction
   1. Second component of the Triad—functional hypothalamic amenorrhea
      a. Most prevalent cause of amenorrhea in the adolescent age group
   2. Other menstrual irregularities included in the spectrum: oligomenorrhea (intervals longer than 35 days), luteal deficiency, and anovulation
   3. There are two types of amenorrhea:
      a. Primary amenorrhea: menstruation cycles not starting by age 15 years
      b. Secondary amenorrhea: absence of ≥3 consecutive months after menarche
   4. Proposed mechanism of functional hypothalamic amenorrhea
      a. Low energy availability → inhibition of hypothalamic gonadotropin releasing hormone (GnRH) → decreased luteinizing hormone (LH) secretion from pituitary → ovarian suppression and decreased estrogen

E. Low bone mineral density (BMD)
   1. Disordered eating and menstrual irregularities with estrogen deficiency predispose women to the third component of the Triad—low BMD

2. International Society for Clinical Densitometry (ISCD) — recommended that the terms osteoporosis and osteopenia not be used in premenopausal women and children unless risk factors are present
   a. Z-scores less than -2.0 to be called "low bone density below the expected range of age" in premenopausal women and "low bone density for chronological age" in children
3. In 2007, the ACSM defined the terms
   a. "Low BMD" as a Z-score between -1.0 and -1.9 with secondary risk factors — chronic malnutrition, disordered eating, hypogonadism, glucocorticoid exposure, and previous fractures
   b. "Osteoporosis" as a Z-score ≤ -2.0 with secondary risk factors stated above
4. Direct correlation between length of amenorrhea and reduction in BMD
   a. Estrogen regulates BMD by limiting bone resorption — estrogen stimulates calcitonin and promotes renal retention of calcium
   b. Rate of bone resorption increased and the rate of bone formation declined within 5 days after energy availability was reduced below 30 kcal kg^{-1} FFM · d^{-1} in exercising women — low enough to suppress estrogen
5. Bone density accrual
   a. Largest increases in BMD in female athletes occur when impact sports are started 5 years before menarche
      i. Sports with a high amount of "irregular weight-bearing" increase bone mineral density
   b. A significant increase in BMD occurs with pubertal growth
   c. At age 12, young girls have 83% of their total body BMD
   d. Two years after menarche, 95% of their BMD has formed
   e. Bone growth in females ceases at approximately age 20
   f. Genetics determine 60–80% of peak bone mass
   g. Lifestyle choices, including diet (energy availability, calcium, and vitamin D) and physical activity (athletes have a 5–15% higher BMD than nonathletes) are also predictors of bone accrual during growth

F. Prevalence
1. 78% of high school athletes have one or more components of the female athlete triad
   a. Disordered eating: 19–60% among all female athletes with higher prevalence in leanness sports
   b. Menstrual dysfunction: 20–66% among all female athletes with runners having the highest prevalence
   c. Low bone mineral density: 10–21% all female athletes
   d. All three components of the Triad: 1–2.6% among high school and college athletes, 4.3% among elite athletes

G. Evaluation of the female athlete triad — refer to Tables 50.1 and 50.2

H. Treatment
1. Interdisciplinary team approach to include the athlete, physician, dietician, athletic trainer/physical therapist, psychologist/psychiatrist, parents, and coaches
2. Disordered eating
   a. Dietician consultation — assess energy balance, focus on achieving a positive energy balance by meal planning (pre/postexercise) and education on energy needs for the athlete
   b. Psychologist and/or psychiatrist for moderate to severe eating disorders
3. Amenorrhea
   a. Rule out medical cause of amenorrhea (see Table 50.1)

Table 50.1 Differential diagnosis for amenorrhea

- Polycystic ovary syndrome[a]
- Hypothalamic amenorrhea[a]
  - Stress
  - Exercise
  - Nutrition related
- Hyperprolactinemia[a]
- Ovarian failure[a]
- Pregnancy/lactation
- Thyroid disease
- Pituitary tumor
- Congenital adrenal hyperplasia
- Genitourinary/anatomic abnormalities
  - Mullerian agenesis
  - Complete androgen resistance
- Turner's syndrome

[a]Top four causes of amenorrhea with the exception of pregnancy.

    b. Correct energy deficits/nutritional issues—reduction of training (-1 day/week), dietician consultation—achieve positive energy balance, increase weight and body fat

    c. Psychologist for stress reduction techniques

  4. Low BMD

    a. Improve by treating the underlying problem—optimize nutritional status (meet calcium and vitamin D recommendations), establish normal menses

    b. Add a weight-bearing and resistive exercise program

I. Return to play

  1. Athletes with the Triad may continue to participate in their sports as long as they have no cardiovascular symptoms—chest pain, shortness of breath, syncope/presyncope, dizziness, etc.

    a. If symptoms are present, the athlete should be held from play and undergo a cardiology consultation

J. Outcomes and future risk

  1. Low bone mineral density may set up the athlete for suboptimal bone mineral density leading to early-onset osteoporosis and/or stress fractures

  2. Infertility—reversible if amenorrhea is exercise related

  3. Athletic amenorrhea has been associated with reduced endothelium-dependent dilation of the brachial artery (endothelial dysfunction)

    a. Endothelial dysfunction is a precursor of early cardiovascular disease, long-term studies have not been completed

K. Prevention

  1. Education of physicians, parents, coaches, athletic trainers, and athletes on the three components of the Triad

  2. Screen for the Triad—preparticipation physical examination, annual physical examination by primary care physician, when athlete is evaluated for other sports-related injuries

  3. Promote healthy eating and exercise habits.

Table 50.2 Evaluation of the female athlete triad

History	Physical examination/diagnostic testing
Menstrual history	Physical examination
• Age of menarche	• Height, weight, vital signs (bradycardia, orthostatic hypotension)
• Date of last menstrual period	
• Number of periods in the last year	• Body habitus, Tanner stage
• Number of days between periods	• Sclera injection
• Symptoms associated with periods	• Dental
• Any missed periods	• Caries, parotid gland enlargement
• Previous or current hormonal therapy	• Thyroid
	• Finger callous, cold/discolored hands and feet
Exercise history	
• Current/previous sports	• Acne, hirsutism
• Time spent exercising (hours/week)	• Pelvic exam
• Exercise intensity	Laboratory tests
• Goals for upcoming events	• Complete metabolic panel
Nutrition history	• Complete blood count with differential
• Weight changes, including athlete's highest and lowest weight	• Erythrocyte sedimentation rate
	• Thyroid function tests
• Ideal weight	• Urinalysis
• Calcium requirements, actual consumption	• Pregnancy test
	• Prolactin level
• Binging or purging behaviors	• Follicle stimulating hormone
• Use of diet pills, laxatives, or diuretics	• Luteinizing hormone
Injury profile	• Free testosterone
• Stress fractures, low-impact fractures	• Dehydroepiandrosterone sulfate
• Other overuse injuries	Other studies
Physical and emotional stressors	• Dual-energy X-ray absorptiometry (DXA)—recommended for athletes with >6 month history of disordered eating, oligomenorrhea, or amenorrhea
Medications and supplements	
Family history	
Review of systems	• EKG—prolonged QT interval may be seen in severe eating disorders
• Symptoms of estrogen deficiency—hot flashes, vaginal dryness, dyspareunia	
	• Pelvic ultrasound—evaluate for polycystic ovarian syndrome
• Symptoms of androgen excess—acne, excessive hair, striae	
	• CT of adrenal glands (rule out adrenal adenoma, adrenal hyperplasia)
• Symptoms of pituitary tumor—galactorrhea, headaches, loss of sense of smell, visual disturbances	
	• MRI brain—evaluate for pituitary source
• Symptoms of cardiac involvement—shortness of breath, chest pain, palpitations, dizziness	

Table 50.3 ACOG committee opinion no. 267

Absolute contraindications to aerobic exercise during pregnancy

Hemodynamically significant heart disease

Restrictive lung disease

Incompetent cervix/cerciage

Multiple gestation at risk for premature labor

Persistent second or third trimester bleeding

Placenta labor during the current pregnancy

Ruptured membranes

Preeclampsia/pregnancy-induced hypertension

Reprinted from *Exercise During Pregnancy and the Postpartum Period.* Used with permission. © American College of Obstetricians and Gynecologists, 2002, Committee Opinion No. 267.

III. Exercise during pregnancy

A. Moderate aerobic and strength training poses no increased risk on the mother or fetus in uncomplicated pregnancies
   1. American Congress of Obstetricians and Gynecologists (ACOG) recommends moderate exercise for 30 min on all days of the week
B. Benefits of exercise
   1. Decreases risk of preeclampsia
   2. May prevent gestational diabetes
   3. Women have more favorable subjective outcomes

Table 50.4 ACOG committee opinion no. 267

Relative contraindications to aerobic exercise during pregnancy

Severe anemia

Unevaluated maternal cardiac arrhythmia

Chronic bronchitis

Poorly controlled type 1 diabetes

Extreme morbid obesity

Extreme underweight (BMI <12)

History of extremely sedentary lifestyle

Intrauterine growth restriction in current pregnancy

Poorly controlled hypertension

Orthopedic limitations

Poorly controlled seizure disorder

Poorly controlled hyperthyroidism

Heavy smoker

Reprinted from *Exercise During Pregnancy and the Postpartum Period.* Used with permission. © American College of Obstetricians and Gynecologists, 2002, Committee Opinion No. 267.

Table 50.5   ACOG committee opinion no. 267

Warning signs to terminate exercise while pregnant

Vaginal bleeding

Dyspnea prior to exertion

Dizziness

Headache

Chest pain

Muscle weakness

Calf pain or swelling (rule out thrombophlebitis)

Preterm labor

Decreased fetal movement

Amniotic fluid leakage

Reprinted from *Exercise During Pregnancy and the Postpartum Period.* Used with permission. © American College of Obstetricians and Gynecologists, 2002, Committee Opinion No. 267.

    C. Women who exercise before and during pregnancy have decreased risk of pregnancy-related low back and pelvic pain

    D. Contraindications to aerobic exercise and when to stop activity—Tables 50.3 through 50.5

    E. Avoid elevated temperature in the first trimester—persistent elevated temperature in the first trimester (time of neural tube closure and organogenesis) has been linked to birth defects

      1. Wear loose-fitting, well-ventilated clothing

      2. Moderate intensity—may base off "talk test," if unable to maintain a conversation intensity may be too high.

Recommended Reading

1. Benjaminse A, Gokeler A, Fleisig G, Sell T, Otten B. What is the true evidence for the gender-related differences during plant and cut maneuvers? A systematic review. *Knee Surg Sports Traumatol Arthrosc.* 2011;19(1):42–54.
2. Borg-Stein J, Dugan S, Solomon J. Special considerations in the female athlete. In: Frontera WR, Herring SA, Micheli LJ, Silver JK, eds. *Clinical Sports Medicine: Medical Management and Rehabilitation.* 2007:87–102. Philadelphia, PA: Saunders/Elsevier.
3. Dugan SA. Sports-related knee injuries in female athletes: What gives? *Am J Phys Med Rehabil.* 2005;84:122–130.
4. Hewett TE, Zazulak BT, Myer GD, Ford KR. A review of electromyographic activation levels, timing differences, and increased anterior cruciate ligament injury incidence in female athletes. *Br J Sports Med.* 2005;39:347–350.
5. Hoch AZ, Pajewske NM, Moraske L, Carrera GF, Wilson CR, Hoffman RG, Schimke JE, Gutterman DD. Prevalence of the female athlete triad in high school athletes and sedentary students. *Clin J Sport Med.* 2009;19(5):421–428.
6. Lynch SL, Hoch AZ. The female runner: Gender specifics. *Clin Sport Med.* 2010;29(3):477–498.
7. Micheo W, Hernandez L, Seda C. Evaluation, management, rehabilitation, and prevention of anterior cruciate ligament injury: Current concepts. *PMR.* 2010;2(10):935–944.
8. Nattiv A, Loucks AB, Manore MM, Sanborn CF, Sundgot-Borgen J, Warren MP. American College of Sports Medicine position stand. The female athlete triad. *Med Sci Sports Exerc.* 2007;39(10):1867–1882.

The Athlete With a Disability

Lucinda T. Myers and Stuart Willick

I. Overview of Musculoskeletal Injuries in the Athlete With a Disability

A. Background
  1. Compared with able-bodied sports, there is a relative paucity of published literature on injuries in athletes with a disability
  2. Available epidemiology literature involves mostly retrospective surveys with athletes self-reporting
  3. Reports are limited to body regions involved rather than specific diagnosis
  4. Overall injury rates are about the same for athletes with and without physical disabilities
  5. However, injury patterns differ by sport and type of disability
  6. Injuries carry greater functional consequences for the athlete with a disability.

B. Brief literature review
  1. Wheelchair athletes versus ambulatory athletes: wheelchair athletes primarily experience upper-limb injury while ambulatory athletes (amputee, visually impaired, and cerebral palsy) more often experience lower-limb injury
  2. Amputees: athletes with upper-limb deficiencies tend to have more cervical and thoracic spine injuries compared with athletes with lower-limb deficiencies who have more lumbar spine injuries
  3. Atlanta Summer Paralympic Games in 1996
    a. Athletes with lower limb deficiencies or with visual impairments sustained more ankle injuries than athletes with other impairments
    b. Incidence of shoulder pain in wheelchair users estimated 30–70%
  4. Winter Paralympic Games in 2002
    a. Nine percent of all athletes sustained an injury; most common diagnoses: sprains (32%), fractures (21%), strains, and lacerations (14% each)
    b. In all, 77% of all injuries were due to an acute traumatic etiology
    c. Injury rates among paralympians were higher in sledge hockey (14%) and alpine skiing (12%), and lower in Nordic skiing (2%)
  5. Prevalence of osteoarthritis in amputees
    a. Amputees have increased prevalence of OA in the contralateral knee, compared with able-bodied persons
    b. It is not known if sports participation increases this risk.

C. Injury prevention considerations should include:
  1. For wheelchair athletes, prescribe a training program directed at strengthening the available trunk muscles, rotator cuff, and scapular stabilizer muscles
  2. Provide wheelchair accessible weight machines or modify free weight program
  3. Encourage a thorough stretching program individualized to the athlete, considering the sport and the physical impairment

4. Include proprioception and balance exercises
5. Do not over-train with one type of exercise; use cross-training programs
6. Proper equipment
7. Proper nutrition
8. Proper technique.

MEDICAL ISSUES UNIQUE TO THE ATHLETE WITH A DISABILITY

I. Autonomic dysreflexia (AD)

  A. Definition/pathophysiology
   1. Occurs in spinal cord injury (SCI), at or above the T6 level
   2. In the absence of cortical regulation, any noxious stimuli below the level of the spinal lesion can result in abnormal sympathetic discharge
    a. Sympathetic surge may cause life-threatening hypertension
    b. Brain detects hypertensive crisis via intact baroreceptors in the neck
    c. A compensatory vagal/parasympathetic response decreases heart rate, cardiac output (CO), and blood pressure (BP)
    d. Vasodilation results from intact parasympathetic nerves above the injury causing intra-cranial vasodilation which evokes headache
    e. Lowered cardiac output is not sufficient to offset the sympathetic surge below the injury level and hypertension persists.
  B. Symptoms and signs of AD include: headache, hypertension, bradycardia, blurred vision, nasal congestion, anxiety, piloerection, flushing, and diaphoresis above level of injury.
  C. Treatment
   1. Remove the inciting noxious stimulus. Etiologies may include: distended bladder, distended or impacted bowel, hemorrhoids, urinary tract infection, tight clothing, gallstones, skin breakdown (including ulcers, blisters, sunburn), acute trauma, deep-venous thrombosis
   2. Sit the athlete up to cause an orthostatic drop in blood pressure
   3. Treat hypertension
    a. Nitropaste to skin is fast acting and can be wiped off when symptoms resolve or hypotension ensues
    b. Oral/IV antihypertensives with rapid onset, short duration may be used.
  D. Boosting
   1. Prohibited form of intentional induction of AD to improve sports performance
   2. Athletes use techniques to produce "controlled" sympathetic surge via purposeful, self-induced AD with noxious stimulus, including:
    a. Clamping urinary catheter
    b. Tightening leg straps
    c. Sticking themselves with sharp objects in an insensate location
   3. Boosting presents a serious health risk to the athlete
   4. Boosting is cheating and is prohibited in sports competition
   5. Athletes are subject to disqualification and long-term sanctions.

II. Orthostatic hypotension

  A. Definition/pathophysiology
   1. Individuals with upper thoracic and cervical SCI may have sympathetic/parasympathetic neuroregulatory impairment
   2. Evoked by athlete sitting up suddenly or during intensive sport competition.
  B. Symptoms and signs may include: lightheadedness, nausea, syncope, tachycardia.
  C. Treatment
   1. Maintain appropriate hydration, nutrition, and salt balance

    2. Elastic leg stockings decrease peripheral vascular pooling
    3. Abdominal binders promote venous return
    4. Place athlete in supine or Trendelenburg position for severe episodes
    5. IV fluids and sympathomimetic agents may be used for BP support only in emergency cases as these interventions are included on the prohibited list of the World Anti-Doping Agency (WADA).

III. Thermoregulation

    A. Pathophysiology in SCI population
        1. Impaired vasomotor control secondary to impaired autonomic function
        2. Lack of muscle mass below the level of the SCI lesion
        3. Decreased input to hypothalamic thermoregulatory centers
        4. Impaired sweating mechanism below the level of the SCI lesion results in less surface area available for cooling via evaporation
        5. Unable to generate sufficient body heat or "shiver" response
        6. Impaired or absent sensation impairs awareness of cold or damp extremities.
    B. Prevention and treatment
        1. Educate swimmers and cold weather athletes on hypothermia
        2. Educate endurance and warm weather athletes on hyperthermia
        3. Avoid dehydration with appropriate fluid repletion
        4. Athletes should wear lightweight, breathable clothing in hot conditions
        5. Athletes should wear layered, breathable clothing in cold conditions
        6. Athletes with impaired sensation should consult their sensate counterparts regarding cold or numb extremities
        7. Cooling systems may be necessary in hot conditions.

IV. Skin breakdown

    A. Pathophysiology
        1. Pressure in insensate, paralyzed locations causes local tissue ischemia
        2. Every pressure sore seen on the skin should be regarded as serious because of the probable damage below the skin surface, hidden from the examiner.
    B. Risk factors
        1. Athletes with SCI can get pressure sores if they have poor compliance with pressure relief techniques and with prolonged sitting for travel or in race chairs
        2. Athletes with severe spasticity are prone to skin breakdown in locations where high muscle tone or contractures cause persistent skin friction
        3. Athletes with amputations are prone to skin issues at the stump site or areas of increased pressure between skin and prosthesis including: pressure sores, abrasions, cerrucous hyperplasia (Choke syndrome), blisters, rashes.
    C. Diagnosis of pressure sores
        1. Press on the red, pink, or darkened area with your finger; skin should blanch
        2. Remove the pressure and the area should return to red, pink, or darkened color within a few seconds, indicating good blood flow
        3. If the area stays white, then blood flow is impaired and damage has begun
        4. Darkly pigmented skin may not have visible blanching even when healthy.
    D. Staging skin breakdown
        1. Stage I: Skin is intact but skin is red, discolored, hardened, and nonblanchable
        2. Stage II: Epidermis is broken, exposed, creating a shallow open bed
        3. Stage III: Open wound extends beyond dermis to the adipose tissue layer; signs of necrosis and infection may be present
        4. Stage IV: Wound extends to muscle and bone with probability of infection.

E. Prevention and treatment
   1. Proper wheelchair positioning and cushion support
   2. Correct fit of adaptive equipment and prosthetics
   3. Compliance with pressure reliefs
   4. Reduce skin moisture by wearing absorbent fabric
   5. The athlete must:
      a. Stay off the area and remove all pressure
      b. Keep the area clean and dry
      c. Eat adequate calories high in protein, vitamins (especially A and C) and minerals (especially iron and zinc)
      d. Maintain adequate hydration
      e. Find and remove inciting factors
      f. Inspect the area at least twice a day.

V. Peripheral nerve injuries

A. Traumatic neuroma
   1. Hyperplasia of nerve fibers and their supporting tissues
   2. Athletes with amputations are at increased risk of developing painful neuromas at their stump site
   3. Diagnosis is usually clinical, supplemented by ultrasonography or MRI
   4. Treatment
      a. Lidocaine patch
      b. Capsaicin cream
      c. Acetaminophen
      d. Nonsteroidal antiinflammatory drugs (NSAIDs)
      e. Corticosteroid injection
      f. Neuropathic agents such as gabapentin or pregabalin
      g. Percutaneous ablation with alcohol injection or radiofrequency energy
      h. Surgical resection last line of therapy as neuromas may re-occur.

B. Peripheral nerve entrapment syndromes
   1. Athletes who use wheelchairs or crutches are at increased risk for development of upper-limb peripheral neuropathies including:
      a. Median neuropathy at the wrist
      b. Ulnar neuropathy at the wrist within Guyon's canal
      c. Ulnar neuropathy at the elbow within the cubital tunnel
      d. Brachial plexopathies and other proximal nerve injuries at the shoulder
   2. Athletes with below knee amputations are at risk for peroneal neuropathy at the fibular head due to improper prosthetic fit
   3. Proper padding and equipment fit is key to prevention
   4. Treatment
      a. Resting wrist splint to keep wrist in neutral position for ulnar or median neuropathy at the wrist
      b. NSAIDs
      c. Corticosteroid injections
      d. Surgical intervention for athletes who fail conservative management.

VI. Osteoporosis

A. Spinal cord injury, polio, and neuromuscular diseases
   1. Low bone density occurs predominantly in pelvis and lower limbs which are chronically nonweight bearing and denervated
   2. Nonweight bearing causes disuse demineralization

3. Imbalanced osteoblastic and osteoclastic activity occurs
4. Increased fracture risk with even relatively minor trauma
5. Parathyroid dysfunction can be seen in chronic SCI.

B. Laboratory studies
   1. The following markers may identify athletes who are at risk for developing osteoporosis: serum calcium, phosphorous, alkaline phosphatase, 1,25−dihydroxyvitamin D, calcitonin, urinary calcium, and hydroxyproline.

C. Diagnostic imaging
   1. Quantitative computed tomography (QCT)
      a. Isolates densitometric and geometric changes in cortical and trabecular components of bone
      b. Allows for volumetric measurements in grams per cubic centimeter, which is the most precise measurement of bone density
   2. Dual-energy radiographic absorptiometry scan
      a. Most commonly used method for evaluation
      b. Records absolute bone mineral densities in various regions of the body.

D. Treatment
   1. Early weight bearing with assisted standing (if possible)
   2. Mechanical stimulus to the bones of the lower extremities
   3. Calcium supplementation, calcitonin, and/or bisphosphonates.

E. Fracture management
   1. Athletes with sensory loss may not report pain after a fracture
   2. Maintain high index of suspicion in setting of osteopenia or osteoporosis even with minimal trauma or normal x-rays
   3. Nondisplaced fractures can be missed on x-rays in setting of low bone density
   4. MRI or CT imaging may be warranted to fully assess possible bone injury.

Recommended Reading

1. Bernardi M, Castellano V, Ferrara MS, Sbriccoli P, Sera F, Marchetti M. Muscle pain in athletes with locomotor disability. *Med Sci Sports Exercise*. 2003;35(2):199−206.
2. Dec KL, Sparrow KJ, McKeag DB. The physically-challenged athlete: Medical issues and assessment. *Sports Med*. 2000;29(4):245−258.
3. Ferrara MS, Peterson CL. Injuries to athletes with disabilities: Identifying injury patterns. *Sports Med*. 2000;30(2):137−143.
4. Klenck C, Gebke K. Practical management: Common medical problems in disabled athletes. *Clinl J Sport Med*. 2007;17(1):55−60.
5. Laskowski ER, Murtaugh PA. Snow skiing injuries in physically disabled skiers. *Am J Sports Med*. 1992;20:553−557.
6. Melzer L, Yekutiel M, Sukenik S. Comparative study of osteoarthritis of the contralateral knee joint of male amputees who do and do not play volleyball. *J Rheumatol*. 2001;28(1):169−172.
7. Webborn ADJ. The disabled athlete. In: Brukner P, Kahn K, eds. *Clin Sports Med*. North Ryde New South Wales, Australia: McGraw-Hill; 2006.
8. Willick S, Webborn N. Chapter 4: Sport medicine. In: Vanlandewijck YC, Thompson WR, eds. *The Paralympic Athlete*. 1st ed. West Sussex, UK: Blackwell Publishing Ltd.; 2011:76−90.

INDEX